Textbook of

Medical Parasitology

The Authors

Dr Sumeeta Khurana is a professor in the Department of Medical Parasitology, Postgraduate Institute of Medical Education and Research (PGIMER), Chandigarh. After completing her MBBS from Indira Gandhi Medical College, Shimla, she pursued her MD in Microbiology from All India Institute of Medical Sciences (AIIMS), New Delhi. She is a Fellow of the Indian Academy of Tropical Parasitology and the International Medical Science Academy, and was a WHO Fellow at Karolinska Institute, Stockholm, Sweden. She is Joint Editor of the Journal of Tropical Parasitology and is on the editorial board of several other journals. She is also a member of various international and national scientific organisations. Dr Khurana has over two decades of teaching experience and has guided several MD and PhD students, undertaken many research projects on parasitic diseases and published over 100 research papers. She has a passion for teaching, gardening and music.

Dr Abhishek Mewara is an associate professor in the Department of Medical Parasitology, Postgraduate Institute of Medical Education and Research (PGIMER), Chandigarh. He has an MBBS degree from Jawahar Lal Nehru Medical College, Ajmer, and an MD in Microbiology from PGIMER, Chandigarh. He is a member of the National Academy of Medical Sciences, the Indian Academy of Tropical Parasitology and many other prestigious academic bodies. Dr Mewara has more than a decade of teaching experience. He has conducted several nationally and internationally funded research projects on parasites and has published nearly 50 papers. He enjoys music, yoga, reading and travelling.

Textbook of

Medical Parasitology

Sumeeta Khurana

Professor, Department of Medical Parasitology

Postgraduate Institute of Medical Education and Research (PGIMER)

Chandigarh

Abhishek Mewara

Associate Professor, Department of Medical Parasitology

Postgraduate Institute of Medical Education and Research (PGIMER)

Chandigarh

Universities Press

TEXTBOOK OF MEDICAL PARASITOLOGY

UNIVERSITIES PRESS (INDIA) PRIVATE LIMITED

Registered Office
3-6-747/1/A & 3-6-754/1, Himayatnagar, Hyderabad 500 029, Telangana, India
info@universitiespress.com; www.universitiespress.com

Distributed by
Orient Blackswan Private Limited

Registered Office
3-6-752, Himayatnagar, Hyderabad 500 029, Telangana, India

Other Offices
Bengaluru, Chennai, Guwahati, Hyderabad, Kolkata
Mumbai, New Delhi, Noida, Patna, Visakhapatnam

ISBN 978 93 89211 89 4

Typeset in Minion Pro 10/13 pt *by*
ELITE Graphics, Hyderabad 500 039

501758

Printed in India at
Rasi Graphics Private Limited
Chennai 600 014

Published by
Universities Press (India) Private Limited
3-6-747/1/A & 3-6-754/1, Himayatnagar, Hyderabad 500 029, Telangana, India

Contents

Foreword

Given the increasing global burden of parasitic infections in terms of morbidity and mortality, there is a pressing need for a resource that integrates the most current information and the essential facts about individual parasites and the approach to the diseases caused by them. The *Textbook of Medical Parasitology*, authored by Dr Sumeeta Khurana and Dr Abhishek Mewara, is one such resource for undergraduate and postgraduate students of human parasitology and clinicians, not only in India but also abroad. This textbook is a handy guide for workers in the field and is aimed at equipping them with the specialised skills, scientific information and research tools that would enable them to understand parasitism as a biological phenomenon and its relevance to human disease. Moreover, the authors have successfully amalgamated the conventional principles with the latest information on medically important parasites in a crisp, lucid style. The book is also well-aligned with the clinical approach prescribed by the new undergraduate medical curriculum. Parasites are individually dealt with according to the body systems they affect, viz. intestinal, blood or tissue parasites, but are grouped according to their taxonomic statuses. Thus, the book has a clinical orientation without compromising on the conventional principles of medical parasitology.

The first section of the book introduces readers to the subject of parasitology and the basic concepts of immunology. Two sections of the book—Sections II and III—deal with individual parasites. In these sections, the general biology of these parasites and the diseases caused by them, their laboratory diagnosis, treatment, prevention and control have been amply elucidated. The text is supplemented with detailed line diagrams, self-explanatory life cycles and microphotographs. Fresh insights into the immunopathogenesis of parasitic infections, newly developed diagnostic modalities and the latest treatment regimens have been compiled in each chapter. Section IV is dedicated to providing a syndromic approach to the subject in alignment with the integrated system-wise curriculum prescribed for undergraduate students of medicine. This section provides an overview of the disease manifestations of various infectious diseases and the relative place of causative organisms—not just parasites, but also bacterial, viral and fungal pathogens—in each of the syndromes. The last section of the book touches upon some important contemporary topics such as medical entomology, zoonotic parasitic infections and the basic concepts of control programmes deployed for parasitic diseases.

In terms of organisation, *Textbook of Medical Parasitology* is well-planned and succinct. The textual material is supported by clinical case studies, illustrations, photographs and descriptive and multiple-choice questions for key point revision and better preparation for the examinations. While the simplified approach to the explanation of concepts is sure to aid in the quick assimilation of knowledge and make this book enjoyable for undergraduate students of medicine, it is also a handy resource for postgraduate students of Medical Microbiology and even clinicians.

I take this opportunity to congratulate the authors on bringing out this book, which integrates pre-clinical and clinical medical sciences. I am certain that it will be useful not only for students of Medical Parasitology but also for policy makers and programme managers working in the areas of prevention and control of infectious diseases.

Prof. R C Mahajan
MD, FAMS, FNASc, FNA, FTWAS
Professor Emeritus
Postgraduate Institute of Medical Education and Research (PGIMER)
Chandigarh

Preface

More than half of the world's population is infected with at least one member of the two large parasite groups—protozoa and helminths. Parasitic diseases affect human health globally. Though the disease burden is greater among the socioeconomically disadvantaged populations of the developing world, the developed countries are not spared. In the modern era of globalisation, parasites previously unknown to some regions are now emerging in such areas due to increased overseas trade and travel.

In their careers, practitioners of medicine encounter a diverse variety of parasitic diseases. Some of these parasites are restricted to specific regions of the world (e.g., *Schistosoma haematobium* in Africa and *Trypanosoma cruzi* in Central and South America), while others are worldwide in distribution (e.g., *Entamoeba histolytica* and *Giardia duodenalis*). Some parasites are well-adapted to the human host and co-exist in a symbiotic relationship with human beings (e.g., *Entamoeba coli*), while others may cause significant damage to the host (e.g., *Entamoeba histolytica* and *Plasmodium falciparum*). Parasitic infections are transmitted to humans by various modes such as the ingestion of contaminated food and water (e.g., *Giardia duodenalis*), through insect vectors (e.g., *Leishmania donovani*), by penetration of skin (e.g., *Strongyloides stercoralis*), etc. A number of parasitic infections are zoonotic, i.e., they involve animal hosts, and are common in people who live in close contact with certain animals (e.g., *Taenia solium* and *Echinococcus granulosus*). Some parasites cause no harm to immunocompetent hosts but may cause pathology in an immunocompromised host, i.e., they are opportunistic parasites (e.g., *Toxoplasma gondii* and *Cryptosporidium parvum*). The numerous parasitic diseases are widespread and pervade all the disciplines of medical sciences. Thus, a medical student should possess in-depth knowledge of parasitic infections to succeed at patient management.

The field of medicine has seen a paradigm shift in the 21st century. The last few decades have borne witness to significant advances in immunological and genomic technologies, which have contributed to our understanding of the transmission, pathogenesis, diagnosis and management of human parasitic diseases. The utility of molecular techniques has now transcended from being limited to research to becoming a part of routine diagnosis. At the same time, traditional techniques such as microscopy remain the mainstay of diagnosis for several parasitic infections. The management of parasitic diseases depends on the few available anti-parasitic drugs with a dearth of newer effective drugs. Further, despite the scientific advances, the quest for safe and effective vaccines against parasites remains a distant dream.

Encouragingly, the application of basic public health measures such as the provision of clean drinking water, adequate sanitation and control of insect vectors significantly helps in the prevention of parasitic diseases. In the last few decades, many international and national control programmes have relied on these simple preventive measures and have been able to bring about a considerable decrease in the burden of parasitic diseases such as malaria, leishmaniasis, filariasis, soil-transmitted helminthiasis, onchocerciasis, schistosomiasis, etc. Notably, the control programmes for Guinea worm have led to the near eradication of this parasite from the face of the earth.

With the rapidly advancing knowledge of the medical sciences, it is daunting, yet essential, for healthcare professionals to keep abreast of the latest developments in the field. This textbook has been prepared with the objective of inculcating a sound and updated understanding of human parasitic diseases from the perspective of not only undergraduate and postgraduate students but also faculty and clinical practitioners.

The textbook has been organised into five broad sections, which are as follows:

- **Section I** deals with the general concepts and immunology of parasitic infections.
- **Sections II and III** deal with the detailed study of protozoa and helminths respectively. Chapters on individual parasites are arranged according to the organ systems they affect (intestine, blood, tissue, etc.) to enable the study of parasites in the context of these organ systems. Each chapter contains up-to-date information about the morphology, life cycle and pathogenesis of individual parasites and the clinical features, diagnosis, management and prevention of the diseases caused by them. Simple line diagrams of parasite morphology, colourful illustrations of life cycles and standard microphotographs for laboratory diagnosis have been provided for easy assimilation of the concepts. Important information has been emphasised in tables, and separate boxes for laboratory diagnosis and treatment have been provided as tools for a quick recap. The core chapters are equipped with clinical cases and learning goals as well as descriptive and multiple-choice questions to help students prepare for their examinations.

- **Section IV** deals with disease manifestations of infections of the major organ systems of the body (with special reference to parasites) in line with the new clinically-oriented medical curriculum. Readers can best use this section while recapitulating the subject as it provides a bird's eye view of the parasites, bacteria, fungi and viruses affecting the various organ systems of the body and the general mechanisms of the disease processes in these organs.
- **Section V** is aimed at introducing readers to the concepts of zoonotic infections and 'One Health'; medical entomology, the knowledge of which is important in understanding vector-borne diseases; and control programmes for parasitic diseases.
- The **three annexures** at the end of the book deal with the approach to the laboratory diagnosis, laboratory procedures and materials required for testing and the drug therapy regimes for various parasitic infections.

The field of medical sciences is evolving by quantum leaps and bounds. With this in mind, we have endeavoured to provide students with an up-to-date textbook of medical parasitology and hope that they will find it a valuable resource. We invite students and teachers to write to us with their feedback and suggestions to help us improve the textbook.

Dr Sumeeta Khurana
MD Microbiology (AIIMS, New Delhi), MNAMS, FIATP, FIMSA
Professor, Department of Medical Parasitology
Postgraduate Institute of Medical Education and Research (PGIMER), Chandigarh
sumeetakhurana@hotmail.com

Dr Abhishek Mewara
MD Microbiology (PGIMER, Chandigarh), MNAMS
Associate Professor, Department of Medical Parasitology
Postgraduate Institute of Medical Education and Research (PGIMER), Chandigarh
abhimewara@yahoo.com

Acknowledgements

Dedicated to The Almighty and my family
— Sumeeta Khurana

Dedicated to my family and friends
— Abhishek Mewara

We take this opportunity to thank the innumerable people who have helped us understand the nuances of parasitology in umpteen ways.

We would like to express our deep gratitude to our teachers and mentors at PGIMER, Chandigarh—Dr R C Mahajan, Dr Nancy Malla, Dr M L Dubey and Dr R Sehgal, as well as our colleagues in the departments of Medical Parasitology, Medical Microbiology and Virology. Our heartfelt thanks to Dr Neelam Taneja, Dr Manisha Biswal and Dr Ritu Aggarwal for providing us with valuable insights and critical reviews of parts of the textbook. We are grateful to Dr Arti Kapil, AIIMS, New Delhi, for constantly encouraging and inspiring us.

We are thankful to the publishers, Universities Press, for the support they extended to us in preparing this book. We would like to thank Dr Sudha Ganesan, Managing Consultant, Medical Publishing, and Ms Malini Gopalakrishnan, Assistant Editor, for working closely with us to help us assimilate and present our thoughts in a way that would most benefit students. We are also grateful to Mr Madhu Reddy, Director, Universities Press, and President, Orient Blackswan Pvt. Ltd, for the valuable insights and guidance he provided throughout.

To our families, whose unflagging love and support are an incredible source of inspiration, we are ever indebted. Last but not least, we would like to thank our students and patients for the innumerable ways in which they teach us every day; we would like them to know that each one of them has contributed to the piece of work.

A number of the colour microphotographs we have used in this book to provide readers with clear visual representations of the parasites discussed herein have been sourced from image libraries of the Centers for Disease Control and Prevention, Atlanta, USA.

Mapping of Textbook of Medical Parasitology to CBME Competencies

Competency	Reference
General microbiology and immunity	
MI1.1	All chapters
MI1.2	Sections II, III and Annexures I and II
MI1.3	Sections II, III and Chapters 56 and 57
MI1.6	Chapters 13 and 17
MI1.7	Chapter 2
MI1.8	Chapters 2 and 54
MI1.10	Chapters 54 and Annexure I
CVS and blood infections	
MI2.4	Chapters 13, 14, 17, 25, 26, 38, 46, 48, 57 and Annexures I and III
MI2.5	Chapters 13, 17, 19 and 33
MI2.6	Chapters 13 and 33
Gastrointestinal and hepatobiliary system infections	
MI3.1	Chapters 4–11, 23–28, 37–39, 42, 46, 47 and Annexures I and III
MI3.2	Chapters 4, 5, 7, 24–28, 37, 39, 42, 47 and Annexures I and II
Musculoskeletal system, skin and soft tissue infections	
MI4.3	Chapters 10, 18, 29, 30, 32–36, 40, 52 and Annexure I
Central nervous system infections	
MI5.1	Chapters 15, 20, 21, 49 and Annexure I
MI5.2	Chapters 13, 19, 21, 31, 40, 49 and Annexure I
Respiratory tract infections	
MI6.1	Chapters 24, 26, 27, 33, 41, 45, 51 and Annexure I
Genitourinary and sexually transmitted infections	
MI7.1	Chapters 12, 46, 50 and Annexure I
MI7.2	Chapters 12, 50, 55 and Annexure I
Zoonotic diseases and miscellaneous	
MI8.1	Chapters 5–7, 10, 13–19, 29–31, 37–46, 56 and Annexure I
MI8.2	Chapters 7–9, 11, 19, 21, 27, 54 and Annexure I
MI8.4	Chapters 13 and 56
MI8.9	Annexures I and II
MI8.10	Annexures I and II
MI8.13	All chapters
MI8.15	All chapters
MI8.16	Chapters, 13, 15, 17, 23–26, 32–35 and 57

Learning Objectives

The following are the broad learning objectives of this book for students of medicine:

Students should know how to	• Describe the various parasitic agents of infectious diseases, their epidemiology, morphology, mode of infection, pathogenesis, and the immunology, clinical manifestations and course of illness, diagnosis, treatment and prevention of the diseases caused by them • Describe parasitic agents of: – **Fever** (e.g., malaria, kala-azar, filariasis) – **Anemia** (e.g., malaria, hookworm) – **Diarrhea/dysentery** (e.g., giardiasis, amoebiasis, cryptosporidiosis) – **Sexually transmitted infections** (e.g., trichomoniasis) – **Congenital infections** (e.g., toxoplasmosis) – **Genitourinary tract infections** (e.g., schistosomiasis) – **Space-occupying lesions (SOL) in the brain** (e.g., neurocysticercosis) – **SOL of the liver** (e.g., amoebiasis, echinococcosis, liver flukes) – **Worm infestations** (e.g., roundworm, hookworm, tapeworm) – **Meningitis/encephalitis** (e.g., free-living amoeba) – **Ocular infections** (e.g., *Acanthamoeba*) – **Respiratory tract infections** (e.g., paragonimiasis) – **Skin/soft tissue infections** (e.g., cutaneous leishmaniasis, larva migrans) • Describe parasitic agents of: – **Opportunistic infections** (e.g., toxoplasmosis, cryptosporidiosis) – **Zoonotic infections** (e.g., toxoplasmosis, trichinellosis, echinococcosis) – **Foodborne infections** (e.g., trichinellosis) – **Emerging infections** (e.g., *Plasmodium knowlesi, Taenia asiatica*) • Choose appropriate test/s for parasitic diseases
Students should know	• The **anti-parasitic drugs**, describe the mechanism of action, mechanism of drug resistance and the principles of antimicrobial susceptibility testing (e.g., malaria) • The various **National Health Programmes** for the prevention and control of parasitic diseases (e.g., malaria, leishmaniasis, filariasis, soil-transmitted helminths) • Methods of collecting various samples for parasitic diseases
Students should show the necessary skills to	• Demonstrate methods of collecting various samples for parasitic infections • Interpret results of laboratory test/s for parasitic infections • Identify and demonstrate diagnostic features of the parasitic causes of infections such as: – Malaria (differentiate between different *Plasmodium* species) – Filariasis (morphological features of microfilaria) – Intestinal parasitic infections (differentiate between morphology of eggs/cysts/worms of various protozoa and helminths in routine stool microscopy)
Students should be able to perform	• Common tests to diagnose parasitic infections (e.g., routine stool microscopy) and identify parasitic agents by microscopy

Chapter 1 Introduction to Medical Parasitology

INTRODUCTION

Human beings are known to harbour around 300 species of helminth worms and over 70 species of protozoan parasites. Approximately 90–100 of these parasite species are known to infect their human hosts; the rest are rare or accidental parasites of humans. While some of these infections are relatively mild, others are significant causes of morbidity and mortality. It appears that human evolution and parasitic infections go hand in hand. Historically, human beings have acquired parasites from animals during their evolution and migration and through agricultural and food practices. The practice of slave trade introduced new parasites to the New World from the Old World. In the modern era, globalisation has resulted in wider dissemination of parasites throughout the world. In recent times, the spread of the human immunodeficiency virus and immunosuppression due to cytotoxic therapy for various conditions such as malignancy and organ transplantations resulted in the establishment of several new opportunistic parasitic infections. A large burden of parasitic diseases is borne by tropical and subtropical countries where the environment is conducive for the growth of parasites. Thus, the fields of **tropical medicine** and **medical parasitology** have co-evolved.

There is a lot to be learned about the history of parasitic infections from ancient textbooks and scriptures. The science of **paleoparasitology**—the study of archaeological material for the presence of helminth worms, eggs or protozoan cysts in naturally or artificially preserved bodies and fossilised or desiccated feces—significantly contributes to the history of science. The first written records of parasitic infections are from a period of Egyptian medicine dating back to 3000–4000 BC; the *Ebers Papyrus* is one such record. In Hindu scriptures such as the *Charaka Samhita* and *Sushruta Samhita*, descriptions of various disease manifestations now known to be caused by parasites can be found. While the large helminths were known to the earliest of human ancestors, protozoa were only recognised much later—after the invention of the microscope and its use by **Antonie van Leeuwenhoek** towards the end of the 17th century. The study of parasitic protozoa only really began two centuries later, following the discovery of bacteria and the introduction of the germ theory by Pasteur and his colleagues at the end of the 19th century. It is not surprising then that the most rapid progress in science and medicine was made in the 20th century. The history of human parasitology revolves around early descriptions of particular diseases and the identification of their parasitic etiology, morphological features, modes of transmission to humans, elaboration of their life cycles, the animals and vector species involved and the establishment of the causal relationship between the parasites and the diseases.

Tropical diseases were first recognised as a distinct branch of medicine when **Sir Patrick Manson**, who is universally regarded as the '**Father of Tropical Medicine**', published the textbook *Tropical Diseases* in 1898. In his book, Manson described diseases caused by parasites, viz. malaria, amoebic dysentery, kala-azar, African trypanosomiasis and schistosomiasis among others. **Karl Asmund Rudolphi**, a professor of anatomy, is credited with being the '**Father of Helminthology**', while **Antonie van Leeuwenhoek** is considered the '**Father of Protozoology and Bacteriology**'. Our understanding of parasitic diseases and their treatment is owed to a fair number of scientists, some of whom received the prestigious Nobel Prize for their noteworthy contributions to the field of parasitology (see box below).

Scientists who received the Nobel Prize for their work in the field of parasitology

- **1902, Sir Ronald Ross:** Discovered the life cycle of the malaria parasite in humans and mosquitoes.
- **1907, Charles Louis Alphonse Laveran:** Demonstrated that the mosquito is the agent of transmission for malaria and identified the malaria parasite.
- **1927, Julius Wagner-Jauregg:** Used malaria-induced fever (malariotherapy) for the treatment of late-stage syphilis.
- **1928, Charles Nicolle:** Discovered that epidemic typhus is transmitted by lice.
- **1993, Kary Mullis:** Developed the polymerase chain reaction (PCR) technique.
- **2015, William C. Campbell and Satoshi Omura, and Tu Youyou:** Campbell and Omura jointly received the honour for the discovery of a novel therapy against infections caused by roundworms (ivermectin). Youyou was recognised for her discovery of a novel therapy against malaria (artemisinin).

MEDICAL PARASITOLOGY

This is a branch of parasitology that deals with the study of parasites that infect and produce disease in humans. Broadly, medical parasitology can be categorised into three branches, which are as follows:

- **Medical protozoology**—deals with the study of protozoa.
- **Medical helminthology**—deals with the study of helminths.
- **Medical entomology**—deals with the study of arthropods and other organisms (non-arthropods such as cyclops) that act as vectors or cause disease in humans.

NOMENCLATURE OF PARASITES

Parasites are named according to the binomial nomenclature put forward by Linnaeus in his *Systema Naturae* in 1735. In this system, each living species is designated a two-part name consisting of a genus name and a species name. Names are typically derived from Greek or Latin and usually attributed to the size and shape of the parasitic forms. Alternatively, they are derived from the names of the discoverer or the geographical area or habitat of the parasite or its host. The genus name of the parasite always begins with a capital letter while the species name is entirely lowercased. The full name of the organism is always italicised, e.g., *Ancylostoma duodenale* (etymology: [from Greek] *ankylos* = hook + *stoma* = mouth and *duodenale* = in the duodenum).

PARASITE

The word parasite originally comes from the Greek word *parasitos*, the literal translation of which is 'eaters at court' (*para* = alongside + *sitos* = food), and which later came to mean organisms that live at another's expense. A parasite is an organism that lives in or on another organism (host) and derives nutrients from it with or without harming the host. These organisms are larger and more complex than bacteria, with a eukaryotic cell structure similar to that of human host cells. Parasites are of the following types:

- **Endoparasite:** These are parasites that live within the body of the host and cause infection. The parasitism may be:
  - **Obligate:** Here, the organism cannot survive without the host (this is true of most parasites).
  - **Facultative:** When the parasite is capable of existing in the free-living state, it is said to be facultative (e.g., *Acanthamoeba*).
  - **Accidental:** Here, a parasite establishes itself in a host other than its normal host. Once there, the parasite may develop further or reach a 'dead end' (e.g., *Toxocara*, a dog roundworm, sometimes infects humans and causes a migrating larva disease called 'visceral larva migrans').
- **Ectoparasite:** These are parasites that live on the body surface of the host. They may cause disease either directly (e.g., scabies and lice) or indirectly by transmitting other microorganisms contained in them (e.g., fleas and ticks). The infection caused by such parasites is termed an **infestation**.

HOST

A host is defined as a living organism that harbours the parasite and provides it shelter and nourishment. Hosts may be of the following types:

- **Definitive host:** This is a host that harbours the **adult** stage of a parasite or in which the parasite can replicate **sexually**. Definitive hosts may be human beings or animals. In the majority of parasitic infections of medical importance, humans serve as the definitive hosts.
- **Intermediate host:** This is a host that harbours the **larval** stage of a parasite or in which the parasite undergoes **asexual** multiplication. For example, human beings act as intermediate hosts in malaria and hydatid disease. Some parasites require two intermediate hosts to complete their larval stages. These hosts are known as the first and second intermediate hosts, respectively.
- **Paratenic host (carrier or transport host):** This is a host in which the larval stage of a parasite remains **viable without developing further**. This larva develops further once it gets transferred to a host that is suitable for its life cycle. A paratenic host is not essential for the life cycle of the parasite. For example, the broad tapeworm, *Diphyllobothrium latum*, exists in the larval form in small fish, which when eaten by a bigger fish, penetrates the intestine of the latter and survives therein without further development; the bigger fish thus serves as a paratenic host to this parasite.
- **Reservoir host:** This is a host that harbours a parasite, maintains the infection pool in the environment and serves as a significant source of infection to other susceptible hosts. Animals, birds and fish serve as reservoirs for parasitic infections.
- **Accidental host:** Humans may act as accidental hosts for parasites that have a natural life cycle in animals. Such an infection may be a dead end for

the parasite as it cannot be transmitted further (e.g., hydatid cysts formed in humans in infections caused by *Echinococcus granulosus*).

VECTOR

This term generally refers to bloodsucking insects or other arthropods that transmit the parasite to the host (e.g., female *Anopheles* mosquitoes [transmit malaria] and sandflies [transmit *Leishmania*]).

HOST–PARASITE RELATIONSHIP

Living organisms associate with each other in numerous ways. The following are the types of relationships two organisms can have:

- **Symbiosis (from Greek; means living together):** It is a close physical association between the two organisms living together.
  - **Commensalism:** It is an association in which only the harboured organism is benefitted but without causing any harm to the host. A commensal is capable of living independently of the host.
  - **Mutualism:** This type of association is beneficial to both organisms. In most cases of mutualism, the host has better fitness in the presence of the partner organism.
  - **Parasitism:** It is an association in which the parasite not only derives benefits from the host but also causes harm to the host. The host, on the other hand, is not benefitted in any way.
- **Carrier state:** This is a state in which a person harbours the parasite without any clinical or sub-clinical disease, and can transmit the parasite to others.
- **Disease:** The disease is the clinical or subclinical manifestation of the infection. It may be mild, moderate or severe and in some cases, may even lead to the death of the host.

MODES OF TRANSMISSION OF INFECTION

Parasites may be transmitted to the host in various ways (Table 1.1). Some of the common modes of transmission are as follows:

- **Oral route:** It is the most common mode of transmission of parasites. Humans acquire infections when they ingest food (vegetables or meat), water or soil contaminated with feces containing the infective stages of the parasite.
- **Vector-borne:** Various parasitic diseases are transmitted by the inoculation of the parasite into the host by bloodsucking insect vectors (e.g., malaria). Some are transmitted through the feces of vectors which get deposited on the host's skin (e.g., *Trypanosoma cruzi*).
- **Penetration of the skin and mucous membranes:** Humans acquire infections when the larval forms of the parasite penetrate through intact skin.
- **Sexual contact:** Parasites that reside in the genitourinary tract are usually transmitted by this mode.
- **Vertical transmission:** Some parasites are transmitted from mother to fetus.
- **Autoinfection:** A number of intestinal parasites are transmitted by an individual to himself from a contaminated hand (external autoinfection) or by reverse peristalsis (internal autoinfection). The parasitic stage excreted in feces must be immediately mature or infectious for such transmission to be viable.
- **Blood transfusion:** Certain parasites can be transmitted during the transfusion of blood or blood products.
- **Organ transplantation:** Some infections may be transmitted from one host to another by organ transplantation.
- **Reactivation of latent infection:** Some infections persist in a host as latent infections, and get activated in the event of an immunodeficient or immunosuppressive state, thus causing disease, e.g., *Toxoplasma* encephalitis in an AIDS patient.

LIFE CYCLE

A parasite may complete its life cycle in one or multiple hosts. Similarly, human beings may act as either definitive or intermediate hosts.

Direct life cycle: When a parasite requires only one host to complete its development, it is said to have a direct life cycle (Table 1.2).

Indirect/complex life cycle: When a parasite requires two hosts (one definitive host and another intermediate) to complete its developmental cycle, it is said to have an indirect/complex life cycle (Table 1.3). Some parasites (especially trematodes) require two intermediate hosts (Table 1.4).

PATHOGENESIS

The parasite may produce disease in the human body by various mechanisms depending on its intrinsic properties and the organ system it affects. The infected individual

Table 1.1 Modes of transmission of parasites

Route	Source of infection/vector/parasite	
Oral route	Contaminated food or hands	Cysts of *Giardia duodenalis* and *Entamoeba histolytica* Oocysts of *Toxoplasma gondii* Ova of *Enterobius vermicularis* Cercariae of *Fasciolopsis buski*
	Soil	*Ascaris lumbricoides* Hookworm *Trichuris trichiura* *Toxocara* spp.
	Water with infected cyclops	*Dracunculus medinensis*
	Meat – cattle	*Cysticercus cellulosae (Taenia saginata)*
	Meat – pig	*Taenia solium* *Trichinella spiralis*
	Meat – pig, dog	*Toxoplasma gondii*
	Fish	*Diphyllobothrium latum* *Clonorchis sinensis* *Heterophyes heterophyes*
	Snail	*Fasciola hepatica*
	Crab/crayfish	*Paragonimus westermani*
Vector-borne	Mosquito	*Plasmodium* spp. Filaria
	Deer fly	*Loa loa*
	Sandfly	*Leishmania* spp.
	Reduviid bug	*Trypanosoma cruzi*
	Tsetse fly	*Trypanosoma brucei*
	Blackfly	*Onchocerca volvulus*
Penetration of the skin and mucous membranes	Filariform larvae of *Strongyloides stercoralis* Filariform larvae of hookworm Cercariae of *Schistosoma* spp. liberated in water from snails	
Sexual contact	*Trichomonas vaginalis* (the parasite most frequently transmitted by sexual contact) Rarely, *Entamoeba histolytica* or *Giardia duodenalis* among homosexuals	
Vertical transmission	*Toxoplasma gondii*	
Autoinfection	*Taenia solium* *Cryptosporidium* spp. *Enterobius vermicularis* *Strongyloides stercoralis* *Hymenolepis nana*	
Blood transfusion	*Plasmodium* spp. *Babesia* spp. *Leishmania* spp. *Trypanosoma cruzi* *Toxoplasma gondii*	
Organ transplantation	*Toxoplasma gondii* *Trypanosoma cruzi*	
Reactivation of latent infection	*Toxoplasma gondii*	

may remain asymptomatic or experience a mild illness. When overtly symptomatic, the disease manifestations may range from acute or immediate manifestations to a chronic illness. The parasite may produce disease by the following mechanisms:

- **Immune response of the body and inflammation:** In response to a parasitic invasion, the human body mounts an immune response in the form of fever and inflammation to either kill the parasite or contain the infection to a limited area of the body. Inflammation

Table 1.2 Parasites that have a direct life cycle

Protozoa	Helminths
• *Entamoeba histolytica* • *Giardia duodenalis* • *Trichomonas vaginalis* • *Balantidium coli* • *Cryptosporidium* spp. • *Cystoisospora belli* • *Cyclospora cayetanensis* • Microsporidia	• *Hymenolepis nana* • *Ascaris lumbricoides* • Hookworm • *Trichuris trichiura* • *Strongyloides stercoralis* • *Enterobius vermicularis*

Table 1.3 Parasites that have an indirect life cycle with two hosts

Parasite	Definitive host	Intermediate host
Leishmania spp.	Human	*Phlebotomus* (sandfly)
Trypanosoma cruzi	Human	Triatomine (reduviid bug)
Trypanosoma brucei	Human	Tsetse fly
Taenia solium (intestinal taeniasis)	Human	Pig
Taenia saginata	Human	Cattle
Trichinella spiralis	Human, pig	Pig, human
Wuchereria bancrofti, Brugia malayi	Human	Mosquitoes
Onchocerca volvulus	Human	*Simulium* (blackfly)
Dracunculus medinensis	Human	Cyclops
Schistosoma spp.	Human	Snail
Fasciola hepatica	Human, sheep, goat, cattle	Snail
Fasciolopsis buski	Human, pig	Snail
Plasmodium spp.	Mosquito (*Anopheles*)	Human
Babesia spp.	Tick	Human
Toxoplasma gondii	Cat	Human, any vertebrate
Echinococcus granulosus	Dog and other canines	Human
Taenia solium (cysticercosis)	Human	Human, pig

Table 1.4 Parasites that have an indirect life cycle with three hosts (human beings are definitive hosts)

Parasite	Definitive host	First intermediate host	Second intermediate host
Clonorchis spp.	Human, dog, cat, pig	Snail	Fish
Opisthorchis spp.	Human, dog, cat, pig	Snail	Fish
Heterophyes heterophyes	Human, dog, cat, fox	Snail	Mullets
Paragonimus westermani	Human, domestic animals	Snail	Crab, crayfish
Diphyllobothrium latum	Human, dog, cat	Cyclops	Fish

of variable intensity is associated with most parasitic infections. Sometimes, the inflammation is intense and leads to pathology.

- **Mechanical damage:** The parasite may cause direct damage to the affected part of the body. For example, the protozoan *Giardia duodenalis* attaches itself to the intestinal epithelium and disrupts the brush border microvilli, leading to the malabsorption of nutrients.
- **Invasion and tissue damage:** The parasite may invade the tissue with the help of enzymes and other mediators. For example, *Entamoeba histolytica* causes tissue lysis by releasing cysteine proteases; this causes abscess formation and necrosis in the liver.
- **Formation of intracellular cysts:** Some parasites reside intracellularly and form cysts therein. For example, the larvae of *Trichinella spiralis* penetrate muscle cells and reside there, as a consequence of which, there is inflammation in the muscles and loss of contractility of muscle fibres.

- **Space-occupying lesions and pressure symptoms:** Some parasites reach the internal organs and form cysts which may increase in size to cause pressure symptoms. For example, the cysts of *Echinococcus granulosus* in the liver may exert pressure on the hepatobiliary ducts and cause jaundice.
- **Obstruction:** The parasite may multiply at a particular site in sufficient numbers to block the lumen of the organ affected. Roundworms are an example of parasites that can cause intestinal obstruction.
- **Nutrient deficiency:** The parasite may cause nutrition deficiency in the host either by robbing its nutrition, by causing malabsorption or by decreasing the production of the essential components in the body. This is especially observed in children in whom there is a heavy burden of intestinal worm infestation over a long period of time.
- **Allergic manifestations:** Several helminthic infections induce allergic immune responses, especially the production of helminth-specific IgE which can cross-react with environmental allergens. Such a manifestation is seen when the larvae of roundworms pass through the lungs and cause allergic responses.
- **Vector bite and skin penetration of parasite:** The bites of insect vectors may introduce parasites into the human body and may be associated with localised features at the site of the bite. Local erythema, nodules or ulcers such as those seen in cutaneous leishmaniasis may be seen at the site of the bite.
- **Migration of parasite in the viscera:** The larvae of the parasite may migrate to various organs as part of their life cycle or at random, and may incite an inflammatory reaction in the affected organs. For example, *Toxocara* spp. are animal parasites that accidentally infect the human host and start migrating inside the human body causing intense inflammation and damage along their path of migration.
- **Tissue changes:** The parasite may elicit certain tissue changes in the affected body part. Filarial worms living in the lymph vessels evoke repeated inflammation of the affected area, leading to permanent changes in the structure of the lymphatics, connective tissue and skin, and finally, cause the enlargement of the affected body part.
- **Neoplastic changes:** The parasite may elicit certain neoplastic changes in the affected body part. For example, the fluke *Clonorchis sinensis* lives in the bile ducts, where it releases proteins that promote the proliferation of the biliary epithelium and stimulate carcinogenesis.
- **Bacterial superinfections:** A few parasites are typically associated with bacterial superinfections. An example is that of *Strongyloides stercoralis* larvae which carry gut bacteria with them during their migration through the gut to the extraintestinal sites, causing abscesses or sepsis.

PRINCIPLES OF LABORATORY DIAGNOSIS

There are many ways to establish the diagnosis of parasitic infections. The following is a list of the common modalities of investigations used for this purpose:

- **Microscopy:** Feces, blood, bone marrow, lymph node, body fluids or biopsy samples can be used as specimens for microscopic studies. The microscopic detection of parasitic stages like trophozoites or cysts, various developmental stages such as amastigotes and schizonts in protozoa or ova, larval forms or adult worms or segments of helminths constitute the most important modality for parasitic diagnosis. These may be demonstrated directly in a wet mount or after staining with dyes.
- **Culture:** Though culture has little bearing on parasitic diagnosis except in the case of a few infections like kala-azar, acanthamoebiasis and trichomoniasis, it has much use in the research on parasites.
- **Antibody detection:** Antibody detection may play a role in some parasitic diseases, especially toxoplasmosis, visceral leishmaniasis, cysticercosis, echinococcosis, etc. Techniques like enzyme-linked immunosorbent assay (ELISA), indirect hemagglutination (IHA), immunochromatography, Western blot or enzyme-linked immunotransfer blot (EITB) may be used to demonstrate antibodies.
- **Antigen detection:** Antigen detection plays an important role in the diagnosis of parasitic diseases, viz. malaria, filariasis, giardiasis, cryptosporidiosis, amoebiasis, trichomoniasis, schistosomiasis, etc. Numerous rapid diagnostic tests (RDT) or immunochromatographic tests (ICT) are available as point-of-care tests for diagnosis as in the case of malaria.
- **Nucleic acid detection:** The detection of parasitic DNA plays an important role in the diagnosis of most parasitic infections and is gradually assuming the status of the new gold standard for the diagnosis of some parasitic infections. It not only helps in diagnosis but also in species differentiation, epidemiology, drug resistance studies, etc. Techniques like polymerase chain reaction (PCR), real-time PCR (RT-PCR) and

loop-mediated isothermal amplification (LAMP) are the favoured modalities.

- **Intradermal skin tests:** Intradermal hypersensitivity reaction may be used for the diagnosis of some parasitic infections like visceral leishmaniasis (Montenegro test), cystic echinococcosis (Casoni test), trichinellosis (Bachman test), etc.
- **Xenodiagnostic techniques:** Laboratory-reared arthropod vectors may be used to isolate the parasite from clinical samples. This technique is useful for infections like Chagas' disease where Triatomine bugs (reduviid bug) are used for this purpose.
- **Animal inoculation:** Experimental animal inoculation is mainly used for research purposes and rarely for diagnosis. Mice, rats, hamsters and guinea pigs are the common experimental models.
- **Radioimaging techniques:** Imaging techniques play a significant role in the diagnosis of several parasitic diseases, and especially in the case of space-occupying lesions, e.g., cysticercosis, echinococcosis and amoebiasis.
- **Indirect tests:** Blood counts, eosinophilia, increased IgE levels, etc., may provide indirect evidence of parasitic infections.

TREATMENT

Though quite a few parasitic infections are self-limiting, some require medical or surgical management (refer to **Annexure III**, *Drug Therapy for Parasitic Infections*).

- **Medical management:** The parasite may require chemotherapy; the choice of drug, dose and duration depend on the parasite and the affected site.
- **Surgical management:** Some parasites require surgical intervention, e.g., the removal of a hydatid cyst from the liver.

MULTIPLE CHOICE QUESTIONS

1. **Who is considered the father of tropical medicine?**
   a. Robert Koch
   b. Antonie van Leeuwenhoek
   c. Patrick Manson
   d. Louis Pasteur
2. **Who was conferred the Nobel Prize in 1902 for the discovery of the life cycle of the malaria parasite in humans and mosquitoes?**
   a. Ronald Ross
   b. Patrick Manson
   c. Robert Koch
   d. Antonie van Leeuwenhoek
3. **A host that harbours the adult stage of parasites or in which the parasites replicate sexually is termed as ________:**
   a. Intermediate host
   b. Definitive host
   c. Paratenic host
   d. Amplifier host
4. **The parasite that is transmitted by sexual contact is ________:**
   a. *Trichophyton rubrum*
   b. *Trichomonas vaginalis*
   c. *Enteromonas hominis*
   d. *Giardia duodenalis*
5. **Which of the following parasites is transmitted by penetration of skin?**
   a. Pinworm
   b. Hookworm
   c. *Entamoeba histolytica*
   d. Tapeworm

CHAPTER 2

Immunology of Parasitic Infections

INTRODUCTION

When two organisms live in intimate association, each responds to the presence of the other. Over the many millennia that parasites and their hosts have **co-existed**, both have **co-evolved** and adapted strategies to successfully survive despite each other—the parasite can chronically establish itself and propagate in the host, and the host can harbour the parasite and yet remain asymptomatic. Sometimes, however, this equilibrium is disrupted enough to cause damage to the host.

Parasites, being eukaryotes, are different from bacteria and viruses in terms of their morphological complexity and the way they interact with their hosts. Some of the significant differences are as follows:

- They are considerably **larger** than bacteria and viruses (ranging from unicellular protozoans to multicellular worms).
- They employ **evolved physical characteristics** to survive (such as the thick cuticles of worms and the formation of highly resistant cysts).
- They have **complex life cycles** consisting of various stages (e.g., ova ⟶ larva [L1 ⟶ L2 ⟶ L3 ⟶ L4] ⟶ adult), with each stage having **a different antigenic repertoire**.
- The different stages **may exist in different body organs** (e.g., the adult *Taenia solium* resides in the intestine, whereas the larval cysts exist in the brain and muscles).
- The different stages may pass through **hosts of entirely different host species** (e.g., *Plasmodium* cycles between humans and mosquitoes).

In order to overcome the adversary, the host employs a variety of defence mechanisms depending on the type of parasite and its life cycle stage. Generally, the host is able to differentiate its own antigens ('**self**') from the parasitic antigens ('**non-self**') and respond in one of the following two ways:

- **Non-specific responses:** These do not depend on the 'specific' recognition of a non-self molecule.
- **Specific responses:** In this type of response, the host recognises a 'specific' non-self molecule.

LINES OF DEFENCE

Fortunately, the human body is equipped with several **defence mechanisms** and has a large **armamentarium** at its disposal to tackle invaders.

1. **The first line of defence** is that of non-specific responses in the form of various physical barriers and **innate immunity** to keep intruders at bay. Innate immunity is present naturally and is not elicited by prior sensitisation to the antigen (e.g., by infection or vaccination). It is a rapid response to foreign invasion and usually sufficient to handle most infections. Some such defences are:
   - **The physical barrier** of intact skin
   - **Antimicrobial secretions such as fatty acids, lysozymes, RNAases** (RNA degrading ribonucleases), **DNAases** (DNA degrading deoxyribonucleases) and α- and **β-defensins,** which inhibit attachment and establishment of the pathogen
   - **Mucus secretion** in the respiratory and gastrointestinal tracts and the vagina
   - **Ciliary activity** in the respiratory tract and the **flushing action** of the urinary tract
   - **Acidic environment** of the stomach and the vagina
   - **Sudden pH change** from the stomach to the intestine
   - **Commensal microorganisms** living in/on the skin, oral cavity, respiratory and gastrointestinal tracts and the vagina, which compete with the pathogens for available attachment sites
   - Immune cells in the body recognise certain structures called **pathogen-associated molecular patterns (PAMP)** which are vital for the pathogens' survival, and mount an attack against organisms carrying these; PAMPs are composed of a combination of carbohydrates, proteins, lipids and nucleic acids
2. **The second line of defence or adaptive immunity** is specifically produced in response to exposure to foreign substances. Once activated against a specific type of antigen, this type of immunity remains throughout life. The adaptive immune system has a '**memory**' of pathogens it has encountered before.

The first- and second-line defence systems differ in their *modus operandi* and have unique sets of tools (Table 2.1). However, to optimise the available toolset, both systems use some common mechanisms.

A general 'strategy' followed by the two defence mechanisms to deal with the infective agent consists of the following steps:

1. Recognise the invader.
2. Communicate with each other and react to the invasion.

Table 2.1 Differences between the innate and adaptive arms of immunity

Innate immunity	Adaptive immunity
Rapid action	**Delayed** action
Conserved patterns of recognition and **fixed** but **broad** range of responses	**Can adapt** to the specific antigen and hence is **highly specific** but with **narrow** range of responses
Does not alter on repeated exposure	**Evolves** with successive infections; helps prevent re-infection and has 'memory'
Chief tools are inflammation, phagocytosis (macrophages, neutrophils, eosinophils, basophils, mast cells and platelets), complement (**alternate pathway**), natural killer cells and cytokines	Chief tools are cytokines, humoral (B cell) and cell-mediated (T cell) responses, specific phagocytosis, and complement (**classical pathway**), in tandem with some tools of innate immunity

3. Develop a 'memory' for subsequent interaction with the immunogen.

MECHANISMS OF RECOGNITION

The human body employs various mechanisms to recognise different types of intruders, mark them for easy identification by the immune cells, communicate with the other wings of defence and recruit defenders at the site of action.

Parasites have characteristic macromolecules on their surface and excrete or secrete unique proteinaceous macromolecules. These substances are referred to as antigens and can be recognised by the host.

Some of the mechanisms of recognition of pathogens by the host immune system are as follows:

- **Pathogen-associated molecules:** Pathogens have certain structures called **pathogen-associated molecular patterns (PAMP)** which are recognised by the host defence.
- **Host-associated receptors:**
  - The host immune system has **pattern recognition receptors (PRR)** complementary to the PAMPs. **Toll-like receptors (TLR)**, a type of PRR present on surfaces of various cells, recognise specific PAMPs. Another set of nucleotide-binding oligomerisation domain-like receptors or **NOD-like receptors (NLR)** are present intracellularly. These are important for mediating the trafficking of various immune chemicals and promoting inflammation.
  - **The complement system** consists of several proteins with a variety of biological activities. These proteins also function as soluble PRRs to mark the pathogen molecule by 'tagging' it (**opsonising**).
  - **Killer activation receptors (KAR)** and **killer inhibitory receptors (KIR)** are receptors present on the cell surfaces of **natural killer (NK)** lymphocytes that also differentiate between self and foreign antigens.
  - **Opsonising antibodies:** Several types of antibodies opsonise parasites by binding to their specific antigens through their **Fab end** (fragment antibody binding region), thus acting as receptors for the cells. The phagocytic cells, in turn, have receptors (**FcR**) **for the Fc** (fragment crystallisable) **end** of these antibodies (Fig. 2.1).
  - **Somatic receptors** are specialised high precision receptors of the adaptive immunity formed on the surface of B and T cells in response to specific parasite antigens.
    - **B cell receptors (BCR):** They are heterodimeric α and β immunoglobulin chains on the surface of B cells.
    - **T cell receptors (TCR):** They are heterodimeric α–β or γ–δ peptide chain pairs present on the surface of T cells.

MECHANISMS AND TOOLS OF COMMUNICATION AND REACTION

Cells of Different Lineages

- **Monocytes/macrophages:** These engulf (phagocytose) and kill parasites by toxic **reactive oxygen intermediates (ROIs)** formed by the reduction of O_2 into superoxide

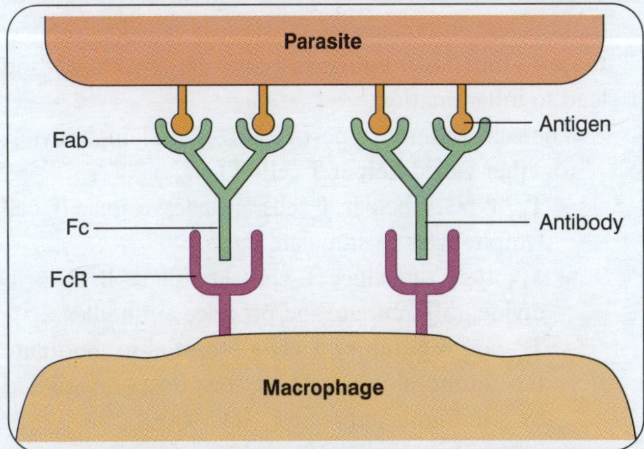

Fig. 2.1 Antibody opsonisation—antibody binding to the parasitic antigen at its Fab end and to the Fc receptor (FcR) of a phagocyte at its Fc end

anions ($^*O_2^-$), hydrogen peroxide (H_2O_2) and hydroxyl radicals (*OH), and by enzymatic digestion (acid hydrolases, myeloperoxidases, lysozymes, lactoferrins, defensins, etc.). Other toxic molecules like nitric oxide (NO) are also involved. Macrophages also secrete other signalling molecules which regulate the inflammatory response.

- **Neutrophils:** These are phagocytic cells that can kill parasites by both ROIs and O_2-independent mechanisms. They have a more intense respiratory burst (i.e., release of ROIs) than macrophages in which highly toxic secretory granules are released upon the parasite.
- **Eosinophils:** The eosinophil counts, along with IgE counts, are generally increased in parasitic infections, especially in those caused by helminths, which cannot be phagocytosed (larger targets). When a threat is encountered, eosinophils rush to the peripheral tissues such as the lungs and gut, where they are more likely to encounter large invaders. In addition to killing parasites by both ROIs and O_2–independent mechanisms, eosinophils release their contents upon the parasite in synchrony with mast cells, thereby killing it.

Eosinophils bind to *Schistosoma* worms coated with IgE/IgG and directly degranulate the major basic protein (MBP), ROIs, histamine, etc., on the surface of the worm.

- **Basophils/mast cells:** These contain a number of preformed mediators and cytokines such as heparin and histamine. In conjunction with eosinophils, these play an important role in killing and expelling worms from the gut.
- **Platelets:** They are capable of killing various types of parasites and exhibit both antibody-dependent and -independent cytotoxicity.
- **T cell lymphocytes:** There are a variety of T cells that release proteinaceous substances called cytokines; these induce an immune response in other cells and lead to inflammation.
  - There are different types of CD4$^+$ T cell lymphocytes, together called **helper T cells (T_h)**.
    - **T_{h1}** type of helper T cells act on cytotoxic T cell lymphocytes to stimulate them.
    - **T_{h2}** type of helper T cells stimulate B cells to divide, differentiate and produce antibodies.
    - **T_{reg}** are **regulatory T cells** essential to modulate the humoral or cellular responses mediated by immunosuppressive cytokines such as interleukin-10 (IL-10) and transforming growth factor β (TGF β). **T_{h3}** are a subset of T_{reg} found in the mucosa and are responsible for **oral tolerance** to the beneficial commensal microbes.
    - **T_{h17}** are proinflammatory cells which act by secreting **interleukin-17**.
  - CD8$^+$ T cell lymphocytes are called **cytotoxic T cells (CTL)**. These directly destroy infected cells with help from T_{h1} cells.
- **B cell lymphocytes/plasma cells:** Proteinaceous immunoglobulins (Ig), i.e., antibodies, are secreted by B cell lymphocytes. B cells mature to become **plasma cells** which secrete the Igs. The B cell response may be independent of or dependent on T cells.
- **NK cells:** These do not express variable receptors like B and T cells. They recognise abnormal-looking cells by detecting alterations in the host cells through KARs and kill the infected cells. NK cells act as the bridge between the innate and adaptive immune systems. NKT cells can act as both helper cells (secreting cytokines that shape responses) and cytotoxic cells (killing target cells).

Antibodies

There are five classes or isotypes of Ig (IgA, IgD, IgE, IgG and IgM) with different polypeptide structures and specialised functions. Antibodies attach to specific sites on the antigen by molecular recognition through the Fab region and usually trigger additional host responses (Fig. 2.2a–d). The following are the most significant functions of antibodies:

- **Neutralisation:** When antibodies bind to the parasite receptor site, they render it ineffective (neutralise the site), thus preventing further spread, blocking escape from lysosomes and overcoming the resistance of the parasite phagosome to fuse with the lysosome.
- **Enhancing phagocytosis:** Antibodies opsonise parasites (**opsonisation**) on their own and also act as co-stimulants for other molecules (such as complement–complement fixation) for recognition by macrophages.
- **Antibody-dependent cell-mediated cytotoxicity (ADCC):** Opsonisation of the parasite is followed by direct killing of the parasite by cytotoxic cells such as macrophages, eosinophils and neutrophils.

Soluble Defence Molecules

Several soluble chemical mediators act as effectors of the defence system as well as signalling molecules for inter- and intracellular communication.

- **Cytokines:** Numerous low-molecular-weight protein molecules secreted by leukocytes and other cells of the

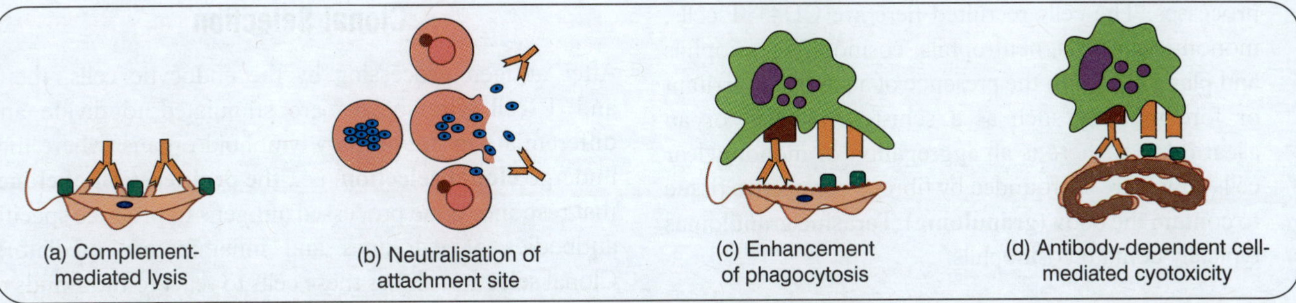

Fig. 2.2 (a), (b), (c) and (d) Mechanisms by which antibodies control parasitic infections

body are involved in cellular division, differentiation and inflammation related to innate as well as adaptive immunity.

- **Type I interferons (IFN I)** α, β **and** γ: IFNα and β are mainly important for viral infections, while IFNγ is produced by activated T cells and NK cells.
- **Interleukins (IL):** Various types of interleukins are produced by T cells, phagocytes and tissue cells, and perform a variety of functions.
- **Colony-stimulating factors (CSF):** These stimulate division and differentiation of different components of the bone marrow and are responsible for controlling the proportions of different types of cells in circulation.
- Many other molecules such as tumour necrosis factor α and β (TNF), transforming growth factor β (TGF) and insulin-like growth factor β (IGF) are also involved in regulating the immune response.

◈ **Complement system:** In the innate immune system, the complement system is activated by the alternative or mannan-binding lectin (MBL) pathway. In the adaptive immune system, it is activated by the classical pathway which is mediated by antigen–antibody complexes. The complement system mediates the killing of pathogens by the following three mechanisms:

- By lysing the pathogen by introducing a **membrane attack complex (MAC)**
- By **activating inflammatory phagocytes** and mediating chemotaxis
- By **opsonising** the pathogen-infected cell and facilitating its destruction

Phagocytosis

It is the process of ingesting particulate bodies akin to endocytosis or pinocytosis. It is a basic but primary line of defence against small foreign invaders like bacteria or protozoan parasites. Several cell types exhibit phagocytosis including polymorphonuclear leukocytes (PMNs), monocytes and macrophages. Phagocytes are strategically located in the tissues close to the capillaries and sinuses to keep 'a watch' for intruders. After engulfment, the foreign material is digested through lysosomal action and oxidative burst. Phagocytosis can occur non-specifically as an innate immune response or as a specific response when facilitated by opsonising antibodies and complement proteins.

> Some parasites have adapted to an intracellular mode of living using a variety of mechanisms to avoid destruction by the host cell. Toxoplasma prevents phagosome–lysosome fusion; *Leishmania* survives inside the fused phagolysosome; *Trypanosoma cruzi* escapes to the macrophage cytoplasm, while *Plasmodium* prefers the immunologically privileged erythrocytes.

Inflammation

It is a non-specific reaction which is biologically characterised by redness, heat, swelling and pain at the site of action. The increased temperature is an indicator to the other immune effectors of the ongoing inflammatory process. The different phases of inflammation are as follows:

◈ **Acute inflammation**, the first phase, lasts for about 2–4 days and is characterised by increased vascular permeability by capillary dilation leading to fluid accumulation or edema. There is an accumulation of PMNs (chiefly) at the site of the invasion or injury guided by chemotactic molecules (**chemokines**), the concentrations of which are found to increase in a gradated manner from the vessels to the tissue site (**chemotaxis**).

◈ **Subacute inflammation**, the second phase, lasts for 3 days to more than a week and is characterised by the presence of mononuclear cells (monocytes and lymphocytes) and fibrocytes which secrete collagen and form a fibrous capsule around the pathogen.

◈ **Chronic inflammation** is the third phase and comes into play if the infection is not cleared by the first two processes. The cells recruited here are CD4$^+$ T cells, mononuclear cells, neutrophils, eosinophils, basophils and plasma cells. In the presence of a persistent irritant or foreign body such as a schistosomal egg or an ascarid larva, there is an aggregation of mononuclear cells which are surrounded by fibrous connective tissue to contain the body (**granuloma**). Parasitic granulomas typically contain eosinophils.

Antigen Processing and T_h Polarisation

Parasitic antigens are ingested and processed by macrophages and other endocytic cells called **antigen-presenting cells (APCs)**. Dendritic cells are the most effective APCs. These APCs present the processed parasite antigens on their surface with the help of **MHC (major histocompatibility complex) molecules** to both B and T cells. This process is required for adaptive immunity.

- **MHC complex:** The human chromosome 6 possesses the genes that code for structural molecules and enzymes—together called the MHC complex—required for antigen processing. There are three classes of MHC complexes with different functions—MHC class I, II and III.
  - **MHC class I** molecules are expressed on most nucleated cells of the human body and present processed antigens in the cytosol to activate CD8$^+$ T cells (cytotoxic T cells).
  - **MHC class II** molecules are restricted to B cells, macrophages and dendritic cells and present exogenous antigens in phagolysosomes to activate CD4$^+$ T cells (T_h).
  - **MHC class III** molecules have diverse functions.
- The antigen processing by APCs also drives the T_h response differentiation into T_{h1} or T_{h2} types (Table 2.2). However, the T_{h1}/T_{h2} responses are not exclusive in action and switch during the course of an infection.

Table 2.2 Differences between T_{h1} and T_{h2} types of cell-mediated immunity

T_{h1} type	T_{h2} type
Combat **intracellular** pathogens	Combat **extracellular** pathogens
Stimulate CMI, cytotoxicity and inflammatory functions	Stimulate **B cells** to produce **antibodies**
Mediated by IL-1 and -2, IFNγ	Mediated by IL-4, -5, -6, -10 and -13
IL-12 required for production of T_{h1} cells	IL-4 important for production of T_{h2} cells

Clonal Selection

After antigen processing by the endocytic cells, the B and T cell lymphocytes are stimulated to divide and differentiate in the primary lymphoid organs, where they undergo **clonal selection**, i.e., **the proliferation of clones** that respond to the processed antigens to produce specific antibodies or cytokines and inflammatory mediators. Clonal selection allows these cells to react to thousands of different types of antigens.

Immunological memory: Some of the clonally selected B and T cells are preserved by the immune system (**memory cells**) in the chance that there is a another infection by the same parasite in the future. The second response is faster as it does not require the initial processing of the antigens (Fig. 2.3).

Humoral Response

Extracellular organisms in the blood, body fluids and the gastrointestinal tract are amenable to the action of antibodies produced by B cell-mediated response through CD4$^+$ T_{h2} cells. The action is predominantly based on opsonisation, phagocytosis and complement-mediated lysis (as is the case with *Trypanosoma brucei*). For intracellular parasites, antibodies are less effective; nevertheless, they are still useful as they limit the further spread of the parasite (e.g., *Trypanosoma cruzi* and *Leishmania*). Different types of antibodies have different roles. Some of these are as follows:

- **IgA** is synthesised in large amounts and secreted in tears, sweat and gastrointestinal, genitourinary and respiratory tract secretions to defend the parts of the body exposed to the external environment. IgA binds

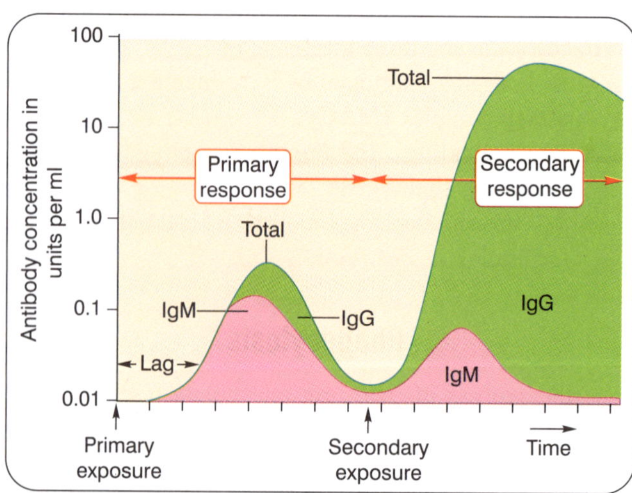

Fig. 2.3 Primary and secondary immune response—concentration and isotypes of antibody response after the first and subsequent encounters with the antigen

to the integument of the parasite along with IgG and attracts eosinophils which attack it through ADCC.

- **IgM** and **IgG** are often considered to be the most important in **protozoan** infections because they bind to parasite-specific antigens on infected cells, promoting phagocytosis, ADCC and complement-mediated lysis. IgG-positive individuals in malaria-endemic areas are temporarily protected against fresh infection.
- **IgE** antibodies, which are usually present in extremely low serum concentrations, are often elevated in **helminth** infections. In response to exposure to the parasites, IgE antibodies join the IgA antibodies on mast cells, inducing degranulation and the release of vasoactive mediators such as histamine and chemotactic factors. IgE also mediates allergic reactions and anaphylaxis (**type I or immediate hypersensitivity**).

IgE first induces inflammation, which damages the surface of the parasite to release antigens, and then activates IgG which causes further damage. T cells process the antigen and stimulate the goblet cells to proliferate and secrete cytokines and mucus which get coated on the surface of the parasite and expel it from the gut. Simultaneously, gut motility is increased by mast cell mediators to facilitate this expulsion.

Cell-Mediated Immune Response (CMI)

Although humoral and CMI are two distinct systems, they are intertwined. The immune response involves both arms to a variable extent. For intracellular parasites (e.g., *T. cruzi* and *Leishmania*), CMI is especially important as antibodies cannot access them. The CMI classically involves T lymphocytes which, by releasing various cytokines, initiate a cascade of reactions, leading to macrophage and CTL activation. Cytokines may also directly damage parasites. The end result is tissue injury by the cytotoxic products and non-specific inflammation which help to eliminate the parasite.

In cutaneous leishmaniasis, T_{h1} cells play a role in limiting the infection, whereas in the severe mucocutaneous variety, T_{h2} response is active with inadequate cellular response.

- **Delayed hypersensitivity** is mediated by $CD4^+$ T_{h1} cells (requiring MHC class II complex), mainly for parasites in phagolysosomes. The activated $CD4^+$ T cells further activate the macrophages either directly or by producing IFNγ. Once activated, the macrophages initiate phagocytosis and the release of various molecules such as TNF, ROIs, NO and destructive enzymes. Macrophages are also activated by IFNγ released from NK cells.
- **Cytotoxic T cell lymphocyte (CTL) activity** is mediated by $CD8^+$ CTLs (requiring MHC class I complex) and is aimed directly at the affected cells with parasites in the cytosol. Membrane damage and apoptosis brought about by these CTLs result in the lysis of the affected cells.

Abnormal Growth Responses

Another response to chronic inflammation caused by parasites is abnormal cell growth. **Hyperplasia**, in which the parasite stimulates the host to produce an increased number of cells, is one such response. For example, when the adult liver fluke, *Fasciola hepatica*, reaches the bile duct, it induces the enlargement of the bile duct epithelium. The fluke then grazes on these cells. **Neoplasia** or cancerous change is also an abnormal growth response. There is a definite correlation between the presence of *Schistosoma haematobium* in the urinary bladder and the occurrence of bladder carcinoma and between *Opisthorchis viverrini* and cholangiocarcinoma.

Concomitant Immunity

In an individual infected with a parasite, there is a 'vaccine-like' partial or complete protection against severe disease or reinfection with the same parasite. This is called **concomitant immunity** or **premunition** or **non-sterile immunity**. In *Schistosoma* infections, an individual infected with an adult fluke becomes immune to infections by cercariae of the same species. Such partial immunity against severe disease is also seen in the case of malaria in hyperendemic regions such as Africa, where the infection is maintained by continuous exposure to the parasite.

PARASITIC COUNTERMEASURES TO COMBAT HOST IMMUNITY

Just as host immunity has evolved through the ages, parasites have also evolved and developed ingenious methods to successfully infect the host by either utilising the host's own machinery or by escaping the immune response mounted by the host. The following are some of the mechanisms by which parasites achieve this:

- **Using host machinery**
  - Using complement for cell entry (e.g., *Leishmania*)
  - By **molecular mimicry** of host molecules (e.g., *Trypanosomes*)

- By acquiring the surface layer of host antigens (e.g., *Schistosoma*)
- **Physical separation** from the immune system protects the parasite from being directly harmed by antibodies, complement, soluble cytokines, phagocytosis and cytotoxicity. Some of the ways in which antibodies achieve this are as follows:
  - **Intracellular location** (e.g., *Toxoplasma, Plasmodium* and *Leishmania*)
  - **Cyst formation** (e.g., *Trichinella,* hydatid cysts and cysticerci)
  - **Nodule formation** (e.g., *Onchocerca*)
  - Residence in the intestine (e.g., tapeworms and nematodes)
- **Manipulating host immunity**
  - By resisting phagocytolysis (e.g., *Leishmania* and *Toxoplasma*)
  - By degrading antibodies (e.g., *Entamoeba histolytica*)
  - By disrupting lymphoid cell function (e.g., *Trichinella*)
  - By downregulating inflammation by **stimulating the release of anti-inflammatory molecules** such as prostaglandins, IL-10 and TGFβ
  - By shifting the balance of immunity to **T_{h2} type** of response
- **Presence of free circulating parasite antigens**—free antigens in the circulation block and consume the antibodies and effector cells. Persistent antigenic stimuli result in **polyclonal activation of B/T cells** and **non-specific hypergammaglobulinemia**, thus causing the exhaustion of the capacity of the immune system to produce effector molecules (e.g., *Leishmania,* trypanosomes and *Plasmodium*).
- **Antigenic variation**—different antigens of the same protein may be expressed in succession by some parasites to confuse the host immunity (e.g., proteins such as *Trypanosoma* VSG, *Plasmodium* PfEMP and *Giardia* VSP).

Helminths and Immune Regulation

The cosmopolitan prevalence of helminth infections reflects their ability to manipulate the host immune system to promote their survival. They do this mainly by suppressing immune responses that could result in their elimination from the host. This downregulation of the immune system by helminths takes effect at multiple levels and is associated with a modified T_{h2} response, i.e., a **modulation towards a T_{h2}/T_{reg} response**. Though such modulation of the immune response has some harmful effects, it also confers some benefits to the host.

- **Beneficial aspects:** Responsiveness to some antigens and autoantigens is decreased and excessive inflammatory reaction is reduced. The host is thus protected against some allergic and autoimmune or chronic inflammatory diseases.
  - **Hygiene hypothesis:** Lower rates of childhood infections in developed countries can be attributed to higher standards of living and public health, antibiotics usage, vaccination, etc. (**improved hygiene**). In these countries, epidemiological studies have indicated a higher incidence of allergies (e.g., asthma, eczema and allergic rhinitis) and autoimmune diseases (e.g., multiple sclerosis and inflammatory bowel disease) than in developing countries where childhood infections are common. This phenomenon of increased incidence of allergic disorders associated with lower incidence of infections is called the '**hygiene hypothesis**'. The reasons for this inverse relationship of hygiene to immune disorders are not completely clear. There is some evidence that helminths can attenuate allergic conditions by modulating the immune response. Other factors associated with developed societies such as pollution, obesity and lifestyle may also have a role in this inverse relationship.
- **Harmful aspects:** The modified immune response hampers protection against other infections as well. This has the following harmful results:
  - Susceptibility as well as severity of other microbial infections increases.
  - Responsiveness to 'bystander' antigens such as vaccines may be decreased and could compromise the vaccine efficacy.
  - A large proportion of individuals may become asymptomatic carriers with depressed immune reactivity to the infecting parasite; this leads to chronicity of the infection. Such chronic infections rob the host of its nutrition and cause growth retardation and long-term morbidity.

Multiple Choice Questions

1. Which of the following is NOT TRUE regarding the T_{h1} type of immune response?
   a. It helps to combat intracellular pathogens.
   b. It is mediated by IL-1, IL-2 and IFNγ.
   c. IL-4 is required for the production of T_{h1} cells.
   d. It stimulates cell-mediated immunity, cytotoxicity and inflammatory functions.

2. There is a definite correlation between the presence of ________ parasite in the urinary bladder and the occurrence of bladder carcinoma.
   a. *Schistosoma haematobium*
   b. *Trichomonas vaginalis*
   c. *Entamoeba histolytica*
   d. *Taenia solium*

3. Antigenic variation as a means of evading the host's immune response is adopted by ________:
   a. Hookworms
   b. *Entamoeba histolytica*
   c. *Trypanosoma*
   d. *Fasciola hepatica*

4. Molecular mimicry of host molecules as a means of evading immune response is adopted by ________:
   a. Trypanosomes b. *Entamoeba histolytica*
   c. Malarial parasite d. Hookworms

5. Intestinal ________ infections are characterised by a predominant IgE response.
   a. Protozoan b. Helminth
   c. Bacterial d. Viral

CHAPTER 3

Protozoa – Introduction and Classification

(*proto* [English] = first + *zoion* [Greek] = animal)

INTRODUCTION

The biological organisation of the living world fundamentally consists of two classes—prokaryotes and eukaryotes. **Prokaryotes** are comprised entirely of bacteria while **eukaryotes** include all other unicellular or multicellular organisms. **Unicellular eukaryotes** are called **protists or protozoa**. **Multicellular eukaryotes** include **metazoa** (all helminths, molluscs, arthropods, fish, amphibians, reptiles, birds and mammals) and plants whose cells are organised with defined functions and division of labour. While helminths have been long known to be associated with human disease, protozoa, being too small to be visible to the naked eye, were not known to exist until Antonie van Leeuwenhoek (1632–1723) invented the microscope. Even then, it was another 200 years before microscopic organisms were associated with diseases in animals and humans.

MORPHOLOGY

Protozoans are highly diverse in their structural organisation. A protozoan is single-celled, ranges in size from 2–250 µm and consists of cytoplasm and nuclear material bound by a limiting membrane and several accessory organelles (Fig. 3.1).

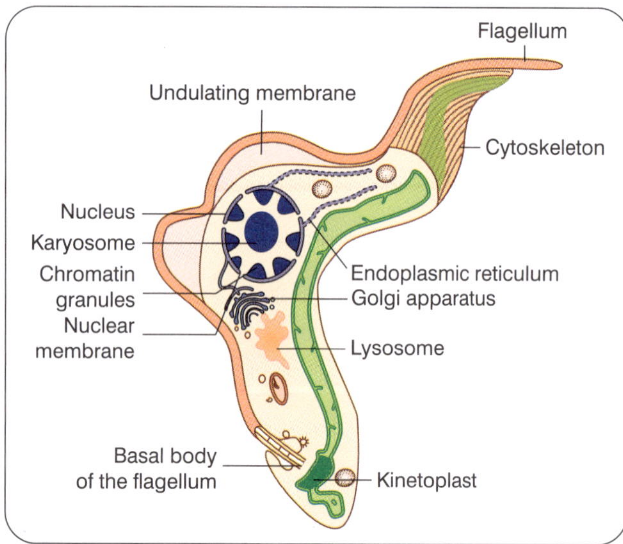

Fig. 3.1 Line diagram of a protozoan cell showing its various organelles

There are two morphologically distinct stages seen in the protozoan life cycle:

- **Trophozoite:** It is the **active** feeding and multiplying stage, usually seen in favourable conditions.
- **Cyst:** It is the **inactive/resting/dormant** stage. A cyst is characterised by a thick cyst wall which allows it to survive harsh environmental conditions.

Nucleus and Cytoplasm

- **Nucleus:** The nucleus contains the deoxyribonucleic acid (**DNA**) of the organism on well-defined **chromosomes**. The structural features of the nucleus often help in the differentiation of the various species. The nucleus is bound externally by a well-defined **nuclear membrane**. The inner aspect of the nuclear membrane is lined with **chromatin granules**, the arrangement and density of which differ within species. The nucleoli exist as conspicuous structures known as **karyosomes** situated inside the nucleus. Their size, shape, density and location (central or eccentric) also differs in different amoebic species. Some protozoans have more than one nucleus—ciliates have two differently sized nuclei, a macronucleus and a micronucleus (e.g., *Balantidium*).
- **Kinetoplast:** In flagellates such as trypanosomes, a non-nuclear DNA-containing body called the kinetoplastid is situated near the kinetosome (the origin of the flagella).
- **Cytoplasm:** The cytoplasm is generally divisible into a clear ectoplasm and granular endoplasm containing a number of structures—the nucleus, Golgi bodies, the endoplasmic reticulum, microtubules, mitochondria, food vacuoles and contractile vacuoles. Numerous structures develop from the cytoplasm such as organelles of locomotion and the cyst wall.
- **Plasma membrane:** The cytoplasm is surrounded by a lipid bilayer interspersed with various membrane glycoproteins.
- **Contractile vacuole:** Located in the cytoplasm, the contractile vacuole has excretory and osmoregulatory functions.
- **Cyst wall:** A thick wall forms in the cystic stage of the parasite's life cycle to bear environmental stress. It is a complex structure that consists chiefly of a filamentous network of N-acetyl-D-galactosamine and cyst wall protein complexes along with cellulose.

Organelles of Locomotion

Broadly, three types of organelles for locomotion are seen in protozoa.

- **Pseudopodia:** These are temporary protrusions of the surface of a cell that assist in movement and feeding (e.g., *Entamoeba*). **Lobopodia** are a type of pseudopodia found in most medically important amoebas; they are finger-shaped and contain both the ectoplasm and endoplasm. **Acanthopodia** are spine-like pseudopodia (as seen in *Acanthamoeba*). Movement occurs due to protoplasmic streaming which is a result of the interaction of microfilaments and myosin (Fig. 3.2a).
- **Flagella:** These are long, delicate, whip-like structures (Fig. 3.2b) consisting of 9+2 arrangement of microtubules that originate from the **kinetosomes** (examples of flagellated protozoa include *Giardia* and *Trypanosoma*). Flagella may be anteriorly, laterally or posteriorly located depending on the position of the kinetosome.
- **Cilia:** The surfaces of some protozoa (like *Balantidium*) are covered with fine, hair-like filaments that have internal structures like those of flagella (Fig. 3.2c); these filaments are called cilia. These appear to move back and forth in unison.

FEEDING AND EXCRETION

The medically important protozoa are **heterotrophic**, i.e., they require energy in the form of complex carbon molecules and preformed nitrogenous amino acids. They employ various strategies to obtain nutrition from the environment. Some of these are as follows:

- Some protozoa have temporary mechanisms for the **ingestion** of food such as **phagocytosis** for particles and **pinocytosis** for fluids (**endocytosis**). Others have a permanent opening like a **cytostome** through which food is engulfed to form a **food vacuole**, inside which digestion takes place (e.g., *Balantidium*).
- **Excretion** takes place through **temporary openings** that extrude undigested products or by **diffusion** of ammonia through the cell membrane into the external surroundings. For intracellular protozoans, waste products **accumulate** in the host cell and are released on the death of the host cell, causing toxic symptoms in the host (as in the case of malaria). Apart from excretion, **contractile vacuoles** also help in osmoregulation by pumping out excess water from the cell.

ENCYSTMENT AND EXCYSTATION

Some protozoa have the property of transforming from an active trophozoite to a dormant cyst to survive extremes of temperature, pH and osmolarity.

- **Encystment** may be induced in conditions such as shortage of food, dehydration and changes in pH, temperature and oxygen concentration. In such situations, a cyst wall is secreted, starch and glycogen are stored for nutrition, the metabolism is downregulated and many organelles are resorbed. A nuclear division may render the cyst with more nuclei than the trophozoite stage. A cyst lacks the ability to grow and multiply; it has an environment-resistant wall and is non-motile. It has to be mechanically transferred from one host to another through water, vegetation, air, fomites, etc.
- **Excystation** occurs when favourable conditions are restored. This stage is characterised by the absorption of water and swelling of the cyst, upregulation of metabolism, dissolution of the cyst wall by protozoan and host enzymes and reorganisation of the cytoplasmic organelles.

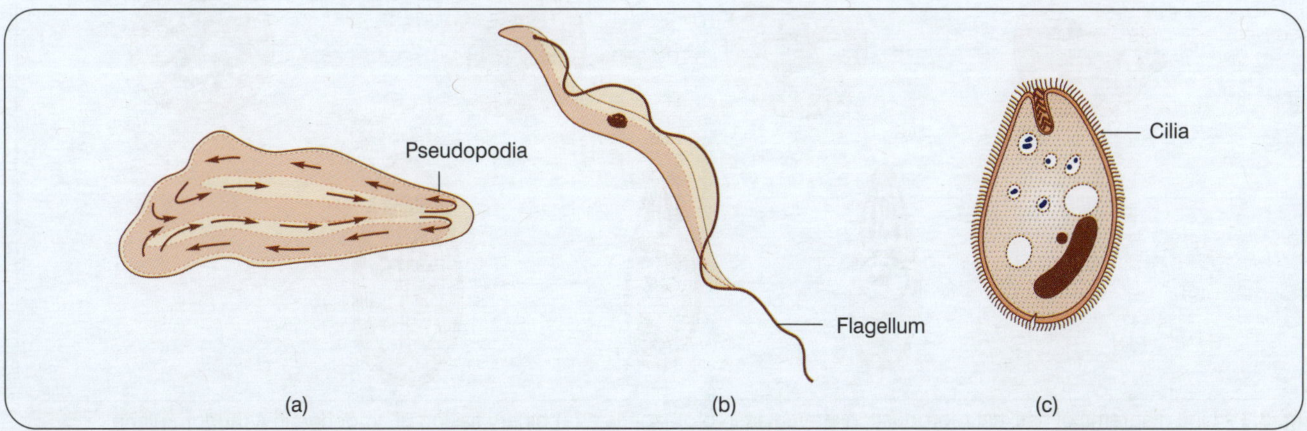

Fig. 3.2 Line diagrams of appendages of locomotion in protozoans: (a) pseudopodia in amoebae, (b) flagella in trypanosomes and (c) cilia in ciliates

REPRODUCTION

Asexual Multiplication

The more common mode of reproduction in protozoa is asexual reproduction. The following are the modes of asexual multiplication seen in protozoans:

- **Binary fission:** In this type of multiplication, each parasite divides in a random (e.g., amoebae, Fig. 3.3a), longitudinal (e.g., *Leishmania*, Fig. 3.3b) or horizontal plane into two roughly equal parts. All cellular structures are duplicated before division.
- **Multiple fission (schizogony/merogony):** In this type of multiplication, more than two daughter cells are produced by repeated division of the nucleus and essential organelles, followed by layering of each nucleus with cytoplasm and a cell membrane. The parent cell is called **schizont or meront** and the daughter cells are called **merozoites**. Finally, the parent cell ruptures and releases the numerous daughter cells (e.g., *Plasmodium*, Fig. 3.3c).
- **Endodyogeny:** Some protozoa multiply by internal budding which results in the formation of two daughter cells (e.g. *Toxoplasma*, Fig. 3.3d).
- **Sporogony:** This type of multiplication is characterised by multiple fission after the formation of the zygote which leads to the generation of **sporozoites**.

Sexual Reproduction

This mode of reproduction is less common in protozoa. The following sexual processes are seen in protozoans:

- **Gametogony (syngamy):** In this type of multiplication, a union of macro- and micro-gametes (female and male) produces a zygote from which daughter cells are produced (e.g., *Plasmodium*).
- **Conjugation:** In this type of multiplication (as in *Balantidium*), two cells temporarily unite to exchange genetic material and subsequently separate. However, the number of cells remains the same after conjugation, and the parasite multiplies by asexual binary fission only.

LIFE CYCLE

- **Single host:** Protozoans like *Entamoeba* and *Giardia* require only one host within which they multiply asexually in the trophozoite stage and get converted to the resting cystic stage to complete their life cycles.

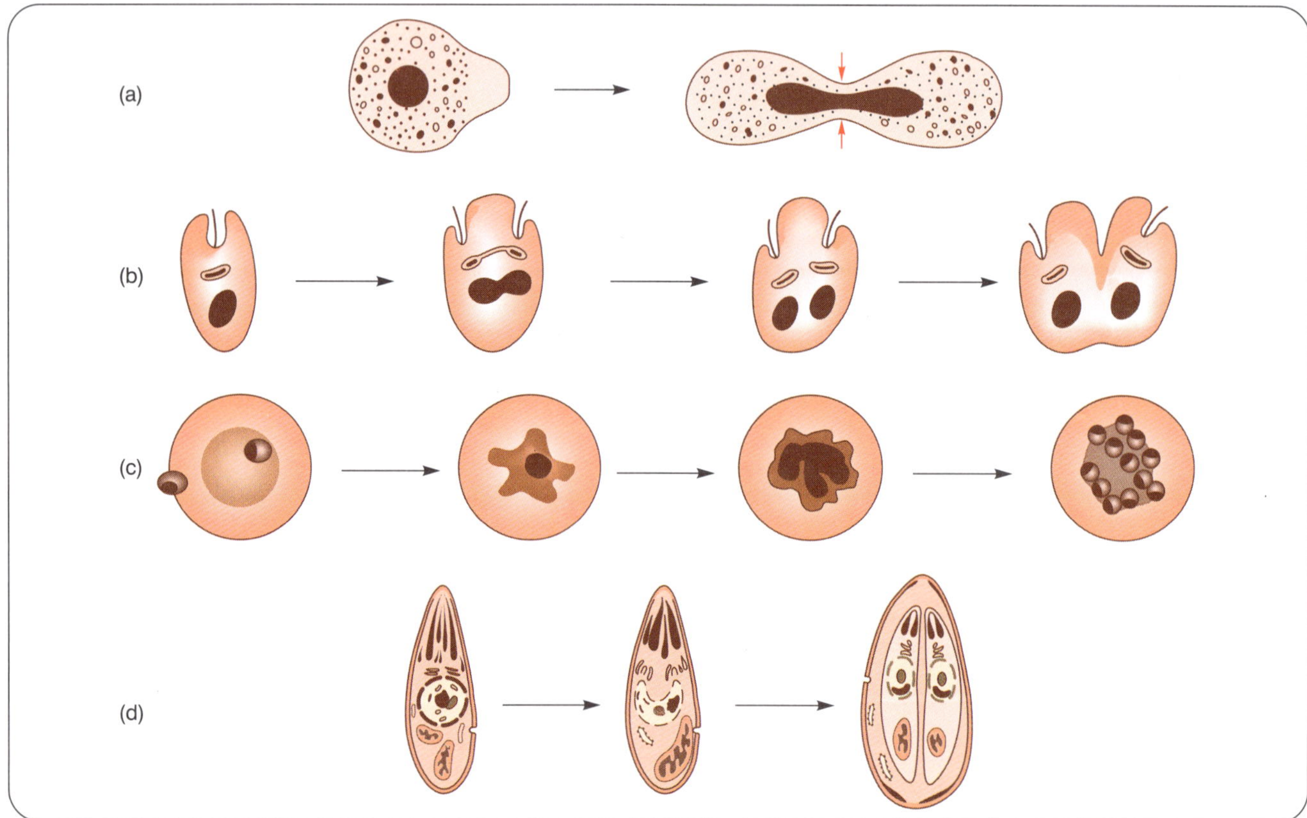

Fig. 3.3 Line diagrams of asexual reproduction strategies in protozoans – (a) binary fission of amoebae in a random plane, (b) binary fission of *Leishmania* in the longitudinal plane, (c) multiple fission (schizogony/merogony) in *Plasmodium* and (d) endodyogeny in *Toxoplasma*

These cysts can survive unfavourable environments and get transmitted from one host to another by various routes.

- **Two hosts:** Some protozoa like *Plasmodium* and *Leishmania* multiply asexually in one host (man) and by sexual means in another host (mosquito or sandfly). This is called **alternation of generation**.

CLASSIFICATION OF PARASITES

The taxonomy of microorganisms has come a long way since **Carl Linnaeus** (in 1758) classified all living things under two kingdoms—Animalia and Plantae—and introduced the concept of lower-level taxonomic categories (class, order, genus and species). In 1998, based on fresh information available at the biochemical and molecular levels, **Thomas Cavalier-Smith classified living things into six kingdoms—Bacteria, Protozoa, Chromista, Plantae, Fungi and Animalia**—effectively separating protozoa from both plant and animal kingdoms. The classification of parasites has evolved extensively since then and continues to do so owing to the sophistication of molecular taxonomic methods and bioinformatics. The Cavalier-Smith classification of 1998 has been adopted in this chapter to maintain consistency with the current medical literature.

Broadly, the **parasites** of human importance belong to three kingdoms—Protozoa, Chromista and Animalia.

- **Kingdom Protozoa:** This kingdom comprises unicellular, eukaryotic, **non-photosynthetic** organisms that lack cell walls and plastids. It consists of two subkingdoms—**Archezoa and Neozoa**. Most medically important parasites belong to seven phyla (Fig. 3.4).
  - **Subkingdom 1 – Archezoa:** This comprises unicellular eukaryotic organisms that have some prokaryotic features in their ribosomes, transfer ribonucleic acid (tRNA) and lack mitochondria, Golgi bodies and some other organelles. *Giardia* and *Trichomonas* belong to this subkingdom.
  - **Subkingdom 2 – Neozoa:** This comprises unicellular eukaryotic organisms that typically

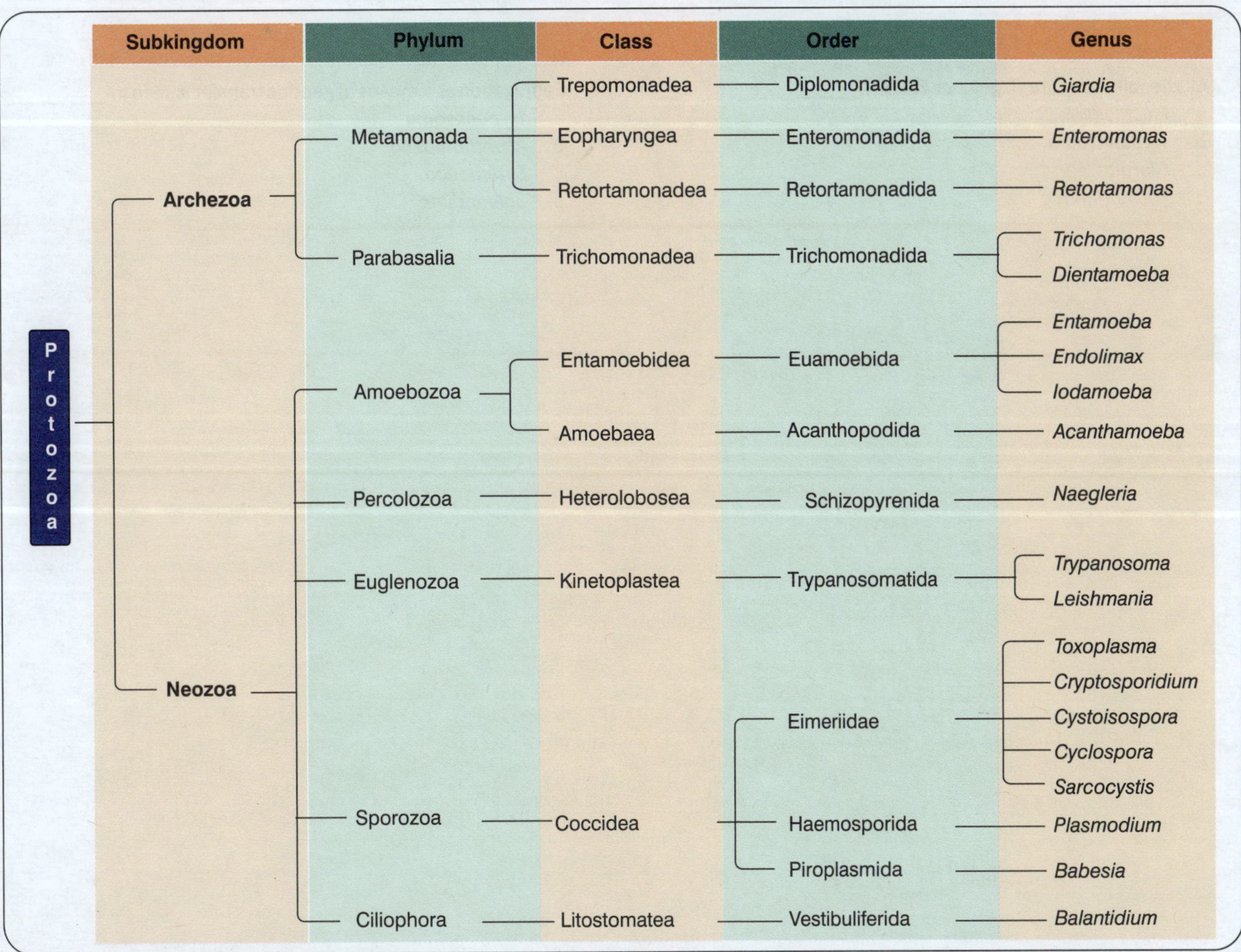

Fig. 3.4 Classification of kingdom Protozoa

possess mitochondria, Golgi bodies and cytoplasmic inclusions including hydrogenosomes and peroxisomes. The majority of parasites of human importance belong to Neozoa.

- **Kingdom Chromista:** This kingdom comprises unicellular, eukaryotic, **photosynthetic**, filamentous or colonial organisms (in part 'algae'), some with a secondary loss of plastids. ***Blastocystis hominis*** is the only medically important human parasite from this kingdom.
- **Kingdom Animalia:** This kingdom comprises multicellular, eukaryotic, **heterotrophic** (those that feed on organic matter and digest it internally) organisms. All medically important **helminths** belong to this kingdom.

Questions

1. Discuss various modalities of reproduction in protozoa.
2. Discuss the organelles of locomotion in protozoa.
3. Discuss encystment and excystation and their importance for protozoa.

Multiple Choice Questions

1. The organs of locomotion in *Balantidium* are _________ :
   a. Flagella
   b. Cilia
   c. Pseudopodia
   d. Fimbria
2. All the following are flagellates EXCEPT _________:
   a. *Plasmodium*
   b. *Trypanosoma*
   c. *Giardia*
   d. *Trichomonas*
3. Alternation of generation is seen in _________ :
   a. *Plasmodium*
   b. *Giardia*
   c. *Entamoeba histolytica*
   d. *Trichomonas vaginalis*
4. Conjugation as a means of genetic transfer is seen in _________:
   a. *Trypanosoma*
   b. *Acanthamoeba*
   c. *Entamoeba*
   d. *Balantidium*

CHAPTER 4

Entamoeba histolytica

([From Greek] *entos* = inside + *amoibos* = changing; *histos* = tissue + *luein* = to dissolve)

Case Study and Learning Goals

A 25-year-old male presents to the emergency department with a history of high-grade fever and pain in the right hypochondrium for the past seven days and complaints of a loss of 10 kg of weight over the last two months. He had bloody diarrhea about 3 months back and is a chronic alcoholic. Ultrasonographic examination reveals a space-occupying lesion measuring 3 cm in the right lobe of his liver. What are the parasitic causes of space-occupying lesions in the liver? How would you approach the laboratory diagnosis in this case? How would you treat this patient?

INTRODUCTION

Amoebae are animalcules that do not have any definitive shape. A number of amoebae are found in the human intestine where they usually exist as commensals, though they may occasionally be implicated in diarrhea. The **only amoeba to have definite pathogenic potential is *Entamoeba histolytica***, a major cause of **bloody diarrhea (dysentery) and extra-intestinal invasive disease** in humans. Amoebae that closely resemble this pathogen are *E. dispar*, *E. moshkovskii* and *E. bangladeshi*. *E. hartmanni*, *E. coli*, *E. gingivalis* (present in the mouth), *Endolimax nana* and *Iodamoeba butschlii* are other members of the family *Entamoebidae* that differ from *E. histolytica* in morphology. These species cause no symptomatology.

The earliest reference to bloody diarrhea containing mucus was found in the Sanskrit astrological treatise, *Bhrigu Samhita,* which dates back to about 1000 BC. Similar medical conditions were mentioned in Assyrian and Babylonian texts dating back to the 6th century BC. Liver abscess was described in the 2nd century BC by Galen and Celsus, though the causative agent, being microscopic, remained elusive for a long time. Much later (in 1873), *E. histolytica* was discovered in Russia by Friedrich Losch, who also established the parasite–disease relationship in dogs experimentally. In 1925, Emile Brumpt suggested that apart from the pathogenic *E. histolytica*, the genus also includes a morphologically similar but non-pathogenic species, *E. dispar*; however, his conjecture was promptly dismissed. Consequently, the presence of similar-looking amoebae continued to be a source of confusion for scientists for many years. It was only after the advent of biochemical techniques that a clear distinction was made between the pathogenic *E. histolytica* as the non-pathogenic commensal *E. dispar* based on the **electrophoretic banding patterns of isoenzymes (zymodemes)**. This distinction was confirmed in the second half of the 20th century by molecular biology techniques.

EPIDEMIOLOGY

E. histolytica is responsible for amoebiasis, a disease that is prevalent across the globe, affecting about 10% of the world's population. The highest burden of the disease is borne by developing countries (as a result of poor hygiene and sanitation), particularly in the tropical and subtropical regions in Central and South America, Africa, the Indian subcontinent and China. Globally, *E. histolytica* is the **second most common parasitic cause of mortality (after malaria)**, accounting for an estimated 55,000 deaths each year. In **India**, amoebiasis affects about 15% of the population and has been reported from across the country.

In addition to being a potentially fatal disease, amoebiasis has important social and economic implications as it requires several weeks of hospitalisation and takes 2–3 months for patients to recover fully—this results in a loss of wages in an already impoverished population.

Risk Factors

The **risk factors** that predispose to increased severity are young age (children, especially neonates are at greater risk), pregnancy, corticosteroid use, alcoholism, malignancy, malnutrition, homosexual activity, immigration and travel. It is one of the most frequently isolated pathogen among **travellers** returning from endemic areas after a long stay.

MORPHOLOGY

E. histolytica has several successive life cycle stages, viz. trophozoite, pre-cyst, cyst and metacyst stages.

Trophozoite (From Greek; *Trophe* = Food + *Zoon* = Animal)

It is **amoeboid** in shape, usually **20–30 µm in size (though it could range from 10–60 µm)** and actively **motile** in fresh stool with short hyaline **pseudopodia** that extend and withdraw (Fig. 4.1a).

- The cytoplasm is visible with a clear, thin ectoplasm on the outside and a granular **'ground-glass'** endoplasm inside.
- Iron hematoxylin staining allows the clear visualisation of the **nucleus**, which is single and spherical with a **compact karyosome** at its centre. Delicate fibrils radiate outwards from the karyosome to the nuclear membrane. The inner surface of the nuclear membrane is lined with **evenly distributed fine chromatin granules**.
- Food vacuoles with **ingested erythrocytes** and bacteria can often be seen.

Cyst (From Greek; *Kystis* = Bladder)

The trophozoites condense to form spheroid **pre-cysts** which mature into cysts measuring **10 × 20** µm in size. Cysts are typically found in formed, i.e., semi-solid, and solid stool (Fig. 4.1b and c).

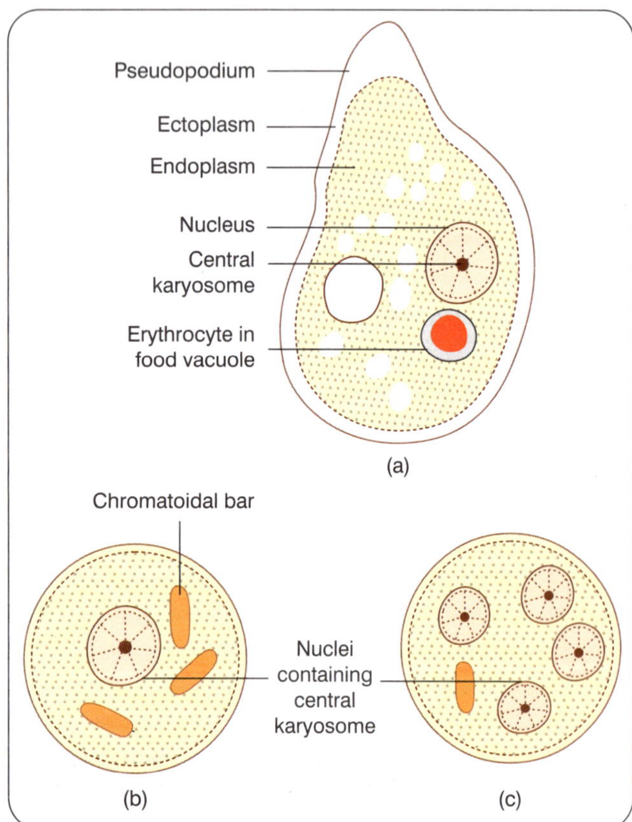

Fig. 4.1 Line diagrams of *E. histolytica:* (a) trophozoite, (b) pre-cyst and (c) cyst

- An early cyst has one nucleus which divides into two or four nuclei **(metacyst)** on maturation.
- The mature cyst has a hyaline cyst wall.
- Glycogen vacuoles and refractive chromatid bars are present in the pre-cyst; these generally disappear on maturation. Glycogen is stained dark brown on iodine staining, whereas chromatid bars remain unstained and appear as clear areas.

LIFE CYCLE (Fig. 4.2a and b)

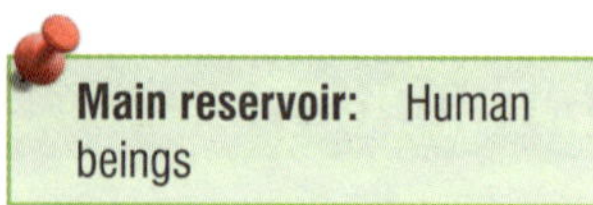

Humans are the only significant reservoir hosts for *E. histolytica*. The **cysts are the infective forms** and are ingested through contaminated drinking water or food or from contaminated hands; they may even be transmitted by sexual contact. The different life cycle phases are as follows:

- **Excystation (conversion of cyst to trophozoite):** After ingestion, the cysts pass through the acidic environment of the stomach and reach the alkaline small intestine, where the cytoplasm and the nuclei divide to form eight small amoebulae or small trophozoites. These migrate towards the caecum and feed and multiply in the crypts of the **large intestine** asexually by simple **binary fission**. They feed on starch, mucosal secretions and bacteria. The pathogenic amoebae can hydrolyse the mucosa and initiate **tissue invasion**.
- **Encystation (conversion of trophozoite to cyst):** As the amoeba move further down the intestinal tract, the contents of the intestine become progressively dehydrated, which stimulates some of the amoeba trophozoites to encyst. The encystation process occurs only in the intestine. Both trophozoites and cysts are released in the feces. Cysts are commonly seen in formed stool but not in dysenteric stool (in which only trophozoites are seen). Trophozoites cannot encyst once they are outside the human body or once they have invaded the tissues. This is the reason for the absence of cysts from liver abscess pus. Cysts are very resistant and can survive in moist, cool environments for days to weeks; they are not killed by routine chlorination, which causes trophozoites to disintegrate within a few hours.

Individuals harbouring the amoebae may continue to pass cysts in their stool. Such individuals are known as **carriers** or **cyst-passers**. They may either be **asymptomatic** or **healthy carriers**. Those who develop clinical disease and subsequently recover are known as **convalescent carriers**.

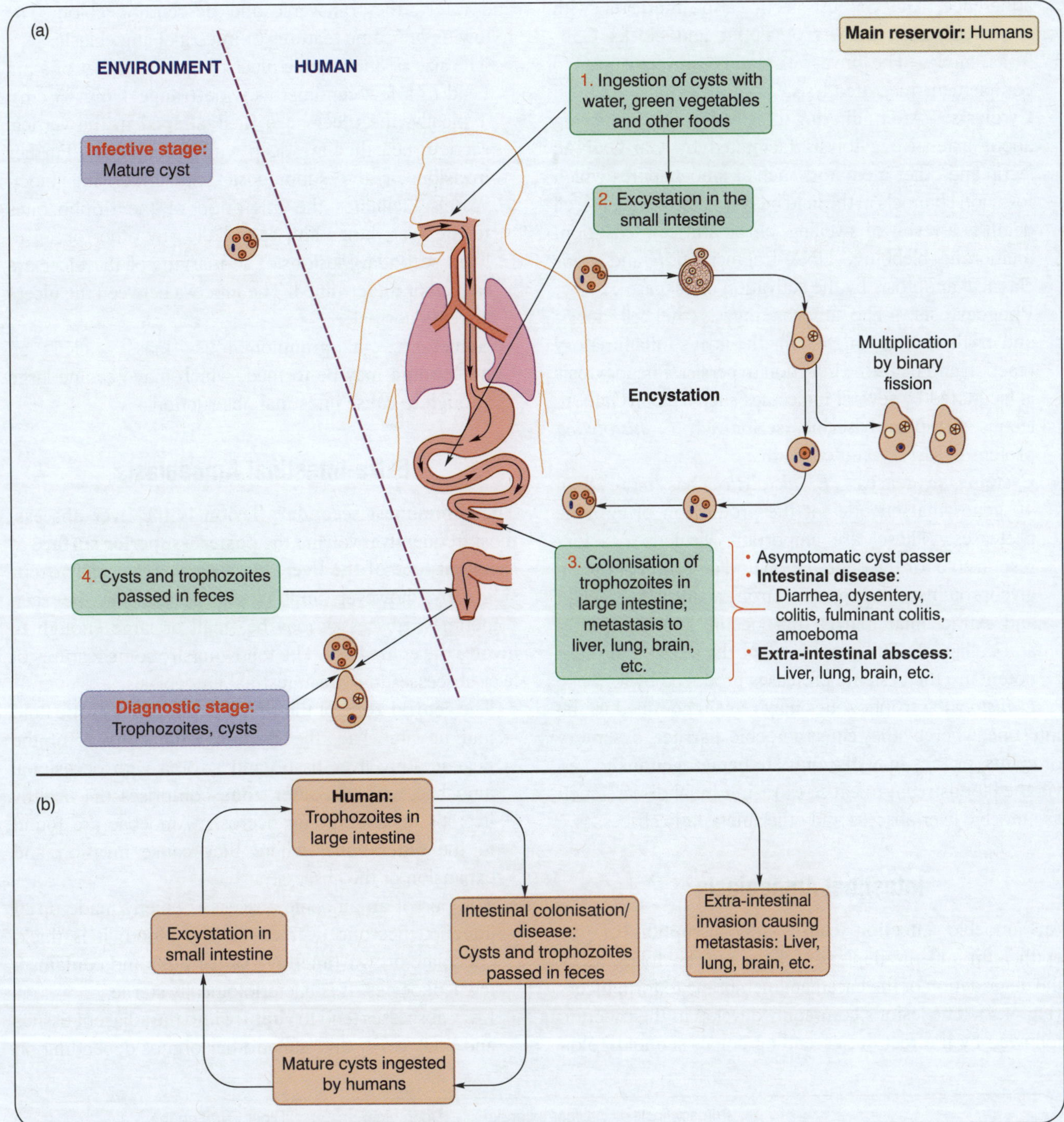

Fig. 4.2 Life cycle of *E. histolytica:* (a) detailed and (b) schematic diagrams

PATHOGENESIS

Human beings are infected with the cystic forms of *E. histolytica*. After excystation, some of the amoebae are successful in colonising the large intestine; the manifestation varies from a carrier state to diarrhea or invasive disease. *E. histolytica* is equipped with several virulence factors that enable it to cause extensive tissue destruction by lysing host cells. The following are the mechanisms of pathogenesis of the infection:

- **Adherence:** The 260 kDa **galactose and N-acetyl-D-galactosamine (Gal/GalNAc) lectin** present on the trophozoite surface facilitate adherence by binding to the human colonic mucin glycoproteins, epithelial cells and other target cells. Although mucin facilitates the binding of the parasite, it also protects the intestinal epithelium from direct lysis. In addition to facilitating adherence, Gal/GalNAc lectin also interferes with the chemotactic activity of TNFα and blocks C5b-9 assembly. The invasive strains are resistant to complement-mediated lysis.

- **Cytolysis:** After adhering to cells, the amoebae bring about extensive cytolysis facilitated by Gal/GalNAc lectin and other mediators such as amoebapores which form ion channels in the lipid bilayer of the host cell. Cell death is a result of swelling, chromatin condensation, membrane blebbing, DNA fragmentation and non-classical apoptosis by the activation of caspase 3.
- **Phagocytosis:** The amoeba ingests the cell debris and erythrocytes, which limits the host's inflammatory reaction and helps the infection to persist. Phagocytosis is facilitated by several molecules such as Gal/GalNAc lectin, phosphatidylserine, serine-rich *E. histolytica* protein (SREHP) and collectins.
- **Cysteine proteases:** *E. histolytica* has more than 40 genes that encode for the production of cysteine proteases. These are important virulence factors responsible for the degradation and digestion of mucin glycoproteins, hemoglobin (iron acquisition), villin and extracellular matrix (fibronectin, laminin, elastin and collagen). The more virulent the strain, the more potent are the cysteine proteases produced by it.

E. histolytica trophozoites may remain confined to the intestine, whereby they cause amoebic diarrhea, dysentery or colitis, or they may **disseminate hematogenously**, i.e., via the bloodstream to cause extra-intestinal disease such as amoebic liver abscess and other metastatic abscesses.

Intestinal Amoebiasis

An amoebic infection causes the disruption of the epithelium and the depletion of the mucus, followed by the degradation of the basement membrane to form ulcers (Fig. 4.3). The lesions commonly develop in the caecum, followed by the rectum, ascending colon, sigmoid colon and rarely, the transverse and descending colon. The following are some features of intestinal amoebiasis:

- The size of an amoebic ulcer ranges from that of a pin head to a few centimetres wide (range 1 mm–3 cm). Typically, the **ulcers are flask-shaped** in the vertical section, i.e., they are deep with broad bases. Further invasion of the submucosa and underlying blood vessels facilitates the migration of the trophozoites to the liver, lungs and essentially any other organ to form secondary lesions. The margins of the ulcer are ragged or undermined. The mucosa between the ulcers appears normal.
- Sometimes, a granulomatous mass called an **amoeboma** may be formed, which may become large enough to cause intestinal obstruction.

Extra-intestinal Amoebiasis

The **commonest secondary lesion is the liver abscess**, most frequently involving the **postero-superior surface of the right lobe of the liver**. Liver abscesses usually occur singularly; however, multiple abscesses may be seen sometimes. Abscesses may be small or large enough to involve the entire liver. The following are some features of liver abscesses in extra-intestinal amoebiasis:

- The **central zone** of the abscess contains necrotic fluid and no amoebae, the **median zone** consists of the degenerating liver tissue and stroma with occasional amoebae, and the **outer zone** comprises the healthy liver tissue undergoing necrosis. Amoebae are found in the outer zone, where they cause invasion and expansion of the abscess.
- The pus of an amoebic abscess is chiefly made up of liquefied necrotic liver tissue and blood; it is thick, chocolate brown (**anchovy sauce pus**) and contains a few leukocytes. It is bacteriologically sterile.
- Liver abscesses tend to **rupture** into the adjacent tissues and body cavity and affect other organs depending on

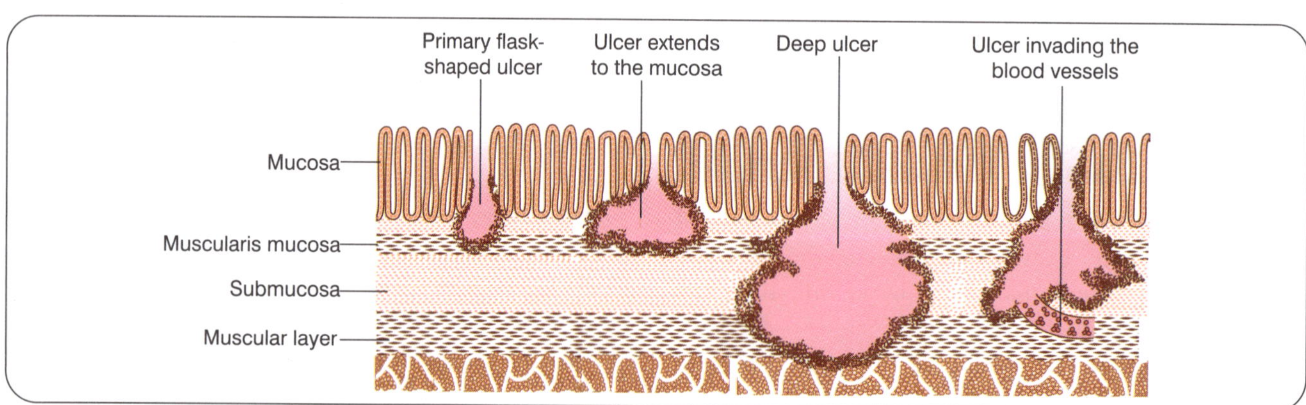

Fig. 4.3 Line diagram showing the characteristics of amoebic ulcers

the location of the abscess and the direction of the rupture (Fig. 4.4). A right-sided abscess may rupture into the lung or right pleural cavity through the diaphragm or subphrenically into the peritoneal cavity. A left-sided abscess may rupture into the stomach, pericardial cavity or the left pleural cavity. An inferior abscess may rupture into the intestine, while a posterior abscess may affect the inferior vena cava. An external rupture may involve the abdominal wall and skin.

- Trophozoites may also be carried via the bloodstream to cause metastatic abscesses anywhere in the body.

CLINICAL FEATURES

The incubation period of *E. histolytica* varies from 1–4 weeks. The most common type of amoebic infection is asymptomatic cyst passage. Even in highly endemic areas, most patients harbour *E. histolytica/E. dispar* cysts asymptomatically. When symptomatic, the clinical features may be of intestinal or extra-intestinal disease.

Intestinal Disease

Asymptomatic disease

Approximately 90% of the infections remain asymptomatic or mildly symptomatic.

Symptomatic disease

- **Diarrhea:** A gradual onset of lower abdominal pain and mild diarrhea is followed by malaise, weight loss and diffuse lower abdominal pain, occasionally progressing to dysentery.
- **Amoebic dysentery:** This is the typical manifestation of intestinal amoebiasis. The onset is usually gradual, and the symptoms include colicky abdominal pain, fever, prostration, bloody diarrhea with mucus and pus cells, and often, weight loss. Though it resembles bacillary dysentery, a few clinical and laboratory features help to differentiate between the two entities (Table 4.1).
- **Amoebic appendicitis:** This entity presents with acute right lower abdominal pain that mimics appendicitis.
- **Amoeboma:** Amoebic infections may present as a palpable abdominal mass that may be confused with carcinoma. It may produce a characteristic napkin-ring constriction of the bowel wall on X-ray.
- **Fulminant colitis or toxic megacolon:** This is a less common entity. The patient presents with intense colicky pain, fever and profuse bloody diarrhea. It is associated with high mortality rates (40%), especially in patients on corticosteroid therapy. For this reason, it is important to exclude amoebiasis in patients with inflammatory bowel disease.
- **Chronic non-dysenteric colitis:** Often resembles inflammatory bowel disease with potentially severe consequences if corticosteroids are administered.

Extra-intestinal Amoebiasis

Amoebic liver abscess (ALA)

Hepatic involvement is the most common extra-intestinal complication of amoebiasis—it is reported in

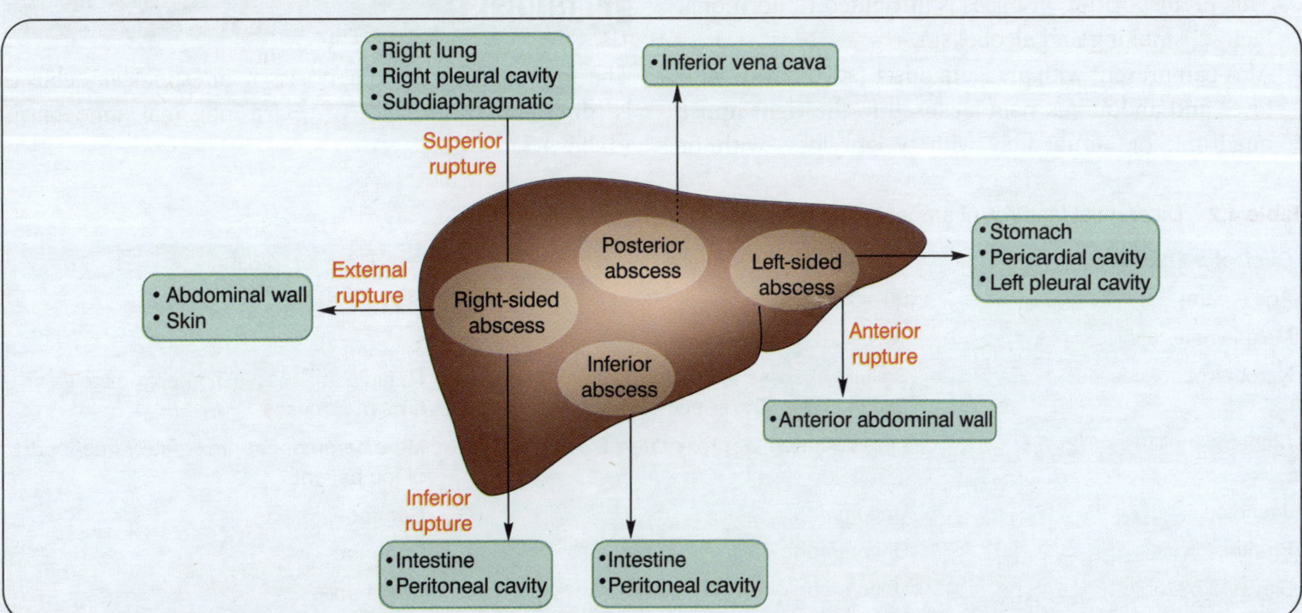

Fig. 4.4 Line diagram showing the various sites of rupture of amoebic liver abscesses

Table 4.1 Differential features of amoebic and bacillary dysentery

Clinical features	Amoebic dysentery	Bacillary dysentery
Onset	Gradual	Acute
Fever	Present in <40%	Almost always present
Abdominal tenderness	Localised to the right upper quadrant of the abdomen or referred to the shoulder	Generalised
Tenesmus	Absent	Present
Stool sample		
Odour	Offensive	Not offensive
Colour	Dark red	Bright red
Nature	Scanty feces mixed with blood and mucus; heme-positive	Blood and mucus with little or no feces
Consistency	Not adherent to container	Adherent to container
Reaction	Acidic	Alkaline

about 2–10% of individuals infected with *E. histolytica* (Table 4.2). It may occur along with colitis but more frequently presents after 2–5 months or even years later. The history of amoebic dysentery is absent in more than half of the cases.

- Amoebic colitis affects both sexes equally; invasive amoebiasis, on the other hand, is much more common in adult males than in females. In particular, ALA is 7–10 times more common in males than females with a predominance among males aged 18–50 years. This predisposition in males is attributed to hormonal factors, smoking and alcoholism.
- ALA can present with an acute onset (<10 days), with fever and abdominal pain localised to the right upper quadrant, or sub-acutely with weight loss, with or without fever or abdominal pain. The pain may radiate to the right shoulder and may be accompanied by a non-productive cough.
- On examination, there is point tenderness over the liver. Hepatomegaly is seen in half of the cases, but jaundice is less common.
- ALA tends to rupture into the adjacent tissues and may affect other body organs.

Pulmonary amoebiasis

In a few patients, the lung may become involved by the extension of the liver abscess through the diaphragm or by direct hematogenous spread from the intestine. The lower part of the right lung is usually involved. A hepato-bronchial fistula may result with expectoration of **chocolate brown sputum** in which amoeba may be demonstrated.

Cutaneous amoebiasis

It occurs by direct extension of an abscess around the anus, a colostomy site or a discharging sinus from an amoebic abscess, leading to extensive necrotic destruction of the skin. The lesion may be mistaken for a condyloma or epithelioma.

Other organ involvement

Less commonly, distant organs may become involved by the hematogenous route or through the lymphatics. Abscesses may develop in the brain, spleen, kidney, genitourinary organs and adrenals. The spread of the infection to the brain is usually fatal.

DIAGNOSIS

The approach to the diagnosis of intestinal amoebiasis is different from that of extra-intestinal amoebiasis (Table 4.3).

Table 4.2 Differential features of amoebic and pyogenic liver abscess

Clinical features	Amoebic liver abscess (ALA)	Pyogenic abscess
Age (years)	20–40	>50
Male:female ratio	10:1	1:1
Number of abscesses	Solitary abscess in 80% of chronic ALA cases and in about 50% of acute ALA cases	Multiple abscesses in approximately 50% of all cases
Diabetes mellitus	Less common, approximately 2% of patients	More common, approximately one-fourth of the patients
Jaundice	Uncommon	Common
Pruritus	Uncommon	Common
Elevated bilirubin	Uncommon	Common
Elevated liver enzymes	Uncommon	Common

Table 4.3 Diagnostic characteristics of various tests for intestinal and extra-intestinal amoebiasis

Test	Intestinal amoebiasis	Amoebic liver abscess	Comments
	Sensitivity		
Microscopy of fecal sample	75–80%	<10%	Cannot differentiate *E. histolytica/ E. dispar/E. moshkovskii*
Microscopy of liver abscess aspirate	Not done	<25%	–
Culture	50%	<25%	Laborious and slow
Antigen detection	30–95% (in fecal sample)	90–100% (in abscess aspirate)	May not be suitable for preserved samples
Serology	>90%	70–80% in acute, and >90% in convalescent sample	Cannot differentiate current from past infection
PCR	90–100%	90–100%	Currently considered the gold standard

Diagnosis of Intestinal Amoebiasis

Lab diagnosis

- **Microscopy:** By visualising trophozoites and cysts
  - Direct microscopy of stool or sigmoidoscopy samples using wet and iodine mounts or permanent staining
  - Histopathology of biopsy samples
- **Culture:**
  - National Institute of Health (NIH) media, Boeck and Drbohlav egg serum medium containing Locke's solution, Balamuth's medium and Diamond's medium
  - Zymodeme/isoenzyme analysis
- **Coproantigen detection:** ELISA and immunochromatographic tests
- **Serology:** Not useful
- **DNA detection:** PCR and real-time PCR

Stool is the specimen of choice. Due to intermittent shedding of amoebae, it is recommended that a minimum of **three samples be collected on consecutive days**. Sigmoidoscopic material may also be useful for investigations. The stool specimen should be examined immediately (within 1–2 hours of collection). Alternatively, it should be preserved in formalin, polyvinyl alcohol or merthiolate iodine until the time of study; refrigeration is not recommended. Prior administration of substances like **kaolin, bismuth, barium sulfate or anti-amoebic drugs interfere with parasite identification**.

Microscopy

- **Wet and iodine mounts:**
  - Direct examination of stool in saline and iodine mount is done to demonstrate trophozoites or cysts. In a fresh sample, the motility of the trophozoite can be appreciated in such a saline mount, while the internal structures of a cyst are better seen when stained with iodine (Fig. 4.5a, b, c and d).
  - **Charcot-Leyden crystals**—diamond-shaped, refractile and clear structures, 5–50 µm in size—are seen in saline preparations. Though these are not pathognomonic of amoebiasis and may be seen in numerous bowel conditions, they help to differentiate amoebic dysentery from bacterial dysentery.
- **Permanent staining: Stool or sigmoidoscopic samples** can also be examined by staining them with permanent stains such as trichrome, iron and hematoxylin, periodic acid Schiff (PAS) and hematoxylin and eosin (H&E) stains. The internal structures of cysts and trophozoites are well demonstrated by permanent stains (Fig. 4.5e, f, g and h).
- **Limitations of microscopy:**
  - Cysts and trophozoites of *E. histolytica* are morphologically indistinguishable from those of non-pathogenic look-alikes—*E. dispar* or *E. moshkovskii*—except for the presence of **ingested RBCs in the trophozoites** of *E. histolytica*. However, this feature may not always be observable. In the absence of ingested RBCs, it is more appropriate to report it as *Entamoeba histolytica/E. dispar/ E. moshkovskii*.
  - A single sample has a poor sensitivity of 25–30%, which can increase to 75–80% when three or more samples are examined.

Stool culture

Entamoeba is usually cultured in a medium containing bacterial associates (**polyxenic**) or one lacking any such associates (**axenic**) but with starch and serum added to provide nourishment to the amoebae.

- A variety of culture media can be used for *Entamoeba* such as National Institute of Health (NIH) media,

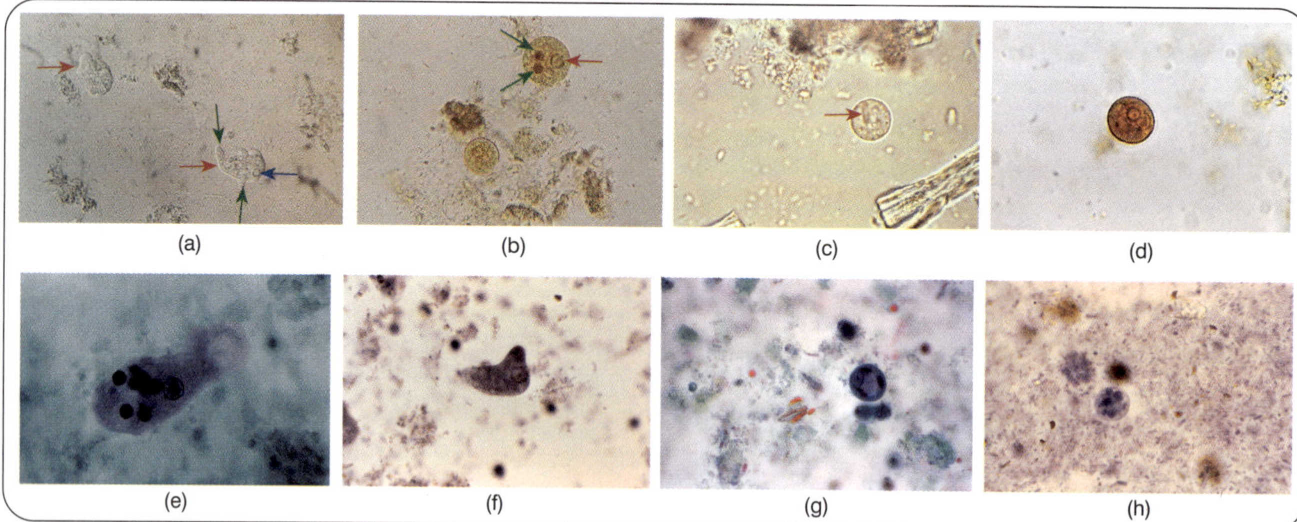

Fig. 4.5 Features of trophozoites and cysts of *E. histolytica:* (a) unstained direct wet mount showing *E. histolytica* trophozoites (red arrow) with nucleus (blue arrow) and pseudopodia (green arrows), (b) a trophozoite of *E. histolytica* in a wet mount stained with iodine showing nuclear morphology (red arrow) and phagocytosed erythrocytes (green arrows), (c) unstained *E. histolytica* cyst displaying a visible chromatoid body (red arrow), (d) iodine-stained *E. histolytica* cyst, (e) trichrome-stained *E. histolytica* trophozoite with phagocytosed erythrocytes seen as dark, round inclusions, (f) iron hematoxylin-stained *E. histolytica* trophozoite, (g) trichrome-stained immature *E. histolytica* cyst containing a single, eccentrically situated nucleus with central karyosome and four darkly stained and bluntly tipped chromatoid bodies and (h) iron hematoxylin-stained *E. histolytica* cyst with four nuclei (*Source [c–h]:* Centers for Disease Control and Prevention [CDC], Public Health Image Library [PHIL], Image IDs 434, 532, 14544, 17554, 16253, 16261)

Boeck and Drbohlav egg serum medium containing Locke's solution, Balamuth's medium and Diamond's medium.

- Stool culture has a low sensitivity of about 50% and is labour intensive and time-consuming (takes 5–10 days), thus is not routinely used for diagnosis. *E. histolytica* cultures are generally reserved for reference laboratories where they are used for characterisation of isolates by techniques such as zymodeme/isoenzyme analysis. Cultures can also be used for drug susceptibility tests and pathogenesis studies.

Zymodeme analysis/isoenzyme analysis: The electrophoretic mobility patterns of some isoenzymes such as **hexokinase, malic enzyme and phosphoglucoisomerase** help in detecting and differentiating various species of *Entamoeba* isolated from cultures. In the pre-molecular era, this method was considered the gold standard for differentiating *E. histolytica* from *E. dispar*. It is, however, time-consuming, difficult to perform and dependent on parasite culture.

Coproantigen detection

Various antigens that are routinely targeted for diagnostic purposes are as follows:

- *E. histolytica*-derived Gal/GalNAc lectin
- Serine-rich *E. histolytica* protein (SREHP)
- Lysine-rich surface antigen
- Lipophosphoglycan (LPG)

Other than stool, antigens may also be detected in aspirates from liver abscesses or serum. Many of these tests can be used to differentiate the pathogenic *E. histolytica* from the non-pathogenic *E. dispar*. Enzyme-linked immunosorbent assay (ELISA) is the most commonly used format to detect the antigens of *E. histolytica*. Immunochromatographic tests (ICT) or lateral flow assays are available for the simultaneous detection of antigens specific to *Giardia lamblia*, *E. histolytica/E. dispar* and *Cryptosporidium parvum* from fecal samples. Antigen detection tests are reported to have variable sensitivity (30–95%) and specificity (80–100%) as compared to both microscopy and the culture of stool samples. Serum samples also show similar sensitivity and specificity.

Serodiagnosis

While amoebic antibody detection test in serum is likely to be positive in extra-intestinal disease, it may or may not be positive in intestinal disease. Moreover, a positive serology cannot differentiate between a past infection and a current one because of the persisting antibodies; thus, it is not useful for diagnosis.

Nucleic acid-based detection

In a modern laboratory, PCR and its various modifications can be used to detect and differentiate between various species of *Entamoeba* using genes coding for 18S RNA, 30-kDa protein, hemolysin (HLY6), cysteine proteinase, SREHP, actin, etc. Molecular tests offer higher diagnostic sensitivity and specificity (90–100%) and allow simultaneous detection and differentiation of *E. histolytica*/*E. dispar*. Multiplex (with more than one gene target) molecular panels for gastrointestinal parasite pathogens such as *Giardia lamblia*, *Cryptosporidium* and *E. histolytica* are also available commercially.

Histopathology

A sigmoidoscopic sample can be used to demonstrate the parasite. PAS staining (organisms appear bright pink with a green-blue background) or H&E staining are often used. Typical flask-shaped ulcers with normal intervening areas are characteristic.

Diagnosis of Amoebic Liver Abscess (ALA)

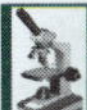

Lab diagnosis

- **Microscopy:** By visualising trophozoites
  - Direct microscopy of aspirated pus and sputum (pulmonary rupture)
- **Culture:**
  - National Institute of Health (NIH) media, Boeck and Drbohlav egg serum medium containing Locke's solution, Balamuth's medium and Diamond's medium
- **Antigen detection:** ELISA and immunochromatographic tests
- **Serology:** Useful in non-endemic areas
  - IgG antibody detection
- **DNA detection:** PCR and real-time PCR
- **Other diagnostic parameters:**
  - Leukocytosis, ↑ alkaline phosphatases
  - Radiology – ultrasonography

Microscopy

Trophozoites may be detected in aspirated liver pus. Though the sensitivity of this method is low (<25%), it is confirmatory. Stool microscopy is usually negative for the presence of parasites.

Culture

This method may be employed; however, it has low sensitivity (<25%).

Antigen detection

Antigen detection by ELISA in the serum of ALA patients is extremely sensitive (90–100%) when performed before treatment. Antigens are usually absent in stool samples collected from ALA patients. The sensitivity of this method is also poor when it is performed on abscess fluid.

Serology

Antibody detection tests are helpful in establishing the diagnosis of ALA in non-endemic areas. However, a positive test does not necessarily mean current infection in an endemic area. Further, seropositivity cannot differentiate between recent and past infections since the antibodies persist even after cure. About 70–80% of cases of acute infection and 90% convalescent samples test positive for antibodies.

Molecular diagnosis

PCR on amoebic liver pus has a sensitivity and specificity of 90–100%. PCR assays targeting *18SrDNA* with species-specific probes are the most common and recommended tests.

Other diagnostic parameters

- Leukocytosis and elevated alkaline phosphatases are characteristically seen in ALA.
- Ultrasonography (USG) of the liver shows the site and number of the abscesses. USG-guided aspiration may be done to establish the diagnosis or to drain the abscess. An amoebic abscess is typically present in the right lobe of liver and is often a solitary lesion. However, imaging cannot reliably distinguish amoebic abscesses from pyogenic abscesses or necrotic tumours.

TREATMENT

Luminal agent (for amoebic dysentery, asymptomatic carriage or coupled with treatment with tissue-active agent in amoebic liver abscess [ALA] or colitis)

Drug of choice

- *Paromomycin:* For adults, 30 mg/kg/day orally in divided doses TDS × 5–10 days; for children, 25 mg/kg/day orally in divided doses TDS × 5–10 days

Alternate drugs

- *Diloxanide furoate:* For adults, 500 mg orally TDS ×10 days; for children, 20 mg/kg/day orally in divided doses – TDS × 10 days
- *Iodoquinol:* 650 mg TDS × 20 days

Tissue-active agent (for amoebic colitis and ALA)

Drugs of choice

- *Metronidazole:* For adults, 750 mg TDS orally or IV × 5–10 days; for children, 50 mg/kg/day orally in divided doses TDS × 10 days
- *Tinidazole:* For adults, 2 g once daily orally × 3–5 days; for children, 60 mg/kg/day orally in divided doses TDS × 5 days

Alternate drug

- *Nitazoxanide:* For adults, 500 mg orally BDS × 3 days; for children >4 years, 200 mg BDS; for children <4 years, 100 mg BDS × 3 days

Patients with invasive disease and ALA require treatment with two drugs—an **amoebicidal tissue-active agent and a luminal cysticidal agent**. Those with asymptomatic amoebiasis may be treated with just a luminal cysticidal agent. More than 90% of the patients respond dramatically to treatment. Broad-spectrum antibiotics may be also be prescribed to treat bacterial superinfection in cases of fulminant amoebic colitis and suspected perforation.

Surgical drainage of liver abscess may occasionally be required in addition to anti-parasitic therapy. Drainage is typically reserved for the following cases:

- When the patient fails to show clinical response to anti-parasitic therapy within 3–5 days
- For abscesses at high risk of rupture such as an abscess larger than 5–10 cm or a left lobe abscess which could rupture into the pericardium or an abscess at risk of imminent rupture
- When the diagnosis is uncertain and where a pyogenic abscess or bacterial superinfection of the ALA is a concern

PREVENTION AND CONTROL

- **Food and water safety** are of paramount importance. Boiling is the most effective method of sterilising fluids. Routinely used doses of chlorine and iodine are too low to kill cysts. The consumption of commonly contaminated foods such as lettuce, mint and coriander in their **raw forms** should be avoided. These vegetables may be washed with a detergent and subsequently soaked in acetic acid or vinegar for 10–15 minutes before consumption.
- Attention to **hand hygiene** is critical. Fecal–oral exposure should be avoided including that which is associated with sexual practices.
- Household contacts of patients with amoebiasis should be screened.
- Patients with amoebic colitis should avoid using anti-motility agents.
- There is no vaccine available for human use to date. Research in the area is being carried out in animal models.

NON-PATHOGENIC OR LESS PATHOGENIC INTESTINAL AMOEBAE

A few other amoebae have the same life cycles and geographical distribution as *E. histolytica*, and have occasionally been implicated in diarrheal diseases; however, the association is not proven. They usually exist as harmless or commensal agents in the gastrointestinal tract. The morphological differences between the trophozoite and cyst stages of these amoebae are presented in Tables 4.4 and 4.5 and Fig. 4.6a–h.

Entamoeba dispar

This intestinal amoeba is morphologically identical to *E. histolytica* and is the more common *Entamoeba* to be found in human feces. It is non-pathogenic. It has long been confused with *E. histolytica,* from which it can be microscopically differentiated based on the presence or absence of ingested RBCs in the trophozoite. Conventionally, zymodeme analysis and more recently, molecular tests targeting small subunit rRNA gene and antigen detection tests are used to differentiate *E. dispar* from the pathogenic *E. histolytica.*

Entamoeba moshkovskii

E. moshkovskii is considered non-pathogenic, with only a few cases of intestinal infections having been reported in children from Bangladesh, Australia and India. It is commonly found in sewage and was first identified in Moscow. This amoeba too is morphologically identical to *E. histolytica*/*E. dispar*. Molecular tests can reliably differentiate it from other similar species.

Entamoeba bangladeshi

E. bangladeshi is another non-pathogenic species morphologically identical to *E. histolytica*. It has been isolated from Bangladeshi infants and children who have diarrhea but more evidence is needed to ascertain whether it has pathogenic potential.

Entamoeba gingivalis

It resides in the oral cavity and although it is often recovered from patients who have pyorrhea alveolaris, it is still considered to be non-pathogenic. No cyst stage is known in the life cycle of *E. gingivalis*. It is the only species known to ingest white blood cells.

Entamoeba coli

It is larger than *E. histolytica* and sluggishly motile. *Entamoeba coli* harbours a single nucleus with an eccentric karyosome. Its cysts have 1–8 nuclei and its chromatid bars have rough, pointed ends. It tends to be commoner in warm climates (Fig. 4.6a–d).

Table 4.4 Differentiating features of the trophozoite stages of amoebae inhabiting the human intestinal tract

Characteristic	*Entamoeba histolytica/ Entamoeba dispar/ Entamoeba moshkovskii*	*Entamoeba hartmanni*	*Entamoeba coli*	*Endolimax nana*	*Iodamoeba butschlii*
Size	10–60 μm but usual range, 20–30 μm	5–12 μm	15–50 μm	6–12 μm	8–20 μm
Motility	Progressive, with hyaline, finger-like pseudopodia; motility may be rapid	Usually non-progressive	Sluggish non-directional, blunt, granular pseudopodia	Sluggish, usually non-progressive	Sluggish, usually non-progressive
Nucleus: Number and visibility	Difficult to see in unstained preparations; 1 nucleus	Usually not seen in unstained preparations; 1 nucleus	Often visible in unstained preparations; 1 nucleus	Occasionally visible in unstained preparations; 1 nucleus	Usually not seen in unstained preparations; 1 nucleus
Peripheral chromatin (stained)	Fine granules, uniform in size and usually evenly distributed; may have beaded appearance	Morphology is similar to *E. histolytica/ E. dispar,* chromatin may appear as a solid ring rather than beaded	May be clumped and unevenly arranged on the membrane or appear as a solid, dark ring	Usually no peripheral chromatin	Usually no peripheral chromatin
Karyosome (stained)	Small, usually compact; centrally located but may also be eccentric	Usually small and compact; may be centrally located or eccentric	Large, not compact; may or may not be eccentric; may be diffuse and darkly stained	Large, irregularly shaped	Large, may be surrounded by refractile granules that are difficult to see ('basket nucleus')
Cytoplasm appearance (stained)	Finely granular, 'ground-glass' appearance; clear differentiation of ectoplasm and endoplasm; small vacuoles may be present	Finely granular	Granular, with little differentiation into ectoplasm and endoplasm; usually vacuolated	Granular, vacuolated	Granular, may be heavily vacuolated
Inclusions (stained)	May contain bacteria; presence of RBCs diagnostic of *E. histolytica*	May contain bacteria; no RBCs	Bacteria, yeasts, other debris	Bacteria	Bacteria

Entamoeba polecki

It was originally found in the intestines of pigs, but has also been recovered from human stool specimens.

Entamoeba chattoni

Entamoeba chattoni is commonly found in wild primates.

Entamoeba hartmanni

In the past, *Entamoeba hartmanni* was considered a small race of *E. histolytica*. However, it is now recognised as a separate species and is found worldwide.

Endolimax nana

The nucleus of *Endolimax nana* has a large, irregularly shaped karyosome with a thin chromatin layer; sometimes, the chromatin layer is absent (Fig. 4.6e and f). It is found worldwide.

Iodamoeba butschlii

It hosts a large karyosome and a characteristically large glycogen vacuole which stains deep brown with iodine stain (Fig. 4.6g and h).

Table 4.5 Differentiating features of the cyst stages of amoebae inhabiting the human intestinal tract

Characteristic	*Entamoeba histolytica/ Entamoeba dispar/ Entamoeba moshkovskii*	*Entamoeba hartmanni (small race Entamoeba)*	*Entamoeba coli*	*Endolimax nana*	*Iodamoeba butschlii*
Size of cyst	10–20 µm	5–10 µm	10–40 µm	5–10 µm	5–20 µm
Shape	Spherical	Spherical	Spherical or oval	Oval	Oval or spherical
Nucleus	1–4 nuclei depending on maturity; nuclear characteristics difficult to see on wet preparation	1–4 nuclei	2–8 nuclei	2–4 nuclei	1 nucleus
Peripheral chromatin in the nucleus (stained smear)	Fine, uniform granules, evenly distributed on the periphery	Fine granules evenly distributed on the periphery	Coarsely granular; may be clumped and unevenly arranged on the periphery	No peripheral chromatin	No peripheral chromatin
Karyosome (stained smear)	Small, compact, usually centrally located	Small, compact, usually centrally located	Large, eccentric	Large, central or eccentric	Large, usually eccentric and refractile
Chromatoidal bodies in cytoplasm (stained smear)	May be present; usually elongated, with blunt, rounded, smooth edges	Usually present; elongate, with blunt, rounded, smooth edges	May be present; splinter-shaped with rough pointed ends	Occasionally present as small granules or inclusions	Absent
Glycogen mass (stained with iodine as reddish-brown mass)	May be diffuse or absent in mature cyst; may be present in early cyst	May or may not be present	May be diffuse or absent in mature cyst	Less common	Large, compact, well-defined mass, very characteristic

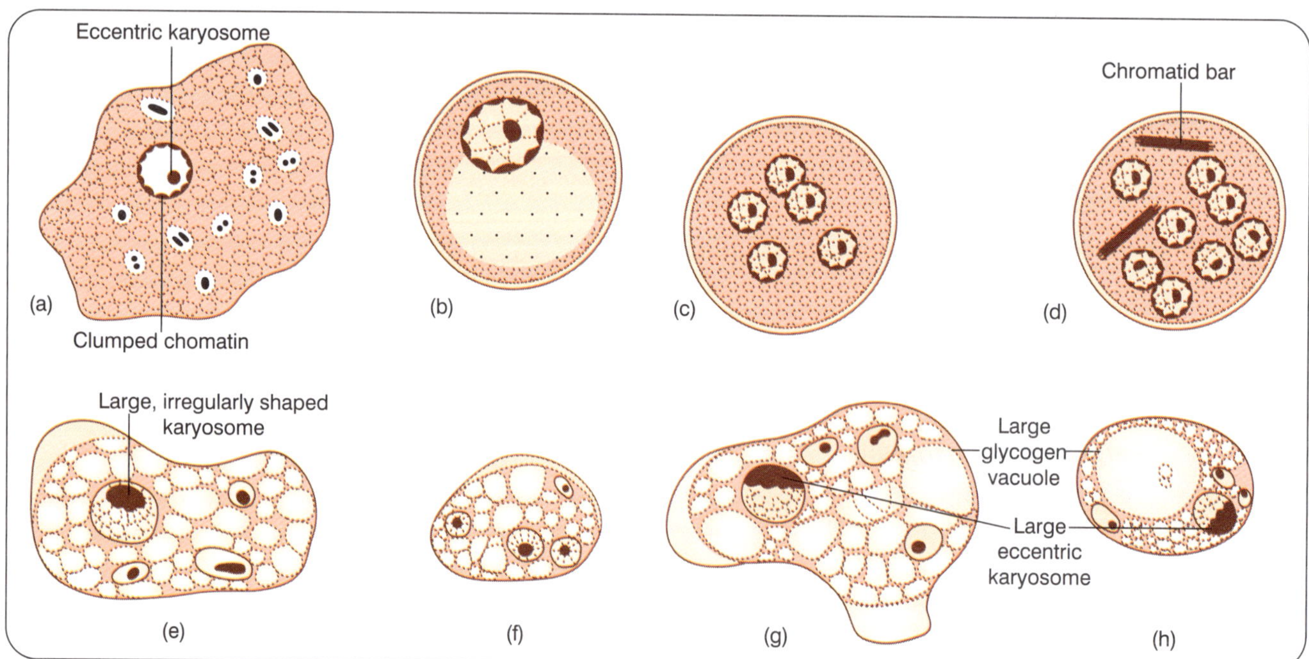

Fig. 4.6 Line diagrams of trophozoites and cysts of non-pathogenic intestinal amoebae: (*a*) trophozoite of *Entamoeba coli* with a single nucleus, eccentric karyosome and unevenly arranged clumped chromatin, (b–d) cysts of *E. coli* with eccentric 1-, 5-, and 8-nuclei with or without roughly pointed chromatid bodies, (e–f) trophozoite and cyst of *Endolimax nana* with a large karyosome and thin chromatin layer and (g–h) trophozoite and cyst of *Iodamoeba butschlii* with a large eccentric karyosome and large glycogen mass

Questions

1. Discuss the diagnosis and management of invasive amoebiasis.
2. Differentiate between amoebic and bacillary dysentery.
3. Differentiate between amoebic and pyogenic liver abscess.
4. List the differential diagnoses of the infective causes of space-occupying lesions (SOL) in the liver.
5. Describe the morphological differentiation of various species of *Entamoeba* with illustrations.

Multiple Choice Questions

1. Excystation of *Entamoeba histolytica* occurs in __________ :
   a. Small intestine
   b. Large intestine
   c. Stomach
   d. In the external environment
2. *Entamoeba histolytica* divides by __________:
   a. Multiple fission
   b. Binary fission
   c. Conjugation
   d. Sporulation
3. Amoebic liver abscess can be diagnosed by all the following EXCEPT __________:
   a. Demonstration of trophozoites in liver abscesses
   b. Demonstration of cysts in liver abscesses
   c. Demonstration of amoebic antigen in liver abscesses
   d. Demonstration of DNA in liver abscesses
4. The commonest site of secondary spread of *Entamoeba histolytica* is __________:
   a. The liver
   b. The lungs
   c. The skin
   d. The brain
5. Amoebic liver abscess most commonly involves the __________ region of the liver.
   a. Postero-superior surface of the left lobe of the liver
   b. Postero-superior surface of the right lobe of the liver
   c. Antero-superior surface of the right lobe of the liver
   d. Antero-inferior surface of the left lobe of the liver
6. *Entamoeba histolytica* typically produces __________ ulcers.
   a. Tumbler-shaped
   b. Flask-shaped
   c. Deep, punched
   d. V-shaped
7. Which of the following statements about amoebic liver abscess is NOT TRUE?
   a. It usually produces a single abscess.
   b. It involves the postero-superior portion of the right lobe of the liver.
   c. Amoebae are best demonstrated in the centre of the necrotic cavity.
   d. It is more common in males than females.
8. Amoebic dysentery is typically characterised by the following features EXCEPT __________:
   a. Onset is usually gradual.
   b. Fever may not be present in half of the infected persons.
   c. Abdominal tenderness is generalised.
   d. Tenesmus is absent.
9. *Entamoeba histolytica* trophozoites can be differentiated morphologically from similar-looking *Entamoebae* on stool microscopy by __________:
   a. Clear differentiation of ectoplasm and endoplasm
   b. Tongue-like pseudopodia
   c. Presence of ingested RBC
   d. Presence of Charcot-Leyden crystals
10. The treatment of choice for uncomplicated amoebic liver abscess is __________:
    a. Metronidazole
    b. Metronidazole plus paromomycin
    c. Paromomycin
    d. Amphotericin B

Chapter 5

Giardia

(*Giardia lamblia* named after scientists Alfred Mathieu Giard and Vilem Dusan Lambl)

Case Study and Learning Goals

A 5-year-old female presents with complaints of on-and-off diarrhea for the last two months. She has been passing greasy and foul-smelling stools several times a day associated with mild abdominal pain and frequent belching that smells like eggs. What are the causes of acute diarrhea? How would you approach the laboratory diagnosis in this case? How would you treat this patient?

INTRODUCTION

Giardia is a **unicellular flagellate** which is a common cause of endemic diarrhea worldwide. It was first discovered in 1681 by **Antonie van Leeuwenhoek** while examining his own diarrheal stools under the microscope. The species of human importance is *Giardia duodenalis* (syn. *G. intestinalis*, *G. lamblia*), which was named after Alfred M. Giard and V. Lambl. *G. duodenalis* also infects other mammals such as cattle, horses, dogs, cats, rats and pigs. Several other species also exist and are harboured by hosts other than humans; these include *G. agilis* (amphibians), *G. ardeae* (birds), *G. muris* (rodents) and *G. varani* (lizards).

Currently, *G. lamblia* is classified into **eight assemblages (A–H)** based on 18S ribosomal RNA gene sequences. These assemblages are widely distributed amongst various mammalian species. Humans are known to be infected by **assemblages A and B**.

EPIDEMIOLOGY

Giardia is a leading but treatable causes of infectious gastroenteritis worldwide. It accounts for **6–8%** of cases of **acute diarrhea** and **11–45%** of those of **chronic diarrhea**. It is frequently implicated in **outbreaks of diarrheal disease**. It is especially prevalent in children in developing countries with an incidence of 2–7% among higher socioeconomic groups, and more in lower socioeconomic settings. The prevalence rates in India range from 4% to as high as 53%.

Transmission

- Though **waterborne** transmission generally causes only sporadic cases, outbreaks associated with contaminated drinking water, swimming pools and recreational waters are also well documented.
- **Foodborne** transmission is associated with foods such as fruits, vegetables, salads, shellfish, oysters, etc. Often, the poor personal hygiene of food handlers is implicated in institutional settings.
- Though this is not entirely clear, **zoonotic transmission** is likely to occur. The infected livestock are known to shed 10^5–10^6 *Giardia* cysts/gram of feces, thereby contaminating the environment.
- **Traveller's diarrhea**—*Giardia* is the **most common parasitic etiology** of diarrhea in travellers visiting endemic areas.

Risk Factors

Risk factors include poor personal hygiene, low socioeconomic status, overcrowding (as in prisons and camps), visiting childcare facilities, immunocompromised states such as hypogammaglobulinemia (IgA deficiency and common variable immunodeficiency), travel to endemic countries (such as South Asia, South-East Asia, North Africa, the Caribbeans and South America), contact with animals, occupations such as sewage cleaning and irrigation and homosexual activity. Reduced gastric acid secretion due to achlorhydria, malnutrition, atrophic gastritis, antacid treatment and surgery also predispose to giardiasis.

MORPHOLOGY

G. duodenalis is a **eukaryote** with distinct nuclei and nuclear membrane, a cytoskeleton and an endomembrane system. However, it is **anaerobic** and lacks mitochondria. It exists in two stages which are as follows:

Trophozoite (Feeding Stage)

- It is **pyriform/pear-/tennis racket-shaped**, bilaterally symmetrical, 10–20 µm × 5–15 µm in size, with two axonemes and four pairs of flagella with 9+2 arrangement of microtubules.
- The flagella help in motility, which is of a characteristically rapid, **tumbling** and spinning type, akin to a **falling leaf**.

- The trophozoite has **two nuclei** (Fig. 5.1a) symmetrically aligned to the long axis. The nuclei are not visible in unstained preparations. The trophozoite also has **two claw hammer-shaped median bodies** and a large concave ventral disc or sucking disc which helps in clasping on to the intestinal epithelium.
- The arrangement of various organelles and flagella gives *Giardia* its typical shape and the name **'the grand old man of the intestine'** (Fig. 5.1b). It appears **spoon-shaped** (Fig. 5.1c) in the lateral view.

Cyst (Dormant Stage)

It is thick-walled, non-motile, round or oval and 11–14 µm × 7–10 µm in size with axonemes and **four nuclei**. It is resilient to chlorination and temperature variations and persists in the environment for several weeks to months.

LIFE CYCLE (Fig. 5.2a and b)

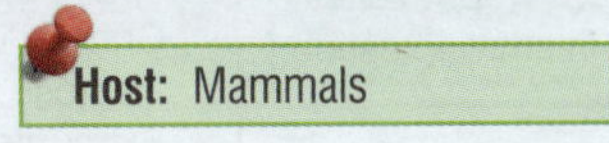

The dormant **quadrinucleate cysts, which are the infective forms** of *G. duodenalis*, are ingested through contaminated drinking water or food. The various phases in its life cycle are as follows:

- **Excystation:** The cyst passes through the acidic environment of the stomach and reaches the small intestine. Once there, excystation occurs within 10 minutes, and two trophozoites emerge from one cyst. The excystation process is stimulated by the low pH of the stomach and facilitated by the pancreatic proteases in the proximal small intestine. The trophozoite actively moves and colonises the intestinal crypts and starts feeding. It reproduces by asexual replication by longitudinal binary fission.
- **Encystation:** On exposure to the mildly alkalotic pH of the biliary juices, some trophozoites undergo encystation in the jejunum. Each cyst contains two trophozoites and four nuclei.

Both cysts and trophozoites are released into the external environment through feces, but only the cyst can survive in the environment and go on to infect another host.

PATHOGENESIS

G. duodenalis **infects the host by the fecal-oral route** through contaminated water and food. It can be transmitted from person to person, and possibly from animals to humans and also vice versa. Its **incubation period is 12 weeks** (the range being 1–45 days) and the infectious dose is **10–100 cysts.**

Mechanism of diarrhea: Peculiarly, *Giardia* **does not invade the epithelium** or **secrete any known diarrheal toxin**. The pathogenesis occurs as follows:

- After excystation, the trophozoites colonise the proximal small intestine by adhering to the brush border of the enterocytes. This is facilitated by the **clasping mechanism of the ventral disc**. The brush border microvilli are thus disrupted (Fig. 5.3a and b).
- In addition, the adherence of the trophozoites to the epithelium is promoted by **N-acetyl-D-galactosamine lectin** (present on the surface of the parasite) which binds to the mucin of the host cells.
- **Increase in the intestinal permeability** is brought about by alteration of the microtubular arrangement and disruption of the tight junctional proteins of the epithelium.
- **Apoptosis** (programmed cell death) is induced in the enterocytes.

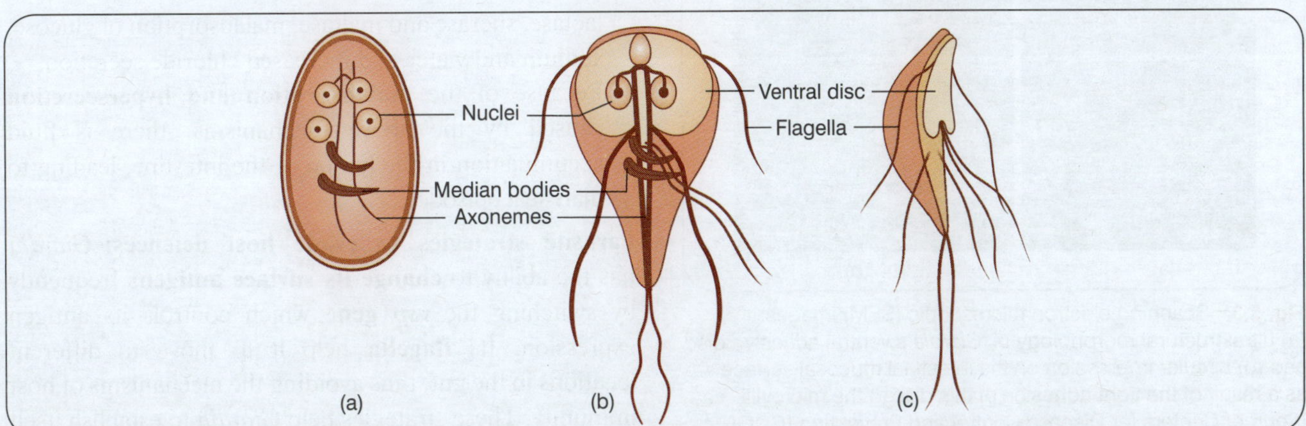

Fig. 5.1 Line diagram of *Giardia duodenalis:* (a) cyst, (b) frontal view of trophozoite and (c) lateral view of trophozoite

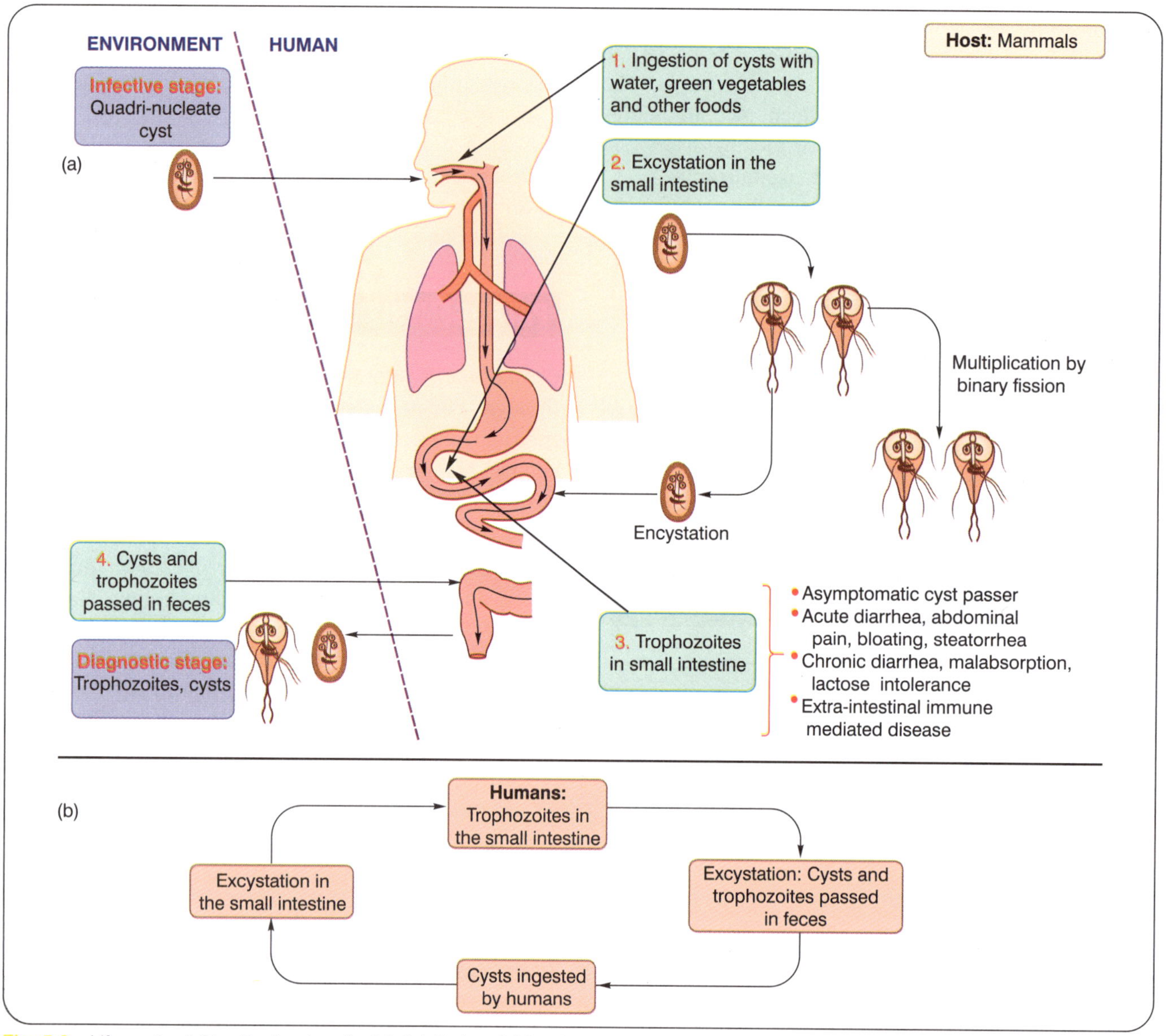

ENVIRONMENT
HUMAN
Host: Mammals
Infective stage: Quadri-nucleate cyst
(a)
1. Ingestion of cysts with water, green vegetables and other foods
2. Excystation in the small intestine
Multiplication by binary fission
Encystation
4. Cysts and trophozoites passed in feces
Diagnostic stage: Trophozoites, cysts
3. Trophozoites in small intestine
- Asymptomatic cyst passer
- Acute diarrhea, abdominal pain, bloating, steatorrhea
- Chronic diarrhea, malabsorption, lactose intolerance
- Extra-intestinal immune mediated disease

(b)
Humans: Trophozoites in the small intestine
Excystation: Cysts and trophozoites passed in feces
Cysts ingested by humans
Excystation in the small intestine

Fig. 5.2 Life cycle of *Giardia duodenalis:* (a) detailed and (b) schematic

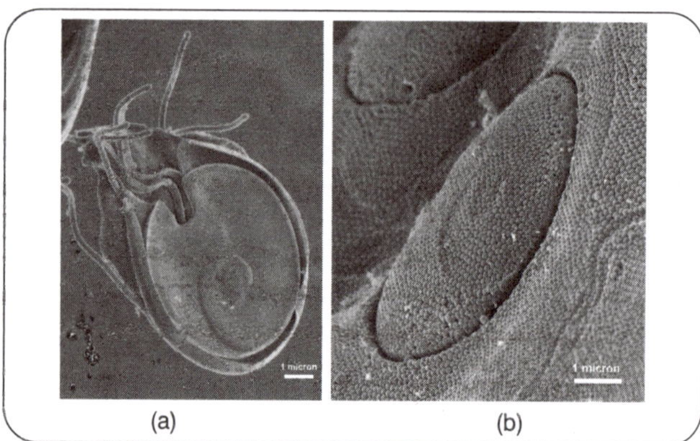

Fig. 5.3 Scanning electron microscopic (SEM) images: (a) ultrastructural morphology of *Giardia*'s ventral adhesive disc and (b) circular impression on the intestinal mucosal surface as a result of the tight adhesion of this disc to the microvilli (*Source:* Centers for Disease Control and Prevention [CDC], Public Health Image Library [PHIL], Image ID 11644)

- As a result of all of the above, there is shortening of epithelial microvilli and loss of epithelial barrier function, reduced activity of disaccharidases such as lactase, sucrase and maltase, malabsorption of glucose, sodium and water and increased chloride secretion.
- Because of the **malabsorption and hypersecretion** caused by the above mechanisms, there is fluid accumulation in the lumen of the intestine, leading to diarrheal episodes.

Parasite strategies to evade host defences: *Giardia* has the ability to **change its surface antigens** frequently by switching the ***vsp* gene** which controls its antigen expression. Its **flagella** help it to move to different locations in the gut, thus avoiding the mechanisms of host immunity. These strategies help *Giardia* to establish itself in the host for long periods and cause chronic diarrhea.

Additionally, soon after establishing in the gut, *Giardia* starts forming **resilient cysts** for further propagation in the environment.

> ***Giardia's*** **genome contains more than 200 copies of *vsp* (variant surface protein) genes.** Only one gene is expressed at any given time; it switches every 6 to 13 generations.

CLINICAL FEATURES

Giardia infections are **asymptomatic in 35–70%** of the infected population, of which 5–15% are cyst passers. In about **25–50%** of the infected, the symptoms may range from **acute self-limiting diarrhea to chronic diarrheal syndrome**. The following are the features of the different clinical manifestations of *Giardia* infections:

- **Acute disease:** It may be associated with abdominal pain, bloating, burping that exudes an **odour of eggs or sulphur**, indigestion and rarely, explosive diarrhea. A diarrheal episode may last for 7–10 days. The stool is often **greasy and foul-smelling** (steatorrhea) without gross pus, blood or mucus.
- **Chronic disease:** There may be malaise, abdominal discomfort, intermittent diarrhea or diarrhea alternating with constipation. Weight loss due to malabsorption is seen in the majority of patients with chronic diarrhea, especially in children living in resource-poor countries. **Malabsorption of vitamins A and B12, iron, zinc, protein, fat and D-xylose is frequently documented**. In over half of the patients, disaccharidase deficiency leads to **lactose intolerance** which may persist for months, even after adequate treatment and clearance of infection. Most often, the condition is clinically confused with irritable bowel syndrome. In children, there may be cognitive decline, lower intellectual quotient (IQ), poor psychosocial development, stunting, nutritional deficiencies and failure to thrive.
- **Extra-intestinal and long-term consequences:** In some patients, giardiasis may be associated with immune-mediated reactive arthritis or urticaria.

DIAGNOSIS

The diagnosis of giardiasis is generally made by the **demonstration of the trophozoites or cysts in the stool** of infected patients. **Stool examination** may be performed on fresh specimens or after preservation with SAF, polyvinyl alcohol (PVA) or 10% formalin. Ideally, **three specimens collected on different days** should be examined to factor in the **intermittent shedding of the cysts**. The intake of antibiotics, enemas, laxatives and barium studies may lead to false-negative results. The sensitivity of this stool examination is as follows:

- Single stool examination: 50–70%
- Three stool examinations: 90%

Lab diagnosis

- **Microscopy:** By visualising trophozoites and cysts
  - Direct microscopy of stool using wet and iodine mount or permanent staining
  - String test: On duodenal samples
  - Histopathology: On duodenal biopsy obtained by endoscopy
- **Coproantigen detection:** ELISA and immunochromatographic tests
- **Serology:** Not useful
- **DNA detection:** PCR
- **Other tests:**
  - Fecal fat analysis
  - Xylose tolerance breath test

Microscopy

- **Wet and iodine mount:** Trophozoites may be found in fresh, watery stool but disintegrate rapidly, whereas cysts are detected in soft and formed stool. Fecal leukocytes and RBCs are characteristically absent. In a fresh sample, the tumbling leaf-life motility of the trophozoite can be appreciated (Fig. 5.4a–d).
- **Permanent staining:** In preserved stool samples, trophozoites and cysts can be examined by staining with permanent stains like trichrome and iron and hematoxylin stains which enhance the internal structures well (Fig. 5.4e and f).

Stool Antigen (Coproantigen) Detection

- ELISA or immunochromatographic/rapid card tests can be used to detect *Giardia* antigens with a sensitivity and specificity approaching 80% and 98% respectively.
- Commercially, panels are also available for the simultaneous detection of *Entamoeba histolytica*, *Cryptosporidium* and *Giardia*.

String Test

A duodenal sample obtained by performing the string test can be subjected to microscopy; this method has a sensitivity of 50–85%.

- The string test (**entero-test**) employs a gelatin capsule containing a nylon string with a weight attached to it. After fixing one end of the string the patient's cheek, he is asked to swallow the capsule. The gelatin dissolves in the stomach

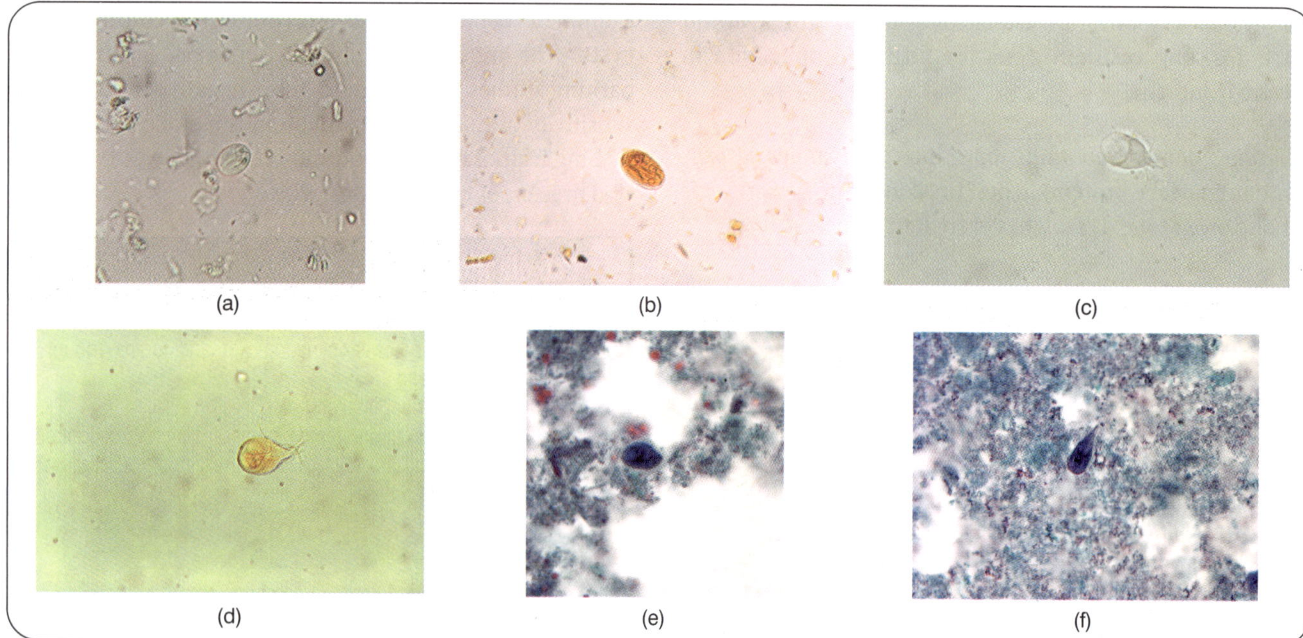

Fig. 5.4 Features of trophozoites and cysts of *Giardia duodenalis*: (a) unstained cyst in a direct wet mount, (b) iodine-stained cyst in a direct wet mount, (c) unstained trophozoite in a direct wet mount with a visible ventral sucking disc, (d) iodine-stained trophozoite in direct wet mount, (e) trichrome-stained dark blue cyst and (f) trichrome-stained dark blue trophozoite (*Source [b–f]:* CDC, PHIL, Image IDs 1945, 3743, 3904, 7832, and 7833)

and the weight carries the string into the duodenum. The string is left in place for 4–6 hours or overnight, and the patient is instructed to fast. After removal, the mucus from the string is examined for trophozoites.

Endoscopy and Biopsy

Duodenal samples can also be obtained by endoscopic aspiration and biopsy. Apart from trophozoites, the duodenal biopsy may also show atrophic microvilli and mild lymphocytic infiltrates.

Serology

Antibody detection is not useful in endemic countries as it cannot differentiate between present and past infection.

Nucleic Acid-Based Detection

PCR may detect parasite concentrations as low as **one parasite/μl** in stool samples. The commonly used gene targets are *SSU rRNA* (small subunit ribosomal RNA), *gdh* (glutamate dehydrogenase), *tpi* (triose phosphate isomerase) and *bg* (beta-giardin) genes.

Other Tests

- Fecal fat analysis with Sudan stain may confirm steatorrhea.
- Disaccharidase deficiency can be diagnosed with a **xylose tolerance breath test** which indicates whether the nutrients are being adequately absorbed or not.

TREATMENT

First-line
- *Tinidazole:* For adults, 2 g orally, single dose; for children, 50 mg/kg single dose
- *Metronidazole:* For adults, 250–500 mg orally TDS × 7–10–14 days or 2 g daily × 3 days; for children, 5 mg/kg TDS × 10–14 days or 35–40 mg/kg daily for 3 days

Second-line
- *Albendazole:* For adults, 400 mg QID × 5 days; for children, 15 mg/kg × 5–7 days
- *Nitazoxanide:* For adults, 500 mg BDS × 3 days; for children, 200 mg BDS × 3 days
- *Paramomycin:* For adults, 500 mg TDS × 5–10 days; for children, 10 mg/kg TDS × 5–10 days

Diarrhea usually resolves within 1–2 weeks of completing the treatment. The cyst excretion ceases as early as 2 days after the initiation of treatment. Up to **20% resistance to metronidazole** is reported. **Metronidazole and tinidazole are not recommended in the first trimester of pregnancy because of potential carcinogenicity to the fetus as reported in rats.**

Several patients may experience symptoms even after adequate therapy; they should be advised to maintain a high fibre diet and to avoid lactose products. Probiotics and prebiotics may be helpful as adjuncts. All infected persons should be treated as the infection may cause malabsorption, which leads to the depletion of nutrients.

PREVENTION AND CONTROL

- Ensuring **clean drinking water, proper disposal of excreta and good hygienic practices like** hand washing and washing and peeling of raw fruits and vegetables are the most effective preventive measures.
- The cysts can be destroyed by hyperchlorination (4–6 mg/l), halogens (2% iodine solution × 30 min), UV rays, boiling (for at least 5 minutes) and sand filtration.
- Those travelling to developing countries and forest areas should consider all water to be potentially contaminated.
- There are no vaccines for humans; however, a killed vaccine is available for dogs and cats.

OTHER FLAGELLATES OF MINOR IMPORTANCE

Dientamoeba fragilis

D. fragilis is a protozoan parasite of the human gastrointestinal tract but its role in the etiology of disease is debatable. It **only exists in the trophozoite stage**; cysts are not formed. The trophozoite ranges in size from 4–20 µm and has one or two nuclei—**bi-nucleate forms are more common** (Fig. 5.5). The nuclei are not visible in unstained preparations, contain no peripheral chromatin, and the **karyosome is fragmented into 3–5 granules**. The motility of this parasite is attributed to its characteristic blunt, fan-shaped pseudopodia. *D. fragilis* does not possess undulating membranes or external flagella like other trichomonads.

Trichomonas tenax

T. tenax is a commensal in the mouth. Some studies point towards its association with periodontal disease.

Other Intestinal Flagellates

Pentatrichomonas hominis, *Chilomastix mesnili*, *Enteromonas hominis* and *Retortamonas intestinalis* can also be recovered from the intestine. These organisms are harmless.

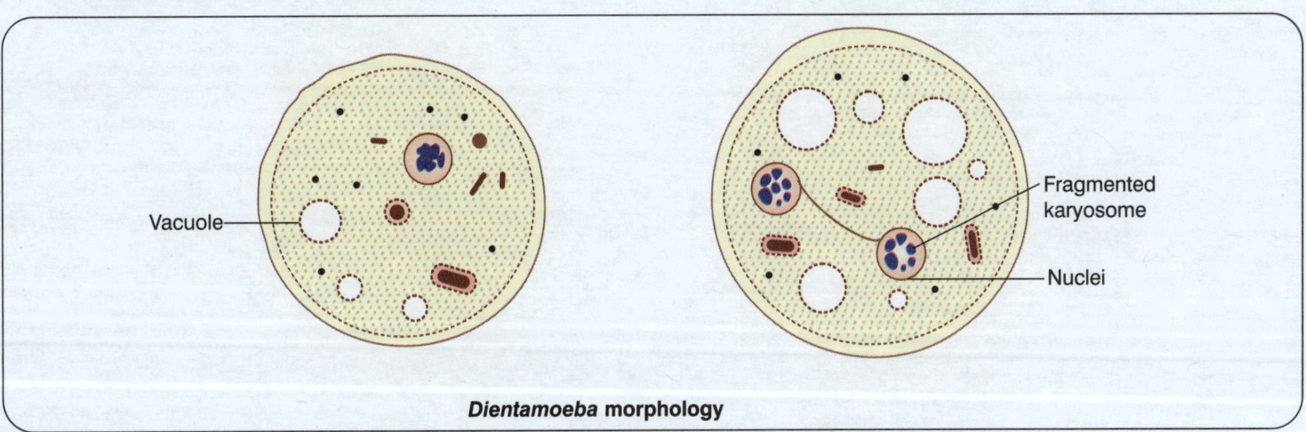

Fig. 5.5 Line diagram of *Dientamoeba fragilis:* Uni- and bi-nucleate forms with fragmented karyosome

QUESTIONS

1. Describe in detail the life cycle and morphology of *Giardia duodenalis* with suitable diagrams.
2. Discuss the clinical features and pathogenesis of giardiasis.
3. Discuss the laboratory diagnosis, management and prevention of giardiasis.

Multiple Choice Questions

1. The trophozoite of *Giardia* has ____________ nuclei.
   a. One
   b. Two
   c. Three
   d. Four
2. The cyst of *Giardia* has ____________ nuclei.
   a. One
   b. Two
   c. Three
   d. Four
3. The trophozoite of *Giardia* is ____________ shaped.
   a. Banana
   b. Pyriform
   c. Round
   d. Coil
4. *Giardia* trophozoite has __________.
   a. Tumbling or falling leaf motility
   b. Jerky motility
   c. Spiralling motility
   d. No motility
5. The stool in diarrhea caused by *Giardia* is typically __________ .
   a. Bloody
   b. Greasy
   c. Rice water-like
   d. None of these
6. Which parasite is the most common cause of traveller's diarrhea?
   a. *Entamoeba*
   b. *Cryptosporidium*
   c. *Giardia*
   d. *Sarcocystis*

Chapter 6

Balantidium coli

([From Greek] *balantion* = sack + *kolon* = terminal intestine)

Case Study and Learning Goals

A 40-year-old male resident of a psychiatric institution presents with bloody diarrhea. The microscopic examination of his stool specimen reveals a large, actively moving organism with a kidney-shaped nucleus. What could be the etiology? How would you approach the laboratory diagnosis in this case? How would you treat this patient?

INTRODUCTION

Balantidium coli is the **only ciliate known to cause human disease**. It is also the **largest protozoan parasite of humans**. It was first recognised in the gastrointestinal tracts of frogs; however, it is just as commonly found in pigs, rodents and many mammals. Human infections caused by *B. coli* were first reported by P. H. Malmsten in 1856. This organism was mistaken to be a species of *Paramecium* until 1863 when F. Stein placed it under the genus *Balantidium*. A recent update in taxonomy recognises the naming of this species as *Balantioides coli* and the clinical disease as balantiosis.

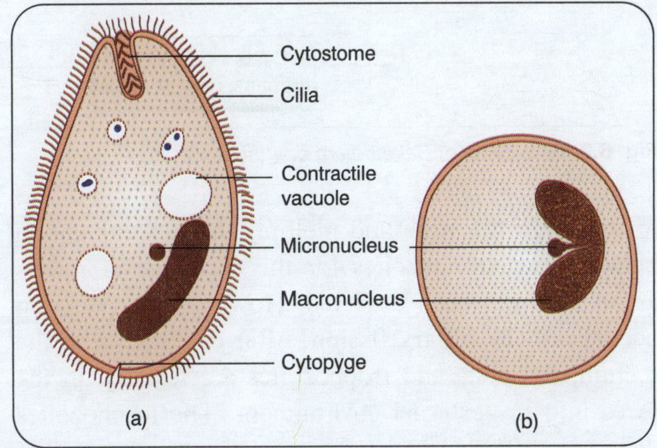

Fig. 6.1 Line diagram of *Balantidium coli*: (a) trophozoite and (b) cyst

EPIDEMIOLOGY

Balantiosis is a less common zoonotic disease seen mostly in populations living in close **contact with pigs**. The organism, though pathogenic, has low virulence. *B. coli* is distributed worldwide. Human infections are chiefly reported from tropical and subtropical regions, especially Latin America, South-East Asia, the Philippines and Papua New Guinea; they are rarely reported in India. **Institutionalised persons** are at high risk of person-to-person transmission, especially those residing in psychiatric units for long periods. **Abattoir workers** and **veterinarians** too stand a higher chance of acquiring the infection.

MORPHOLOGY

B. coli exists in both trophozoite and cyst forms (Fig. 6.1a and b).

Trophozoite

It is ovoid with a pointed anterior and a round posterior end. It is **30–200 µm long** and **30–100 µm wide** and actively motile with the help of short **cilia**. Other features of the trophozoite are as follows:

- It has two nuclei—a large **horseshoe-/kidney-/bean-shaped macronucleus** and a small, round micronucleus.
- A funnel-shaped cytostome is present anteriorly for the ingestion of food. Posteriorly, a small excretory opening called the cytopyge is present.
- Two contractile vacuoles are present in the cytoplasm to maintain osmotic balance. These contain ingested bacteria and debris.

Cyst

The cysts are ovoid and **40 × 60** µm in size. They have two nuclei and are surrounded by a thick wall.

LIFE CYCLE (Fig. 6.2)

Pigs are the reservoir hosts of *B. coli*; 40–100% of the pig population is infected with this organism. Humans acquire the infection by **ingesting cysts** through contaminated food and water. When the cysts reach the small intestine, they liberate trophozoites which migrate

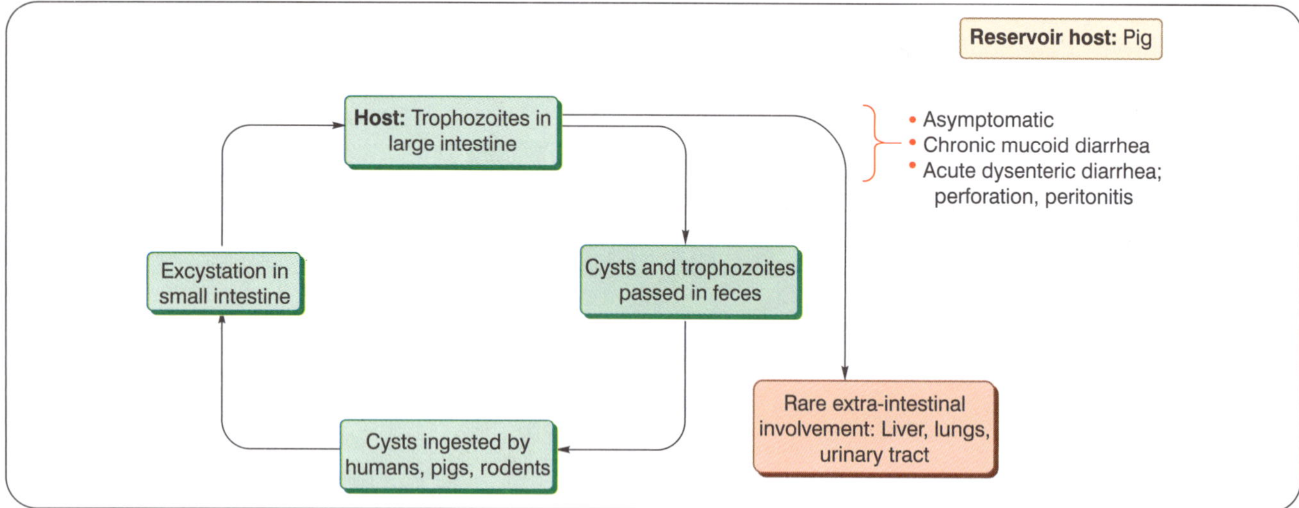

Fig. 6.2 Life cycle of *Balantidium coli* (schematic)

to the **large intestine** and multiply there. Conjugation between two trophozoites for the exchange of nuclear material has been observed. However, reproduction occurs only by **binary fission**. After encystation in the rectum, the cysts and trophozoites are released in the feces into the external environment. The trophozoites disintegrate fairly quickly, whereas the **cyst is capable of infecting other hosts**.

PATHOGENESIS

Usually the affected site is the large intestine, i.e., the colon and rectum; however, the terminal ileum may also be involved in rare cases. Extra-intestinal spread is rare. *B. coli* can produce proteolytic enzymes capable of digesting the intestinal epithelium and forming **wide-mouthed ulcers**. In fulminant cases, necrosis and sloughing of the mucosa are seen with an occasional perforation of the intestine.

CLINICAL FEATURES

Typically, most infected individuals remain **asymptomatic**.

Chronic disease: In symptomatic disease, a chronic course is more common, characterised by abdominal pain, intermittent **mucoid diarrhea** (rarely bloody) and weight loss.

Acute disease: Occasionally, an **amoebic dysentery-like severe disease** is seen with the passage of blood and mucus, fever, intestinal colic, severe dehydration and renal insufficiency. Extensive disease may lead to fulminant colitis, perforation, peritonitis and renal failure. Rarely, **extra-intestinal involvement** of the liver, lungs, pleura and urinary tract is reported, especially in immunocompromised patients.

DIAGNOSIS

The laboratory diagnosis largely depends on the demonstration of the parasite in stool specimens. Owing to the intermittent excretion of the parasite, multiple samples should be examined to improve the detection rates.

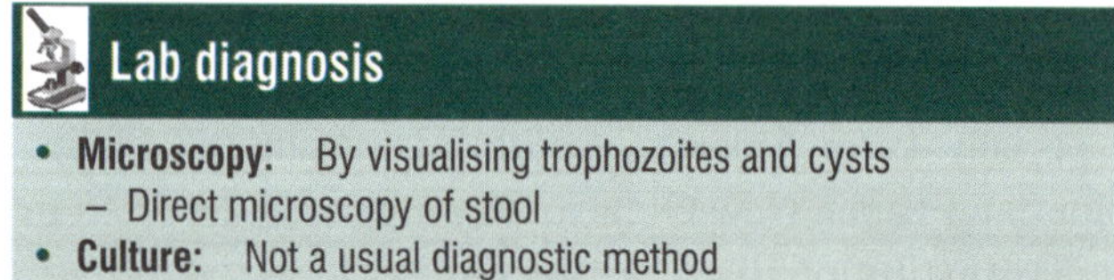

Lab diagnosis

- **Microscopy:** By visualising trophozoites and cysts
  - Direct microscopy of stool
- **Culture:** Not a usual diagnostic method

Microscopy

Wet mount: In a saline wet mount of a fresh stool specimen, the trophozoite may be identified based on its large size and **spiralling or rotational motility** (Fig. 6.3a). Cysts (Fig. 6.3b) are found in semiformed or formed stool. A phase-contrast microscope is helpful in viewing the internal structures of unstained parasites.

Stained smears: Though Lugol's iodine (1:5 to 1:100 dilution) or hematoxylin and eosin stain can be used to stain the specimen, these darken the cytoplasm, thereby obscuring the internal details.

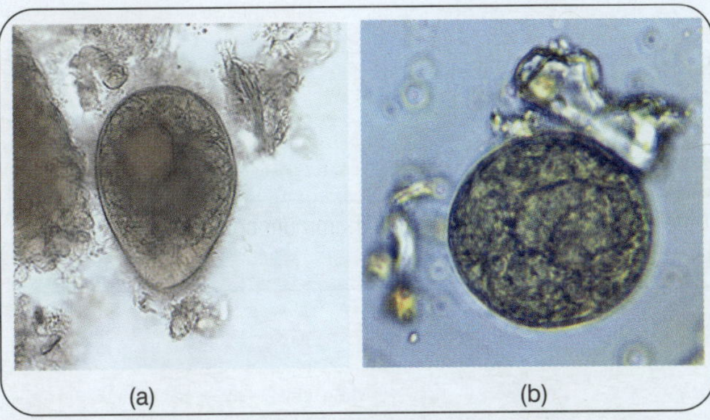

Fig. 6.3 Features of trophozoites and cysts of *Balantidium coli:* (a) trophozoite in a wet mount showing cilia and (b) cyst with a conspicuous kidney-shaped nucleus (*Source:* Centers for Disease Control and Prevention, DPDx)

Stool Culture

Culture is normally not attempted. However, if required, *B. coli* may be cultured on the same media as those used for *Entamoeba histolytica*.

TREATMENT

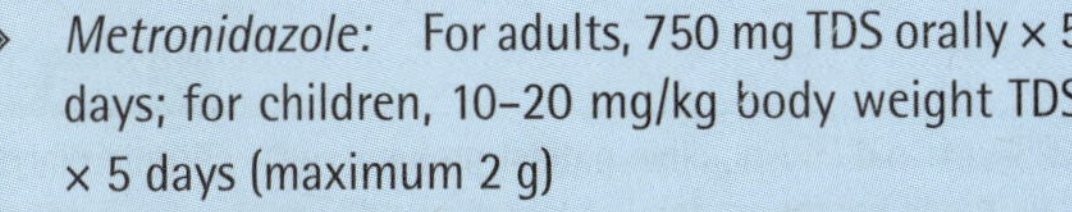

Drug of choice

- *Metronidazole:* For adults, 750 mg TDS orally × 5 days; for children, 10–20 mg/kg body weight TDS × 5 days (maximum 2 g)

Alternate drug

- *Tetracyclines:* For adults, 500 mg QID × 10 days; for children, 10 mg/kg QID × 10 days

PREVENTION AND CONTROL

- Provision of clean, uncontaminated water for drinking is the most crucial preventive measure. Boiling or filtering of water is more effective than treatment with chlorine, which is ineffective against cysts at the concentrations normally used for water treatment.
- Avoiding the use of night soil or activated sludge as fertiliser breaks the chain of transmission.

Questions

1. Discuss the clinical presentation of balantiosis.
2. Discuss the diagnosis and management of balantiosis.

Multiple Choice Questions

1. Which of the following is the main reservoir host for *Balantidium coli*?
   a. Human being
   b. Monkey
   c. Pig
   d. Cattle
2. Which of the following can cause dysentery?
   a. *Giardia*
   b. *Ascaris*
   c. *Entamoeba dispar*
   d. *Balantidium coli*
3. Which of the following is the largest protozoan parasite to inhabit the gastrointestinal tract of humans?
   a. *Cystoisospora belli*
   b. *Entamoeba histolytica*
   c. *Balantidium coli*
   d. *Giardia*
4. Which is the natural host for *Balantidium coli*?
   a. Cattle
   b. Pig
   c. Rodent
   d. Human being
5. The only parasite that has cilia and causes infection in human beings is __________:
   a. *Trichomonas*
   b. *Giardia*
   c. *Leishmania*
   d. *Balantidium*

Chapter 7

Cryptosporidium

([From Greek] *cryptos* = hidden + *spora* = seed)

Case Study and Learning Goals

A 25-year-old HIV-positive patient presents with chronic diarrhea. What are the parasitic causes of diarrhea in immunocompromised patients? How would you approach the laboratory diagnosis of this case? How would you treat this patient?

COCCIDIAN PROTOZOA

A few coccidian protozoans including *Cryptosporidium*, *Cystoisospora* and *Cyclospora* are important **diarrheal pathogens**. These parasites have fairly similar morphologies (including a **complex of apical structures [apicomplexans]** for entry into host cells), life cycles and clinical presentations. However, they differ in their epidemiological aspects. They are important **opportunistic pathogens of immunocompromised hosts**. Some of them also have a tendency to cause **waterborne or foodborne outbreaks**.

INTRODUCTION

Cryptosporidium has been recognised as an **opportunistic pathogen** of young children and immunocompromised adults and is listed as an **AIDS-defining illness**. Two species commonly cause human infections – ***C. hominis***, which is found mainly in humans, and ***C. parvum***, which is found in cattle and humans. The species were initially named on the basis of their host species. However, with the help of molecular studies, several genotypes and occult species infecting humans, animals, reptiles, birds and fishes are now recognised.

Cryptosporidium was first reported in 1907 by Ernest Edward Tyzzer in the stomach of an autopsied mouse. The name *Cryptosporidium parvum* was coined in 1912. It was long associated with diarrhea in animals; it was first reported in humans in 1976 in a child who presented with diarrhea. The first case of cryptosporidiosis in a homosexual man with an HIV infection was reported in 1982. Subsequently, the association between cryptosporidiosis and AIDS was noted in several cases. Since then, *Cryptosporidium* has been recognised as an important opportunistic parasite.

EPIDEMIOLOGY

Cryptosporidiosis is of significant public health importance due to the unavailability of effective treatment and on account of its ability to spread through the water supply (outbreak potential), its wide host range and the variety of possible modes of its transmission (person-to-person, waterborne, animal-to-human and foodborne).

Cryptosporidium has many remarkable characteristics which are critical to its epidemiology and spread of infection. Its oocysts are very hardy (they survive even in seawater); they are chlorine- and acid-resistant, relatively small and fully infectious when shed, and the infectious dose is very small (<10 to 100 oocysts). Moreover, they can complete their life cycles in a single host.

Risk Factors

The major risk factors are the ingestion of contaminated drinking or recreational water, contact with infected persons or animals, immunocompromised status and travel to endemic areas.

- **Children:** In developed countries, cryptosporidiosis occurs in up to 7% of immunocompetent children who have diarrhea; the corresponding percentage in developing countries is 12%. Cryptosporidium has now been recognised as the **second most common cause of moderate to severe diarrhea in children globally after rotavirus** and is associated with increased risk of death in children <2 years of age.
- **Immunocompromised patients:** Patients who have AIDS, those who have malignancies including hematological malignancies (T cell deficiencies like SCID and CD40 ligand deficiency, i.e., hyper IgM syndrome), those receiving chemotherapy, those on hemodialysis, and bone marrow and solid organ transplant recipients are more prone to severe disease. In developed countries, cryptosporidiosis occurs in 14% of patients with AIDS with diarrhea, while in developing countries, it occurs in 24% of such patients.
- **Outbreaks:** *Cryptosporidium* has been responsible for numerous outbreaks in developed countries. Most of

the outbreaks have occurred due to the contamination of drinking or recreational waters. In 1993, a large-scale waterborne outbreak of cryptosporidiosis occurred in Milwaukee, USA, affecting more than 400,000 people. This outbreak was a harbinger of the significant emergence of *Cryptosporidium* spp. as a major human pathogen.

- **Traveller's diarrhea:** *Cryptosporidium* is a significant cause of diarrhea in travellers returning from endemic areas.

MORPHOLOGY

There are various stages in the life cycle of *Cryptosporidium*, namely oocyst, sporozoite, trophozoite, meront, merozoite, macro- and micro-gametes and zygote. However, only the oocysts are recovered from stool specimens. Other life cycle stages can be seen in intestinal biopsies.

Oocysts

They are round, refractile, 4–6 μm in size, **acid-fast** and should be differentiated from other acid-fast structures (Fig. 7.1a, b and c and Table 7.1). Each mature oocyst contains four slender fusiform **sporozoites**.

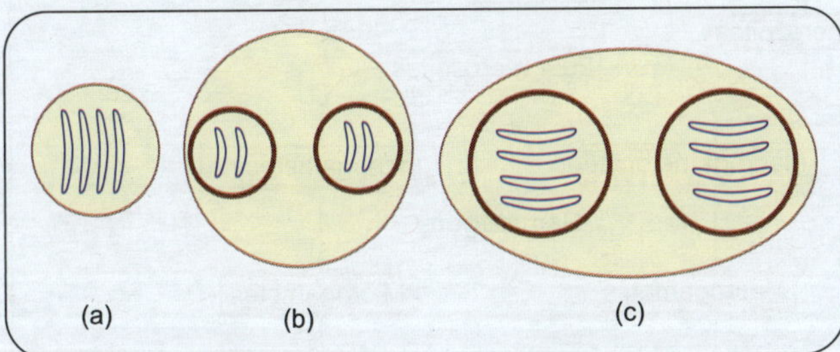

Fig. 7.1 Line diagrams of coccidian oocysts: (a) *Cryptosporidium* oocyst (4–6 μm) with four sporozoites, (b) *Cyclospora* oocyst (8–10 μm) with two sporocysts, each containing two sporozoites and (c) *Cystoisospora* oocyst (20–30 μm) with two sporocysts, each containing four sporozoites

LIFE CYCLE (Fig. 7.2a and b)

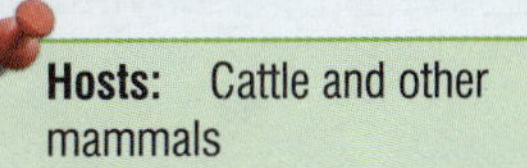

Human beings are infected by the ingestion or inhalation of the oocysts. Though several animals are known to act as reservoirs of *Cryptosporidium*, it can complete its life cycle in a single host. The various phases in its life cycle are as follows:

- After uptake, the oocysts **excyst** in the intestine to liberate four motile sporozoites which attach to the brush border epithelium of the intestine (or respiratory epithelium/biliary tract) with the help of their apical poles. A cytoskeletal rearrangement is induced in the host cell, and a parasitophorous vacuole located at the microvillous surface of the host cell is formed around the sporozoite.
- The sporozoite is converted into a trophozoite which, in turn, grows to form two types of meronts which reproduce by asexual multiplication; this is known as **merogony (schizogony)**.
  - **Type I meronts** produce eight merozoites, which can invade more epithelial cells to continue the asexual reproductive cycle.
  - **Type II meronts** produce four merozoites, which initiate the sexual cycle known as **gametogony** by forming micro- and macro-gametes.
- The gametes fertilise to form zygotes, which form two types of oocysts – thin-walled and thick-walled.
  - The **thin-walled oocysts** are unique in their ability to re-initiate the invasion of host cells (autoinfection), undergo **sporogony** and continue the intestinal life cycle of the parasite. Autoinfection is the key factor in the maintenance of chronic infection in an immunocompromised individual.
  - The **thick-walled oocysts** undergo **sporogony** within the intestine to form four sporozoites and are ready to be immediately infective when released into the environment with the host's feces. These oocysts persist for a long time in water.

Table 7.1 Comparative morphological features of intestinal coccidian parasites

Parasite	Size (μm)	Shape	Number of sporozoites per oocyst	Infectivity of oocyst when excreted	Acid-fast staining	Autofluorescence
Cryptosporidium	4–6	Round	4	Infective	Yes	No
Cystoisospora	20–30 × 10–15	Elliptical	8 (2 sporocysts with 4 sporozoites each)	Infective after 1–2 days	Yes	Yes
Cyclospora	8–10	Spheroidal	4 (2 sporocysts with 2 sporozoites each)	Infective after 7–15 days	Variable	Yes

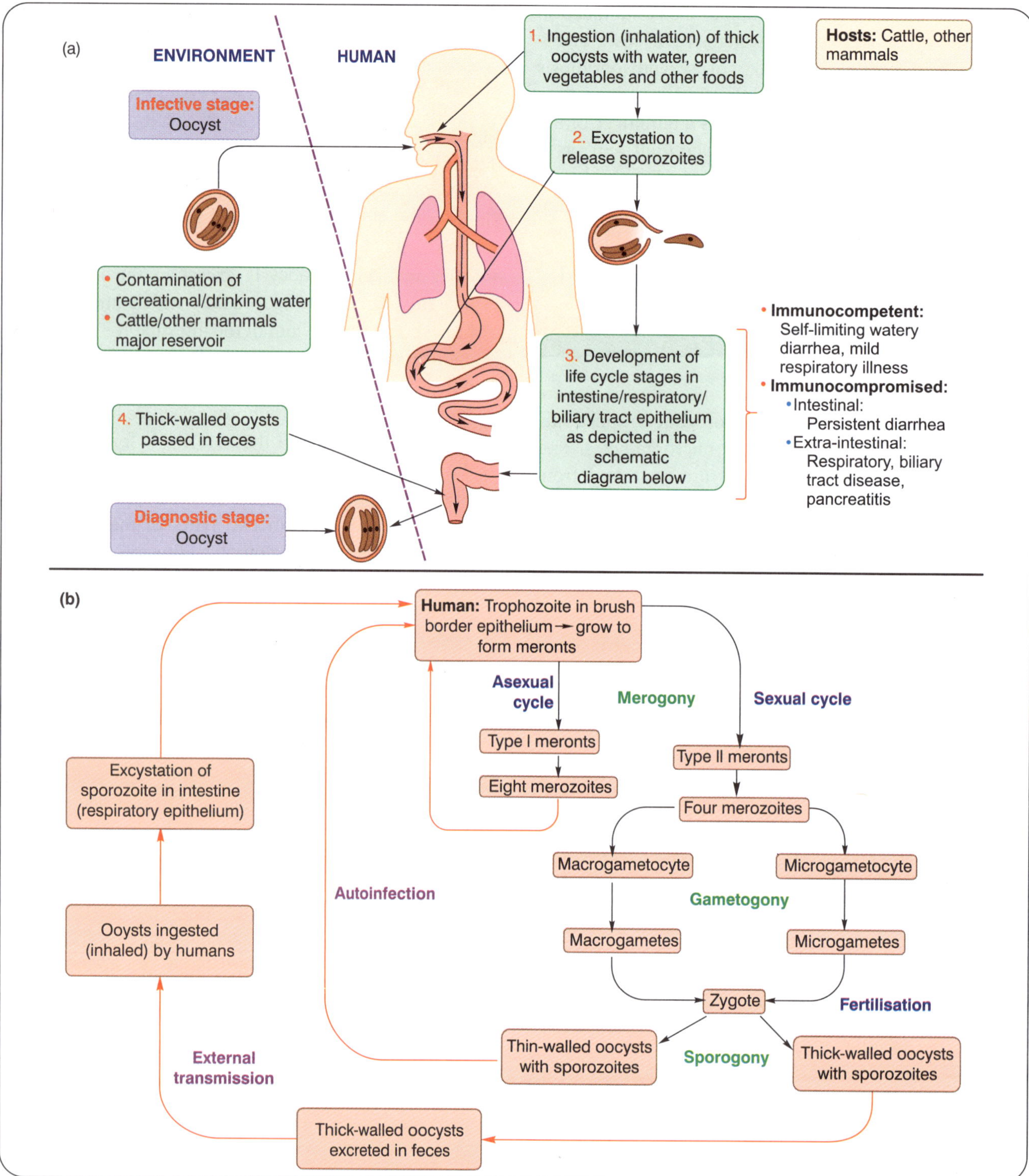

Fig. 7.2 Life cycle of *Cryptosporidium*: (a) detailed and (b) schematic

PATHOGENESIS

The gastrointestinal tract is the most affected since *Cryptosporidium* multiplies in the brush border epithelium of the intestine. However, the respiratory and biliary tracts are also infected in an immunocompromised host.

The following are the mechanisms of pathogenesis of the infection:

- The heaviest infection is seen in the distal jejunum and ileum. On infection of the host cells, the parasite induces the activation of the transcription factor NF-κB which inhibits the cell apoptosis.

- An enterotoxin has been implicated (though yet unproven) in the pathogenesis of cryptosporidial diarrhea.
- Typically, there is partial villous atrophy, crypt hyperplasia and infiltration of the lamina propria by inflammatory cells in the gastrointestinal tract. Malabsorption of disaccharides, vitamin B12, bile acids and fatty acids, and decreased absorption of fluids and electrolytes due to increased permeability lead to nutrient deficiency.
- The respiratory tract shows infiltration of the lamina propria by inflammatory cells, loss of cilia, hyperplasia and hypertrophy of the epithelial cells.

CLINICAL FEATURES

The incubation period ranges from 3–14 days. The clinical manifestations vary according to the immune and nutritional status of the host. Most infections are asymptomatic. When symptomatic, there is profuse watery diarrhea in both immunocompetent and immunocompromised hosts. This diarrhea may be indistinguishable from any other acute non-bloody diarrheal illness except that cryptosporidiosis is more likely to become persistent, typically resulting in weight loss.

Cryptosporidiosis is now recognised as an important etiological agent of the following:

- **Self-limiting diarrhea in an immunocompetent host**
- **Persistent diarrhea in children**
- **Chronic diarrhea in an immunocompromised host**

The features of *Cryptosporidium* infection in an **immunocompetent** host are as follows:

- The infection is usually asymptomatic in adults.
- When symptomatic, it is a significant cause of persistent diarrhea in children <5 years of age, and also causes traveller's diarrhea.
- This diarrhea can be of sudden onset and is generally watery and voluminous with a frequency of 3–6 times a day (often more). Sometimes, it is explosive, foul-smelling and mucoid.
- The illness usually lasts 1–2 weeks, although it may last for a month or longer in some patients. It is associated with an increased risk of mortality in children. It causes growth failure, neurocognitive impairment and contributes significantly to malnutrition in children.
- Other acute symptoms are malaise or fatigue, anorexia, pyrexia, abdominal pain, nausea or vomiting and cramps with considerable weight loss.
- Pus, blood and fecal leukocytes are typically absent in the stool.

The features of *Cryptosporidium* infection in an **immunocompromised** host are as follows:

- Cryptosporidiosis is more severe in HIV-seropositive patients and frequently causes chronic diarrhea. The patient passes copious amounts of watery stools (as much as 17 litres). Such an infection can cause mortality, particularly in those with low $CD4^+$ counts (<150/mm^3). It is listed as an **AIDS-defining illness (clinical category C)** by the CDC (Centres for Disease Control and Prevention, USA).
- Extra-intestinal involvement of the biliary tract (sclerosing cholangitis), gallbladder, liver, pancreas and respiratory system is also seen in patients who have AIDS.

DIAGNOSIS

The approach to the diagnosis of cryptosporidiosis is chiefly based on the detection of the parasite or its antigen or nucleic acid. Stool is the specimen of choice. Oocyst excretion is intermittent and thus, multiple fecal samples (either fresh or fixed in 10% formalin) may be necessary for diagnosis. **Concentration techniques** involve either floatation, e.g., in Sheather's sugar solution, zinc sulphate or saturated sodium chloride solution, or sedimentation with formalin-ether.

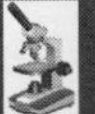

Lab diagnosis

- **Microscopy:** By visualising oocysts
  - Modified acid-fast stain, fluorescent stain
  - Histopathology: Of biopsy sample
- **Coproantigen detection:** ELISA and immunochromatographic tests
- **Serology:** Not useful
- **DNA detection:** PCR, real-time PCR, LAMP and multiplex assays

Microscopy

- **Wet mount:** The oocysts are refractile (shiny) structures but are difficult to visualise in unstained wet preparations because of their small size.
- **Modified acid-fast or Kinyoun staining:** Oocysts are **acid-fast**, i.e., they retain the **bright red colour** of primary carbol fuchsin staining on secondary decolourisation with 1% sulphuric acid or acid alcohol. Oocytes appear as round, red-coloured structures, 4–6 μm in size against a background of blue (methylene blue) or green (malachite green) counterstain. *Cryptosporidium* oocysts must be differentiated from

yeasts and the larger oocysts of *Cyclospora* (8–10 µm) (Fig. 7.3a).

- **Fluorescent stain:** Auramine-rhodamine, auramine-phenol, auramine-carbol fuchsin and acridine orange can be used. The major advantage of these stains is rapid screening and higher detection efficacy though the specificity is low.
- **Direct fluorescent antibody staining:** Staining with specific fluorescent-labelled monoclonal antibodies is more sensitive and specific to detect *Cryptosporidium* oocysts.

Coproantigen Detection

Oocyst antigen-capture methods such as enzyme immune assays or immunochromatographic lateral flow assays may be used. Commercial kits for *Cryptosporidium* are available in ELISA and immunochromatographic formats. ELISA kits have sensitivities ranging from 60–100% with excellent specificity.

Serodiagnosis

Antibody detection is only used for sero-epidemiological purposes; it is not helpful in diagnosis.

Nucleic Acid-Based Detection

PCR-based methods for the detection of *Cryptosporidium* DNA are more sensitive, take less time and can play an important role in outbreak situations when species and genotype identification is important. Multiplex gastrointestinal parasite panels that include *Cryptosporidium* are commercially available but are expensive.

Histopathology

Biopsy samples stained with hematoxylin and eosin reveal the intracellular life stages of *Cryptosporidium* in the brush border of the epithelium of the small intestine (Fig. 7.3b).

TREATMENT

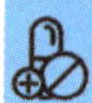

Drug of choice
- *Nitazoxanide:* For adults, 500 mg BDS orally × 3 days; for children >4 years, 200 mg BDS × 3 days, and for <4 years, 100 mg BDS × 3 days

Alternate drug
- *Paromomycin:* 25–35 mg/kg/day orally × 14 days

For HIV-AIDS patients
- Anti-parasitic drugs not efficacious
- HAART with a protease inhibitor in addition to nitazoxanide is recommended

Supportive management
- Replacement of fluids and electrolytes is critical

No anti-parasitic drug has proven effective against cryptosporidiosis in severely immunocompromised patients. Highly active anti-retroviral therapy (HAART) with a protease inhibitor as part of the regimen of initial therapy in addition to nitazoxanide is considered the best

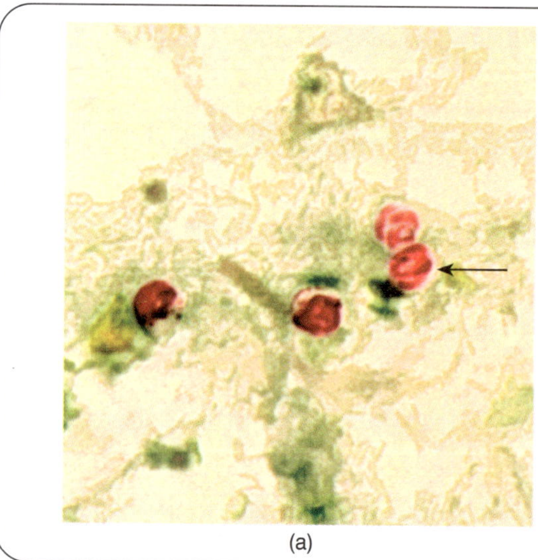

(a)

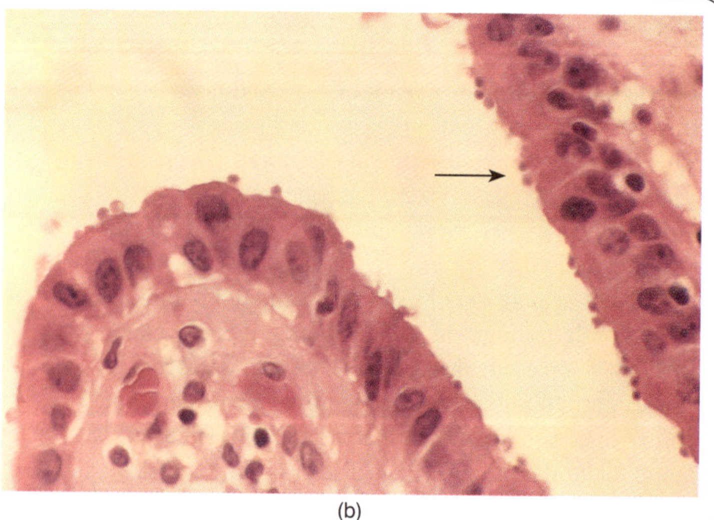

(b)

Fig. 7.3 Features of oocysts of *Cryptosporidium*: (a) modified acid-fast method showing bright red oocysts with elongated sporozoites and (b) histopathology of gallbladder tissue from an AIDS patient showing *Cryptosporidium* lining the luminal surface of the epithelial cells (*Source:* Centers for Disease Control and Prevention [CDC], Public Health Image Library [PHIL], Image IDs 7829 and 968)

approach for such patients. The infection responds best to an improvement in the host's immune status.

PREVENTION AND CONTROL

- The most significant preventive measure is improvement in quality of **water, sanitation and household hygiene and animal control**.
- Health education and increased awareness are also important.
- Those travelling to endemic countries should only consume boiled or bottled water.
- Filtration is effective only with filters that have a pore size of 1 μm.
- There is no vaccine available for the disease.

QUESTIONS

1. Discuss the diagnosis and management of cryptosporidiosis.
2. Discuss opportunistic intestinal parasitic infections.

MULTIPLE CHOICE QUESTIONS

1. The drug of choice for cryptosporidiosis in children is ____________.
   a. Albendazole
   b. Nitazoxanide
   c. Metronidazole
   d. Cotrimoxazole
2. Which of the following is TRUE about cryptosporidiosis?
   a. It is an AIDS-defining illness.
   b. It occurs only in immunocompromised children.
   c. It responds best to fluconazole.
   d. It affects the central nervous system.
3. Which of the following statements about *Cryptosporidium* is FALSE?
   a. The oocyst is an acid-fast structure.
   b. The oocyst is bigger than an RBC.
   c. It is a significant cause of diarrhea in children below 5 years of age.
   d. It causes an AIDS-defining illness.
4. The oocyst of *Cryptosporidium* ____________:
   a. Contains eight sporozoites.
   b. Contains four sporozoites.
   c. Is bigger than an RBC.
   d. Has autofluorescence property.
5. *Cryptosporidium* infection can be prevented by all the following EXCEPT ____________:
   a. Consumption of properly washed food and safe water
   b. Boiling water
   c. Avoidance of walking barefoot
   d. Avoidance of recreational water

Chapter 8

Cystoisospora

([From Greek] *kystis* = bladder + *isos* = identical + *spora* = seed)

Case Study and Learning Goals

A 25-year-old HIV-positive male presents with diarrhea of 4 weeks' duration. The stool microscopy reveals 20 μm long, elliptical parasitic oocysts. What are the parasitic causes of chronic diarrhea? What other staining would you like to do in this case? How would you treat this patient?

INTRODUCTION

The coccidian parasites of the genus *Cystoisospora* that infect mammals were earlier classified under the **genus *Isospora***. However, they have now been reclassified as members of the genus *Cystoisospora* based on genetic studies. **The only *Cystoisospora* species reported to cause disease in humans is *C. belli***. It was first identified as a human pathogen among military personnel during World War I, and hence the name *belli* (from *bellum* [Latin] meaning war).

EPIDEMIOLOGY

Although *Cystoisospora* are distributed worldwide, they are predominantly found in tropical regions and in developing countries (especially South-East Asia, Africa, the Middle East and South America). *C. belli* chiefly causes diseases in immunosuppressed patients but can also infect immunocompetent persons; however, the disease in such persons is quite mild. Prevalence rates ranging from 4–15% have been reported in HIV-infected patients. It has also been implicated in traveller's diarrhea. However, unlike *Cyclospora*, it is not implicated in large outbreaks.

Risk Factors

Immunosuppression as in AIDS, lymphoblastic leukemia, adult T cell leukemia, lymphoma, lymphoproliferative disorders and being a transplant recipient is the most significant risk factor for *Cystoisospora* infections. Individuals who have malabsorption syndrome, those who spend a considerable amount of time at daycare centres or psychiatric institutions, and those who travel to endemic areas are also very susceptible.

MORPHOLOGY

Like *Cryptosporidium, C. belli* exists in various life cycle stages, of which only the immature oocysts are recovered in stool specimens.

Oocyst

The oocysts are **elliptical** and **20–30 μm × 10–15 μm** (Fig. 8.1a) in size. They are **acid-fast** and should be differentiated from other acid-fast coccidian parasites. The immature oocyst containing a single sporoblast is excreted in the stool; it then divides into two sporoblasts, each of which matures into a sporocyst. Each sporocyst contains four fusiform sporozoites (Fig. 8.1b–d).

LIFE CYCLE

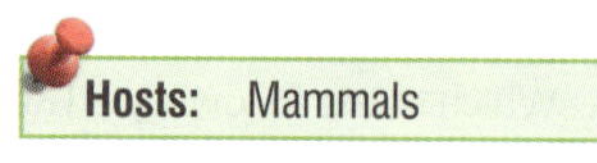

Human infections are caused by the **ingestion of the mature sporulated oocysts** of *C. belli*. The oocysts excyst in the proximal small intestine to liberate sporozoites which follow an intracellular life cycle like that of *Cryptosporidium*. **Immature unsporulated oocysts with a single sporoblast are liberated** from the intestine; these sporulate externally in 1–2 days to become infective. *C. belli* can complete its life cycle in a single host.

In immunocompromised individuals, the sporozoites may migrate to extra-intestinal sites such as the lymph nodes, liver and spleen, where they may remain dormant in a cyst-like structure and cause extra-intestinal disease later.

PATHOGENESIS

Infection is acquired by the ingestion of water or food contaminated with oocysts. The virulence factors of the parasite are unknown. However, it is indicated that direct invasive cell damage and inflammation play a role in the pathogenesis. *C. belli* primarily infects the duodenal and jejunal epithelium which shows villous atrophy, crypt hypertrophy, collagen deposition in the lamina propria and eosinophilic infiltration.

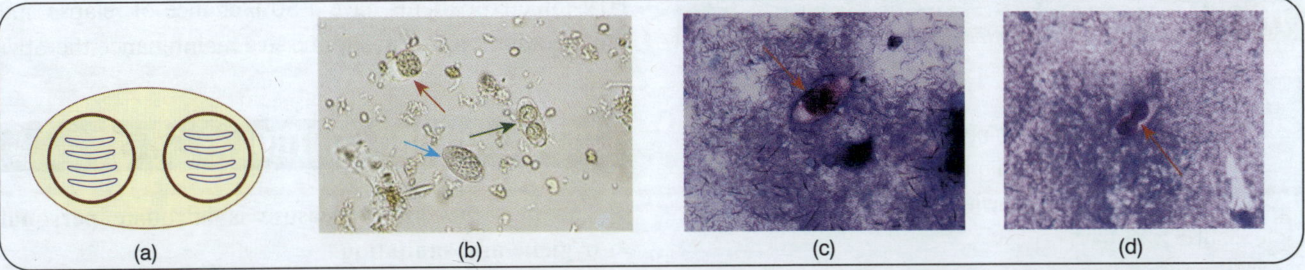

Fig. 8.1 Features of *Cystoisospora belli*: (a) a line diagram of an oocyst (20–30 μm) with two sporocysts, each containing four sporozoites, (b) oocysts in a wet mount in three different stages of sporulation—unsporulated (lower, blue arrow), single sporoblast (top, red arrow) and two sporocysts (right, green arrow), (c) an oocyst with a single sporoblast in a stool sample stained with modified acid-fast stain and (d) an oocyst with two sporocysts in a stool sample stained with modified acid-fast stain

CLINICAL FEATURES

The incubation period of *C. belli* ranges from 2–14 days. It infects both immunocompetent and immunosuppressed patients. The following are some clinical features of the disease:

- In the **immunocompetent**, the disease is usually mild and is characterised by fever, nausea, vomiting and **self-limiting watery diarrhea**.
- In severely **immunocompromised** patients, **chronic diarrhea** which may last months to years is often reported and has been associated with muscle wasting and atrophy, and sometimes, death. Extra-intestinal disease has also been reported atypically.
- Patients with malabsorption syndrome, particularly malnourished children, are also at increased risk of chronic cystoisosporiasis.

DIAGNOSIS

The approach to the diagnosis of the disease is primarily based on the demonstration of oocysts—either immature or mature, containing two sporocysts. Oocyst excretion is intermittent and thus, multiple fecal samples (either fresh or fixed in 10% formalin) may be necessary for diagnosis. Sensitivity can be improved by concentration techniques like Sheather's sugar flotation, or sedimentation with formalin-ether. Rarely, a biopsy of the small intestine may be required.

Lab diagnosis

- **Microscopy:** By visualising immature or mature oocysts
  - Direct microscopy of stool
  - Acid-fast staining
  - Histopathology: Of small intestinal biopsy
- **DNA detection:** PCR, real-time PCR, multiplex PCR

Microscopy

- **Wet and iodine mount:** Direct examination of stool in normal saline is useful since oocysts are large and have a characteristic morphology (Fig. 8.1b). Charcot-Leyden crystals derived from eosinophils are also found in the stools of these patients.
- **Modified acid-fast stains:** The oocysts are acid-fast to 1% sulphuric acid or acid alcohol, and appear bright red against a blue or green background (Fig. 8.1c and d).
- **Fluorescent stains:** Auramine-rhodamine, auramine-phenol, auramine-carbol fuchsin and acridine orange can be used, the main advantage of these stains being rapid screening.
- **Autofluorescence:** In unstained preparations, autofluorescence can be observed under 330–380 nm ultraviolet filter.

Serodiagnosis

This is generally not helpful.

Nucleic Acid-Based Detection

Both conventional PCR and real-time PCR targeting 18S rDNA show excellent sensitivity and specificity. Multiplex PCR panels for simultaneous detection of several enteric pathogens are now available commercially.

Histopathology

Histological samples stained with hematoxylin and eosin reveal the intracellular life stages of *Cystoisospora* in the brush border epithelium of the small intestine.

Other Diagnostic Parameters

Peripheral eosinophilia, which is generally seen in helminthic infections, is a distinctive feature of *Cystoisospora* infection.

TREATMENT

Drug of choice

- *Trimethoprim–sulphamethoxazole (TMP-SMX)*: For adults, 160/800 mg QID × 10 days followed by suppressive therapy with TMP-SMX 160/800 mg BDS × 21 days

Alternate drugs

- *Pyrimethamine*: 75 mg/day along with folinic acid 25 mg/day × 7–10 days
- *Ciprofloxacin*: 500 mg BDS × 7 days

HIV-infected patients have a 50% chance of relapse and thus require long-term suppressive maintenance therapy.

PREVENTION AND CONTROL

- The best preventive measure is adequate **personal hygiene and sanitation.**
- Thorough washing of vegetables and fruits and sterilisation of water generally prevent fecal-oral transmission from contaminated food, water and possibly, environmental surfaces.

QUESTIONS

1. Discuss the diagnosis and management of cystoisosporiasis.
2. Differentiate between *Cryptosporidium*, *Cyclospora* and *Cystoisospora*.

MULTIPLE CHOICE QUESTIONS

1. Autofluorescence is a feature of ___________ oocysts excreted in stool samples.
    a. *Cryptosporidium*
    b. *Cystoisospora*
    c. *Microsporidia*
    d. *Giardia*
2. The drug of choice for the treatment of *Cystoisospora* infection is ___________.
    a. Trimethoprim–sulphamethoxazole
    b. Albendazole
    c. Nitazoxanide
    d. Amphotericin
3. Which of the following statements about *Cystoisospora* is TRUE?
    a. It is NOT an AIDS-defining illness.
    b. It affects the central nervous system.
    c. It produces acid-fast oocysts.
    d. The oocysts are immediately infectious when excreted.
4. Which of the following is TRUE about the mature oocysts of *Cystoisospora belli*?
    a. They are elliptical, measure 10–20 µm in size and contain one sporocyst with 8 sporozoites.
    b. Oocysts are immediately infectious when excreted.
    c. They are spherical, 6–10 µm in size and contain one sporocyst with four sporozoites each.
    d. They are elliptical, measure 20–30 × 10–15 µm in size and contain two sporocysts with four sporozoites each.
5. Which of the following statements about *Cystoisospora* infection is TRUE?
    a. It leads to large outbreaks linked to the ingestion of contaminated food.
    b. It causes self-limiting diarrhea in immunocompetent patients.
    c. The diagnosis is made by serological tests.
    d. There are many species of *Cystoisospora* that cause human infections.

Chapter 9

Cyclospora

([From Greek] *kuklos* = circle + *spora* = seed)

Case Study and Learning Goals

A 25-year-old male who recently returned from Peru presents with diarrhea of 3 weeks' duration. He has a history of eating raw raspberries in Peru. What are the parasitic causes of diarrhea associated with travel to the developing countries? How would you approach the laboratory diagnosis in this case? How would you treat this patient?

INTRODUCTION

Cyclospora cayetanensis is an **opportunistic parasite** of immunocompromised individuals, especially AIDS patients. It has also been reported to have caused a number of outbreaks involving both immunocompromised and immunocompetent hosts. Co-infection with *Cyclospora*, *Cryptosporidium* and other parasites is frequently reported. About 20 species of *Cyclospora* have been identified worldwide, of which only *C. cayetanensis* has been described as a pathogen in humans. It is closely related to the animal coccidian parasite, *Eimeria*.

C. cayetanensis was first recognised by Richard Ashford in Papua New Guinea in 1979. However, it received attention only in 1986 when it was found in the stool of HIV-positive patients; it was named in 1992. The increased use of acid-fast staining for the diagnosis of *Cryptosporidium* played an important role in the identification of the other acid-fast oocysts including *C. cayetanensis*.

EPIDEMIOLOGY

C. cayetanensis is worldwide in distribution but more common in the tropical and subtropical regions of the world. The disease is endemic in Haiti, Guatemala, Peru and Nepal; those who **travel** to these areas are at an increased risk. Outbreaks related to food imported from these areas are frequently reported in the developed world.

Parasitic causes of traveller's diarrhea

- *Cryptosporidium parvum*
- *Entamoeba histolytica*
- *Giardia duodenalis*
- *Cyclospora cayetanensis*

Risk Factors

Consumption of untreated water and berries, a lack of adequate sanitation, immunocompromised status and travel to endemic regions are among the risk factors.

- **Raspberries** are characterised by fine, hair-like projections that facilitate the entrapment of the 'sticky' *Cyclospora* oocysts. California strawberries, Florida blueberries, Guatemala blackberries and Guatemala/Chile raspberries as well as other fresh produce such as basil and lettuce, when eaten raw, are frequently implicated in *Cyclospora* infections.
- *Cyclospora* oocysts are unsporulated when excreted (unlike those of *Cryptosporidium*) and require 7–15 days to sporulate. However, these oocysts are hardy and highly resistant to common disinfectants used in food and water processing.

MORPHOLOGY

C. cayetanensis also exists in various life cycle stages like *Cryptosporidium*. Only the immature oocysts are recovered from stool specimens.

Oocysts

The oocysts are spheroidal and **8–10** µm in size with membrane-bound refractile globules. They are variably acid-fast, and contain two sporocysts—each 4 µm in size and containing two fusiform sporozoites (Fig. 9.1a and b). The oocyst shows auto-fluorescence under UV light, unlike *Cryptosporidium parvum* (Fig. 9.1c).

LIFE CYCLE

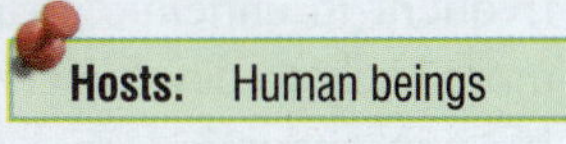

Humans are the only known hosts for *C. cayetanensis*. It resides in the jejunum and follows a similar intracellular life cycle as that of *Cryptosporidium* except that **unsporulated oocysts liberated** from the intestine require 7–15 days to sporulate before becoming infective, unlike *Cryptosporidium* oocysts which are ready to infect as soon

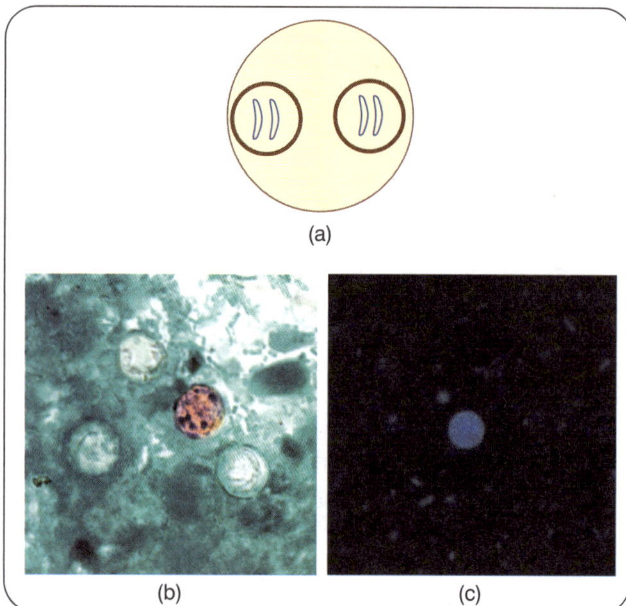

Fig. 9.1 Features of *Cyclospora cayetanensis*: (a) a line diagram of an oocyst (8–10 μm) with two sporocysts, each containing two sporozoites, (b) oocyst from a stool sample fixed in 10% formalin solution showing variable acid-fastness among the four oocysts with modified acid-fast stain and (c) an oocyst showing autofluorescence (*Source:* Centers for Disease Control and Prevention [CDC], Public Health Image Library [PHIL], Image ID 7827 and CDC, DPDx)

as they are excreted. *Cyclospora* can complete its life cycle in a single host.

PATHOGENESIS

Human beings acquire the infection by the ingestion of contaminated food and water. *Cyclospora* primarily infects the intestinal epithelium, which shows inflammation, partial villous blunting and crypt hyperplasia. There is malabsorption of D-xylose and weight loss. The virulence factors of the parasite are unknown.

CLINICAL FEATURES

The incubation period is about 3–10 days. *Cyclospora* infection may be asymptomatic or symptomatic.

- Asymptomatic infection or mild disease is more frequent in endemic areas, where young children are more likely to develop clinical symptoms than adults.
- In non-endemic areas, the infections are almost invariably symptomatic.
  - There may be acute and persistent diarrhea, which may be preceded by a flu-like illness.
  - There may be chronic watery diarrhea, nausea, flatulence, fatigue, abdominal cramping, low-grade fever and weight loss. Post-infection fatigue may persist for a long period.
- The disease is more **severe and prolonged in HIV/AIDS**, with about 50% relapse even after treatment. The average duration of diarrhea for HIV-positive patients is longer than that for HIV-negative patients (6 months vs. 2 months) and may be life-threatening in the former group.

DIAGNOSIS

The mainstay of diagnosis is the detection of oocysts in stool samples. Sometimes, a jejunal biopsy may have to be performed.

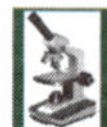

Lab diagnosis

- **Microscopy:** By visualising oocysts
  - Direct wet mount of stool
  - Modified acid-fast stain
  - Autofluorescence
- **Histopathology:** Jejunal biopsy
- **DNA detection:** PCR

Microscopy

- **Wet mount:** Unsporulated oocysts (8–10 μm) can be observed in wet preparations by light, phase contrast and epifluorescence microscopy. They are approximately twice the size of *Cryptosporidium* oocysts (4–6 μm).
- **Modified acid-fast or Kinyoun staining:** Oocysts are variably acid-fast, i.e., some are acid-fast, some take on a lighter colour and others remain unstained (Fig. 9.1b).
- **Autofluorescence:** The oocysts fluoresce white-blue when the wet mount is examined under an epifluorescence microscope using a 330–380 nm excitation filter or fluorescent blue-green when an excitation filter of 450–490 nm is used (Fig. 9.1c).

Nucleic Acid-Based Detection

PCR on fecal samples is a more sensitive diagnostic tool and especially useful in outbreak investigations as compared to conventional microscopy.

Histopathology

Histological examination of intestinal biopsies may show villous atrophy, acute and chronic inflammatory changes in the lamina propria and *Cyclospora* in the supranuclear area inside the enterocytes.

TREATMENT

Drug of choice

- *Trimethoprim-sulphamethoxazole (TMP-SMX):* For adults, 160/800 mg BDS × 7–10 days; for children, 5/25 mg/kg BDS × 7–10 days
- Recurrent symptomatic cyclosporiasis in AIDS patients may be treated with secondary prophylaxis with TMP-SMX three times a week indefinitely

Alternate drug

- *Ciprofloxacin:* 500 mg BDS × 7 days in patients allergic to sulfonamides

Supportive management

- Electrolytes and fluids

PREVENTION AND CONTROL

- The most significant preventive measure comprises adequate **hygiene, food washing and sanitation.**
- **The safety of imported foods** should be monitored.
- **Secondary prophylaxis** should be administered to AIDS patients with recurrent cyclosporiasis.

QUESTIONS

1. Describe the life cycle and morphology of *Cyclospora* with suitable diagrams.
2. Discuss the clinical features, laboratory diagnosis, management and prevention of cyclosporiasis.

MULTIPLE CHOICE QUESTIONS

1. All the following are features of oocysts of *Cyclospora* excreted in feces EXCEPT ______ :
   a. Autofluorescence
   b. Acid-fastness
   c. Spindle shape
   d. Unsporulated when freshly excreted in feces
2. The etiological agent of diarrhea outbreaks characteristically associated with Guatemala raspberries is ______ .
   a. *Cryptosporidium*
   b. *Cystoisospora*
   c. *Cyclospora*
   d. *Cryptococcus*
3. Which of the following statements about *Cyclospora* infection is TRUE?
   a. It causes disease in both immunocompetent and immunocompromised individuals.
   b. It causes bloody diarrhea.
   c. The infection frequently disseminates to other body organs.
   d. The treatment of choice for cyclosporiasis is albendazole.
4. Which of the following statements about *Cyclospora* infection is FALSE?
   a. It may present as acute disease to chronic diarrhea.
   b. It is an AIDS-defining illness.
   c. Drug of choice is trimethoprim-sulphamethoxazole.
   d. It is an important causative agent of traveller's diarrhea.
5. Each sporulated oocyst of *Cyclospora* contains ______ :
   a. Two sporozoites
   b. Two sporocysts containing two sporozoites each
   c. Two sporocysts containing four sporozoites each
   d. Eight sporozoites

CHAPTER 10

Sarcocystis

([From Greek] *sarx* = meat + *kystis* = bladder)

Case Study and Learning Goals

A 25-year-old male presents to the clinic with muscular pain and weakness. He lived in Malaysia during the past year and is a meat-eater. What are the parasitic causes of myositis? How would you approach the laboratory diagnosis in this case? How would you treat this patient?

INTRODUCTION

Sarcocystis are coccidian parasites found in the striated muscles of mammals, birds and reptiles. There are more than 150 species of *Sarcocystis* that are known to infect various animals. However, only a few species, viz. ***S. hominis, S. suihominis*** and ***S. lindemanni*** cause human disease. Until their life cycles were elucidated, these parasites were thought to belong to the genus *Isospora* due to the structural similarity between the sporocysts of the two genera. Unlike other coccidia, *Sarcocystis* have an obligatory two-host life cycle.

The *Sarcocystis* cysts were first described by Johannes Friedrich Miescher, who observed them in the muscles of a mouse. The life cycle of this parasite, which involves a herbivore and a carnivore, was elucidated by M. Rommel and A. O. Heydorn in 1972.

EPIDEMIOLOGY

Sarcocystosis is a zoonotic disease with a wide range of animal reservoirs. Several ruminants serve as intermediate hosts and thereby, as sources of human infection. *Sarcocystis* causes two types of clinical entities – intestinal and extra-intestinal sarcocystosis.

- **Intestinal sarcocystosis:** It is a mild disease acquired by eating raw meat. It has been most frequently reported from European countries, viz. France, Germany, Poland, etc. *S. hominis* and *S. suihominis* are the main infecting agents.
- **Extra-intestinal (muscular) sarcocystosis:** It is caused by various zoonotic species of *Sarcocystis* and is acquired through water or food contaminated with oocysts. Rarely described until recently, it has now become clinically relevant, particularly in travellers, due to a series of outbreaks reported from Malaysia in which *S. lindemanni* was incriminated.

MORPHOLOGY

Oocyst

It is found in the intestine of the definitive hosts. Oocysts are spherical, each measuring **15–20 μm × 15–20 μm**. Each oocyst contains **two sporocysts** enclosed by a fragile cyst wall (Fig. 10.1a).

Sporocyst

It is oval, measuring **15–20 μm × 8–10 μm**. Each sporocyst contains **four sporozoites**.

Tissue Cyst

It is also known as a **sarcocyst**, a **zoitocyte** or a **Miescher's** cyst. These cysts are found in the muscles of intermediate hosts (Fig. 10.1b). They are elongate, spindle-shaped cysts, **100–350 μm** in size, containing numerous **bradyzoites**, each measuring 7–16 μm.

LIFE CYCLE

> **Definitive hosts:** Human beings
> **Intermediate hosts:** Cattle, pigs and human beings (accidental)

Humans serve as definitive hosts for *S. hominis* and *S. suihominis* when they consume the sarcocyst-containing meat of infected cattle and pigs (intermediate hosts). Alternatively, humans may serve as **accidental 'dead-end' intermediate hosts** on consuming contaminated food or water containing sporocysts excreted by infected carnivores.

In the natural life cycle of the parasite, human infections are caused by the **ingestion of tissue sarcocysts** in **undercooked meat**. The cysts get digested in the stomach and small intestine to liberate bradyzoites which enter the intestinal epithelial cells and undergo **gametogony**

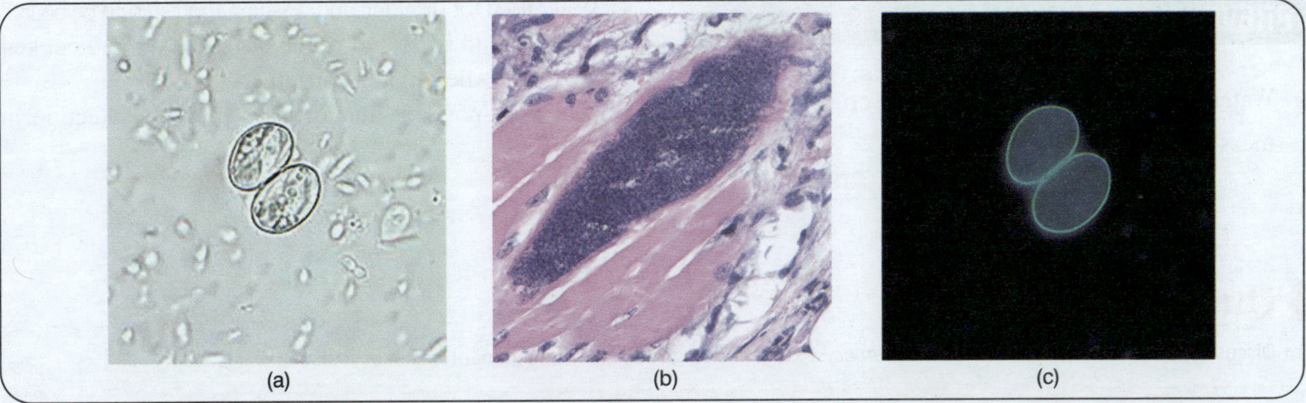

Fig. 10.1 Features of *Sarcocystis* species: (a) sporulated oocyst in an unstained wet mount, (b) a sarcocyst in muscle tissue with numerous bradyzoites stained with H&E and (c) a sporulated oocyst showing autofluorescence under UV microscopy (*Source:* Centers for Disease Control and Prevention [CDC], DPDx)

to differentiate into macro- and micro-gametocytes. The gametes fuse to form oocysts which sporulate in the intestine and are released with feces into the external environment, either as oocysts or as single sporocysts.

The intermediate hosts (cattle and pigs) are infected by the ingestion of the sporocysts which rupture in the intestine to liberate the sporozoites. These sporozoites penetrate the intestine and enter the endothelial cells of the arteries to form 1st generation schizonts, and subsequently, 2nd generation schizonts in the capillary endothelium throughout the body. The schizonts liberate merozoites, which enter the **skeletal and cardiac muscles cells and occasionally the brain**, where they generate numerous bradyzoites by repeated binary fission to form a **sarcocyst or tissue cyst**.

CLINICAL FEATURES

Intestinal sarcocystosis: It is self-limiting and is usually asymptomatic. Patients may present with nausea, abdominal pain and diarrhea. The symptoms appear earlier after the ingestion of beef (about 3–6 hours) than they do when pork is ingested (about 24 hours).

Extra-intestinal (muscular) sarcocystosis: Though it is usually asymptomatic, this type of sarcocystosis may cause muscle pain, weakness or **myositis**, depending on the size of the cyst. A history of travel or residence in a tropical country, especially in South-East Asia may point to the diagnosis.

DIAGNOSIS

Eliciting a history of the consumption of undercooked meat is of value in diagnosing sarcocystosis. The examination of stool samples or a muscle biopsy can help confirm the diagnosis (Fig. 10.1a and b).

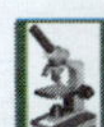

Lab diagnosis

- **Intestinal sarcocystosis:** By visualising oocysts or sporocysts
  - Stool microscopy
  - UV microscopy
- **Muscular sarcocystosis:**
  - Histopathology: Of muscle biopsy

Microscopy

- **Wet and iodine mount:** Direct examination of stool in saline and iodine mount helps in the identification of oocysts or sporocysts (Fig. 10.1a). Unlike the oocysts of *Cystoisospora belli* to which the oocytes of *Sarcocystis* resemble in size, the latter are fully developed when passed in feces.
- **Ultraviolet microscopy:** The oocysts autofluoresce under ultraviolet light (Fig. 10.1c).

Histopathology

A muscle biopsy may reveal tissue cysts containing numerous bradyzoites (Fig. 10.1b).

TREATMENT

- No specific treatment is recommended for *Sarcocystis* infection.
- Cotrimoxazole, furazolidone and albendazole have been used, but their efficacy is not clear.
- Corticosteroids may provide symptomatic relief in myositis.

PREVENTION AND CONTROL

- Water and food hygiene are the most crucial preventive measures.
- Water used for drinking and washing food should be boiled.
- Meat should be stored in the deep freezer and cooked thoroughly before it is consumed.
- Proper disposal of human feces prevents infection in animals.

QUESTIONS

1. Discuss the morphology and life cycle of *Sarcocystis* and the diagnosis and management of sarcocystosis.

MULTIPLE CHOICE QUESTIONS

1. Intestinal sarcocystosis may develop from _____________ :
   a. The consumption of undercooked or raw infected meat
   b. The consumption of food and water contaminated with sporocysts
   c. Blood transfusion
   d. Mother-to-child transmission
2. Extra-intestinal sarcocystosis may develop from _____________ :
   a. The consumption of undercooked or raw infected meat
   b. The consumption of food and water contaminated with sporocysts
   c. Blood transfusion
   d. Mother-to-child transmission
3. Which of the following statements about *Sarcocystis* is FALSE?
   a. It has an obligatory two-host cycle.
   b. It is a parasite that chiefly infects animals.
   c. It only causes infections in immunocompromised patients.
   d. It infects the red blood cells.
4. Intestinal sarcocystosis is diagnosed by the _____________ :
   a. Identification of sarcocysts in stool samples
   b. Identification of sporocysts/oocysts in stool samples
   c. Identification of bradyzoites in stool samples
   d. All of the above
5. *Sarcocystis* infection can be prevented by _____________:
   a. Avoidance of ingestion of raw or undercooked meat
   b. Avoidance of walking barefoot
   c. Safe blood transfusion
   d. Safe sex

CHAPTER 11

Microsporidia

([From Greek] *micros* = small + *spora* = seed)

Case Study and Learning Goals

A 25-year-old male who has AIDS presents with watery diarrhea of 6 months' duration and wasting. What are the parasitic causes of diarrhea in HIV patients? How would you approach the laboratory diagnosis in this case? How would you treat this patient?

INTRODUCTION

Microsporidia are a group of ubiquitous **intracellular parasites** that infect an **extensive range of hosts** including arthropods, fish, amphibians, reptiles, birds and animals. More than 1,400 species belonging to over 200 genera have been described so far, of which around 15 species have been identified as human pathogens (see box). The taxonomic status of microsporidia is in a state of flux, shifting between protozoa and fungi. Conventionally, they are considered protozoa and dealt with by diagnostic parasitology laboratories.

Microsporidia species of human importance

- The majority of human infections are caused by *Enterocytozoon bieneusi*, followed by *Encephalitozoon* species (*E. cuniculi*, *E. hellem* and *E. intestinalis*).
- The less frequently reported genera are *Microsporidium sensu stricto*, *Trachipleistophora*, *Nosema*, *Pleistophora*, *Vittaforma*, *Anncaliia* and a few others.

In 1857, Karl Wilhelm Von Naegeli studied a microsporidia outbreak in silkworms which was also subsequently investigated by Louis Pasteur in 1865. The parasitic group did not receive much attention as a human pathogen and was only sporadically documented until the AIDS epidemic in the 1980s, after which more and more species causing fulminant disease in immunocompromised individuals began to come to light.

EPIDEMIOLOGY

Both vertebrates and invertebrates serve as reservoirs of infection. Species of microsporidia that infect humans have been identified in water sources as well as in wild, domestic and food-producing farm animals, implicating them in **waterborne**, **foodborne** and **zoonotic transmission.**

Microsporidia have emerged as **opportunistic pathogens** globally, especially in the severely immunocompromised, and more specifically, in AIDS patients and transplant recipients. It is also known to cause diseases in immunocompetent individuals, especially travellers and the elderly.

MORPHOLOGY

Microsporidia species are unicellular. Their most observed life stage is that of spores.

Spores

These are ovoid and quite small—**1–4** µm in size. They lack mitochondria, peroxisomes and Golgi bodies. The following are some features of the spores of microsporidia:

- The spore wall has two layers—the outer layer is composed of keratinaceous proteins and the inner layer contains chitin. The plasma membrane lies inside the spore wall.
- Each spore contains a **coiled polar filament or tubule**. On contact with the host cell, germination ensues, whereby the polar filament rapidly uncoils and extrudes from the spore wall. After complete eversion, the filament forms a hollow tube which facilitates the transfer of the infective sporoplasm into the host cell (Fig. 11.1a and b). In some species, the polar tube punches a hole in the host membrane to facilitate penetration, while in others, the host cell membrane expands and engulfs the sporoplasm.

LIFE CYCLE (Fig. 11.2)

Hosts: Arthropods, fish, amphibians, reptiles, birds and mammals

The **infection is acquired by the ingestion of the highly resistant spores**, and possibly by inhalation. The

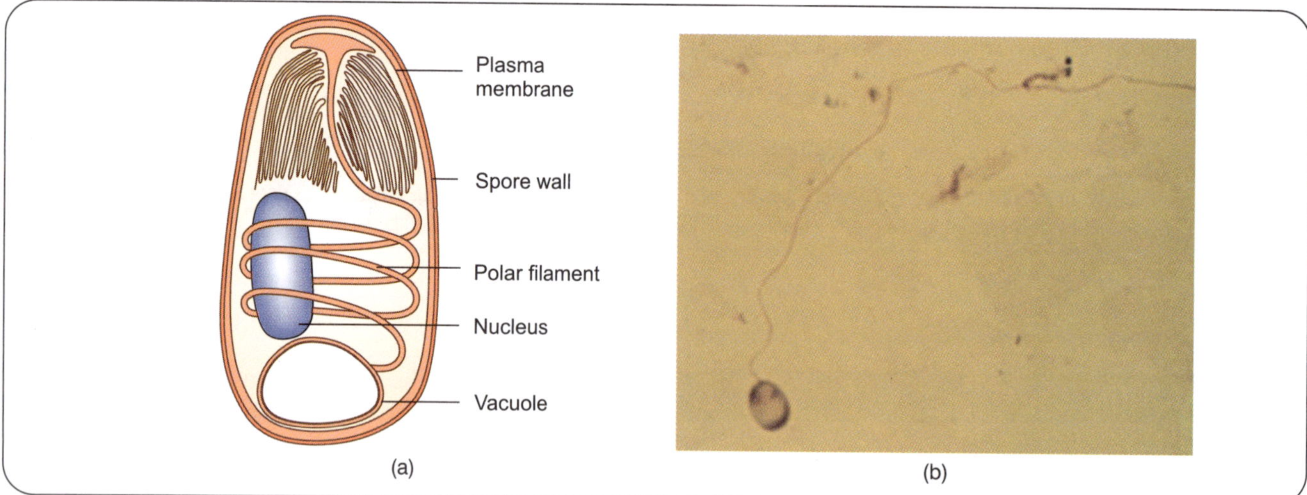

Fig. 11.1 Features of microsporidia: (a) ultrastructural details of a spore and (b) a spore with the polar tube extruding from it (*Source:* Centers for Disease Control and Prevention, DPDx)

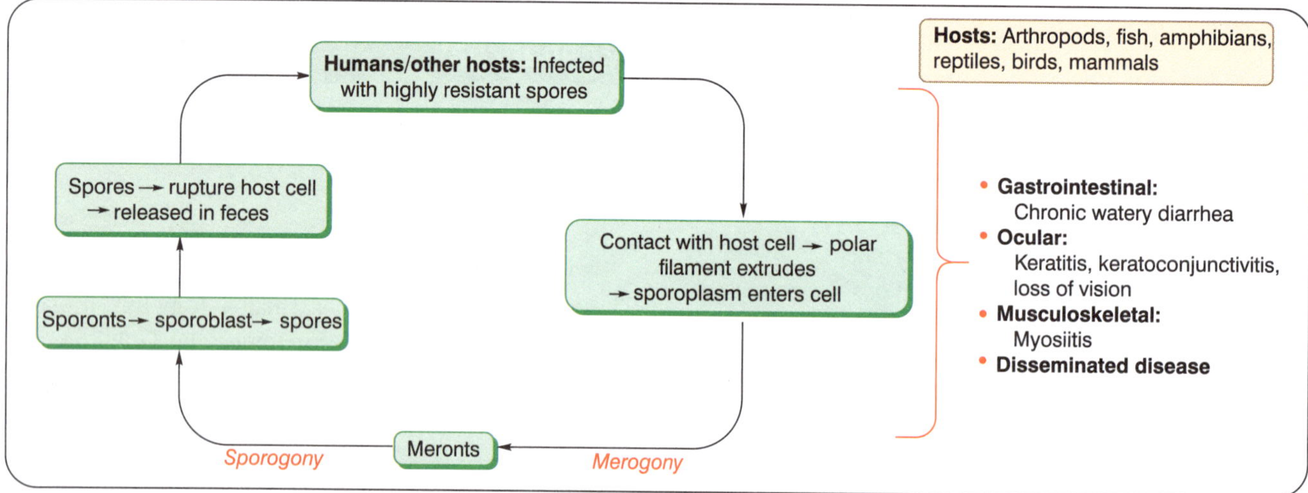

Fig. 11.2 General life cycle of microsporidia (schematic)

spore introduces its contents into the host cell through its polar filament. Depending on the species, the sporoplasm is located either in the host cytoplasm (as in *Enterocytozoon*) or in a parasitophorous vacuole (as in *Encephalitozoon*). It undergoes **merogony** by binary or multiple fission and forms **meronts**. The meronts undergo **sporogony** and produce **sporonts** which give rise to **sporoblasts**. The sporoblasts start producing **spores** which increase in number and finally rupture the host cell before getting released from it. These highly resistant spores are released along with the host's feces into the external environment, from where they may be ingested by another host.

PATHOGENESIS

- **Gastrointestinal:** *E. bieneusi* causes villous blunting, sloughing and crypt hyperplasia, leading to malabsorptive diarrhea due to the decreased surface area and decreased functionality of the villi. *E. intestinalis* causes invasive disease. It is found in a variety of cells, which facilitates its dissemination to other visceral organs. Affected areas show necrosis and mucosal erosion.
- **Ocular:** Microsporidia that infect the eye are not invasive, and remain on the epithelial surface. Punctate keratitis and conjunctivitis are usually seen. The eyes could also be involved in disseminated infection. Usually, the affected individuals are immunocompromised. However, the use of contact lenses or trauma to the cornea and exposure to mud predispose the immunocompetent too.

CLINICAL FEATURES

The clinical manifestations of microsporidiosis are quite diverse, depending on the species and route of infection

(Table 11.1). Currently, microsporidia are considered common agents of self-limiting or asymptomatic infections of the gastrointestinal tract in immunocompetent hosts. In an immunocompromised host, however, the infection has a prolonged and severe course. Disseminated infections can be life-threatening. The following are the features of different clinical manifestations of microsporidial infections:

Gastrointestinal disease: Of all of the manifestations of microsporidiosis, *E. bieneusi*- or *E. intestinalis*-associated diarrhea is the most common. Chronic diarrhea over several months is associated with wasting and cholangiopathy mimicking cycloisosporiasis and cryptosporidiosis in AIDS patients, especially when the CD4 counts fall below 100/mm^3. Diarrheal stools are watery and are not accompanied by blood or fever. Hepatic, pancreatic and renal involvement may occur in immunocompromised patients. It is also reported as a cause of diarrhea in travellers and the elderly.

Ocular disease: Infections of the cornea (keratitis) and conjunctiva (keratoconjunctivitis) are seen in both immunocompetent (usually following corneal trauma or the use of contact lens) and immunocompromised individuals and may lead to blindness.

Musculoskeletal, renal, hepatic or pulmonary disease: Some species preferentially infect the musculoskeletal organs, the lungs or the kidneys.

Disseminated disease: In immunocompromised patients, some species may cause disseminated disease, i.e., involving multiple organs.

DIAGNOSIS

The approach to the diagnosis of microsporidial infections relies on the demonstration of the parasite (Fig. 11.3a–f) or its DNA in the clinical samples. Stool is the specimen of choice for gastrointestinal infections, whereas corneal scrapings (Fig. 11.3a and b) are examined for ocular infections. Body fluids, biopsy or impression smears (prepared by pressing the glass slide directly on the lesions) may also be used.

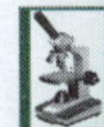

Lab diagnosis

- **Microscopy:** By visualising spores
  - Modified trichrome/fluorescent chitin staining of stool or corneal scrapings
  - Histopathology: Of biopsy sample
  - Electron microscopy
- **Antigen detection**
- **Culture:** On Vero, RK-13 and MRC-5 cell lines
- **DNA detection:** PCR and real-time PCR

Microscopy

- **Modified trichrome stain:** Various modifications of the trichrome stain like chromotrope 2R-based Weber method (Fig. 11.3c) or Ryan's stain (Fig. 11.3d) are useful. Microsporidia spore walls stain bright pinkish-red against a green or blue background. Often, a more darkly stained band or belt-like structure is seen along the diagonal or equatorial aspect of the spore (Fig. 11.3b).
- **Fluorescent chitin stains:** Calcofluor white and Uvitex 2B staining are sensitive and rapid methods for detecting microsporidia spores in stool, intestinal fluid, biopsy imprints and tissue specimens (Fig. 11.3e).
- **Other stains:** Giemsa-stained stool smears show oval spores with light grey-blue cytoplasm and intensely purple band-like nuclear structures (Fig. 11.3a). Modified acid-fast stain may be useful for corneal scrapings since microsporidia are acid-fast.

Electron microscopy

In the past, this was considered the gold standard for the identification of microsporidia. However, it requires rigorous and invasive sampling in addition to technical expertise. Moreover, the results cannot be obtained rapidly, and are difficult to interpret. For

Table 11.1 Microsporidia species affecting different organ systems

Organ system	Species involved
Gastrointestinal tract	*Enterocytozoon bieneusi* (90%), *Encephalitozoon intestinalis*
Lungs	*E. bieneusi, Trachipleistophora anthropopthera*
Central nervous system	*Encephalitozoon cuniculi*
Eyes	*Microsporidium* spp., *Nosema ocularum, Encephalitozoon hellem, Trachipleistophora hominis, Anncaliia algerae, Vittaforma corneae*
Muscles	*Anncaliia vesicularum, A. algerae, Pleistophora ronneafiei, T. hominis*
Disseminated	*Anncaliia connori, E. cuniculi, T. anthropopthera, E. hellem*

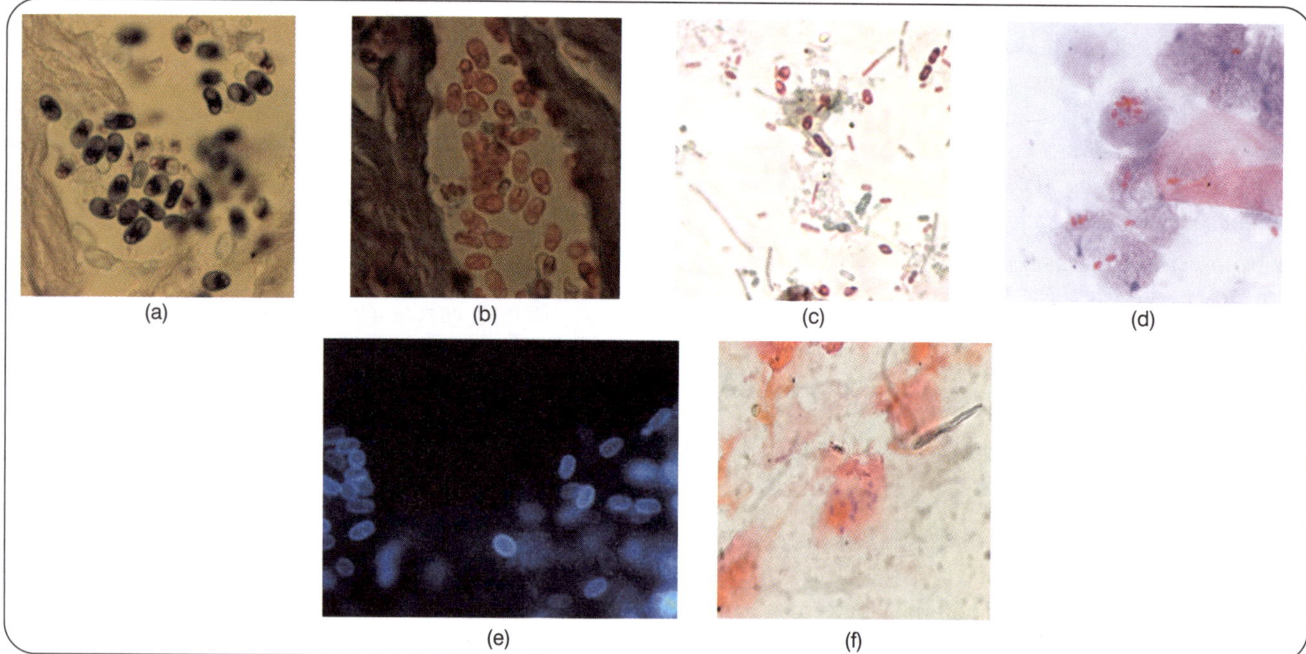

Fig. 11.3 Features of microsporidia: (a) microsporidia spores from a corneal section, stained with Giemsa, (b) microsporidia spores from a corneal section stained with trichrome stain, (c) microsporidia stained with chromotrope 2R, (d) *Encephalitozoon cuniculi* spores from urine stained with Ryan's modified trichrome, (e) *Encephalitozoon intestinalis* stained with calcofluor white and (f) microsporidia stained with Gram stain (*Source:* CDC, DPDx)

these reasons, electron microscopy has been replaced by molecular techniques for species identification and confirmation.

Histopathology

Microsporidia may be detected intracellularly in various tissue sections stained with hematoxylin and eosin.

Antigen Detection

Various immunofluorescence assays are available for the detection of microsporidia using monoclonal or polyclonal antibodies.

Cell Culture

Microsporidia may be cultured in mammalian cell lines like monkey or rabbit kidney (Vero, RK13) or human fetal lung fibroblast cell lines (MRC-5). However, cell cultures are labour intensive.

Nucleic Acid-Based Detection

PCR and its various modifications are currently the gold standard for the diagnosis and speciation of microsporidia, replacing electron microscopy as the preferred diagnostic method. Specific probes have also been used for in situ hybridisation on tissue samples.

TREATMENT

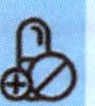

Intestinal microsporidiosis

Drugs of choice

- For *E. bieneusi*: Oral fumagillin, 20 mg TDS
- For other species: Albendazole, 400 mg orally BDS, continued until CD4 count >200 cells/mm^3 or at least 6 months after the initiation of HAART
- Supportive fluid management and antimotility agents

Ocular infections

- Topical fumagillin in saline (final concentration of 70 µg/ml) plus oral albendazole until resolution of ocular lesions
- Topical voriconazole 1% plus topical moxifloxacin with oral albendazole

Highly active antiretroviral therapy (HAART) should be prescribed for all AIDS-associated microsporidia infections; immune restoration with an increase in CD4 count to >100 cells/mm^3 leads to the resolution of the disease.

PREVENTION AND CONTROL

- HAART should be initiated before the patient becomes severely immunosuppressed.
- Food and water hygiene and avoiding undercooked food are crucial in prevention.

Questions

1. Discuss the diagnosis and management of intestinal microsporidiosis.
2. List the causes of infective keratitis.

Multiple Choice Questions

1. The presence of a polar tubule or polar filament is characteristic of:
   a. *Cryptosporidium*
   b. *Plasmodium*
   c. *Leishmania*
   d. Microsporidia
2. The drug of choice for *Enterocytozoon bieneusi*-induced diarrhea is:
   a. Chloroquine
   b. Fumagillin
   c. Amphotericin
   d. Ampicillin
3. Most of the gastrointestinal infections caused by microsporidia are attributed to:
   a. *Vittaforma* spp.
   b. *Enterocytozoon bieneusi*
   c. *Encephalitozoon hellem*
   d. *Encephalitozoon intestinalis*
4. The morphological form demonstrated in most tissues for the diagnosis of microsporidial infections is:
   a. Oocyst
   b. Spore
   c. Ovum
   d. Sporocyst
5. Microsporidial infections are more frequently reported in AIDS patients with CD4 count less than:
   a. 500
   b. 800
   c. 100
   d. 1,000

Chapter 12

Trichomonas

([From Greek] *thrix* = hair + *monas* = single unit)

Case Study and Learning Goals

A 25-year-old female presents with vaginal discharge and vulval pruritus. What are the infectious causes of vaginal discharge? How would you approach the laboratory diagnosis in this case? How would you treat this patient?

INTRODUCTION

Trichomonas vaginalis is a flagellate parasite which commonly resides in the genital and urinary tracts of men and women. It was first discovered in purulent vaginal secretions and secretions from the male urogenital tract in 1836 by Alfred Francois Donne who also named the organism in 1837.

EPIDEMIOLOGY

Trichomonas vaginalis is a cosmopolitan parasite which affects all ethnic groups. It is considered the **most common sexually transmitted infection (STI) in the world after viral STIs**.

- *T. vaginalis* affects approximately 20% of women in the reproductive age group in Africa and the Americas and about 8% of women in South-East Asia, Europe and the Eastern Mediterranean and Western Pacific regions.
- *T. vaginalis* is reported to be the etiology of 10–20% of all cases of non-specific urethritis in males.
- It is also an important cause of complications in pregnancy, is associated with cervical cancer and predisposes to HIV infection.

MORPHOLOGY

T. vaginalis exists **only in the trophozoite** stage; it **cannot form cysts**. Certain structures called **pseudocysts** have been observed, which do not have the true cyst wall, but are spherical, immotile and resistant to adverse environmental conditions such as osmotic lysis, detergent treatment and acidic pH.

Trophozoite

It is **pyriform or pear-shaped**, is **7–25 × 5–15** μm **(the average being 10 × 7** μm**) in size** and has a conspicuous nucleus (Fig. 12.1). Its motility is defined by jerky,

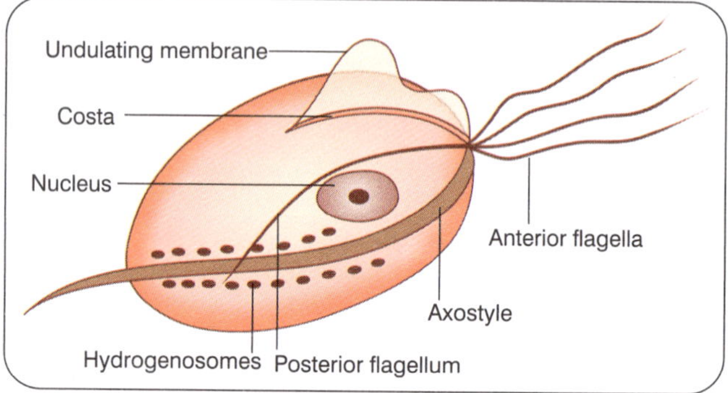

Fig. 12.1 Line diagram of *Trichomonas vaginalis* trophozoite

rapid movements. The following are some characteristic features of *T. vaginalis* trophozoites:

- Four anterior flagella (present in a tuft-like arrangement) and one posterior flagellum originate from the kinetosome.
- Two more structures originate from the kinetosome—an undulating membrane running along the posterior flagellum, spanning about half the length of the cell, and a costa.
- A rigid structure called the axostyle runs from the anterior to the posterior end of the trophozoite. It probably helps the parasite to anchor itself to the vaginal epithelium.
- A conspicuous feature of *T. vaginalis* is the absence of mitochondria. Instead, hydrogenosomes are present, which perform the metabolic functions.

LIFE CYCLE (Fig. 12.2)

Hosts: Human beings

The trophozoite of *T. vaginalis* resides in the **urogenital tract of humans**—in the vagina and urethra in females and the prostate, seminal vesicles and urethra in males. It is primarily **anaerobic**. Usually, the acidic pH (4.0–4.5) of the normal vagina inhibits its growth. However, once it establishes itself, it disrupts the natural lactic acid-producing bacterial flora; as a result, the pH increases

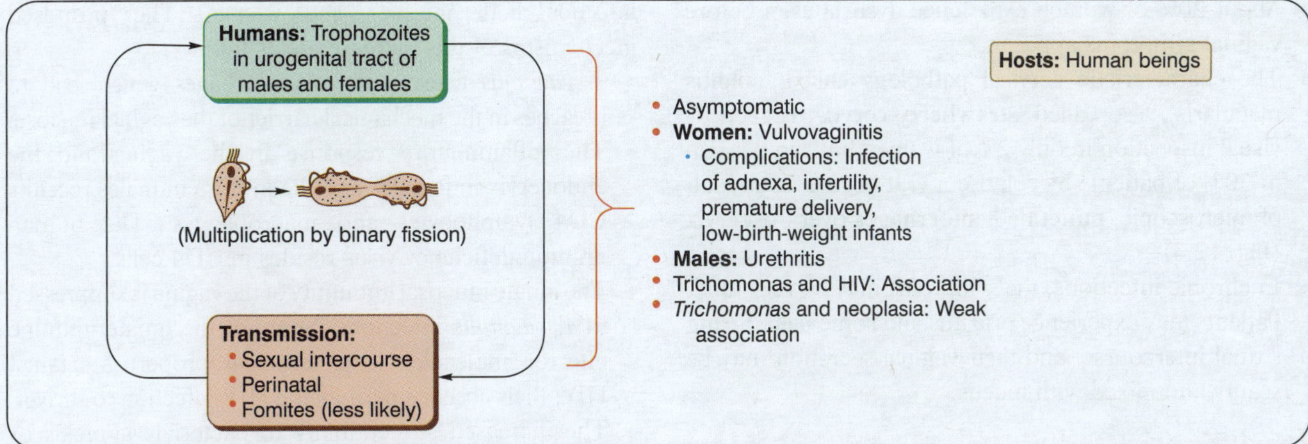

Fig. 12.2 Life cycle of *Trichomonas vaginalis* (schematic)

to 5.0–6.0, which is more favourable for the growth of *T. vaginalis*. It feeds on bacteria, leukocytes and cell exudates.

T. vaginalis divides by **binary fission** to maintain its population; there is **no cystic stage** in its life cycle. Humans usually transmit *T. vaginalis* by **sexual intercourse**, though it has also been found in neonates born to infected mothers. Fomites are also rarely implicated in transmission. It is possible that the pseudocyst stage may play a role in the non-sexual mode of transmission, though this has not yet been proven.

PATHOGENESIS

Most strains of *T. vaginalis* have low pathogenicity, and hence most infected persons remain asymptomatic. A few strains, however, induce itching and inflammation. After a few days of infection, the vaginal epithelium shows degeneration and leukocytic infiltration resulting in micro-ulcers in the genital mucosa with intense inflammation. The mechanism of pathogenesis of the infection is as follows:

- **Binding to host cells:** The parasite binds to the vaginal epithelial cells with the help of adhesins and cysteine proteases.
- **Tissue damage and cytopathic effects:** The pathogenicity of *T. vaginalis* mainly involves tissue damage and cytopathic effects which are chiefly caused by cysteine proteases though the secretion of cell-detaching factors is also implicated. The cumulative effect is the degradation of laminin, vitronectin and other components of the extra-cellular matrix, hemolysis of RBCs and damage of the host cell membranes.
- **Degradation of normal flora:** The normal vaginal flora is disrupted and the vaginal pH markedly increases to >5. *T. vaginalis* infections are commonly associated with vaginal dysbiosis, i.e., imbalance of the normal vaginal microbial flora. Bacterial vaginosis is an example of one such condition characterised by a major shift from the dominant lactobacilli to anaerobic bacterial species in the vagina.
- **Evasion of immune response:** *T. vaginalis* evades the host's immune response by coating its surface with host proteins and by degrading immunoglobulins and complement.

CLINICAL FEATURES

The incubation period of *T. vaginalis* ranges from 4–28 days.

Asymptomatic Infection

Most infected men (75%) and women (25–50%) are asymptomatic, and harbour *T. vaginalis* in their genital tracts. Women may carry the infection for as many as 3–5 years, serving as carriers who are capable of transmitting the infection.

Symptomatic Infection in Women

The vagina, urethra and endocervix are the most likely sites of infection. The following are some features of the infection:

- The chief presenting feature is vulvovaginitis, characterised by **frothy, green and malodourous profuse vaginal discharge** (seen in 50% of cases). Other features may be vulval itching, dysuria or abdominal pain.
- The symptoms may be cyclical, and often appear or worsen during and after menstruation.

- About 20% of women experience dysuria even before vaginal symptoms appear.
- The characteristic cervical pathology called 'colpitis macularis', also called '**strawberry cervix**', is seen by visual inspection in only 2% of women but can be seen in 50% of patients by colposcopy. It occurs as a result of microscopic, **punctate hemorrhages** over the cervix (Fig. 12.3).
- In chronic infections, the symptoms may be very mild. Patients may experience pruritus and some pain during sexual intercourse, and their vaginal secretion may be scanty and mixed with mucus.

Complications

- Infections of the adnexa, the Skene's and Bartholin's glands and the endometrium may occur.
- Vaginitis emphysematosa, in which gas-filled blebs develop in the vaginal walls, is a rare complication.
- Serious consequences, such as infertility, premature rupture of the placental membranes, premature delivery, low-birth-weight infants and neonatal death are also associated with infection.

Symptomatic Infection in Men

Infections in the male may be asymptomatic or may present as self-limited, persistent or recurring urethritis. *T. vaginalis* has been detected in 10–20% of male subjects with non-specific urethritis. Prostatitis and epididymitis have also been reported.

T. vaginalis and HIV

T. vaginalis infection is associated with an increased predisposition to human immunodeficiency virus (HIV) infection both in men and women. The proposed mechanisms of this increase are as follows:

- *T. vaginalis* causes micro-hemorrhages which lead to breaches in the mechanical barrier of the vaginal mucosa.
- The inflammatory response in the vagina and the endocervix in females and the urethra in males recruits CD4 lymphocytes and macrophages. The human immunodeficiency virus resides in CD4 cells.
- The innate mucosal immunity of the vagina is suppressed in *T. vaginalis* infections. Some of the innate immune effector molecules have virucidal properties against HIV; their absence permits the HIV infection to thrive.
- The increased susceptibility to bacterial vaginosis or persistence of abnormal vaginal flora increases the risk of contracting an HIV infection.

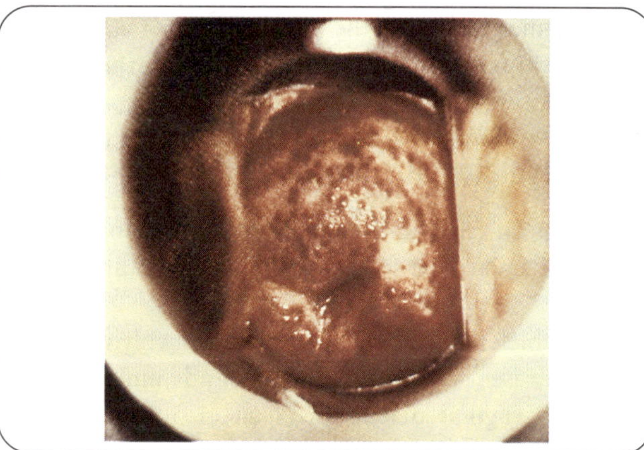

Fig. 12.3 Intravaginal colposcopic view of strawberry cervix, a characteristic pathology of *Trichomonas vaginalis* infection (*Source:* Centers for Disease Control and Prevention [CDC], Public Health Image Library [PHIL], Image ID 5240)

T. vaginalis and Neoplasia

There is a weak association between trichomoniasis and **cervical dysplasia**. Sero-epidemiologic evidence indicating an association between *T. vaginalis* and prostate cancer suggests that the infection may increase the risk of more aggressive cancer.

DIAGNOSIS

The appropriate clinical specimens for the diagnosis of trichomoniasis in women are endocervical swabs, urine and vaginal fluid; in men, urethral discharge, urine, prostate secretions or semen may be used. Vaginal secretions can be obtained from the fornices of the vagina and the lateral vaginal wall using a plastic loop or swab.

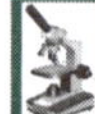

Lab diagnosis

- **Microscopy:** By visualising trophozoites
- **Culture:**
  - Diamond's TYI liquid broth medium, cysteine-peptone-liver-maltose medium and Feinberg–Whittington medium
  - InPouch TV kit
- **Antigen detection:** ELISA and point-of-care immunochromatographic tests
- **Serology:** Not useful
- **DNA detection:** PCR, real-time PCR, Xpert TV and FilmArray

Microscopy

- **Wet mount:** The collected secretions are suspended in normal saline and subjected to light microscopic examination under a high-power field (40×) to look for the characteristic motile trophozoites of *T. vaginalis*. The sensitivity of microscopy ranges from 40–80%. The specimen must be examined within 10–20 minutes of sample collection, after which time the motility may be lost, making it difficult to differentiate the trophozoites from the similar-looking neutrophils (Fig. 12.4a).

- **Stained smears:** Smears may be stained with Papanicolaou or Giemsa stain (Fig. 12.4b). Fluorescent stains like acridine orange may also be used. These organisms may be difficult to recognise in permanent stains as they may not preserve their typical pear-shaped morphology.
- **Direct fluorescent antibody test:** This method is more sensitive than wet mount but is also more expensive.

Culture

It is considered the **gold standard** for the diagnosis of *T. vaginalis* infections.

- It is most important that the specimen be collected correctly, immediately inoculated into the proper medium, and incubated appropriately.

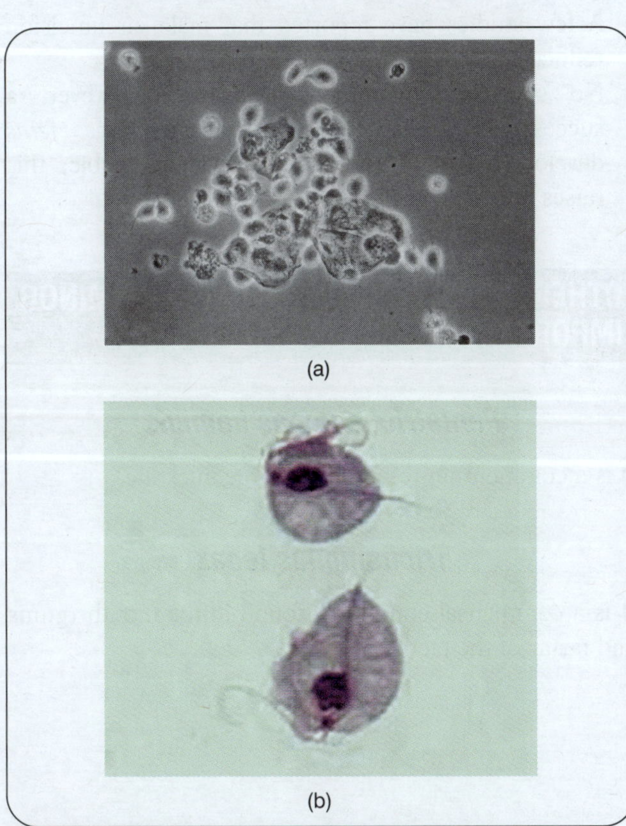

Fig. 12.4 Features of trophozoites of *Trichomonas vaginalis*: (a) a wet mount of vaginal discharge showing numerous trophozoites and (b) two trophozoites in a vaginal smear stained with Giemsa (*Source:* CDC, PHIL, Image ID 14500 and CDC, DPDx)

- The media most suitable for culture are Diamond's TYI liquid broth medium, cysteine-peptone-liver-maltose medium and Feinberg–Whittington's medium.
- Culturing has the advantage of higher sensitivity (75–85%) and specificity (100%) than microscopy.
- Its drawbacks are its higher cost and its long turnaround time (3–7 days).

InPouch TV kit (BIOMED Diagnostics, USA) is a self-contained culture system which serves as a specimen transport container, a growth chamber during incubation and a 'slide' for microscopy. Once it is inoculated, it does not need to be opened for examination; a parasite growth is obtained in five days. This kit is reported to be superior to other available culture methods.

Antigen Detection

Commercial rapid (provides the result in 10 minutes) immunochromatographic (dipstick) antigen detection-based tests like OSOM *Trichomonas* Test (Sekisui Diagnostics, USA) and XenoStrip-*Tv* (Xenotope Diagnostics Inc., USA) have high sensitivity and specificity. They are available as point-of-care tests (they can be performed wherever the patient is, e.g., at the patient's bedside or in the clinic).

Serodiagnosis

This is not of much use and cannot differentiate between past and current infections.

Nucleic Acid-Based Detection

Nucleic acid amplification tests (NAATs) have been validated and are commercially available for use on different samples including urethral, vaginal, endocervical and urine samples. The PCR amplification of *18S rRNA* and *pfoB* gene of *T. vaginalis* has also been shown to have results comparable to culture. DNA probe-based tests are also available for the detection of *T. vaginalis*.

- A real-time PCR based automated system, Xpert TV assay (Cepheid, USA), is available for the detection of *T. vaginalis*. It is a rapid test (with a turnaround time of <1 hour), with a sensitivity of 95% and a specificity of 95–100%.
- Recently, a fully automated multiplex PCR system, FilmArray (BioFire Diagnostics, USA), has been developed for the simultaneous detection of multiple sexually transmitted pathogens. It has the potential to provide rapid and accurate results.

Other Diagnostic Parameters

- The presence of pus cells in the vaginal fluid
- Elevated pH of >5 (this differentiates it from candidal vaginosis where pH is <4.9, but not from bacterial vaginosis)
- Whiff test is carried out by adding potassium hydroxide to the vaginal fluid for the olfactory detection of amines which give off a typical fishy odour; this test is positive in about 75% patients but is also positive in cases of bacterial vaginosis

TREATMENT

Oral therapy
- Drug of choice
  - *Metronidazole:* 2 g as a single dose or 500 mg BDS × 7 days
  - *Tinidazole:* 2 g as a single dose

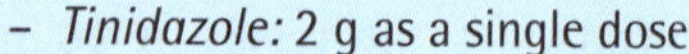

Topical therapy
- *Metronidazole:* 500 mg vaginal tablets OD × 10 days or high-dose metronidazole, 750 mg combined with miconazole vaginal suppository BDS × 7 days

WHO recommends a **syndromic approach** to the management of STIs including trichomoniasis, especially in resource-poor settings. The ideal approach, however, is screening for trichomoniasis wherever facilities are available followed by the treatment of the positive cases. **Sexual partners should be treated simultaneously.**

Resistance

Clinical resistance of *T. vaginalis* to metronidazole is reported in 4–10% cases; resistance to tinidazole is seen in 1%. Resistance is relative and can be overcome with higher doses of oral metronidazole.

Topical Therapy

The major limitation of vaginal administration of drugs for the treatment of trichomoniasis is the inability of the drug to reach infected organs other than the vagina (the cervix and Bartholin's, Skene's and periurethral glands). However, topical therapy may be useful during pregnancy, during which time the oral drugs may produce severe side effects, or when the patient is allergic to metronidazole.

Follow-up

Recurrent or persistent infections are very common—the patient may be reinfected by an untreated sexual partner or occasionally, may be infected with an antimicrobial-resistant strain of *T. vaginalis*. For this reason, it is recommended that patients who receive treatment be re-tested three months after the initial treatment.

PREVENTION AND CONTROL

- The most important preventive measure is the use of condoms or barrier methods.
- Sexual partners should be treated simultaneously since males are frequently asymptomatic.
- A few studies have reported that male circumcision reduces the chances of infection.
- No successful vaccine is available. However, a successful vaccine against *Tritrichomonas fetus* developed for cattle is commercially available; this raises hopes for a possible human vaccine.

OTHER INTESTINAL FLAGELLATES OF MINOR IMPORTANCE

Pentatrichomonas hominis

It is a commensal present in the large intestine.

Trichomonas tenax

It is a commensal commonly found in the mouth (gums and tartar of the teeth).

Questions

1. Discuss the diagnosis and management of trichomoniasis.
2. List the differential diagnosis of the infective causes of vaginitis.

Multiple Choice Questions

1. What percentage of males infected with *Trichomonas vaginalis* are symptomatic?
   a. 100%
   b. 20–25%
   c. 75%
   d. 2%
2. Strawberry cervix is a pathognomonic sign of __________infection.
   a. *Candida tropicalis*
   b. *Trichomonas vaginalis*
   c. *Neisseria gonorrhoeae*
   d. *Treponema pallidum*
3. The most common non-viral sexually transmitted infection in women is ______________.
   a. Trichomoniasis
   b. Chlamydiasis
   c. Gonorrhea
   d. Candidiasis
4. *Trichomonas vaginitis* is associated with a change in vaginal pH to ___________.
   a. More than 5
   b. Less than 3
   c. Less than 5
   d. More than 3
5. The treatment of choice for trichomoniasis is ______________ ___________.
   a. Amphotericin B
   b. Fluconazole
   c. Oral metronidazole or tinidazole
   d. Cotrimoxazole

CHAPTER 13

Plasmodium

(*Plasmodium* [Greek] from *plasma* = formed structure; *falciparum* [Latin] from *falx* = sickle + *parus* = like another; *vivax* [Latin] from *vivo* = live + *ax* = inclined to; *malariae* [Italian] from *mala aria* = bad air)

Case Study and Learning Goals

A 40-year-old male presents to the emergency with high-grade fever associated with chills and rigors for the last five days. His fever rises in the evening and subsides after profuse sweating and is followed by extreme fatigue and sleepiness. What are the parasitic causes of fever? How would you approach the laboratory diagnosis in this case? How would you treat this patient?

INTRODUCTION

Of all the microbial scourges to affect human beings, malaria is one of the worst, with the greatest morbidity and mortality. Human malaria is caused by **five species** of the apicomplexan parasite ***Plasmodium* – *P. vivax*, *P. falciparum*, *P. malariae*, *P. ovale*,** and the fifth and emerging species, ***P. knowlesi*.** The bite of the **female *Anopheles* mosquito** is the mode of transmission of these parasites to human beings. Most malarial deaths are attributed to *P. falciparum*.

Given that malaria poses a significant healthcare burden globally, it has been targeted for elimination and eradication. The intense and combined efforts of more than a hundred countries have been devoted to trying to meet this ambitious goal with measures such as improved diagnosis, combination drug therapy and mosquito control using tools like insecticide-treated nets, sprays, repellents, etc. As a result, there has been a significant decline in the number of cases and deaths. However, malaria control still presents a considerable challenge due to the widespread endemicity of the disease and its vector, the parasite's resistance to drugs, the lack of newer drugs and the absence of an effective vaccine.

EPIDEMIOLOGY

Malaria has shaped human history and culture since antiquity. It has changed the outcomes of wars and aided

A Brief History of Malaria

The earliest reference to the typical fever associated with malaria was made in 2700 BC in China. Mentions of the classical features of malaria have also been found in Greek, Roman, Indian, Assyrian, Arabic and other ancient medical literature. It was only after the 'germ theory' of the causation of infections was proposed that the knowledge of the enigmatic malaria fevers progressed from speculations of their **association with marshy swamps, heat, and 'bad breath'**, to the detailed study of the causative agent and its vectorial transmission. Our current knowledge of malaria is credited to umpteen scientists who devoted their life's work to the study of this disease. **Alphonse Laveran** was the first to observe the malaria parasite in blood (in 1880) and describe the ex-flagellating male gametocytes, female gametocytes, trophozoite and the schizont stage. In 1891, **D. L. Romanowsky** developed a staining method with methylene blue and eosin which allowed other scientists to describe the parasite morphology better. Based on his experience with filarial worms, **Patrick Manson** indicated for the first time (in 1894) that mosquitoes could possibly be the vectors of the malarial parasite. Taking up the mantle from Manson, **Ronald Ross** worked on this puzzle for several years; finally, in 1897, after observing the growth of oocysts on the gut wall of a mosquito that had fed on a malaria patient, he established the role of mosquitoes as vectors of the malarial parasite. For his work, Ross was awarded the **Nobel Prize in 1902**. Around the same time, **G. B. Grassi, A. Bignami** and **G. Bastianelli** described the developmental stages of the malarial parasite in mosquitoes. In due course, the various stages of the parasite's complex life cycle were elucidated through the painstaking efforts of numerous scientists. In 1947, Henry Shortt and Cyril Garnham demonstrated that the parasite develops in the liver before appearing in the blood. It was another four decades before Wojciech Krotoski (in 1982) demonstrated the dormant stages of *P. vivax* in the liver. The drug currently used for malaria treatment across the world—**artemisinin**—was discovered by **Youyou Tu in 1971**. Her discovery was based on a 1,700-year-old recipe prescribed by Ge Hong for a juice extracted from the leaves of the **qinghao** (*Artemisia annua*) plant which could treat fever. For her discovery, Youyou was awarded the **Nobel Prize in 2015**.

the rise and fall of empires. It has been a major deterrent for crusaders aspiring to colonise malaria-endemic regions. **Even in modern times, malaria is one of the world's leading killers**, claiming the life of one child every two minutes. Children under five years of age are at the greatest risk of the life-threatening complications of malaria. More than 220 million cases of malaria are reported every year worldwide, with more than four lakh deaths, most of which are children. Malaria is most prevalent in the tropical regions of the world, viz. **Africa** and the **South-East Asia Region (SEAR)**. The disease is also widespread in the Eastern Mediterranean, Western Pacific and Central and South American regions (Fig. 13.1).

- The World Health Organization (WHO) estimates that 92% of malaria cases and 93% of deaths due to malaria are reported from Africa, followed by the South-East Asia Region (SEAR)—from where about 5% of the cases are reported—and the Eastern Mediterranean Region with 2% of the world's cases.
- Six countries account for >50% of all malaria cases globally—Nigeria, the Democratic Republic of the Congo, Uganda, Cote d'Ivoire, Mozambique and Niger.
- India accounts for close to 4% of the global burden of malaria; the majority of the malaria cases reported from the SEAR.

The mortality rates of malaria have decreased dramatically over the past two decades due to highly effective control programmes implemented in several countries. However, it continues to pose a heavy burden on tropical countries and is a threat to non-endemic countries and a danger to travellers to the endemic areas.

Distribution of Species

- ***P. falciparum* is the most common *Plasmodium* species worldwide**; it is found predominately in Africa, the north-eastern and eastern parts of the Indian subcontinent, East Asia and Oceania.
- ***P. vivax* is the most common *Plasmodium* species in the Indian subcontinent** as well as East Asia, Oceania and Central and South America.
- ***P. ovale*** causes a small percentage of infections, mostly in Africa. It has two morphologically identical sympatric species – *P. ovale curtisi* and *P. ovale wallikeri*.
- ***P. malariae*** is a less common species of *Plasmodium* predominantly reported from sub-Saharan Africa.
- ***P. knowlesi*** is the simian malaria parasite; it is chiefly found in Malaysia, and to a lesser extent in other parts of South-East Asia.

Precipitating Factors

The following factors are associated with an increase in the cases of malaria:

- Heavy rains following a period of drought.
- The migration of refugees or workers from a non-endemic region to an area of high transmission.
- Breakdown in malaria control and prevention services because of calamities like military conflicts or civil disorder.

Epidemiology in India

Malaria is a significant public health problem in India. The majority of cases are reported from the **eastern and**

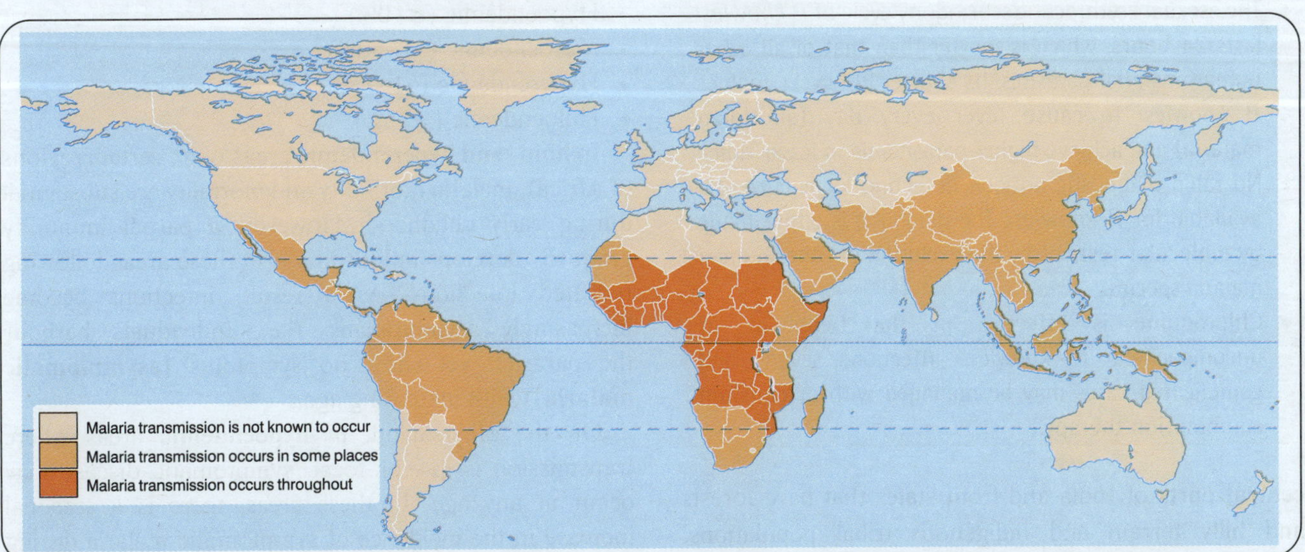

Fig. 13.1 Geographical distribution of malaria (*Source:* Adapted from Centers for Disease Control and Prevention [CDC])

Plasmodium knowlesi

- *P. knowlesi* causes malaria in long-tailed or pig-tailed **monkeys** (genus *Macaca*).
- It is an emerging agent of human malaria and the **fifth *Plasmodium* species known to cause the disease in humans.** It is an example of host-switching from monkeys to humans as an ongoing process of evolution.
- The first human case was reported in 1965 in an American who had travelled to Malaysia. The parasite was, however, considered a concern to human health only after a large number of cases from Malaysia (between 2000 to 2002), which were first identified as *P. malariae* with atypical presentations, were confirmed as *P. knowlesi* with the help of molecular tests.
- It is **mainly reported from Malaysia,** and to a lesser extent from other parts of South-East Asia including Thailand, Cambodia and Vietnam. It has also been reported in individuals who travel to these countries.
- Humans get infected when they enter the forest or forest fringe areas where monkey hosts and *Anopheles* vectors co-exist. Currently, there is no definitive proof of human ⟶ mosquito ⟶ human transmission of *P. knowlesi.*
- In India, *P. knowlesi*-specific gene sequences have been detected in stored blood samples taken from human malaria patients from the Andaman and Nicobar Islands.
- The diagnosis of *P. knowlesi* infection is challenging as it has many morphological features which make it difficult to differentiate it microscopically from *P. falciparum* and *P. malariae.* Like *P. falciparum,* the **early stages of *P. knowlesi* appear ring- and *applique*-like** with one or two chromatin dots. On the other hand, the **late stages of this parasite have a band-like appearance** similar to *P. malariae.*
- The asexual erythrocytic schizogony cycle of *P. knowlesi* lasts **24 hours,** which is shorter than that of all other human malarial parasites. Its shorter life cycle enables *P. knowlesi* to **cause fever every day (quotidian malaria)** and achieve higher parasitemia in lesser time.
- No rapid diagnostic antigen detection kit is currently available for *P. knowlesi.* The diagnosis is either made by **molecular tests** or by the exclusion of other human malaria species.
- **Chloroquine** is effective in the treatment of uncomplicated *P. knowlesi* infection; severe and complicated cases may be managed with **artemisinin combination therapy.**

central parts of India and from states that have forests and hilly terrain and indigenous tribal populations, viz. **Odisha** (most affected), Chhattisgarh, Jharkhand, Madhya Pradesh, Maharashtra, and some north-eastern states like Tripura, Meghalaya and Mizoram. **Currently, the majority of malaria cases in India are caused by *P. vivax*.** In fact, India contributes to about half of the total global burden of *P. vivax*-related infections. *P. falciparum* runs a close second and predominates the eastern and north-eastern states. The two major vector species known to transmit malaria in India are *Anopheles culicifacies* and *A. stephensi*. The less common vector species found in India are *A. fluviatilis*, *A. minimus* and *A. dirus*. Though cases of malaria are reported all the year round, it peaks during and after the rainy season corresponding to increased mosquito breeding and transmission. As a result of continued efforts over several decades, the incidence of the disease and related deaths has considerably reduced in the recent years. India is now poised for malaria elimination by 2030.

Classifying the Magnitude of the Endemicity of Malaria

The distribution of malaria is complex and varies considerably in different geographical areas. Various criteria have been used to classify the endemicity of malaria.

I. Endemicity based on rates of parasitemia or palpable spleen rates

Conventionally, endemicity is defined in terms of the **rates of parasitemia** (percentage of children in whom blood films are positive for the malaria parasite) **or palpable spleens** (percentage of children with enlarged spleens) **in children between 2 and 10 years of age**. On this basis, endemicity of regions is classified as:

- Hypoendemic (<10%)
- Mesoendemic (11–50%)
- Hyperendemic (51–75%)
- Holoendemic (>75%)

In **holo- and hyperendemic areas** (e.g., certain regions of Africa), malaria morbidity and mortality are substantial during early childhood. However, a partial immunity gradually develops in individuals in these areas following repeated infections. As a result, infections become increasingly asymptomatic (i.e., individuals harbour the parasite, yet show no symptoms **[asymptomatic malaria]**) with increasing age.

On the other hand, in **hypoendemic** areas where transmission is low or focal, symptomatic disease may occur at any age. In these areas, there is a seasonal increase in the incidence of symptomatic malaria during the rainy season coinciding with increased mosquito breeding. In such areas, increased transmission could result in epidemics with high mortality.

II. Endemicity based on transmission pattern

Another way to understand malaria endemicity is to classify regions as having **stable or unstable malaria depending on the transmission pattern**.

- **Stable malaria** is seen in regions of intense transmission throughout the year as seen in the western and eastern parts of Africa and the north-eastern parts of India. In these areas, severe disease is usually seen in children, while adults acquire some immunity against severe disease.
- **Unstable malaria** is seen in regions like the north-western parts of India and the Americas where malaria transmission is seasonal, and all age groups are affected.

III. Endemicity based on phasing requirement of elimination programmes

The **annual parasite incidence (API)** (API = [confirmed cases during one year/population under surveillance] × 1000) is used as the primary criterion for classifying geographical regions for the purpose of phasing malaria elimination programmes (Table 13.1).

MORPHOLOGY AND LIFE CYCLE

> **Definitive host:** Female *Anopheles* mosquito
> **Intermediate hosts:** Humans and monkeys (*P. knowlesi*)

Plasmodium species have the morphological features of **apicomplexans**, i.e., a cell body containing an **apical complex consisting of conoid, polar rings, rhoptries, dense granules and micronemes which assist in the invasion of the host cells.** The parasite goes through numerous life cycle stages in its human and mosquito hosts—trophozoite, schizont, merozoite and gametocyte in humans, and ookinete, oocyst and sporozoite in mosquitoes. These life forms have typical morphological features that can be visualised on staining with a suitable Romanowsky stain according to the species of the parasite. These features help in their microscopic identification (Table 13.2; Fig. 13.2a–t and 13.3a and b).

Infection

The majority of human infections are transmitted by the **female *Anopheles* mosquito (definitive host),** which injects the sporozoite into the human host along with its saliva while drawing its blood meal. Rarely, the infection may be transmitted via blood transfusion or transplacentally from mother to fetus.

The sporozoites enter the bloodstream and migrate to the liver within minutes. After reaching the liver, they actively invade the hepatocytes and differentiate to initiate the liver stage schizogony.

Pre-erythrocytic Schizogony

The **asexual** multiplication of the parasites starts in the **hepatocytes.** A single cycle of schizogony releases several thousands of **cryptozoites or merozoites** in 6–12 days, depending on the species. These merozoites **enter the bloodstream** to infect the RBCs.

Latent/dormant stage: A fraction of the merozoites develop into forms known as **hypnozoites** (as they are hidden). These have the capacity to infect more hepatocytes and continue liver schizogony and thereby, to persist in a dormant state and cause a relapse of the disease at a later date. ***P. vivax* and *P. ovale*** are known to exist in the hypnozoite form, which is responsible for **relapses.** *P. falciparum,* on the other hand, does not exist in the hypnozoite form.

Erythrocytic Schizogony

After merozoites enter the bloodstream, they initiate the blood cycle by actively penetrating the RBCs. Once internalised, they exist in a parasitophorous vacuole in the RBC cytoplasm, where they differentiate into ring forms.

Table 13.1 Classification of Indian states and UTs based on API for malaria elimination programmes

Category	Criteria
Category 0: Prevention of re-establishment phase	States/UTs with 0 indigenous cases of malaria
Category 1: Elimination phase	States/UTs (including their districts) reporting API <1 case per 1,000 individuals at risk
Category 2: Pre-elimination phase	States/UTs with API <1 case per 1,000 individuals at risk where some districts have API ≥1 case per 1,000 individuals at risk
Category 3: Intensified control phase	States/UTs with API ≥1 case per 1,000 individuals at risk

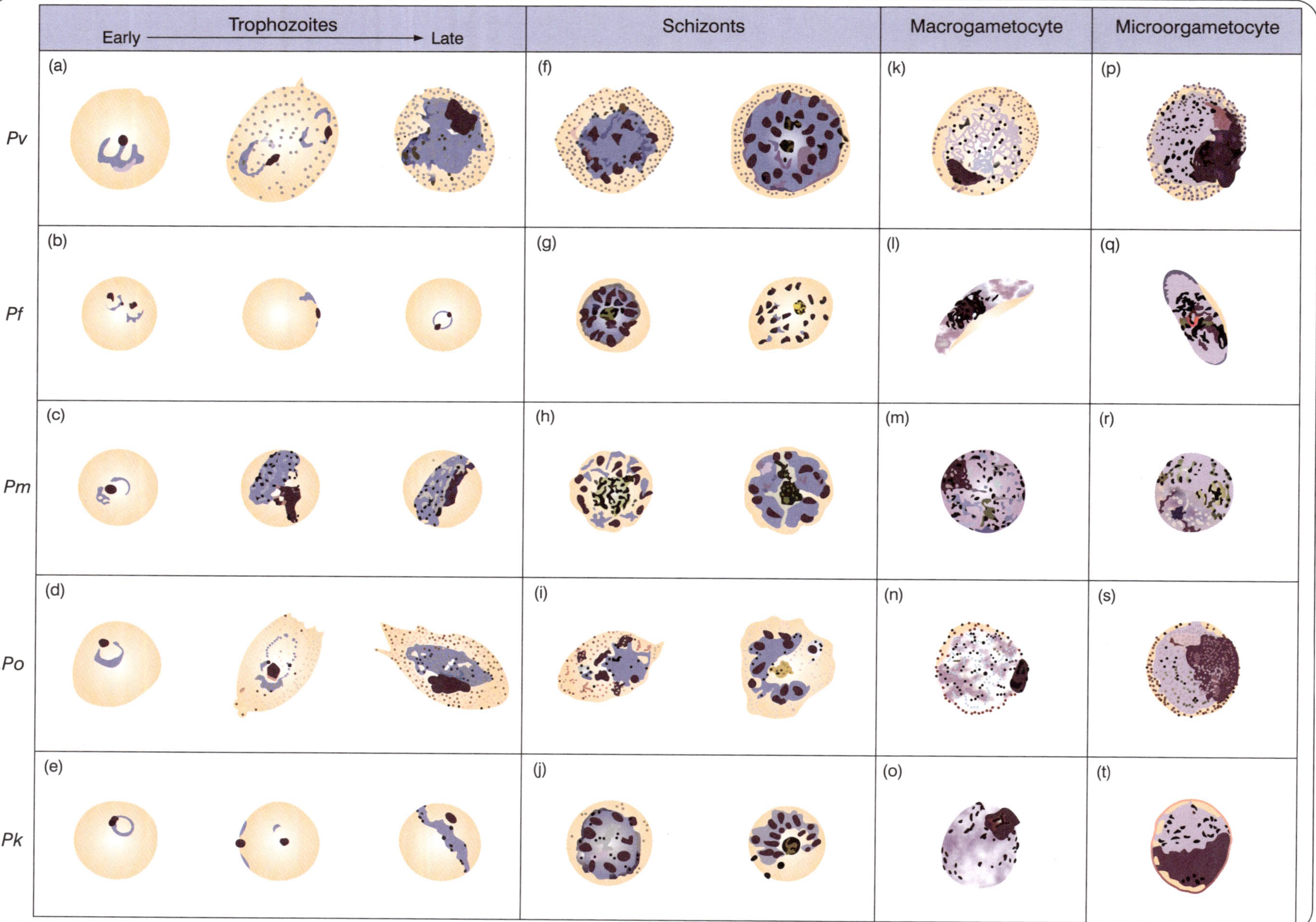

Fig. 13.2 Morphological representations of the different blood stages of *Plasmodium vivax (Pv), P. falciparum (Pf), P. malariae (Pm), P. ovale (Po) and P. knowlesi (Pk)* (rows 1–5 respectively) as appear on staining with Romanowsky stains: (a–e) trophozoites, (f–j) schizonts, (k–o) macrogametocytes and (p–t) microgametocytes

Table 13.2 Morphological features of the different stages of the human malarial parasites on staining with Romanowsky stains and features of their life cycles

Morphological features	*P. vivax*	*P. falciparum*	*P. malariae*	*P. ovale*
RBC shape	Enlarged	Normal	Normal	Enlarged, oval, fimbriated with irregular edges
Stippling in RBC	Schüffner's dots, eosinophilic	Maurer's dots and clefts, basophilic	Ziemann's dots, fine	Schüffner's dots, eosinophilic
Multiple infections in RBC	Common	Very common, *accolle* or *applique* forms	Rare	Rare
Type of RBC infected	Reticulocytes, young RBCs	All ages	Old RBCs	Young RBCs
Young trophozoite	2.5 μm, small and large rings, one red dot of chromatin	1.25–1.5 μm, small delicate rings, one or two red dots of chromatin	2.5 μm, small rings, one large red dot of chromatin	2.5 μm, small and large rings, one large red dot of chromatin
Mature trophozoite	Amoeboid, irregular, vacuolated	Ring forms, 1/4th of RBC	Oval, band forms	Oval, elongated
Schizont	9–10 μm, 12–24 merozoites	4.5–5 μm, 18–24 merozoites (rare in peripheral blood)	6.5–7 μm, 6–12 merozoites	6.2 μm, 6–12 merozoites
Macrogametocyte	11–15 μm, spherical or oval, compact eccentric chromatin	10–15 μm, crescentic (banana-shaped), pointed ends, compact eccentric chromatin	10–12 μm, spherical, compact eccentric chromatin	10–12 μm, spherical or oval, compact eccentric chromatin
Microgametocyte	9–11 μm, spherical or oval, diffuse chromatin	7–10 μm, crescentic (banana-shaped), round ends, diffuse central chromatin	8–10 μm, spherical, diffuse granular chromatin	8–10 μm, spherical or oval, diffuse chromatin
Life cycle features				
Incubation period (in days)	14 (12–17)	11 (9–14)	28 (18–35)	14 (13–15)
Pre-erythrocytic schizogony, number of merozoites produced by each schizont	8 days, 12,000	6 days, 40,000	7–12 days, 2,000	9 days, 15,000
Hypnozoites	Yes	No	No	Possible
Erythrocytic schizogony (in hours)	48	48	72	48
Parasitemia (per mm³ of blood)	20,000	1,00,000–5,00,000	6,000	9,000

Note: *P. knowlesi* has several morphological features that make it difficult to differentiate it microscopically from *P. falciparum* and *P. malariae*. Like *P. falciparum*, the early stages of *P. knowlesi* appear ring- and *applique*-like with one or two chromatin dots. On the other hand, the late stages of this parasite have a band-like appearance similar to *P. malariae*. Its asexual erythrocytic schizogony cycle takes 24 hours, which is shorter than that of all other human malarial parasites. This enables *P. knowlesi* to achieve higher parasitemia in lesser time.

Trophozoite

The early signet ring-shaped forms (0–5 hours) differentiate into **young trophozoites** and subsequently, **late trophozoites** (10–40 hours), which become elongated, amoeboid, irregular or band-shaped. The following are features of this stage:

- The cytoplasm of the trophozoite stains blue with a bright red nuclear chromatin mass.
- A few hours after ingesting the cytoplasm (containing hemoglobin), the digested product of hemoglobin, i.e., the malarial pigment hemozoin, appears in the trophozoite as yellow, brown or black dots.
- The shape and size of the RBCs may change during the trophozoite's growth.
- During this stage, the cytoplasm of RBCs develops various types of granules which give it a reddish-yellow to red dotted or stippled appearance, e.g., Schüffner's dots in *P. vivax*.

Schizont

The fully grown trophozoite may become larger than the RBC and start dividing **asexually** by schizogony or merogony into several daughter cells called merozoites.

The following are features of this stage:

- The size and structure of the schizont and the number of merozoites it contains vary with species.
- Schizonts can be found at various stages of division.
- On the cyclical completion of schizogony—which takes 24/48/72 hours, depending on the species—the RBC ruptures to release its contents, i.e., merozoites, hemozoin pigment and cellular debris into the host blood. This is the cause of malaria fever.

Merozoite

These are oval or round and appear as red chromatin dots embedded in the cytoplasm of the schizont. The merozoites released by the rupture of RBCs infect fresh RBCs and continue the schizogonic cycle or are phagocytosed by the host immune cells.

Gametogony

A small proportion of the merozoites prepare for the **sexual cycle** and differentiate into gametocytes, which further mature in the capillaries of the internal organs, spleen and bone marrow.

Gametocyte

Gametocytes have a compact cytoplasm and do not divide. They exist as macrogametocytes (female) and microgametocytes (male), and mature in about 96 hours.

- **Macrogametocytes:** These are larger than microgametocytes and have a compact, small nucleus and cytoplasm that stains deep blue. Their chromatin is compact and eccentric. They exist in larger numbers than microgametocytes.
- **Microgametocytes:** These are smaller than macrogametocytes. Their relatively large and diffuse nucleus stains red, and their cytoplasm stains pale blue. Their chromatin is diffuse.

The time of appearance of gametocytes after the detection of asexual stages in the peripheral blood varies with the species, ranging from 4–6 days in *P. vivax* and *P. ovale* to 10–14 days in *P. falciparum* and *P. malariae*.

Transmission to Mosquitoes

The **mature gametocytes found in the peripheral blood** are ready to be taken up by mosquitoes. The minimum number of gametocytes required to be present in the peripheral blood to efficiently infect mosquitoes is approximately 12. The further development of these gametocytes depends on several factors such as the species of the mosquito, temperature, humidity, etc.

Fertilisation

In the midgut of the female *Anopheles* mosquito, each microgametocyte develops into 4–8 whip-like filamentous microgametes which break out of it by a process known as **exflagellation**. On the other hand, each macrogametocyte develops into one macrogamete. The two gametes fuse to form a diploid zygote in 20 minutes to 2 hours.

Ookinete

In 12–24 hours, the **zygote** elongates and transforms into an ookinete form measuring 20 × 4 µm in size. The ookinete burrows into the midgut wall and develops into an oocyst in about 40 hours.

Oocyst

The oocyst is a round structure, 6–12 µm in size, usually found between the intestinal epithelium and the basal lamina of the gut. Hundreds of oocysts may be present in the stomach wall of a mosquito.

Sporogony

The oocysts divide **asexually** to become multinucleated, grow to 40–60 µm in size and generate haploid sporozoites. Oocysts mature in about 10 days and rupture in the hemocele of the mosquito to liberate up to 1,000 sporozoites each.

Sporozoite

It is slender, spindle-shaped, about 11–12 × 1–2 µm in size and motile (Fig. 13.3a).

- After the rupture of the oocysts, the sporozoites are distributed to various tissues of the mosquitoes with a predilection towards the salivary gland cells and finally reach the salivary ducts.
- The **sporozoite is the infective stage for humans**; it awaits the mosquito's next blood meal to continue its life cycle.

PATHOGENESIS

The disease manifestations of malaria are attributed to a cumulative effect of the parasite and host factors. The various mechanisms in the pathogenesis of malaria are as follows:

- **Intracellular niche:** The malaria parasite lives inside the immunologically privileged RBCs which lack most cellular organelles.

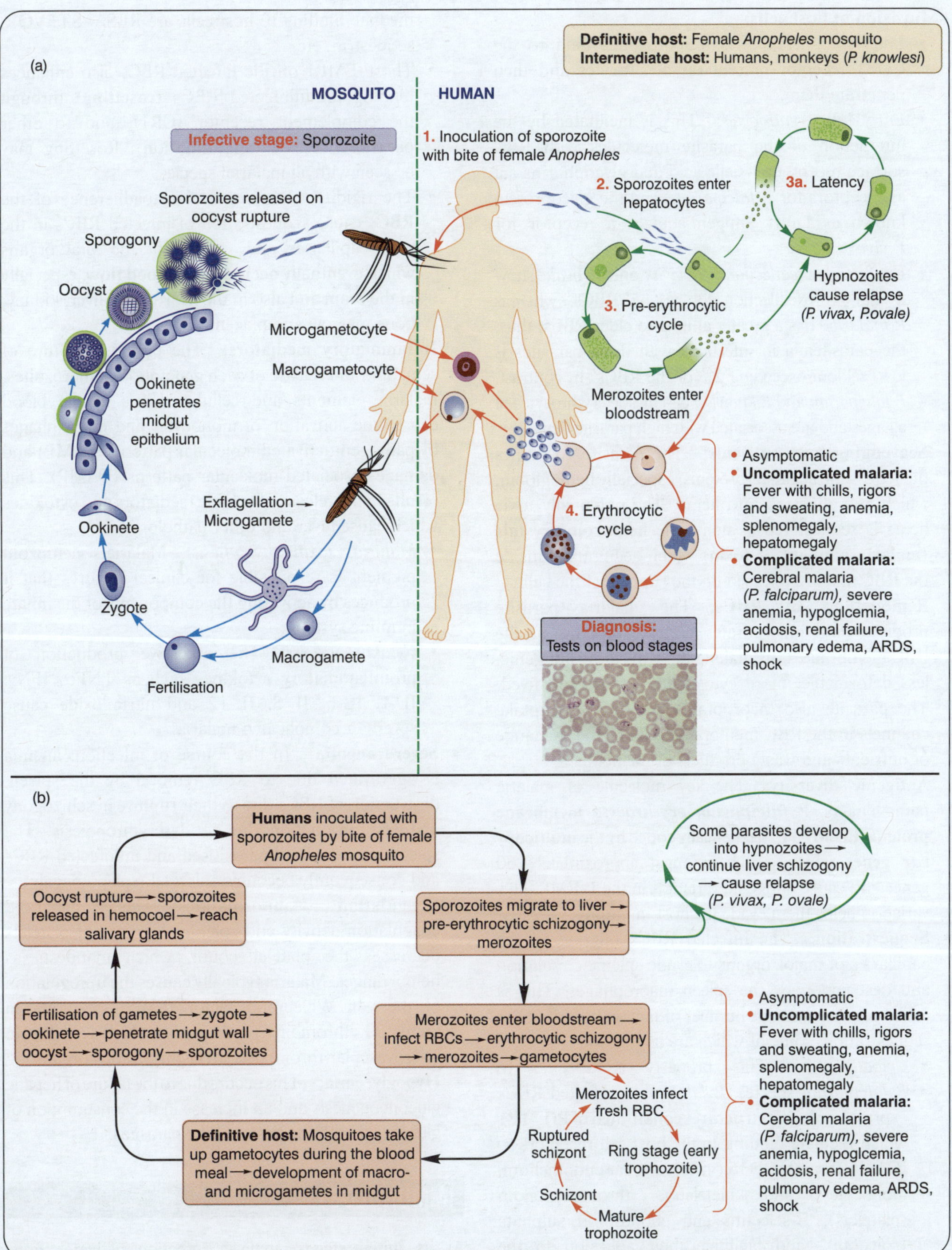

Fig. 13.3 Life cycle of *Plasmodium* spp.: (a) detailed and (b) schematic (*Source [inset]:* CDC, Public Health Image Library [PHIL]; Image ID 2305)

- **Invasion of host cells:**
  - *Entry into hepatocytes:* Sporozoites bind to the CD81 receptor present on hepatocytes and then penetrate them.
  - *Entry into erythrocytes:* This is facilitated by the interaction of the parasite molecules with RBC surface receptors—sialic acid and glycophorins act as receptors for *P. falciparum*, and the glycoprotein known as Duffy antigen acts as a receptor for *P. vivax*.
  - *Erythrocyte predilection:* *P. vivax* and *P. ovale* show a marked predilection for young RBCs, whereas *P. malariae* has a greater affinity to older RBCs; thus, the parasitemia in infections with these parasites is low, seldom exceeding 2% of the RBCs. In contrast, *P. falciparum* and *P. knowlesi* can invade erythrocytes of all ages and are associated with high parasite densities.
- **Scavenging host nutrients:** The parasite consumes the RBC's intracellular proteins, especially hemoglobin, which gets digested into heme. The potentially toxic heme is sequestered as non-toxic **hemozoin crystals** (**malaria pigment or toxin**) which accumulate inside the RBC and are released on the rupture of the cell.
- **Remodelling of RBCs:** The malaria parasite produces and incorporates parasite proteins in the RBC membrane, thus making the RBC more antigenic, less deformable, more cytoadherent and short-lived. The parasite also incorporates new nutrient uptake channels in the RBC membrane to allow the exchange of nutrients and waste products of metabolism.
- **Antigenic diversity:** The key molecule of malaria pathogenicity, ***P. falciparum erythrocyte* membrane protein (PfEMP1)**, is genetically coded by the **multicopy *var* genes** which switch amongst approximately 60 genes and cause antigenic variation in the PfEMP. This variation helps them evade the host immunity.
- **Sequestration:** The infected RBCs migrate to the capillaries of major organs to evade splenic circulation and destruction by the spleen macrophages. This is called sequestration. A number of factors contribute to sequestration, some of which are as follows:
  - *Cytoadherence:* This property is specific to *P. falciparum* species. *P. falciparum*-infected RBCs express **knob-like structures constituted of PfEMP1** which mediate binding to the host cell receptors—ICAM1 (brain), CD36 (microvascular endothelium, monocytes and platelets), thrombospondin (platelets), E-selectins and chondroitin sulphate (placenta)—and facilitate their adhesion to the vascular endothelium. The other allied parasite proteins expressed on the surface of RBCs which mediate binding to host cells are RESA, STEVOR, sequestrin, etc.
  - The PfEMP1 on the infected RBCs also enhances binding to uninfected RBCs (**rosetting**) through the complement receptor (CR1), and to other parasitised RBCs (**agglutination**). Rosetting may be seen with all malarial species.
  - The rigidity, clumping and cytoadherence of the RBCs cause sequestration of infected RBCs in the microcapillaries and venules of the vital organs which eventually **occludes the blood flow**, especially in the brain and also in the heart, lung, liver, kidney, bone marrow and placenta.
- **Inflammatory mediators:** The periodic rupture of schizonts and release of each generation of merozoites, malaria pigments and cellular debris in the blood causes the activation of monocytes and macrophages by pathogen-activated molecular patterns (PAMP) and damage-associated molecular patterns (DAMP). This results in the release of soluble mediators and cytokines which cause fever and other pathology.
  - *Malaria toxin hypothesis:* Malarial hemozoin pigment is responsible for clinical features that it produces by activating the components of the innate immune system.
  - *Cytokine storm:* The excessive production of proinflammatory cytokines such as TNFα, IFNγ, IL-1, IL-6, IL-8, IL-12 and nitric oxide cause severe or complicated malaria.
- **Severe anemia:** In the course of infection, anemia is aggravated due to RBC removal by the spleen, destruction of RBCs due to their rupture in schizogony and less production due to dyserythropoiesis. The spleen removes both parasitised and uninfected RBCs and consequently becomes enlarged (splenomegaly).
- **Coagulation abnormalities:** The enhanced coagulation activity and splenic clearance of platelets decreases the platelet count, which manifests as hemorrhages. Malaria typically causes the upregulation of the von Willebrand factor (VWF), resulting in increased thrombin production, which results in microvascular thrombosis involving various organs.
- **Hypoglycemia:** This occurs due to the failure of hepatic gluconeogenesis and an increase in the consumption of glucose by both the host and the parasites.

IMMUNOLOGY

At its initial stages, malaria infection activates non-specific defence responses. Subsequently, the infection is controlled by strain-specific immunity which inhibits the invasion of RBCs and multiplication of the parasite. In due course, exposure to numerous antigens and strains confers protection on the host from high-level parasitemia and disease but not from infection.

Innate Immunity

- Natural killer (NK) cells are the earliest source of IFNγ in malaria and have a crucial role in controlling acute parasitemia. The polymorphisms of NK cell receptors and some other genes influence the immune response to malaria.
- Innate immune response also influences the nature and magnitude of the acquired immunity to malaria.

Acquired Immunity

- Acquired immunity is crucial for malaria in high-transmission areas. Both humoral and cellular immunity are necessary for protection. A polyclonal rise in IgM, IgG and IgA levels is seen in immune individuals, though antibodies do not confer complete protection. T helper (T_h) and T follicular helper (T_{fh}) cells that drive the production of high-affinity antibodies are considered important for acquired immunity to malaria.
- After repeated bouts of subclinical or clinical malaria, an individual develops a partially protective immunity known as **premunition or concomitant immunity**. Such individuals still develop malaria but may not develop severe disease. Such protection is specific for both the species and the strain of the infecting parasite. In regions with **stable and intense transmission**, especially Africa, a state of **asymptomatic parasitemia** without illness is quite common, especially in adults and older children.
  - Newborns in these regions are protected during the first few months of life, presumably due to transplacentally transferred maternal antibodies. However, after a few months, when the maternal antibodies wane off, these infants become susceptible to malaria and its severe complications. Such children acquire protective immunity over the next few years with gradual exposure to the parasite.
  - Women who have developed protective immunity against malaria tend to lose this protection during pregnancy.
  - Individuals who leave endemic areas and move to non-endemic areas rapidly lose their protective immunity. This suggests that continuous antigenic exposure is required for such protection.

In areas with **low transmission**, infections are infrequent, and hence individuals in such areas have **no protective immunity**. Infections are therefore seen among all age groups, and there is a risk of epidemics in these areas.

Factors Contributing to Incomplete Immunity

The following factors contribute to incomplete immunity against malaria:

- The absence of major histocompatibility complex (MHC) antigens on the surface of infected RBCs prevents direct T cell recognition and development of immunity.
- The enormous diversity of *Plasmodium* antigens on the RBC surface that keep changing in the course of infection hinder the development of immunity.

HUMAN FACTORS ASSOCIATED WITH MALARIA

Genetic Factors

Certain genetic factors may provide a biological advantage and **protect the host** against certain types of malaria. They are as follows:

- Individuals who have the sickle cell trait (heterozygotes for the abnormal hemoglobin gene – HbS), which is most predominant in Africa, are relatively protected against severe *P. falciparum* malaria.
- Some blood cell disorders, e.g., hemoglobin C, thalassemias, fetal hemoglobin in adults, HbE, hereditary ovalocytosis and G6PD deficiency are more prevalent in malaria-endemic areas and offer some protection from malaria.
- Individuals who do not have the Duffy blood group show some resistance to infection by *P. vivax*.
- Various genetic determinants like HLA-BW53 may also provide some protection against severe malaria.

Risk Groups

Children, pregnant women, immunocompromised and splenectomised patients, individuals who travel to endemic areas, immigrants and even healthy people who have not had prior contact with *Plasmodium* are especially vulnerable to malaria.

CLINICAL FEATURES

The clinical manifestations of malaria depend on the past immune status of the host. In areas with intense malaria transmission (e.g., some parts of Africa and North-Eastern states of India), asymptomatic parasitemia is usual in adults and severe malaria occurs only in early childhood.

Incubation period: The interval between the infective mosquito bite and the first appearance of clinical symptoms varies with the species of the parasite (Table 13.2).

Acute Disease

Fever: Malaria is a common cause of fever in tropical countries. The initial symptoms are non-specific and include general lethargy, headache, abdominal discomfort and muscle aches followed by fever. Fever is typically associated with chills and rigors. The **classical febrile paroxysm of malaria** synchronises with the erythrocytic schizogony and comprises of three successive stages—**cold, hot** and **sweating stages**.

- The cold stage lasts for 15–60 minutes. The patient feels very cold and experiences intense shivering.
- The hot stage lasts for 2–6 hours. The patient feels extremely hot and the fever rises to 40°C or higher.
- The sweating stage is the last stage of the paroxysm. The patient sweats profusely and the fever comes down rapidly; this is usually followed by a deep sleep.

Usually, the fever is irregular at first and may become periodic later in the course of the disease. In *P. falciparum* malaria, it may never become regular. The periodicity is approximately:

- 24 hours in quotidian malaria by *P. knowlesi* (fever recurs every day).
- 48 hours in tertian malaria by *P. vivax, P. falciparum* and *P. ovale.*
- 72 hours in quartan malaria by *P. malariae.*

Anemia: It is quite common among young children and pregnant women.

Splenomegaly: In non-immune individuals with acute malaria, the spleen enlarges over a period of several days to become palpable. On the other hand, splenomegaly is seen in a high proportion of otherwise healthy individuals in malaria-endemic areas; this is probably due to repeated infections.

Severe and Complicated Malaria

P. vivax, P. ovale and *P. malariae* infections are usually not fatal, though 'cerebral vivax malaria' is increasingly being reported now. In contrast, falciparum malaria is a potentially lethal disease which can progress rapidly to severity. When appropriately treated, uncomplicated falciparum malaria has a mortality rate of <0.1%. However, once vital organ dysfunction sets in, or the percentage of infected erythrocytes increases to >2%, the risk of mortality rises sharply. The following are the manifestations of severe malaria:

- **Cerebral malaria (CM):**
  - Though cerebral malaria is usually associated with *P. falciparum*, other species may also cause CM.
  - The development of CM is much more common in children under five years of age who live in areas of high transmission as compared to adults. In low transmission areas, however, all age groups are affected. It is estimated that approximately 1% of children infected with *P. falciparum* develop CM.
  - The chief symptoms of CM include headache, muscle pain, abrupt onset of convulsions and altered state of consciousness. The clinical features may resemble sepsis. Generalised seizures are specifically associated with falciparum malaria and may forewarn the development of cerebral malaria. Coma is a characteristic and ominous feature of cerebral malaria and has been associated with death rates of 15–20% even after treatment. It manifests as diffuse symmetric encephalopathy; focal signs are unusual. Clinically, CM-induced coma is defined as a major unarousable coma persisting for >30 minutes after generalised convulsion.
  - Residual cognitive, behavioural, motor or neurological sequelae are more common in children.
  - The presence of **retinopathy** is highly suggestive of intracerebral parasite sequestration and is a poor prognostic indicator of CM.

Pathogenesis of cerebral malaria

The various mechanisms of cerebral malaria are as follows:

- The **sequestration** of parasitised RBCs in brain capillaries causes blockage and hypoxia. The PfEMP1 knobs expressed on the RBC surface enhance the binding of parasitised RBCs to the cerebral vascular endothelium.
- **Coagulation abnormalities** result in microvascular thrombosis.
- **Cytokine storm** due to the sequestration and rupture of parasitised RBCs in the cerebral microvasculature leads to endothelial damage.
- **Immune cell/platelet accumulation** which results in endothelial lesions of the blood-brain barrier contributes to brain pathology like edema, ischemia and hemorrhages.

- **Severe anemia:** It is quite common among young children. Severe anemia is often seen as a combined result of the increased destruction and decreased production of RBCs. Such anemia is usually normocytic and normochromic.

- **Coagulation abnormalities:** Especially seen in falciparum malaria, coagulation abnormalities manifest as bleeding from the gums, nose and gastrointestinal tract and/or disseminated intravascular coagulation.
- **Hypoglycemia:** It is associated with a poor prognosis, especially in children and pregnant women. This complication may be compounded by the administration of quinine, which is a powerful stimulant of pancreatic insulin secretion. Hypoglycemia leads to nervous system dysfunction.
- **Acidemia/acidosis:** Acidosis results from the accumulation of organic acids like lactic acid. It is a consistent feature of malaria. The rise in the level of lactic acid is directly proportional to disease severity. It manifests as laboured and deep breathing—often termed 'respiratory distress'—and is an important cause of mortality.
- **Renal failure:** Acute kidney injury is common in severe falciparum malaria and is attributed to erythrocyte sequestration and agglutination in the kidney.
- **Pulmonary edema/respiratory distress syndrome:** It is associated with high mortality. It is especially seen in pregnant women who contract falciparum malaria.
- **Algid malaria:** It is a rare complication of malaria characterised by peripheral circulatory failure, hypotension, profound shock and hypothermia with cold, clammy skin. Algid malaria is associated with the superadded gram-negative septicemia.
- **Liver dysfunction:** Mild hemolytic jaundice is common in malaria; severe jaundice is associated with *P. falciparum* infections. It is attributed to a host of factors, namely decreased gluconeogenesis, reduced liver blood flow, increased clearance of drugs, increased synthesis of clotting factors, etc.
- **Blackwater fever:** Sometimes, massive intravascular hemolysis leading to hemoglobinuria and the passage of dark red to black urine is seen in malaria when G6PD-deficient individuals (though it is seen sometimes even in patients with normal G6PD) receive antimalarial treatment with quinine or artemisinin derivatives. It is usually not associated with renal failure though renal function may be impaired.

Chronic Complications of Malaria

- **Hyperactive malarial splenomegaly (tropical splenomegaly syndrome):** It occurs in people living in malaria-endemic areas in tropical Africa and Asia as the result of an abnormal immunologic response to repeated malaria infections. It is characterised by massive splenomegaly, hepatomegaly, marked rise in serum IgM (due to polyclonal B cell activation) and antimalarial antibody titres, hepatic sinusoidal lymphocytosis and peripheral B cell lymphocytosis. The blood smear for malaria is usually found to be negative. Antimalarial chemoprophylaxis is advised to people who have hyperreactive malarial splenomegaly and live in endemic areas.
- **Quartan malarial nephropathy:** It is a chronic complication seen with *P. malariae* (and possibly with other malarial species). It is a result of injury caused to the renal glomeruli by soluble immune complexes resulting in nephrotic syndrome.
- **Burkitt's lymphoma:** The prevalence of Burkitt's lymphoma, which is strongly associated with Epstein-Barr virus, is considerably high in high malaria-transmission areas of Africa. It is postulated that malaria-related immune dysregulation provokes infection with lymphoma viruses.

Malaria in Special Situations

- **Malaria in pregnancy:** Malaria during pregnancy leads to a loss of pre-existing immunity. It leads to maternal anemia and sequestration of parasites in placental capillaries. Malaria in early pregnancy may lead to abortions. In areas of high malarial transmission, it is associated with fetal distress, premature labour, stillbirth or low birth weight of newborns. This association is reflected in high infant and maternal mortality rates.
- **Malaria in children:** Most of the deaths from falciparum malaria are reported in young African children. Convulsions, coma, hypoglycemia, metabolic acidosis and severe anemia are relatively common among children with severe malaria.
- **Transfusion malaria:** Malaria can be transmitted by blood transfusion, needlestick injury or organ transplantation. The incubation period of such infections is often short because of the absence of the pre-erythrocytic stage.

Recrudescence and Relapse

Recrudescence: Sometimes, after the primary episode of ***P. falciparum* and *P. malariae*** infections, there may be a period of latency during which the patient is asymptomatic. During this period, a **few parasites may persist** in numbers too small to produce fever or be detected by microscopy. In such cases, the parasite continues to replicate in small numbers, as a result of which, a fresh malarial episode occurs about 6–8 weeks after the primary episode. Such a recurrence is called recrudescence. In *P. falciparum* infections, recrudescences occur for 1–2 years, whereas in *P. malariae* infection, they may keep occurring for many years. Recrudescence may be due to the waning of the host's immunity or antigenic variation of the parasite.

Relapse: In ***P. vivax* and *P. ovale*** infections, **hypnozoites remain dormant** in the liver. These may get activated later and initiate fresh erythrocytic cycles and new episodes of malarial fever. Such relapses occur usually between six months to five years after the primary episode. **Radical treatment by primaquine is essential to prevent relapses.**

DIAGNOSIS

The diagnosis of malaria depends on the detection of malarial parasites, their antigens or their nucleic acids in the patient's blood (Table 13.3). Traditionally, the microscopic examination of stained blood smears is considered the **gold standard** for malaria diagnosis.

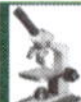

Lab diagnosis

- **Microscopy:** By visualising the blood stages of the parasite
  - Thin blood film
  - Thick blood film
  - Fluorescent microscopy
- **Antigen detection:** By performing rapid diagnostic tests (RDTs)
  - HRP2, LDH and aldolase-based RDTs
- **Serology:** Antibody detection is not useful for diagnosis
- **Culture:** Not useful for routine diagnosis
- **Quantitative buffy coat (QBC) test**
- **DNA detection:** PCR, real-time PCR and LAMP

Microscopy

Malarial parasites can be demonstrated microscopically in suitably stained peripheral blood smears (Fig. 13.4–13.6).

Advantage: Peripheral blood smear preparation is simple, rapid and inexpensive. Further, this method also serves to **differentiate *Plasmodium* species and quantitate** the parasites, and thus helps in guiding the management of the patient.

Disadvantage: It is labour intensive and requires an experienced microscopist.

Specimen

Blood obtained by pricking a finger or earlobe or the great toe in infants and smeared on a slide is the ideal sample because the density of parasites is greater in these capillary-rich areas. Blood obtained by venipuncture

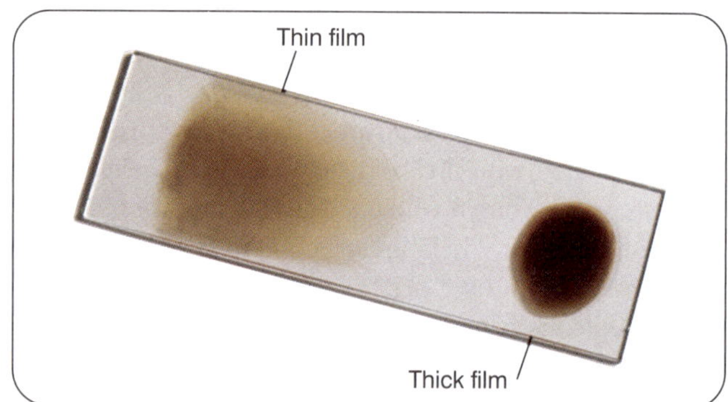

Fig. 13.4 Thin and thick films of peripheral blood for malaria microscopy (*Source:* CDC, PHIL, Image ID 5896)

Table 13.3 Comparison of diagnostic tests available for the detection of malaria

Feature	Microscopy			Antigen detection by rapid diagnostic test (RDT) kits	Culture	Nucleic acid amplification-based tests
	Thick smear Giemsa stain	Thin smear Giemsa stain	Fluorescent stain			
Sensitivity	5–10 parasites/μl	100–200 parasites/μl	100–200 parasites/μl	5–10 parasites/μl	—	1–10 parasites/μl
Species differentiation	Difficult	Easy	Sometimes difficult due to non-specific fluorescence	Easy	Only *P. falciparum* can be cultured; stringent culture conditions required	Easy
Time	6–8 hours	1–2 hours	30 minutes–1 hour	15–20 minutes	5–10 days	1–2 days
Expertise required	Expert microscopist required	Expert microscopist required	Expert microscopist and sophisticated microscope required	Very little training required	Very laborious; expertise required	Laborious; sophisticated equipment and expertise required
Cost	Low	Low	Low	Higher than microscopy but cost-effective	High	High

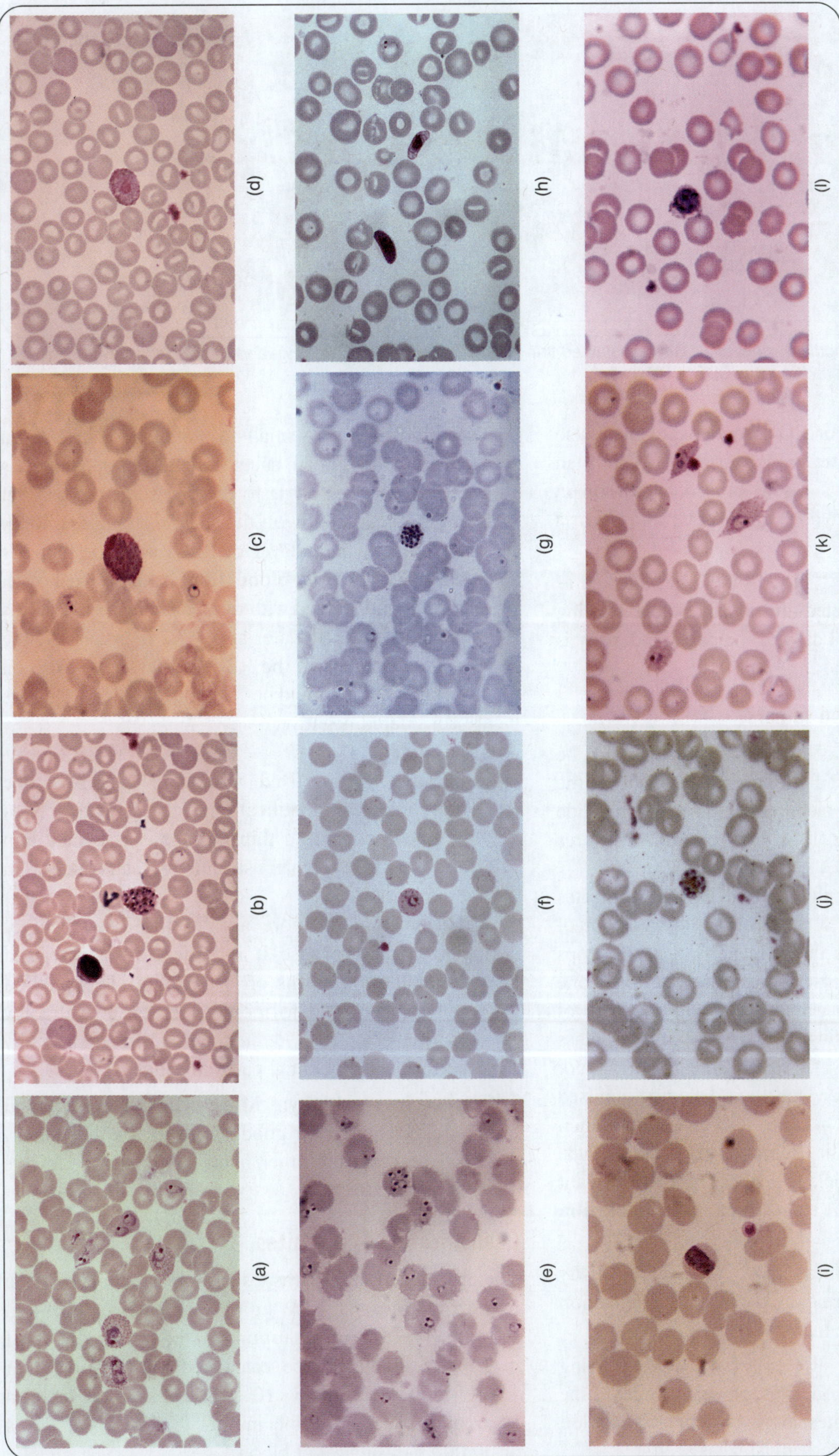

Fig. 13.5 Features of malarial parasites in Giemsa-stained thin peripheral blood films: (a) *Plasmodium vivax* trophozoite with Schüffner's dots, (b) *P. vivax* schizont with 20 merozoites, (c) *P. vivax* macrogametocyte, (d) *P. vivax* microgametocyte, (e) multiple *P. falciparum* ring-form trophozoites within RBCs, small chromatin dots and *accole* forms, (f) *P. falciparum* ring stage with Maurer's dots, (g) *P. falciparum* schizont (rarely seen in peripheral blood), (h) *P. falciparum* macrogametocyte (right) with microgametocyte (left), (i) *P. malariae* band-shaped trophozoite, (j) *P. malariae* schizont with 10 merozoites, (k) *P. ovale* trophozoites in fimbriated ovoid RBCs with Schüffner's dots and (l) *P. ovale* schizont (*Source:* CDC, PHIL; Image IDs 2305, 4974, 5015, 4976, 4884, 2710, 5854, 2704, 639, 12102, 20396 and 20393)

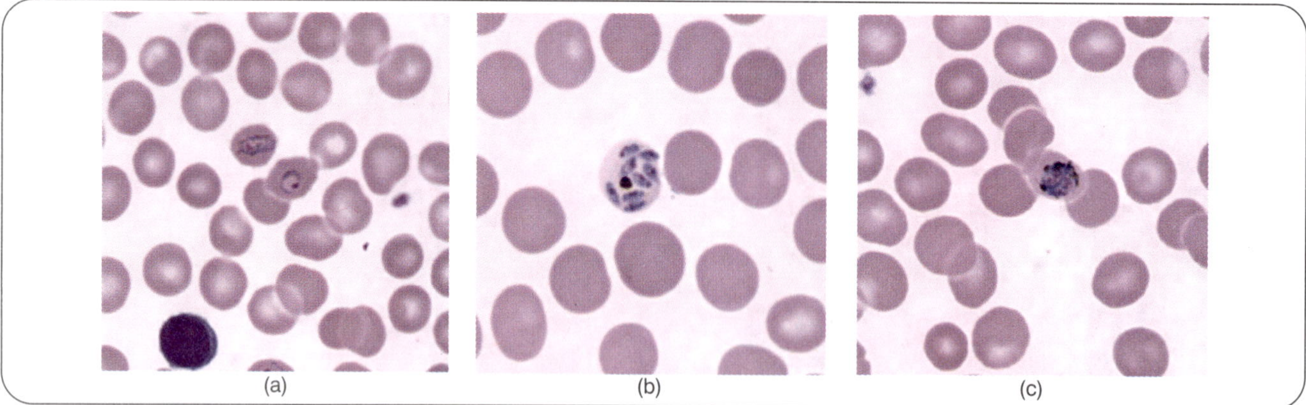

Fig. 13.6 Features of *Plasmodium knowlesi* in Giemsa-stained thin peripheral blood films: (a) ring- and band-shaped trophozoites, (b) schizont and (c) gametocyte (*Source:* CDC, DPDx)

and collected in heparin or EDTA anticoagulant is also acceptable if it can be examined shortly (within an hour) after being drawn so as to prevent alteration in the morphology of white blood cells (WBC) and malaria parasites.

Ideal time to draw blood: Blood should be collected as soon as malaria is suspected and ideally before starting the patient on antimalarial drugs. The parasite density is maximum during this period.

Types of peripheral blood smears

Two types of smears of the specimen should be prepared—thin and thick. Both smears are made at the same time from capillary blood either on the same slide or on different slides (Fig. 13.4; also refer to Annexures I and II).

- **Thick blood film:** A thick blood film concentrates the layers of RBCs on a small surface by a factor of 20 to 30. To prepare a thick smear, 3–4 small drops of blood are first placed close together (to form one large drop) on a clean glass slide. The large drop of blood is then spread using the corner of another glass slide to get about a half-inch square smear. This film of blood is dried completely and then dehemoglobinised (Annexures I and II). This unfixed preparation is then stained with one of the Romanowsky's stains, viz. Giemsa, Leishman's, Field's, Wright's or JSB (Jaswant Singh and Bhattacharji) stain. [**Note: The thick film should not be fixed.**]

  Advantage: Thick smears have greater sensitivity than thin smears and are more useful for the detection of low levels of parasitemia.

  Disadvantage: The lysis of RBCs during the dehemoglobinisation process can make the identification of parasites more difficult. Speciation may be difficult if only the ring stage is seen.

- **Thin blood film:** A small drop of blood is taken on a clean glass slide. Then, using the edge of a second glass slide held at a 45° angle to the first slide, the drop of blood is spread gently on the slide in a single, smooth stroke to get a monolayer of RBCs until the blood is exhausted. The **thin blood film is then fixed with methanol** and stained with diluted Giemsa or Wright's stain using buffered water at pH 7.2 to emphasise the parasite inclusions in the RBCs. At least 200–300 oil immersion fields should be examined before the smears are considered negative.

  Advantage:
  - Because of the fixed monolayer of RBCs, the morphological identification of the parasite species is much easier on a thin film than on a thick film and provides greater specificity than thick film examination.
  - This method is more apt for the assessment of parasitemia because it is easier to visualise and count the organisms on a thin film. This method can also be used to monitor response to therapy (particularly for *P. falciparum* infections) by performing sequential parasite counts.

Difference in sensitivity: More than 200 parasites/µl of blood are required for good results with a thin smear. A thick smear, on the other hand, can detect as few as 5–10 parasites/µl.

Quantification of parasites

The quantification of parasites is done by comparing the number of parasites to the number of RBCs or WBCs in a smear. The approximate numbers of parasites present in 1 µl of blood can be calculated by assuming that 1 µl of blood contains 5×10^6 RBCs. Based on such an assumption, 1% parasitemia implies 1 parasite/100 RBCs or 50,000 parasites/µl of blood.

Quantification of parasitemia

- *RBC-based method:* Performed on a thin film
  - Count the parasitised RBCs in 40 fields in a 100× oil immersion objective (10,000 RBCs considering about 250 RBCs/field).
  - Divide the number by 100 to get percentage of parasitised RBCs/µl of blood.
  - The final result is the **percentage of RBCs infected.**
- *WBC-based method:* Performed on a thick film
  - Count the number of parasites (N) against 100 WBCs.
  - Repeat in two more areas and calculate the average, N (N=Parasites counted against 100 WBCs).
  - Calculate the number of parasites/µl by the formula: (Patient's WBC count [TLC]× N)/100.
  - The final result is the **number of parasites/µl of blood.**

The quantification of parasites is helpful to:

1. Assess the severity of infection—the WHO considers falciparum parasitemia to be heavy and associated with poor prognosis when >5% of RBCs (>2,50,000 parasites/µl) are parasitised
2. Monitor response to antimalarial treatment

In *P. falciparum* malaria, sequestration interferes with the true estimation of parasitemia as only the younger ring forms of the asexual parasites are present in the peripheral blood.

Fluorescent microscopy

Certain fluorescent dyes have an affinity for the nucleic acid in the parasite nucleus, and when excited by UV light at an appropriate wavelength, cause the nucleus to fluoresce. In contrast, mature RBCs do not have a nucleus, and therefore, do not interfere with the fluorescence. Acridine orange (AO) and benzothiocarboxypurine (BCP) exhibit apple green or yellow fluorescence at 490 nm.

Advantage: It is a rapid method of staining and examination.

Disadvantage: These stains are non-specific and stain nucleic acids from all cell types. Thus, expertise is required to distinguish the parasite's nucleus from other fluorescent structures.

Automated microscopy

A commercially available digital automated system (Parasight malaria, Sight Diagnostics Ltd., Israel) has been developed that detects, speciates and even quantitates malaria parasites with greater speed and better consistency than conventional microscopy.

Quantitative Buffy Coat (QBC)

This technique is based on microhematocrit centrifugation. In the system known as quantitative buffy coat (QBC) or QBC II (Becton Dickinson, USA), a commercially available acridine orange-coated capillary tube with an internal float is used to separate layers of WBCs and platelets from RBCs using centrifugation of whole blood (Fig. 13.7). The parasites concentrate below the WBC layer, appearing mainly in the upper layer of RBCs and can be viewed through the capillary tube using a special objective (paralens) with a fluorescence microscope.

Disadvantage: The QBC fluorescence method requires specialised equipment, and cannot distinguish between species, especially if only the ring stage is seen.

Antigen Detection

The detection of specific malaria antigens in blood is useful for malaria diagnosis. Most commercially available test formats are in the form of **rapid strip tests** or **rapid diagnostic tests (RDTs).** Some of the antigens used in such tests are as follows:

- **HRP-2 (histidine-rich protein)** is a water-soluble protein produced at the asexual stages and by the young gametocytes of ***P. falciparum*** (not *P. vivax*). It is expressed in abundance on the surface of the RBC membrane. The disadvantage of this antigen is that RDTs based only on HRP-2 antigen cannot detect infections caused by *P. vivax*, *P. ovale* or *P. malariae*.

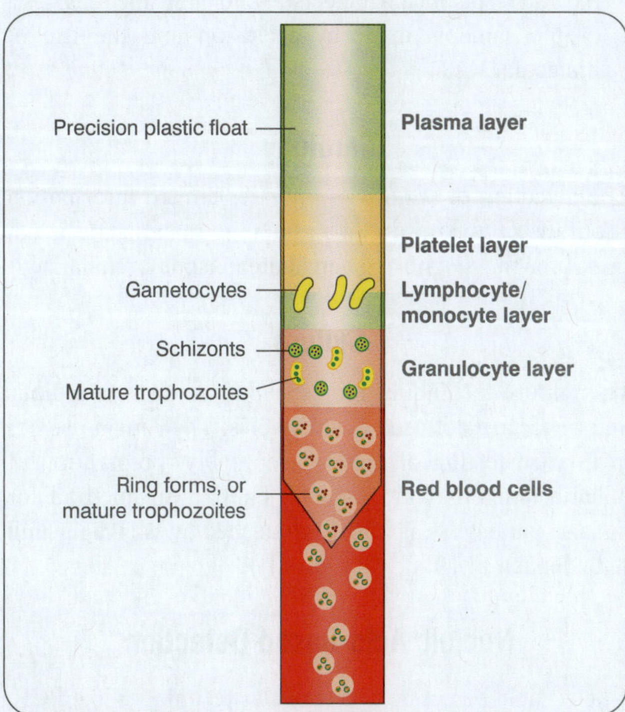

Fig. 13.7 Quantitative buffy coat for malaria detection

- **pLDH (lactate dehydrogenase)** is an enzyme in the glycolytic pathway of the malaria parasite. It is produced both by the sexual and asexual forms of malaria parasites. Different isomers of pLDH exist for each of the four *Plasmodium* spp. infecting humans, and their detection is useful in the diagnosis of malaria and species identification.
- **Aldolase**, an enzyme, is also utilised as a target antigen for malaria diagnosis and speciation.

Advantage:
- Antigen detection has comparable or marginally lower sensitivity than microscopy and is capable of detecting >100 parasites/μl (0.002% parasitemia).
- It produces rapid results (within 15 to 20 minutes).
- It can be performed in the field or at the bedside.
- A combination of antigens can be used to differentiate between various species of *Plasmodium* in a single test kit.
- In India, the National Vector Borne Disease Control Programme (NVBDCP) recommends that bivalent RDT, which can differentiate between *P. vivax* and *P. falciparum*, should be used for rapid diagnosis in areas where microscopy is not available. However, all RDT results should be confirmed by microscopy, when available.

Disadvantage:
- Some of the commercially available kits lack the desired sensitivity and specificity.
- The shelf life of the kit is lower at high temperatures and humidity.
- No RDT specifically detects *P. knowlesi*; the diagnosis of the same is made by exclusion and the use of molecular tests.

Serology

The detection of antibodies provides limited information about the past exposure of a person to malaria and is not useful for the diagnosis of an acute episode of malaria.

Culture

The culture techniques for *Plasmodium* are very tedious and hence are not used for diagnosis. Their main use lies in in vitro testing of drug susceptibility, preparation of malaria antigens and research. The culture method for malaria parasites was initially described by **W. Trager and J. B. Jensen** in 1976 (Annexure II).

Nucleic Acid-Based Detection

Nucleic acid detection by molecular techniques like PCR, real-time PCR and LAMP are increasingly being used not just for diagnosis but also for the detection of drug resistance genes. These methods have the advantage of being extremely sensitive and thus, are useful for the detection of low-level parasitemia.

Other Diagnostic Parameters

Fundoscopy

The examination of the fundus of the eye can be quite useful since **malaria-induced retinopathy has unique features** and has been significantly associated with mortality in children who have cerebral malaria. The use of fundoscopy can and should be used to aid both diagnosis and prognosis.

TREATMENT

The various classes of drugs used as anti-malarial agents act on **different stages of the life cycle** of the parasite and have different mechanisms of action (Table 13.4). No drug has yet been identified that is active against sporozoites; neither is any **single drug known to be effective against all liver and blood stages**. An important factor to be taken into consideration is the **drug sensitivity** of the parasite to the chosen drug. This varies for different geographical regions. An effective drug regimen for malaria is essentially a **combination of different drugs** with complementary activity, specific to the geographical region of the world.

The treatment of malaria in a country depends on the country-specific guidelines based on the local drug susceptibility patterns of the parasites in that country. In India, malaria treatment is governed by national guidelines for treatment (currently in accordance with the **National Drug Policy on Malaria, 2013**) (Table 13.5). This policy is subject to change periodically with the evolution of drug resistance and the availability of newer drugs/combinations.

The following are some guidelines for the treatment of malaria in India:
- The production and sale of **artemisinin monotherapy have been banned in India** to prevent the emergence of resistance to artemisinin derivatives.
- Artemisinin-based therapy is contraindicated in the first trimester of pregnancy.
- Primaquine is contraindicated in pregnant women and in individuals with G6PD deficiency.
- Primaquine is used for both *P. vivax* and *P. falciparum*, but with different aims:
    - In vivax malaria, primaquine is used to **kill the hypnozoites to prevent relapse**.

Table 13.4 Properties of antimalarial drugs

Class	Drug	Stage of action			Affected pathways/mechanism of action	Drug resistance gene markers*
		Liver hypnozoite stage	Blood asexual stage	Blood gametocyte stage		
Endoperoxide	Artemisinin and its derivatives, artesunate, artemether and arteether	–	+	+	Alkylation and oxidative damage of multiple protein and lipid targets, thereby triggering a stress response in parasite	*Pfkelch13*
4-Aminoquinolones	Chloroquine	–	+	+/–	Heme-detoxification in digestive vacuole	*Pfcrt, Pfmdr1*
Aryl-amino alcohols	Quinine	–	+	+/–	Inhibition of hemoglobin import and/or heme-detoxification	*Pfcrt, Pfmdr1*
	Mefloquine	–	+	–		*Pfmdr1*
	Lumefantrine	–	+	–		*Pfcrt, Pfmdr1*
Antifolates	Pyrimethamine	–	+	–	Folate biosynthesis	*Pfdhfr*
	Sulfadoxine	–	+	–		*Pfhdps*
Naphthoquinones	Atovaquone	–	+	+/–	Mitochondrial electron transport chain required for pyrimidine biosynthesis	*Pfcytb*
8-Aminoquinolones	Primaquine, tafenoquine	+	–	+	Unknown	None

**P. falciparum* chloroquine resistance transporter gene – *Pfcrt*; *P. falciparum* cytochrome b – *Pfcytb*; *P. falciparum* dihydrofolate reductase – *Pfdhfr*; *P. falciparum* dihydropteroate synthase – *Pfdhps*; *P. falciparum* kelch 13 – *Pfkelch13*; *P. falciparum* multidrug resistance gene – *Pfmdr1*

Table 13.5 Treatment of malaria as prescribed by the National Drug Policy, 2013

Uncomplicated malaria	
P. vivax	***P. falciparum***
Chloroquine: 25 mg/kg divided over 3 days (10 mg/kg on day 1, 10 mg/kg on day 2 and 5 mg/kg on day 3) + **Primaquine (PQ):** 0.25 mg/kg daily for 14 days to prevent relapse	*Indian states other than the north-eastern states* **Artemisinin combination therapy (ACT): Artesunate** 4 mg/kg/day × 3 days and **sulfadoxine** 25 mg/kg – **pyrimethamine** 1.25 mg/kg × 1 day (ACT–SP*) + **Primaquine:** 0.75 mg/kg administered as a single dose on day 2
	North-eastern states of India where there is resistance to SP **Artemether** 20 mg along with **lumefantrine** 120 mg (ACT–AL) + **Primaquine:** 0.75 mg/kg administered as a single dose on day 2
	Pregnant women 1st trimester: **Quinine** 10 mg/kg TDS × 7 days 2nd and 3rd trimesters: **ACT** as per geographical location
Severe and complicated malaria	
Initial parenteral treatment for at least 48 hours – choose one of the following four options:	**Follow-up treatment** – when the patient can take oral medication following parenteral treatment:
Quinine salt: 20 mg/kg on admission as IV infusion or divided IM injection, followed by maintenance dose of 10 mg/kg, 8 hourly; infusion rate should not exceed 5 mg/kg/hour	**Quinine:** 10 mg/kg TDS with doxycycline 100 mg ODS or clindamycin (in pregnant women and children under 8 years of age); to complete 7 days of treatment
Artesunate (AS): 2.4 mg/kg IV or IM administered on admission, then at 12 hr and 24 hr, then once a day	**Full oral course of area-specific ACT:** *In north-eastern states:* ACT–AL for 3 days + PQ single dose on 2nd day *In other states:* ACT–SP for 3 days + PQ single dose on 2nd day
Artemether (ATM): 3.2 mg/kg IM administered on admission, then 1.6 mg/kg per day	
Arteether: 150 mg IM daily × 3 days; for adults only (not recommended for children)	

  - In falciparum malaria, primaquine is used for its **gametocidal effect; this helps to prevent transmission**.
- *P. ovale* infections should be given the same treatment as *P. vivax* and *P. malariae* as *P. falciparum* infections.

Drug Resistance in Malaria

Drug resistance should be suspected in cases where the patient fails to show clinical improvement or parasitological response (i.e., decreased parasitemia in the blood within 72 hours) despite complete treatment and no history of vomiting or diarrhea. Such cases, which do not respond to ACT, should be treated with oral quinine with tetracycline/doxycycline and reported to the concerned district/state malaria officer.

Falciparum malaria

Antimalarial drug resistance has emerged as one of the greatest challenges facing malaria control today. The drug resistance in *P. falciparum* is widespread and is described against all the available drugs though there are geographical variations in its resistance. Most of the drug resistance in malaria has emerged in the South-East Asian region, especially the Thailand–Cambodia border, and then spread to other regions. Partial resistance to artemisinins has emerged in the Greater Mekong Subregion. Concomitant emergence of resistance to drugs that are given in combination with the artemisinin compound is now causing ACT regimens to fail in several areas.

Vivax malaria

Only sporadic cases of resistance to chloroquine and/or primaquine have been reported in some areas.

Mechanism of drug action and resistance (Table 13.4)

Chloroquine

Mechanism of action: The malarial parasite has a digestive vacuole within which the breakdown of hemoglobin and detoxification of heme to hemozoin occurs. Chloroquine concentrates up to several 1,000-fold in this digestive vacuole due to:

- Protonation and ion trapping of chloroquine aided by the low pH of the vacuole
- Active uptake of chloroquine by membrane transporters of the parasite
- Binding of chloroquine to a specific receptor in the vacuole

Mechanism of resistance: Chloroquine resistance is associated with a decrease in the amount of chloroquine accumulation in the food vacuole due to an **increased efflux** of the drug. This is attributed to a point mutation in the gene which encodes the PfCRT protein (*P. falciparum* chloroquine resistance transporter gene—*Pfcrt*) in the parasite. Point mutations in a gene coding another protein PfMDR1 (*P. falciparum* multidrug resistance gene—*Pfmdr1*) have also been implicated.

Quinine, mefloquine and lumefantrine

Mechanism of action: These drugs act by inhibiting hemoglobin import and/or heme-detoxification.

Mechanism of resistance: It is similar to the resistance of parasites to chloroquine. Resistance to these drugs is attributed to point mutations in the *Pfcrt* and *Pfmdr1* genes.

Sulfadoxine and pyrimethamine (SP)

Mechanism of action: Both dihydropteroate synthase (DHPS), an enzyme unique to the parasite, and dihydrofolate reductase (DHFR), which is present in the host as well as the parasite are essential for folate biosynthesis in the parasite cytosol. SP targets these two enzymes and inhibits the synthesis of folate in the parasite.

Mechanism of resistance: Pyrimethamine and sulfadoxine resistance is associated with point mutations in the *Pfdhfr* and *Pfdhps* genes respectively.

Artemisinins (ARTs) – artesunate, artemether, arteether and dihydroartemisinin

Since the half-lives of artemisinin and its derivatives are very short (1–2 hours), they are combined with a longer-acting partner drug with a different mechanism of action.

Mechanism of action: A heme-iron-catalysed break of the endoperoxide bridge of the drug leads to widespread alkylation and oxidative damage of multiple protein and lipid targets in the parasite.

Mechanism of resistance: Point mutations in the gene coding for the Kelch propeller domain of the K13 protein are associated with artemisinin resistance.

Tests for drug resistance

In vivo tests

In vivo tests are those tests that are **performed on a living body**. Patients with clinical malaria are given antimalarial treatment under observation and are monitored for either failure to clear parasites or for the reappearance of parasites. Based on in vivo tests, WHO has classified response to treatment as shown in the box below.

WHO classification of response to treatment (*Source:* Methods for surveillance of antimalarial drug efficacy, World Health Organization, 2009)

Early treatment failure (ETF):

- After starting treatment, severe malaria or dangerous clinical signs on days 1, 2 or 3 along with parasitemia
- Parasitemia on day 2 higher than what it was on day 0, irrespective of axillary temperature
- Parasitemia on day 3 with axillary temperature ≥37.5°C
- Parasitemia on day 3 ≥25% of what it was on day 0

Late clinical failure (LCF):

- Danger signs of severe malaria in the presence of parasitemia on any day between day 4 and 28 (or day 42) in patients who do not previously meet any of the criteria of ETF
- Parasitemia on any day between day 4 and 28 (or day 42) with axillary temperature ≥37.5°C in patients who do not previously meet any of the criteria of ETF

Late parasitological failure (LPF):

- Presence of parasitemia on any day between day 7 and 28 (or day 42) with axillary temperature <37.5°C in patients who did not previously meet any of the criteria of ETF or LCF

Adequate clinical and parasitological response (ACR):

- Absence of parasitemia on day 14 or 28, irrespective of fever, without previously meeting any criteria of early and late treatment failure

In vitro or ex vivo tests

These are tests done in a **non-living setting (in vitro) or outside the living body but in a live system (ex vivo)**. In such tests, blood samples are obtained from malaria patients, and the malaria parasites are exposed to different concentrations of antimalarial drugs in the laboratory to measure their sensitivity against these drugs.

Molecular markers of drug resistance

Molecular techniques such as PCR or DNA sequencing of drug resistance genes can pinpoint the mutations responsible for drug resistance in blood taken from malaria-infected patients (Table 13.4).

PREVENTION AND CONTROL

Chemoprophylaxis

Chemoprophylaxis should be administered only to selective groups in high *P. falciparum*-endemic areas and travellers to these areas.

- When persons from non-endemic (malaria) regions travel to endemic regions, they are at risk of acquiring malaria infection, and since they are not immune to the disease, it can become severe. Therefore, all travellers to such areas should be advised to use appropriate chemoprophylaxis and personal protection measures for prevention. Even first- and second-generation immigrants living in non-endemic countries who return/travel to their countries of origin should be prescribed chemoprophylaxis, especially when traveling during peak malaria season. Members of the military and paramilitary forces who are stationed in malaria-endemic areas for long periods should also receive chemoprophylaxis.
- The chemoprophylaxis is started 2–20 days before departure to a malaria endemic area and continued for the duration of stay and for 1–4 weeks after return. The choice of drugs depends on the *Plasmodium* species and drug resistance prevalent in the region. Since no one chemoprophylaxis regimen provides 100% protection, other personal protective measures should also be taken. Various drugs for malaria chemoprophylaxis are listed in Table 13.6.

Table 13.6 Drugs used for malaria chemoprophylaxis

Drug	Adult dose	Pediatric dose	Remarks
Atovaquone plus Proguanil	250 mg atovaquone and 100 mg proguanil once daily	62.5 mg atovaquone and 25 mg proguanil daily	Contraindicated in pregnancy and lactation
Chloroquine	300 mg once weekly	5 mg/kg weekly (max. 300 mg)	Long-term safety known; chloroquine resistance reported from most parts of the world; contraindicated in epilepsy and psoriasis
Doxycycline	100 mg once daily	1.5 mg base/kg once daily (max. 100 mg)	Contraindicated in pregnancy and lactation
Mefloquine	250 mg once weekly	5 mg/kg weekly	Contraindicated in first trimester of pregnancy, breast feeding, patients receiving β-blockers, epilepsy, psychosis and heart blocks

Intermittent Preventive Treatment

Intermittent preventive treatment in pregnancy (IPTp) is a full therapeutic course given to pregnant women living in malaria endemic areas of the sub-Saharan Africa to be given at routine antenatal care visits, regardless of whether the recipient is infected with malaria, since the disease is associated with increased morbidity and severity in the pregnant women and adverse effects on the developing fetus. The WHO recommends at least three doses of sulphadoxine–pyrimethamine as IPTp.

Malaria Control Strategies in India

In line with the WHO Global Technical Strategy for Malaria 2016–2030, India has formed a **National Framework for Malaria Elimination (NFME)** 2016–2030. The goal of this framework is to eliminate malaria in this country, i.e., zero indigenous cases across the country by 2030. The **Directorate of National Vector Borne Disease Control Programme (NVBDCP)** is the central nodal agency for the prevention and control of vector borne diseases (VBDs) like **malaria**, dengue, lymphatic filariasis, kala-azar, Japanese encephalitis and chikungunya in India. Malaria control strategies implemented by NVBDCP consist of:

- **Early case detection and prompt treatment:** This is the main strategy in malaria control. All suspected cases of malaria must be confirmed by parasitological diagnosis within 24 hours of fever and treated accordingly. Diagnosis may be made by microscopy or using bivalent RDTs which detect both *P. vivax* and *P. falciparum* antigens in areas where microscopy is not available. Radical treatment is necessary for all the cases of *P. vivax* malaria to prevent continued transmission of malaria.
- **Vector control:** Mosquitoes in the community can be controlled with a combination of modalities:
  - *Chemical agents:* Chemicals with insecticidal and larvicidal property may be used to control mosquito breeding. Indoor residual spraying (IRS), i.e., spraying the walls inside the house with insecticides (for adult mosquitoes), and the use of abate (for larvae) help in source reduction.
  - *Biological agents:* Larvivorous fishes like *Gambusia* and larvicidal bacteria like *Bacillus thuringiensis* may be used in ornamental tanks, ponds, etc.
  - *Personal protective measures against mosquito bites:*
    - Use of mosquito repellent creams, liquids, sprays, etc.
    - Use of protective wire mesh or nets for the doors and windows of houses
    - Use of insecticide-treated bed nets (ITN)/long-lasting insecticidal nets (LLINs)
    - Wearing clothes that cover the body to the maximum extent
- *Environment management, source reduction and community awareness:*
  - Elimination of mosquito breeding areas such as potholes, uncovered water reservoirs, puddles, etc., is most crucial.
  - The Swachh Bharat Mission advocates for a standard of cleanliness and hygiene, and thereby, the elimination of breeding grounds for mosquitoes.

Malaria Vaccine

The world's first malaria vaccine to show a potential to boost malaria control against *P. falciparum* is **RTS,S/AS01**.

- In Phase III of clinical testing in seven African countries, the vaccine was found to bring down the number of malaria cases by 40%, and life-threatening, severe malaria by 30%.
- It has been recommended for pilot implementation in a few countries of Africa with moderate-to-high malaria transmission. It is to be added as a complementary malaria control tool and not replace the recommended preventive, diagnostic and treatment approach of malaria control.
- The WHO-coordinated pilot programme is a collaborative effort with the health ministries of various governments, PATH—a non-profit organisation and GlaxoSmithKline (GSK)—the vaccine developers and manufacturers who are donating the vaccines for this pilot project.

Constituents: The primary component of this vaccine is a **hybrid pre-erythrocytic stage** recombinant protein vaccine expressed in *Saccharomyces cerevisiae*. A chemical adjuvant (AS01) is used to boost the immune response. The main components of the vaccine are:

- R – the central repeat region of *P. falciparum* circumsporozoite protein (CSP)
- T – T cell epitopes of CSP
- S – hepatitis B surface antigen

Dosage: It is administered intramuscularly to **children up to 2 years of age in four doses**—three doses are administered between 5 and 9 months of age and the fourth dose is administered around the second birthday.

Questions

1. Discuss the diagnosis and management of uncomplicated malaria.
2. Differentiate between *Plasmodium vivax, P. falciparum, P. ovale* and *P. malariae.*
3. Write a short note on *Plasmodium knowlesi* malaria.
4. List the differential diagnosis of infective causes of hepatosplenomegaly.
5. Discuss the pathogenesis of cerebral malaria and its management.
6. Discuss the control programme for malaria in India.
7. Write short notes on blackwater fever and severe malaria.
8. Discuss the global epidemiology of malaria.
9. Discuss drug resistance in malaria.
10. Write a short note on the malaria vaccine.
11. Write a short note on tropical splenomegaly syndrome.

Multiple Choice Questions

1. Which of the following scientists has been conferred the Nobel Prize for their work on malaria?
   a. Patrick Manson
   b. Louis Pasteur
   c. Ronald Ross
   d. Alphonse Laveran
2. The most common species of malaria in the world is ___________:
   a. *Plasmodium vivax*
   b. *Plasmodium falciparum*
   c. *Plasmodium malariae*
   d. *Plasmodium ovale*
3. The fifth emerging species of malaria is ___________:
   a. *Plasmodium vivax*
   b. *Plasmodium falciparum*
   c. *Plasmodium knowlesi*
   d. *Plasmodium ovale*
4. The infective stage of the malaria parasite in humans is the ___________:
   a. Gametocyte
   b. Sporozoite
   c. Merozoite
   d. Schizont
5. Relapse occurs in infection with which of the following malaria species?
   a. *Plasmodium vivax*
   b. *Plasmodium falciparum*
   c. *Plasmodium malariae*
   d. *Plasmodium knowlesi*
6. Recrudescence occurs in infections with which of the following malaria species?
   a. *Plasmodium vivax*
   b. *Plasmodium falciparum*
   c. *Plasmodium knowlesi*
   d. *Plasmodium ovale*
7. The ookinete in the life cycle of the malaria parasite is formed in ___________:
   a. The hindgut of the *Anopheles* mosquito
   b. The midgut of the female *Anopheles* mosquito
   c. The RBC of human beings
   d. The human liver
8. Which malaria parasite species has banana-shaped gametocytes, *accolle* forms and *applique* forms?
   a. *Plasmodium vivax*
   b. *Plasmodium falciparum*
   c. *Plasmodium malariae*
   d. *Plasmodium knowlesi*
9. The periodicity of fever in *Plasmodium falciparum* is every ___________:
   a. 24 hours (quotidian)
   b. 48 hours (tertian)
   c. 72 hours (quartan)
   d. No periodicity
10. The migration of infected RBCs in malaria to capillaries is known as ___________:
    a. Rosetting
    b. Sequestration
    c. Maurer's phenomenon
    d. Endobolisation
11. Individuals who have thalassemia, sickle cell disease or G6PD deficiency are protected against which disease?
    a. Typhoid
    b. Malaria
    c. Trypanosomiasis
    d. Schistosomiasis
12. Tropical splenomegaly syndrome is associated with ___________:
    a. Malaria
    b. Kala-azar
    c. Enteric fever
    d. Tuberculosis
13. The gold standard of malaria diagnosis is ___________:
    a. Demonstration of parasite in blood film
    b. Culture of parasites
    c. DNA detection in blood
    d. Rapid immunochromatographic tests (RDT)
14. Chloroquine acts on the __________ stage of the malaria parasite's life cycle.
    a. Blood asexual stages
    b. Hypnozoite liver stages
    c. Gametocytes
    d. All the above

15. The choice of treatment for uncomplicated *Plasmodium falciparum* malaria in India (except in north-eastern states) is ________________.
    a. Artemisinin combination therapy: artesunate + sulfadoxine–pyrimethamine (ACT–SP) PLUS primaquine
    b. Artemisinin alone
    c. Chloroquine alone
    d. Artemisinin combination therapy: Artesunate + sulfadoxine– pyrimethamine (ACT–SP) PLUS chloroquine
16. The mutation in the __________ gene is responsible for drug resistance against chloroquine in the malaria parasite.
    a. *Pfcrt* and *Pfmdr1*
    b. *Pfdhps*
    c. *Pfdhfr*
    d. *Pfkelch13*
17. The mutation in the__________ gene is responsible for decreased efficacy against artemisinin in the malaria parasite.
    a. *Pfcrt, Pfmdr1*
    b. *Pfdhps*
    c. *Pfdhfr*
    d. *Pfkelch13*
18. Histidine-rich protein antigen (HRP-II) is used in the immunochromatographic test for the detection of __________:
    a. *Plasmodium vivax*
    b. *Plasmodium falciparum*
    c. *Plasmodium malariae*
    d. *Plasmodium knowlesi*
19. All the following are features of stable malaria EXCEPT ________:
    a. Intense transmission throughout the year
    b. Seen in western and eastern Africa and north-eastern parts of India
    c. Severe disease usually seen in adults
    d. Partial immunity to malaria
20. The following features are characteristic of *Plasmodium vivax* blood stages EXCEPT __________:
    a. Enlarged RBC
    b. Schüffner's dots in infected RBC
    c. Most parasites are sequestered in internal capillaries
    d. Reticulocytes, young RBCs infected

CHAPTER 14

Babesia

(Named after the scientist Victor Babes)

Case Study and Learning Goals

A 25-year-old male develops fever with chills one month after receiving a blood transfusion. On investigation, a Giemsa-stained peripheral blood film shows intraerythrocytic trophozoites in a tetrad-like arrangement. List the parasites affecting the hemopoietic system. How is this parasite transmitted to humans? How would you treat the patient?

INTRODUCTION

Babesia are **tick-borne** apicomplexan protozoa that **multiply in blood** like the malaria parasites but are **non-pigmented** and have no **pre- or exo-erythrocytic forms.** More than a hundred species are known to infect vertebrate animals but only a few have been documented to cause human infections. These chiefly include *B. microti, B. divergens, B. duncani, B. venatorum*, as well as several other genetically related species namely, *B. divergens*-like, *B. duncani*-like and *B. microti*-like species.

Babesia species was first discovered in 1888 by Victor Babes in cattle in Romania. In 1893, T. Smith and F. L. Kilbourne identified it as the cause of Texas redwater fever of cattle and implicated ticks in the transmission of the disease. Though human infection was first documented in 1957, it was only sporadically reported thereafter. In recent times, however, babesiosis has emerged as a significant public health problem, especially in the USA.

EPIDEMIOLOGY

Babesiosis is an **emerging zoonosis**. Most cases of babesiosis are reported in the north-eastern and mid-western regions of the USA. Reports of such infections have exponentially increased in the past five decades. Babesiosis also occurs sporadically in Europe and Asia. *B. microti* (with rodents as its natural hosts) is most common in the USA, while *B. divergens* (with cattle as its natural hosts) is almost entirely restricted to Europe.

Unlike the malaria parasite, *Babesia* spp. is maintained in a **natural tick–animal reservoir host cycle**. Humans are accidental hosts. The infection is transmitted through the bite of an infected tick, and occasionally through **blood transfusion**. It is now recognised as the most common transfusion-transmitted pathogen in the USA. In rare cases, transmission may occur perinatally or through organ transplantation.

MORPHOLOGY

The various developmental forms of *Babesia* are trophozoites, merozoites, gametocytes, gametes, zygote and sporozoites.

Trophozoite

It is the intra-erythrocytic form of *Babesia.* There are two lineages of this stage—a small type (1–2.5 µm) and a large type (2.5–5 µm). It is usually pear-shaped, but the absence of a parasitophorous vacuole (unlike the malaria parasite) makes it quite pleomorphic. The apical complex contains organelles like rhoptries and micronemes. The trophozoites divide by binary fission to produce pairs or tetrads (**'Maltese cross formation'**). This characteristic arrangement of the trophozoites is helpful in the diagnosis of babesiosis.

LIFE CYCLE (Fig. 14.1a and b)

Definitive hosts: *Ixodes* ticks
Intermediate hosts: Rodents and wild animals (reservoirs)
Amplifying hosts: Deer

The *Ixodes* tick is the definitive host and vector of *Babesia*, and rodents and other wild animals are the intermediate hosts and reservoirs. Deer act as amplifying hosts for *Babesia* by providing ticks with ample breeding grounds on their body and blood meals; however, they seem to be safe from infection.

The various stages in the life cycle of *Babesia* are as follows:

- The infection begins with the bite of a tick, which introduces the infective **sporozoites** along with the saliva into the intermediate host.
- The sporozoite directly penetrates the cytoplasm of the host RBC with the help of its apical complex without forming a parasitophorous vacuole. Once inside the

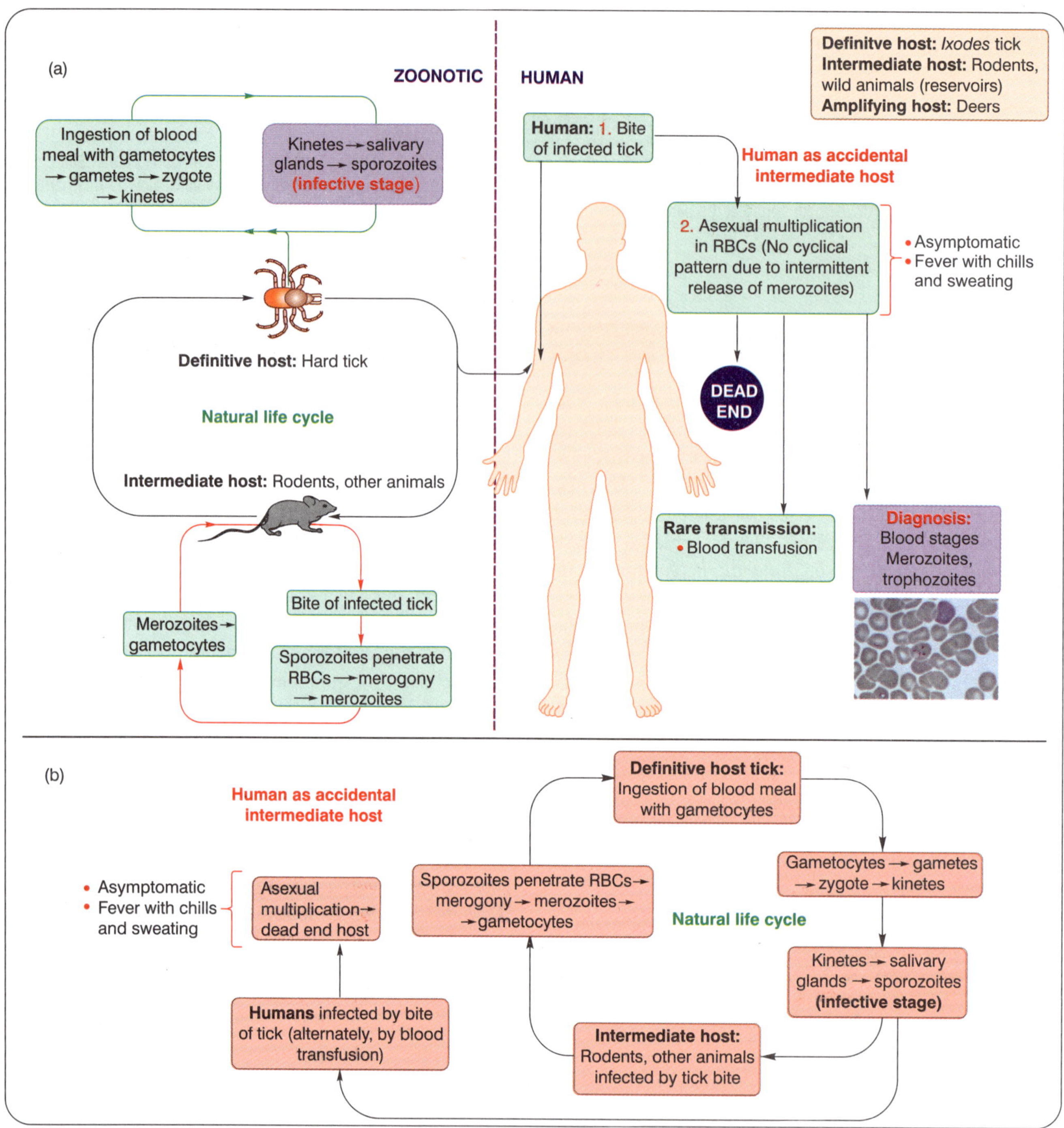

Fig. 14.1 Life cycle of *Babesia* spp.: (a) detailed and (b) schematic (*Source [inset]:* Centers for Disease Control and Prevention [CDC], Public Health Image Library [PHIL]; Image ID 11090)

cytoplasm, sporozoites undergo asexual multiplication (merogony) to form **merozoites**, which invade fresh RBCs and continue to multiply. Merozoites are released intermittently, and thus the associated fever does not have a cyclical pattern. Some trophozoites form **gametocytes** which cannot be distinguished from trophozoites by light microscopy.

- Once the tick ingests gametocytes during its blood meal, the parasite's sexual cycle begins and **gametes** are formed. These gametes fuse to form a **zygote** in the midgut. The zygote divides into primary **kinetes** which reach the hemolymph and invade various tissues of the tick. Subsequent to this, they form secondary kinetes. These reach the salivary glands and undergo sporogony to start the production of **sporozoites**. Transovarial transmission is also seen in the large *Babesia* species.
- **Humans are accidental hosts** who get infected when they are bitten by infected nymphs and adult female

ticks. The asexual multiplication of the parasite occurs in human RBCs but gametocytes are not formed. Thus, humans are essentially the dead end of the natural life cycle of the parasite. However, it is possible for some transmission to occur from a tick biting an infected person or through blood transfusion.

PATHOGENESIS

The pathogenesis of *Babesia* depends on its ability to invade RBCs. The multiplication of trophozoites in the RBCs eventually causes the intermittent lysis of the latter, which results in hemolytic anemia, jaundice and hemoglobinuria. In addition, there is a release of pro-inflammatory cytokines which may cause direct cell damage as well as fluid extravasation and thereby, hypotension and shock. Patients who have undergone splenectomy, immunocompromised individuals and the elderly have limited capacity to clear the infection and are prone to severe disease.

CLINICAL FEATURES

The incubation period is 1–4 weeks after a tick bite and 1–9 weeks after transfusion of contaminated blood products.

Asymptomatic Infection

About a fifth of adults and half the children infected do not show any symptoms, i.e., they have have asymptomatic parasitemia.

Symptomatic Infection

The clinical manifestations of symptomatic disease range from **mild illness** to a **fulminating, fatal disease.**

Patients usually present with a gradual onset of malaise and fatigue followed by a combination of symptoms such as fever with chills and sweating, fatigue, anorexia, headache and myalgia. There may be hepatosplenomegaly, mild to moderate hemolytic anemia and raised liver enzymes. **The cyclical pattern of repetitive febrile episodes noted in malaria is absent in babesiosis** (Table 14.1). Other features of infection are as follows:

- Patients may also experience nausea, abdominal pain, vomiting, depression, cough and arthralgia.
- The symptoms usually resolve in 1–2 weeks but anemia and fatigue may persist for several months.

Severe Disease

Fulminant disease resulting in prolonged convalescence or death is reported in about 3–10% of cases. The mortality rate can be as high as 20% in patients who acquire the infection through blood transfusion. Individuals who have primary or acquired immunodeficiency or HIV/AIDS, those who have had splenectomies, those who are the extremes of ages (neonates and the elderly) and those with comorbidities are at the greatest risk of severe disease. These patients may present with **complications** such as acute respiratory distress syndrome, pulmonary edema, disseminated intravascular coagulation, congestive heart failure, renal failure, coma or splenic rupture.

B. divergens **is associated with more severe disease than** ***B. microti*****.**

Table 14.1 Difference between babesiosis and falciparum malaria

Feature	Babesiosis	*P. falciparum* malaria
Geographical area	North-eastern and mid-western parts of the United States; less commonly, Europe	Mostly, Africa and South-East Asia
Vectors	*Ixodes* tick	*Anopheles* mosquito
Blood stages	Absence of hemozoin pigment	Hemozoin pigment present
Gametocytes in blood	Same as asexual forms, no banana-shaped forms	Banana-shaped gametocytes
Ring stage	Pear-shaped and present as tetrads in 'Maltese cross' arrangements	Circular; single or multiple rings
Fever	No cyclical pattern due to intermittent release of merozoites	Cyclical pattern due to synchronous release of all the merozoites at once
Parasitemia	Usually low	May be very high
Risk factors	Blood transfusion, immunocompromised state, history of splenectomy	No predisposition for the immunocompromised
Treatment	Chloroquine not effective, atovaquone plus azithromycin is the first line of treatment	Chloroquine or the more current artemisinin combination therapy (ACT) are effective

DIAGNOSIS

The diagnosis of *Babesia* infections is largely based on epidemiological and medical history, physical examination and confirmatory laboratory tests. The laboratory diagnosis is made by demonstrating the parasite in a peripheral blood smear or by molecular tests.

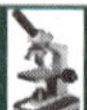

Lab diagnosis

- **Microscopy:** By visualising trophozoites in blood
  - Direct microscopy of peripheral blood film
  - Histopathology: Of biopsy
- **Serology:** IFA, ELISA and western blot
- **DNA detection:** PCR and real-time PCR
- **Animal inoculation:** In mice and hamsters
- **Other diagnostic parameters:**
  - Anemia and thrombocytopenia
  - ↑ LDH
  - Proteinuria and ↑ BUN and creatinine

Microscopy

Trophozoites of *Babesia* may be identified on Giemsa- or Wright-stained thin blood smears (Fig. 14.2a, b and c). These trophozoites are generally seen as ring forms resembling the rings of early-stage *Plasmodium falciparum* trophozoites.

- Multiple thin blood smears should be examined in the early stage of the illness as parasitemia is often low at presentation.
- *Babesia* are distinguished from *P. falciparum* based on the following features:
  - Absence of hemozoin pigment
  - Lack of banana-shaped gametocytes
  - Presence of tetrads (the **'Maltese cross' appearance is pathognomonic**)

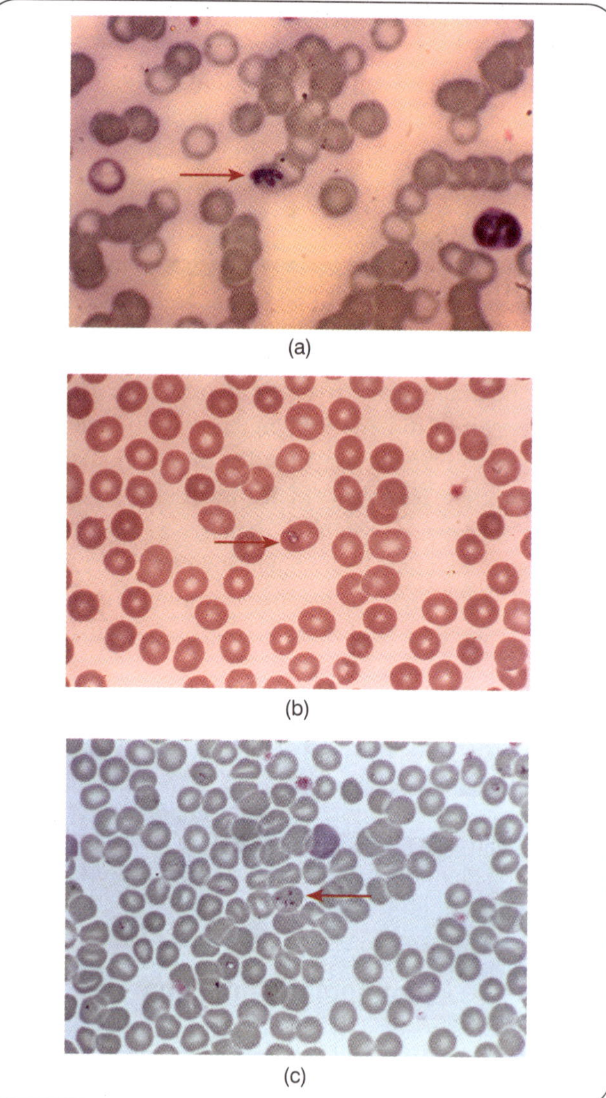

Fig. 14.2 Trophozoites of *Babesia* spp. in blood films resembling those of *Plasmodium* except that they are more pleomorphic, vacuolated and do not produce pigment: (a) tetrad trophozoite, (b) two vacuolated trophozoites and (c) dividing tetrad (*Source:* CDC, PHIL, Image IDs 16362, 15961 and 11090)

Serodiagnosis

The indirect immunofluorescence assay (IFA) is the most widely used serologic test for *Babesia*. ELISA and western blot are also favoured diagnostic modalities. A four-fold rise in *Babesia* IgG titre in acute and convalescent sera confirms recent infection, whereas a single positive test is not confirmatory as it cannot distinguish recent from past infection.

Nucleic Acid-Based Detection

PCR and real-time PCR are more sensitive than blood smears and also provide a molecular characterisation of the *Babesia* species.

Animal Inoculation

The diagnosis can also be confirmed by injecting the patient's blood intraperitoneally into small laboratory animals like mice or hamsters. However, this approach is less sensitive, more time-consuming and more costly.

Other Diagnostic Parameters

The following are also indicators of babesiosis:

- Anemia and thrombocytopenia
- Elevated LDH
- Proteinuria and elevated BUN and creatinine

TREATMENT

First-line drugs (atovaquone plus azithromycin)
- *Atovaquone:* For adults, 750 mg BDS; for children, 20 mg/kg (maximum 750 mg/dose) BDS × 7–10 days
- *Azithromycin:* For adults, 500–1,000 mg on day 1, then 250–1,000 mg × 7–10 days; for children, 10 mg/kg (maximum 500 mg/dose) on day 1, then 5 mg/kg (maximum 250 mg/dose) × 7–10 days

Alternate drugs (quinine plus clindamycin)
- *Quinine:* For adults, 650 mg TDS; for children, 8 mg/kg (maximum 650 mg/dose) TDS × 7 days orally
- *Clindamycin:* For adults, 1.2 g BDS IV or 600 mg TDS orally × 7–10 days; for children, 20–40 mg/kg/day orally in three divided doses × 7 days

In patients with persistent or relapsing disease, a course of at least six weeks is recommended. Treatment is indicated in symptomatic patients or in asymptomatic patients who have a positive blood smear or PCR for >3 months.

PREVENTION AND CONTROL

- Areas where **ticks, deer and mice** are known to thrive, like areas with tall grasses, bushes and forests should be avoided.
- **Protective clothing** sprayed with diethyltoluamide (DEET), dimethyl phthalate or permethrin is helpful in prevention.
- After visiting a bushy area, a thorough search should be carried out to find and remove ticks as soon as possible. Embedded ticks are best removed by using tweezers to grasp the mouth part of the tick without squeezing its body.
- **Those with a history of babesiosis are permanently deferred from donating blood.**
- Although a few vaccines are available for use in cattle, no vaccine is yet available for use in humans.

QUESTIONS

1. Discuss the clinical features, diagnosis and management of babesiosis.
2. Differentiate between the morphological stages of *Plasmodium falciparum* and *Babesia* seen in blood smears.

MULTIPLE CHOICE QUESTIONS

1. Babesiosis is transmitted by the bite of a __________:
   a. Tick
   b. Mite
   c. Bed bug
   d. Louse
2. The vector (*Ixodes*) that transmits babesiosis is also the vector for __________:
   a. Leptospirosis
   b. Lyme's disease
   c. Listeriosis
   d. Plague
3. The treatment of choice for babesiosis is __________:
   a. Chloroquine
   b. Artemisinin
   c. Atovaquone plus azithromycin
   d. Primaquine plus azithromycin
4. Babesiosis is endemic in __________:
   a. Western Africa
   b. Eastern Africa
   c. South-East Asia
   d. North-eastern and mid-western parts of the USA
5. The 'Maltese cross' arrangement of trophozoites is characteristic of __________:
   a. *Babesia microti*
   b. *Trypanosoma cruzi*
   c. *Plasmodium knowlesi*
   d. *Plasmodium malariae*
6. *Babesia* are distinguished from *Plasmodium falciparum* by all the following EXCEPT __________:
   a. Absence of hemozoin pigment
   b. Lack of banana-shaped gametocytes
   c. Presence of ring forms in RBC in tetrads ('Maltese cross')
   d. Presence of band forms

CHAPTER 15

Trypanosoma brucei

([From Greek] *trypanon* = piercing structure + *soma* = body; *brucei* named after the scientist David Bruce)

Case Study and Learning Goals

A 36-year-old male from Gambia presents with lethargy, excessive sleeping during the day and restlessness during the night. He also has a history of on-and-off fever for the last one year. On examination, he is found to have altered mental status and cervical lymphadenopathy. How would you approach the laboratory diagnosis in this case? How would you treat this patient?

GENERAL FEATURES OF HEMOFLAGELLATES

As the name indicates, hemoflagellates live in blood and tissues. Of this group, two genera have significance in human health and disease—*Trypanosoma* and *Leishmania*. The natural transmission of these parasites is by insect vectors. The general cellular organisation follows the scheme of protozoan morphology (Fig. 15.1; also refer to **Chapter 3,** *Protozoa—Introduction and Classification*) and is as follows:

- The nucleus has a central karyosome, the nuclear membrane is lined with chromatin granules and the cytoplasm contains the endoplasmic reticulum, Golgi apparatus and lysosomes.
- A **single flagellum** arises from an invagination of the plasma membrane known as the flagellar pocket. It is either short or runs along the length of the parasite's body. Nearly the entire length of the flagellum lies in a groove and is attached to the cell membrane with filaments. When the flagellum moves, this attachment also moves in tandem, giving it the appearance of an **undulating membrane**.

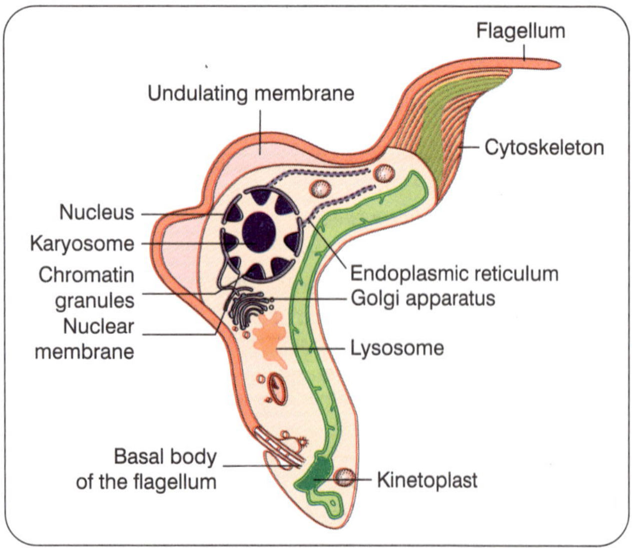

Fig. 15.1 Line diagram of the trypomastigote of *Trypanosoma* spp.

- Below the base of the flagellum lies the **kinetoplast**, which is composed of maxicircles and minicircles of mitochondrial DNA.

The hemoflagellates exist in various intermediate forms depending on the specific biological requirements of the transmission cycle. All these forms may individually multiply by binary fission. The intermediate forms are as follows:

- **Amastigote:** This form exists in vertebrate hosts. It is ovoid with a prominent nucleus and a short flagellum which cannot be seen with light microscopy (Fig. 15.2a).
- **Promastigote:** The parasite exists in this form in insect vectors. It has an elongated body with a long, free flagellum (Fig. 15.2b).
- **Epimastigote:** This form also exists in insect vectors. The epimastigote has an elongated body with a flagellum that arises more posteriorly, but anterior to the nucleus. An undulating membrane is present in this form (Fig. 15.2c).
- **Trypomastigote:** It is pleomorphic and has many intermediate forms which may be seen in both the vertebrate hosts and the insect vector. The cell body is longer with the flagellum and undulating membrane more elongated than they are in other forms (Fig. 15.2d). The kinetoplast and point of origin of the flagellum lie posterior to the nucleus.

The development of hemoflagellates in insects follows one of the following two schemes:

- **Salivaria (anterior station):** After the trypomastigote is ingested by the insect, it develops in the midgut and subsequently migrates to the salivary glands of the insect, e.g., *T. brucei*. In such a scheme, the **insect bite** transmits the parasite to the vertebrate host.
- **Stercoraria (posterior station):** After getting ingested, the trypomastigote develops in the insect's intestine and is excreted with its feces, e.g., *T. cruzi*. Here, transmission occurs when the bite wound is contaminated with the **insect's feces**.

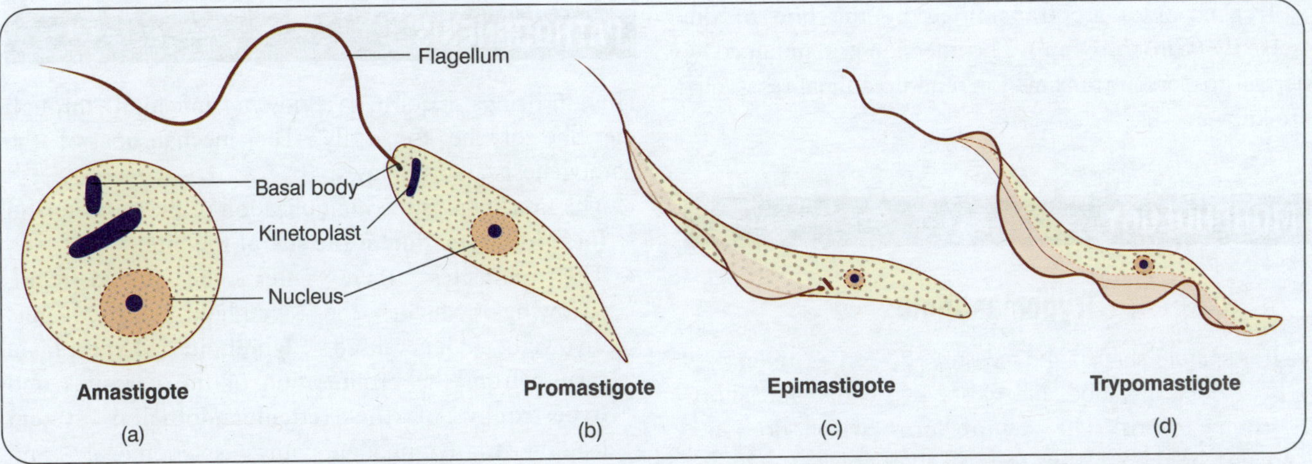

Fig. 15.2 Line diagrams of the morphological stages of hemoflagellates: (a) amastigote, (b) promastigote, (c) epimastigote and (d) trypomastigote

TRYPANOSOMA

INTRODUCTION

Trypanosomes are hemoflagellates of the family *Trypanosomatidae.* These parasites live in the blood and tissues of their vertebrate hosts. They cause two distinct and geographically restricted diseases in humans. These diseases are now included in the WHO's list of **neglected diseases** targeted for elimination.

- **Human African trypanosomiasis (HAT) or sleeping sickness:** This disease is caused by a group of trypanosomes referred to as the *Trypanosoma brucei* complex which is prevalent only in the African continent.
- **American trypanosomiasis or Chagas' disease:** The American trypanosomes include *Trypanosoma cruzi* and *T. rangeli* (non-pathogenic), both of which are prevalent only in South America.

In rare cases, *T. evansi* and a few other zoonotic species are also implicated in human infections. Many other species cause diseases in animals, especially in the African region.

India: Human trypanosomiases of neither of the species present in Africa and America nor their vectors are found in India. However, a few cases of infections caused by ***T. evansi*** (which causes *'surra'* in horses) in veterinarians and some that are caused by *T. lewisi* (of rodent species) and *T. congolense* are reported from various parts of India.

TRYPANOSOMA BRUCEI

INTRODUCTION

Human African trypanosomiasis (HAT) or sleeping sickness is caused by 'Old World trypanosomes'—the *T. brucei* complex which has three morphologically indistinguishable subspecies, namely *T. brucei rhodesiense*, *T. brucei gambiense* and *T. brucei brucei*; of these, only the first two cause HAT.

The lethargy-causing disease was first described in African people by the English surgeon John Atkins in 1721 and by Thomas Winterbottom in 1803. In 1881, Griffith Evans found the parasite in the blood of horses and camels suffering from *surra*. Gustave Simo (1891) was the first to find trypanosomes in human blood. A disease of cattle called *'nagana'*, which is similar to *surra*, was investigated in 1894 by David Bruce who demonstrated that the parasitic forms found in the blood of cattle and horses are the causative agents of the disease and that the tsetse fly may be transmitting it. He also observed that this disease was like the lethargy-causing human disease. In 1909, F. K. Klein demonstrated the importance of the tsetse fly in the life cycle of the parasite.

EPIDEMIOLOGY

Sleeping sickness chiefly affects economically disadvantaged populations in remote rural areas of Africa. It is recognised as a public health problem and is now targeted for elimination by the WHO. The species comprising the *T. brucei* complex differ in their geographical distribution.

- *T. brucei rhodesiense:* Causes sleeping sickness in Eastern Africa.
- *T. brucei gambiense:* Causes sleeping sickness in Western Africa.
- *T. brucei brucei:* It does not cause human disease but causes *'nagana'* in cattle.

Trypanosomes are **transmitted by the bite of the tsetse fly (*Glossina* spp.)**. The infection is maintained by person-to-person transmission, and no animal reservoirs are known.

MORPHOLOGY

Trypomastigote

- It is spindle-shaped and measures 20 × 1–2 μm in size.
- It divides in blood and exists as slender and short, stumpy forms. The stumpy form, which does not divide, is the infective form of the parasite, ready for transmission to the tsetse fly.

Variable surface glycoprotein (VSG) coat: It is a 12–15 nm thick layer of antigenically variable glycoprotein molecules on the plasma membrane which helps the parasite to evade the host immunity. This variation in antigens is achieved by **periodic switching of the *VSG* gene**, whereby only one of the thousand *VSG* genes is expressed at any given time.

LIFE CYCLE (Fig. 15.3a and b)

The various stages in the life cycle of *T. brucei* are as follows:

Vertebrate hosts: Humans and other animals
Insect vector: Tsetse fly

Human cycle: Humans acquire the infection through the **bite of a tsetse fly** which inoculates the human host with the **infective metacyclic trypomastigotes** present in its saliva. The metacyclic trypomastigotes enter the **skin**, undergo morphological differentiation and multiply locally; they can be found in the wound aspirate. These trypomastigotes then enter the **bloodstream, lymph nodes and tissue spaces** and multiply there, after which they can be found in the blood, cerebrospinal fluid and aspirates from tissues and enlarged lymph nodes. The multiplication occurs by binary fission to form slender as well as stumpy intermediate forms. The stumpy forms do not divide and are capable of infecting the tsetse fly.

Vector cycle: When a tsetse fly bites an infected person, the ingested stumpy trypomastigotes transform into procyclic trypomastigotes in the **midgut** of the fly. These then migrate from the midgut to the **salivary glands** (salivaria) where they develop into epimastigotes, which form non-dividing infective metacyclic trypomastigotes in 3–4 weeks. Once infected, a tsetse fly remains infected for life.

PATHOGENESIS

Human beings acquire *Trypanosoma* infections through the bite of the tsetse fly. The mechanisms of the pathogenesis are as follows:

- The first stage is the multiplication of the parasite and **local inflammation at the site of the bite.**
- The parasites then enter the bloodstream, following which, the lymphoid tissue gets involved. Generalised **lymphoid hyperplasia** results from the proliferation of the parasites and **hypertrophy of the reticuloendothelial system** leading to lymphadenopathy, splenomegaly and hypergammaglobulinemia.
- The VSG on the plasma membranes of trypanosomes undergo antigenic variation due to the **periodic switching of the VSG gene** every 5–7 days. This property enables trypanosomes to evade the host immunity. This switching stimulates the production of a different set of antibodies with each antigenic variation and results in hypergammaglobulinemia.
- Human immune mechanisms cannot eliminate all the parasites in the body. Immunopathological phenomena such as autoimmune reactions, thrombocytopenia, disseminated intravascular coagulation and immunosuppression are observed.
- The multiplication of the parasite causes waves of parasitemia and associated **toxemia**. The **invasion of the tissues** causes damage to the endothelial cells of the blood vessels along with granulomatous inflammation and hemorrhages.
- The **invasion of the CNS** is marked by progressive leptomeningitis and inflammation.

CLINICAL FEATURES

The incubation period of trypanosomes ranges from 1–3 weeks. In general, the disease caused by ***T. brucei gambiense* follows a chronic course with slow progression**, whereas that caused by ***T. brucei rhodesiense* runs an acute course with rapid progression** and early death resulting from the involvement of the central nervous system (Table 15.1). If left untreated, both the diseases are fatal.

Chancre: After inoculation into the skin, the metacyclic trypomastigotes multiply and stimulate a local inflammation. A nodule or chancre (measuring 3–4 cm) develops at the site after a few days and resolves spontaneously within 1 to 2 weeks. However, there may be asymptomatic parasitemia for months.

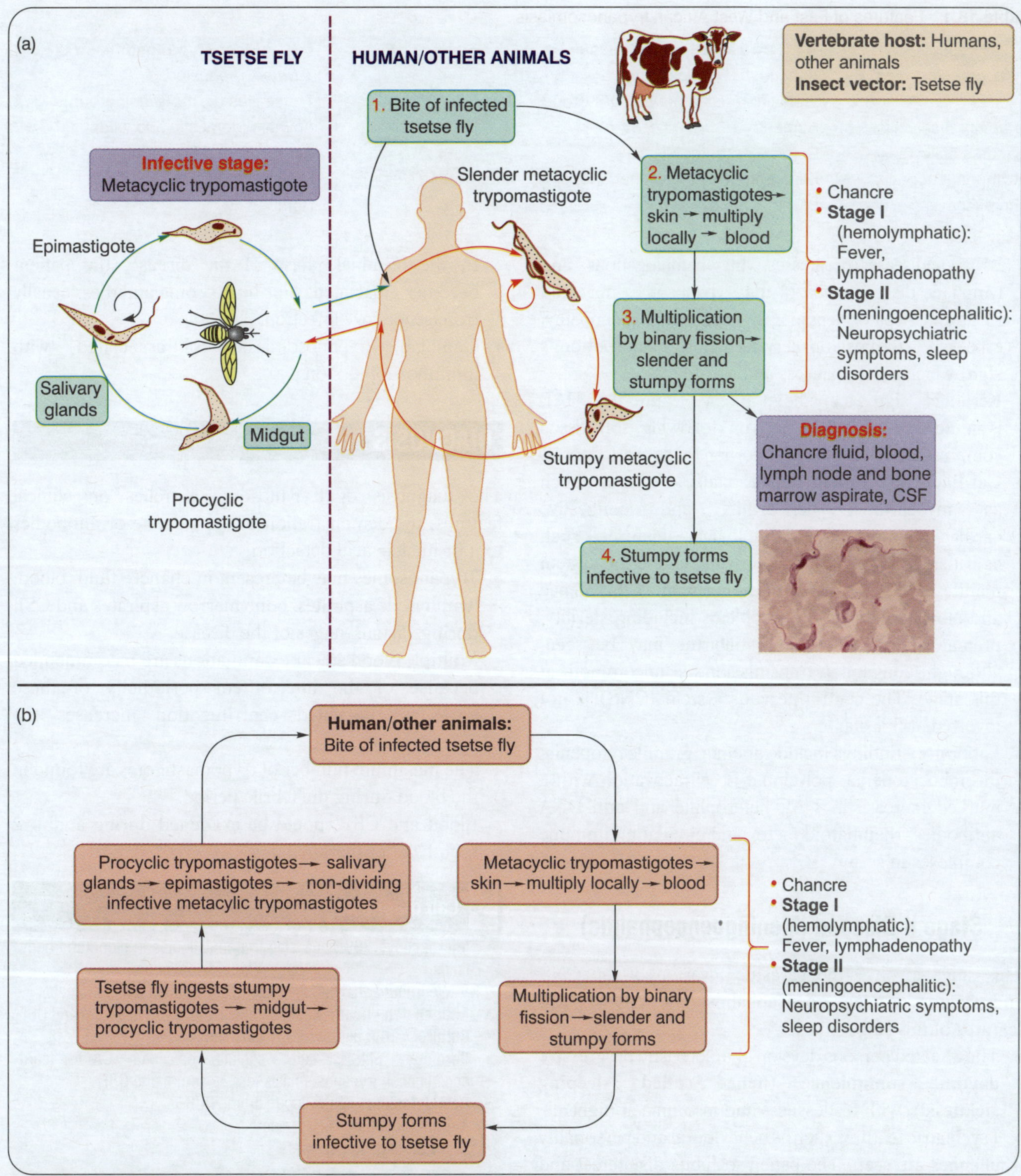

Fig. 15.3 Life cycle of *Trypanosoma brucei*: (a) detailed and (b) schematic (*Source [inset]:* Centers for Disease Control and Prevention [CDC], Public Health Image Library [PHIL]; Image ID 14822)

Stage I Disease (Hemolymphatic)

Classically, symptoms of the early stage tend to be non-specific. The following are features of this stage:

- The disease develops 1–3 weeks after the bite of a tsetse fly. Its symptoms may include headache, malaise, arthralgia, weight loss, fatigue and intermittent fever with rigors, which are often confused with the symptoms of malaria.

Table 15.1 Features of East and West African trypanosomiasis

Features	West African trypanosomiasis	East African trypanosomiasis
Geographical area	*Trypanosoma brucei gambiense*	*T. brucei rhodesiense*
Vector	Tsetse flies (*Glossina palpalis* group)	Tsetse flies (*G. morsitans* group)
Primary reservoir	Humans	Animals (domestic and wild)
Course of illness	Chronic – months to years	Acute – over a few months
Lymphadenopathy	Frequent, cervical lymphadenopathy (Winterbottom's sign)	Minimal (axillary and inguinal)
Parasitemia	Low	High

- As the disease progresses, the hematogenous and lymphatic dissemination of the trypanosomes may lead to fever, hepatosplenomegaly and lymphadenopathy, especially in the posterior cervical region (**Winterbottom's sign**) which is soft, painless and non-tender.
- **Kerandel sign**, a pathognomonic feature of HAT, is a delayed sensation of pain following soft tissue compression that is out of proportion to the exerted force.
- **Cardiac involvement** may cause features such as myocarditis, pericarditis and congestive cardiac failure. Ophthalmological features such as iritis, keratitis and conjunctivitis; endocrine system manifestations like menstrual abnormalities, impotence and alopecia and fertility problems including sterility, prematurity, abortion and stillbirths may be seen, although congenital transmission is uncommon at this stage. The central nervous system (CNS) is **not** involved at this stage.
- Laboratory findings include anemia, granulocytopenia, thrombocytopenia, polyclonal B cell activation with a marked increase in IgM, heterophile and anti-DNA antibodies, rheumatoid factor and circulating immune complexes in serum.

Stage II Disease (Meningoencephalitic)

This stage involves the parasitic invasion of the CNS and progressive meningoencephalitis. The following are features of this stage:

- The affected persons develop characteristic progressive **daytime somnolence (hence called 'sleeping sickness')**, with restlessness and insomnia at night.
- Psychiatric features such as behavioural and personality changes are seen. The patient exhibits disinterest and indifference to the environment and antisocial or aggressive behaviour. Sudden anger and episodes of confusion or delirium are common.
- Myelitis, myelopathy, muscle fasciculation and peripheral motor neuropathy might occur; headache is common. Peripheral reflexes may become positive.
- Trypomastigotes are found primarily in the frontal lobes, pons and medulla. There is progressive leptomeningitis.
- In the terminal phase of the disease, the patient becomes emaciated, slips into a coma and dies, usually from secondary infection.
- Gambian trypanosomiasis is associated with immunosuppression.

DIAGNOSIS

The diagnosis of trypanosomiasis relies on clinical features, the demonstration of the parasite or antibodies to it or nucleic acid detection.

- Trypanosomes may be present in chancre fluid, blood, lymph node aspirates, bone marrow aspirates and CSF during various stages of the disease.
- Multiple blood smear examinations are recommended because of the intermittent periodicity of these parasites. Repeated centrifugation increases the detection rate.
- The maximum number of trypomastigotes are found in the blood during the febrile period.
- Blood and CSF should be examined during and 1–2 months after therapy.

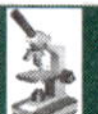

Lab diagnosis

- **Microscopy:** By visualising trypomastigotes in blood and body fluids
  - Wet mount, thin and thick blood films, fluids and buffy coat
- **Antigen detection:** Rapid card test and ELISA in serum and CSF
- **Culture:** KIVI (kit for in vitro isolation)
- **Serology:** ELISA, latex agglutination and CATT (card agglutination trypanosomiasis test) in serum and CSF
- **DNA detection:** PCR and real-time PCR
- **Animal inoculation:** In mice
- **Other diagnostic parameters:**
  - CSF: ↑ proteins, lymphocytosis, ↑ pressure, Mott cells

Microscopy

- **Wet mount:** Highly motile trypomastigotes may be demonstrated on wet mounts of blood or aspirates.
- **Thin and thick films:** Giemsa staining may be performed on fixed thin and thick blood smears or aspirates to demonstrate trypomastigotes (Fig. 15.4).

- **Buffy coat preparations:** Since parasitemia is often low, buffy coat preparations can be used to enhance the sensitivity of detection. The trypomastigotes get concentrated in the buffy coat layer.
- **Microhematocrit centrifugation:** Blood concentration techniques such as using a QBC capillary tube coated with acridine orange are recommended.
- **Mini anion exchange centrifugation:** In this method, trypomastigotes are separated from venous blood using anion exchange chromatography.
- **CSF examination:** The centrifuged deposit of the CSF is examined for the presence of **Mott cells (also called morula or mulberry cells)**. Mott cells are abnormal plasma cells containing large eosinophilic inclusions. Other CSF findings include increased protein level, lymphocytosis and increased pressure.

Serodiagnosis

Antibody detection tests are available in various formats like latex agglutination, card test, ELISA, etc. IgM detection in serum and CSF is of diagnostic value. A simple and rapid card agglutination trypanosomiasis test (CATT) for *T. brucei gambiense* is available for the detection of antibodies in serum. This test, which is highly sensitive but not very specific, is used by field workers in endemic areas for screening. In those found positive, blood and CSF are collected to search for parasites and arrive at a final diagnosis.

Antigen Detection

A simple and rapid card indirect agglutination test is available for the detection of the antigen in serum and CSF in endemic areas. ELISA assays are also available. Antigen detection test in CSF is especially useful to stage the disease. Antigen detection tests are also useful to monitor response to treatment as antigens rapidly clear up post therapy.

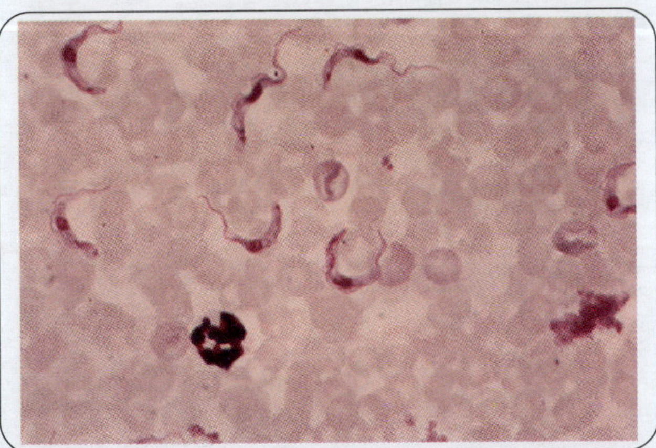

Fig. 15.4 Flagellated trypomastigotes of *Trypanosoma brucei* in a Giemsa-stained thin film blood smear (*Source:* CDC, PHIL, Image ID 14822)

Culture

Samples may be inoculated into KIVI (kit for in vitro isolation) which allows for trypomastigotes to be recovered in 7–10 days. However, culture is not routinely performed, and is only used as a standard for the evaluation of other diagnostic tests.

Nucleic Acid-Based Detection

A number of nucleic acid amplification methods such as PCR, LAMP, NASBA (nucleic acid sequence-based amplification) and FISH (fluorescence in situ hybridisation) are used for diagnosis. These methods reportedly have the ability to detect even a few parasites with excellent sensitivity and specificity reaching 98%. Molecular methods also help to genetically characterise the morphologically similar parasites.

Animal Inoculation

Inoculation of the sample in a mouse model has good sensitivity for the isolation of *T. brucei rhodesiense* but not for *T. brucei gambiense*. However, this method is not commonly employed.

TREATMENT

Trypanosoma brucei gambiense

Early stage (when the CNS is not involved)

- *Pentamidine isethionate:* 4 mg/kg/day IM × 10 days

Late stage (with CNS involvement)

- *Nifurtimox–eflornithine combination therapy (NECT):* Nifurtimox 15 mg/kg/day orally in three divided doses × 10 days PLUS eflornithine 400 mg/kg/day IV × 7 days

Trypanosoma brucei rhodesiense

Early stage (when the CNS is not involved)

- *Suramin:* For adults, 20 mg/kg IV; for children, 10–15 mg/kg IV; the doses are given on days 1, 3, 7, 14 and 21; a test dose is administered before starting the treatment to rule out hypersensitivity to the drug

Late stage (with CNS involvement)

- *Melarsoprol:* 2.2 mg/kg/day IV × 10 days

The treatment of trypanosomiasis is based on symptoms, laboratory findings and whether or not there is CNS involvement. An accurate diagnostic staging to determine whether the disease is early- or late-stage HAT is a crucial issue because the drugs prescribed for the late-stage disease are very toxic.

All drugs currently used for the treatment of HAT are **donated to WHO for free distribution** by the manufacturers, Sanofi and Bayer. All treated patients should be followed-up with twice a year for at least 2–3 years.

PREVENTION AND CONTROL

- **Vector control** should be done by reducing vegetation around human settlements, spraying insecticides and using fly traps.
- **Personal protection** measures such as wearing protective clothing (long-sleeved shirts and long pants) or khaki or olive-coloured clothing (the tsetse fly is attracted to bright and very dark colours) and using insect repellents are also effective.
- Prophylactic treatment should be administered to domestic animals (for Rhodesian trypanosomiasis).
- The WHO assists **National Sleeping Sickness Programmes (NSSCP)** in implementing disease control activities and capacity building through in-service training and workshops at national and international levels. As part of this assistance, the WHO also provides reagents and equipment for screening and diagnosis and drugs for the treatment of trypanosomiasis.
- No vaccine is available yet, the extensive antigenic variation of trypanosomes being the major challenge in preparing an effective vaccine.

Questions

1. Discuss the diagnosis and management of African sleeping sickness.
2. Differentiate between East and West African sleeping sickness.

Multiple Choice Questions

1. Sleeping sickness is caused by ___________:
   a. *Trypanosoma rangeli*
   b. *Trypanosoma brucei*
   c. *Trypanosoma cruzi*
   d. *Trypanosoma amazonensis*
2. Humans acquire *Trypanosoma brucei* infection by the bite of the ___________:
   a. Sandfly
   b. Cat flea
   c. Tsetse fly
   d. Reduviid bug
3. The drug of choice for early-stage *Trypanosoma brucei* infection without CNS involvement is ___________:
   a. Suramin
   b. Ivermectin
   c. Nifurtimox
   d. Miltefosine
4. All the following are features of East African trypanosomiasis EXCEPT ___________:
   a. It is caused by *Trypanosoma brucei rhodesiense.*
   b. It runs an acute disease course of a few months.
   c. Lymphadenopathy is minimal.
   d. Parasitemia is low.
5. Which of the following is NOT a feature of *Trypanosoma brucei* infection?
   a. A chancre is formed at the site of inoculation.
   b. The early stage is characterised by hemolymphatic involvement.
   c. The late stage involves the central nervous system.
   d. The early stage is characterised by megaesophagus and organomegaly.

CHAPTER 16

Trypanosoma cruzi

([From Greek] *trypanon* = piercing structure + *soma* = body; *cruzi* named after the scientist Oswald Cruz)

Case Study and Learning Goals

A 40-year-old male from Brazil presents with fever, headaches and myalgia for the last four days. On examination, he is found to have tender hepatomegaly and his echocardiography shows signs of acute myocarditis. What are the parasitic causes of cardiomyopathy? How would you approach the laboratory diagnosis in this case? How would you treat this patient?

INTRODUCTION

American trypanosomiasis or Chagas' disease is a **zoonotic** disease caused by *Trypanosoma cruzi*, the 'New World trypanosome'. It affects the heart and gastrointestinal tract and is also a significant threat to immunocompromised individuals.

The earliest evidence of Chagas' disease was found in Peru and Chile in mummified bodies dating as far back as 2000 BC. During the period from 1907 to 1912, the Brazilian scientist **Carlos Chagas** described in detail the disease, its causative parasite and its transmission by a bug. Emile Brumpt demonstrated the transmission of Chagas' disease through the feces of the bug in 1912.

EPIDEMIOLOGY

Though Chagas' disease is most common in Brazil and parts of Mexico, the number of cases being reported from non-endemic areas is rising due to population migration. The **triatomine reduviid bug** or **the kissing bug,** which transmits the parasite, thrives in poor housing conditions like mud walls, thatched roofs and surrounding wilderness. The vector species chiefly belong to genera *Triatoma*, *Rhodnius* and *Panstrongylus*. Dogs, cats, raccoons, armadillos, opossums and rodents are important reservoirs of infections.

MORPHOLOGY

The general morphology of *T. cruzi* follows that of trypanosomes (please refer to **Chapter 15,** *Trypanosoma brucei*). The principal difference between *T. cruzi* and other trypanosomes is that it exists in two forms in the human body—trypomastigote and amastigote. The African trypanosomes (*T. brucei*) do not exist in the amastigote stage in humans. However, both species exist in the epimastigote form in their insect vectors.

Trypomastigote

This form is **extracellular** and found circulating in the blood (see Fig. 15.2d in Chapter 15).

- It is spindle-shaped, 16–20 × 2–3 μm in size, with a pointed posterior end. It has a characteristic C or U shape when visualised in peripheral blood films. The kinetoplast is the largest of all trypanosomes and is terminal. The free part of its flagellum extends 2–10 μm beyond the cell body.
- It exists in blood in both long and short forms.
- Trypomastigotes do not divide.

Amastigote

This is an **intracellular** form (see Fig. 15.2a in Chapter 15) found in the reticuloendothelial cells of the lymph nodes, spleen, liver, bone marrow and skeletal, cardiac and smooth muscles, as well as in epidermal cells.

- It is 2–6 μm in size with a large nucleus and a rod-shaped kinetoplast. It is indistinguishable from the L–D bodies of leishmaniasis.
- On entering the cells, the amastigote loses its flagellum and undulating membrane.
- Amastigotes divide by binary fission to form a **pseudocyst**.

Both amastigote and trypomastigote forms are released on the rupture of the cell.

LIFE CYCLE (Fig. 16.1a and b)

Vertebrate hosts: Humans and other animals
Insect vector: Triatomine bug

The various stages in the life cycle of *T. cruzi* are as follows:

Human cycle: The reduviid bug bites human beings when they are sleeping, releasing its saliva into the bite wound; this simulates an itching reaction. The bug also defecates at the site of the bite. Humans acquire the *T. cruzi* infection when the **metacyclic trypomastigotes present in the bug's feces**

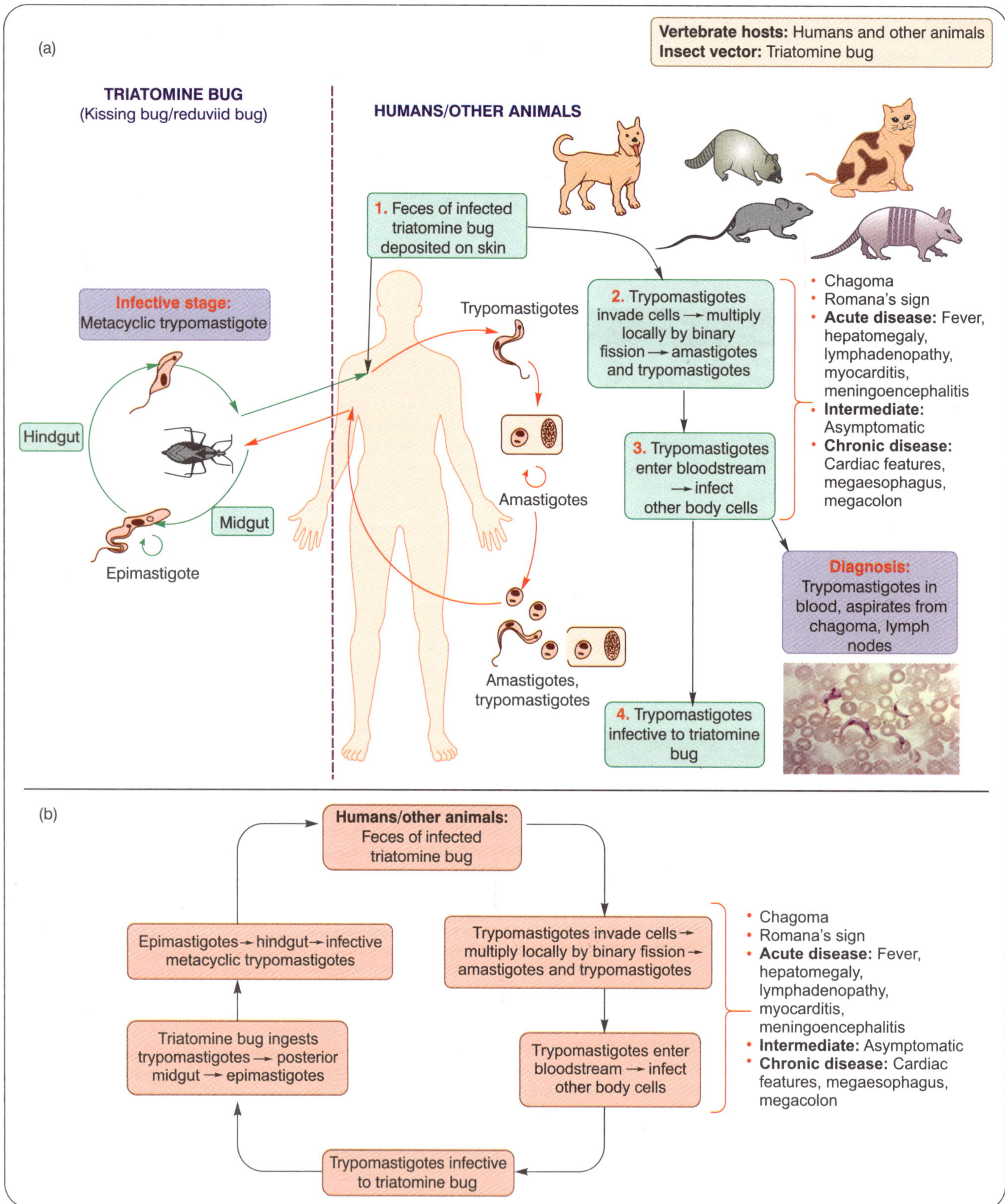

Fig. 16.1 Life cycle of *Trypanosoma cruzi*: (a) detailed and (b) schematic (*Source [inset]:* Centers for Disease Control and Prevention [CDC], Public Health Image Library [PHIL], Image ID 21029)

get rubbed into the bite wound when it is scratched by the host. **Other modes of infection** are as follows:

- Exposure of the mucosa of the eyes and mouth to the feces of the bug
- Accidental ingestion of the bugs or food contaminated with the bug's feces
- Congenital transmission across the placenta or transmission through blood transfusion and

organ transplantation, especially that of the heart

Once the trypomastigotes enter the skin, they are either ingested by the histiocytes or they actively invade the cells, where they metamorphose into **amastigotes**. They continue to multiply locally until the cells reach maximum capacity. Some amastigotes transform into **trypomastigotes**, hence both amastigotes and trypomastigotes are released when the cell ruptures. The amastigotes infect fresh cells and continue the multiplication cycle, while the trypomastigotes enter the **bloodstream** and lymphatics and propagate the infection to other parts of the body. Two forms of trypomastigotes, long and short, are found in the blood. The short, stumpy forms are infective to the insect vector.

Vector cycle: The reduviid bug gets infected by biting an infected person, or rarely, by cannibalising infected bugs. On ingestion, the stumpy trypomastigotes metamorphose into **epimastigotes** which multiply in the posterior part of the bug's midgut. Infective **metacyclic trypomastigotes** develop in the **hindgut** (stercoraria) in 8–10 days.

PATHOGENESIS

The mechanisms of pathogenesis of *T. cruzi* infections are as follows:

- At the site of entry, amastigotes undergo local multiplication in the subcutaneous tissue. This causes inflammation, blockage of the capillaries and edema, and produces a lesion called **chagoma**.
- The amastigote forms can multiply in any cell but have a **predilection for cells of the reticuloendothelial system, cardiac, skeletal and smooth muscle and neuroglia**. Inflammation and pseudocyst formation occur in the affected tissues. The rupture of the **pseudocyst leads to acute inflammation and degeneration of the ganglions** of the adjacent nerve cells. Up to 80% of the ganglions in the heart are lost in the process. This results in the loss of tone of the cardiac muscles and insufficiency of heart function.
- The inflammation, fibrosis and degeneration of nerve ganglions lead to **hypertrophy, loss of tone and flabbiness of the affected organs**. The heart may be enlarged (**megacardia**) with thinning of the myocardium, especially at the apex. The autonomic ganglia of the esophagus and colon become degenerated, resulting in **megaesophagus** and **megacolon** and subsequent loss of peristaltic function.

Autoimmune hypothesis: *T. cruzi* antigens may cross-react with mammalian antigens **(molecular mimicry)**. This theory is supported by the fact that autoreactive antibodies have been detected in infected patients.

CLINICAL FEATURES

The average incubation period of *T. cruzi* is 1–2 weeks. The disease is most common and most severe in children below 5 years of age. The disease syndrome can evolve as acute, intermediate or chronic types.

Chagoma: This is an erythematous subcutaneous nodule which develops at the site of inoculation along with regional lymphadenopathy. It commonly occurs on the face, is painful and gradually subsides over 2–3 months. Subcutaneous edema of the face, legs and feet may be also seen.

Romana's sign: This refers to unilateral edema affecting the eyelids along with conjunctivitis (Fig. 16.2). It occurs when the route of inoculation of the parasite is ocular.

Acute Stage

This stage lasts for 4–8 weeks, after which, the patient either recovers spontaneously or develops chronic infection. The acute symptoms are seen in <1% patients and are characterised by:

- High fever which may be intermittent or continuous
- Myalgia and erythematous rash
- Hepatosplenomegaly and lymphadenopathy
- Acute myocarditis and CNS involvement including meningoencephalitis

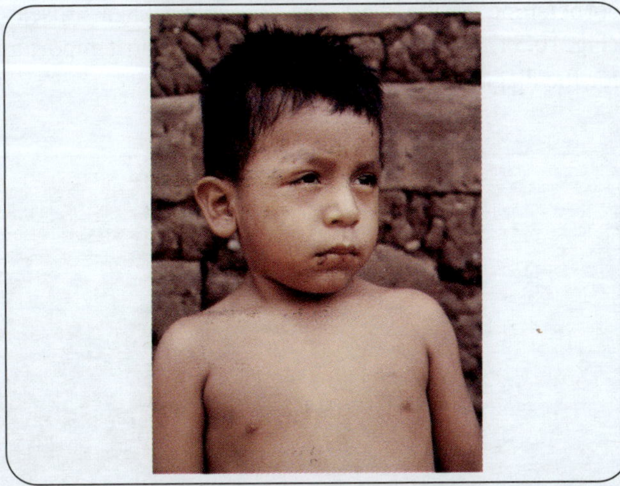

Fig. 16.2 Romana's sign—a child from Panama suffering from Chagas' disease manifesting with the swelling of the right eyelid (*Source:* CDC, PHIL, Image ID 15814)

Intermediate Stage

This stage is asymptomatic. However, the sub-patent parasites in the patient's blood may be transmitted to another person by blood transfusion at this stage.

Chronic Stage

Approximately 30% of patients develop chronic Chagas' disease. It manifests years or decades after the initial infection. The clinical presentations are related to the damage sustained during the acute stage of the disease, the state of the host's immune system and the inflammatory response. The features of this stage are as follows:

- Cardiac features are the most common; these include arrhythmias, chest pain, syncope, cardiomegaly (megacardia), etc. Cardiomyopathy may manifest as sudden death.
- Dilatation of the digestive tract, mainly the megaesophagus, manifests as dysphagia, chest pain and regurgitation. Megacolon manifests as abdominal pain and chronic constipation.

Immunocompromised Patients

HIV-infected patients who have a past history of *T. cruzi* infections are at **risk of reactivation** of Chagas' disease. These patients develop severe multifocal or diffuse meningoencephalitis with numerous tissue parasites. Meningoencephalitis is a rare event in patients who do not have AIDS.

DIAGNOSIS

The **microscopic** demonstration of trypanosomes is the cornerstone of the diagnosis of **acute** Chagas' disease (Fig. 16.3a and b), whereas **serology** is the most important for the diagnosis of **chronic** Chagas' disease.

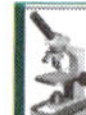

Lab diagnosis

- **Microscopy:** By demonstrating trypomastigotes; it is important in acute disease
- **Antigen detection:** Chemiluminescence immunoassay (CLIA)
- **Culture:** Novy-MacNeal-Nicolle (NNN) medium
- **Serology:** ELISA is useful to diagnose chronic stage and for blood bank screening; radioimmunoprecipitation assay (RIPA) and trypomastigote excreted-secreted antigen immunoblot (TESA-blot) for confirmatory diagnosis
- **DNA detection:** PCR and real-time PCR
- **Xenodiagnosis:** Of reduviid bugs
- **Animal inoculation:** In rats, mice or guinea pigs
- **Others diagnostic parameters:**
  - Chest X-ray and ECG for cardiomyopathy
  - Endoscopy for megaesophagus

Microscopy

- **Wet mount:** Trypomastigotes are present in the blood in acute infections and can be viewed microscopically in wet mounts. The circulating parasite levels decrease rapidly within a few months and are undetectable during the chronic phase. Because of the overlap of the geographic distribution of the two species, *T. rangeli* trypomastigotes (non-pathogenic) have to be differentiated from those of *T. cruzi* (Table 16.1).
- **Stained smears:** Aspirates from chagomas and enlarged lymph nodes can be examined for amastigotes and trypomastigotes by Giemsa staining.

Antigen Detection

Immunoassays are available to detect antigens in the urine and sera of patients with congenital infections and chronic Chagas' disease. A chemiluminescence immunoassay (CLIA) has been developed for blood bank screening and the monitoring of response to treatment.

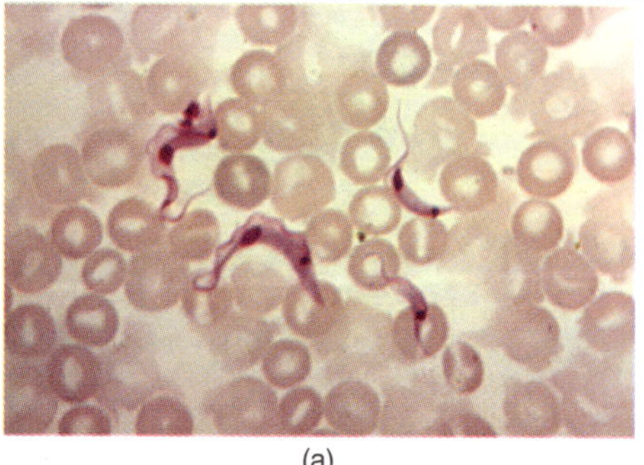

(a)

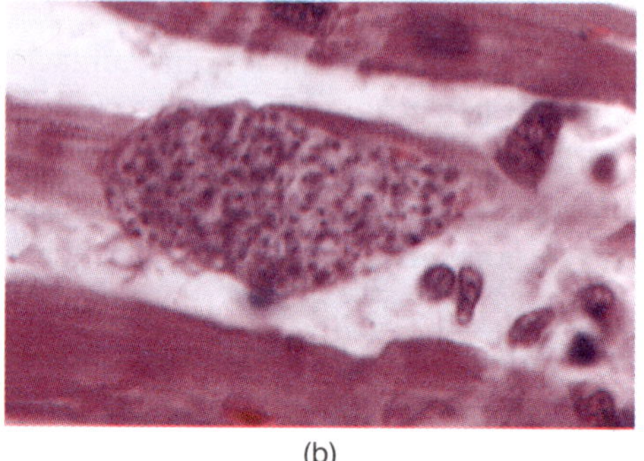

(b)

Fig. 16.3 Features of *Trypanosoma cruzi*: (a) flagellated trypomastigotes, long (left) and short (right) type and (b) a cluster of amastigotes within a striated muscle cell (*Source:* CDC, PHIL, Image IDs 21029 and 21025)

Table 16.1 Differences between *T. cruzi* and *T. rangeli*

T. cruzi	*T. rangeli*
Pathogenic	Non-pathogenic
15–20 μm long	30 μm long, more slender
C- or U-shaped	Not C- or U-shaped
Kinetoplast: Large and terminal	Kinetoplast: Small and subterminal
Primary reservoirs: Opossums, dogs, cats and wild rodents	Primary reservoirs: Wild rodents

Culture

Blood is inoculated in Novy-MacNeal-Nicolle (NNN) medium, incubated at 25°C and observed for the epimastigote forms of *T. cruzi* for up to 30 days before being considered negative. Though more sensitive than microscopy, this method does not help in early diagnosis.

Serodiagnosis

Chronic *T. cruzi* infection is usually diagnosed by detecting IgG antibodies. A highly sensitive antibody-detection ELISA has been developed for blood bank screening and to monitor patients who are undergoing chemotherapy. However, most of these serological tests have low specificity due to cross-reaction with *Leishmania* or treponemes. Various reference tests have also been promoted for confirmatory diagnosis such as radioimmunoprecipitation assay (RIPA) and trypomastigote excreted-secreted antigen immunoblot (TESA-blot), but these also have limited utility.

Nucleic Acid-Based Detection

PCR is useful for the diagnosis of chronic Chagas' disease and neonatal disease and for the monitoring and assessment of patients who have received therapy. It is an efficient modality to differentiate *T. cruzi* from *T. rangeli*. It is reported to have better sensitivity than both microscopy and culture.

Xenodiagnosis

It is especially useful for the diagnosis of chronic disease. Trypanosome-free reduviid bugs are allowed to feed on individuals suspected of having Chagas' disease. If the organisms are present in the blood meal, the parasites multiply and can be detected in the bug's intestinal contents after a few weeks. The time required for this modality limits its usefulness for diagnosing acute disease.

Animal Inoculation

If available, laboratory animals (rats, mice or guinea pigs) can be inoculated with a sample from the patient, and the animal's blood can be observed for trypomastigotes.

Other Diagnostic Parameters

- **Radioimaging and electrocardiography (ECG):** Chest X-ray and ECG are useful for the diagnosis and prognosis of cardiomyopathy.
- **Endoscopy:** The visualisation of megaesophagus also has diagnostic value.

TREATMENT

A few drugs have been attempted for the acute stages with variable efficacy. There is no effective treatment for the chronic stage.

Acute stage
- *Benznidazole:* 5-10 mg/kg/day in 2 divided doses orally × 2-3 months
- *Nifurtimox:* For adults, 8-10 mg/kg/day orally × 3 months; for children 15-20 mg/kg/day × 3 months

PREVENTION AND CONTROL

- **Vector control** using insecticide sprays inside houses is of considerable value.
- **Personal protection** such as insect repellent and mosquito nets should be used.
- **Screening of blood and organ donors** should be done stringently.
- Screening and diagnosis should be done routinely in pregnant women and their children.

Questions

1. Describe briefly the life cycle of *Trypanosoma cruzi*.
2. Discuss the diagnosis and management of Chagas' disease.

Multiple Choice Questions

1. Chagas' disease is caused by __________:
   a. *Trypanosoma rangeli*
   b. *Trypanosoma brucei*
   c. *Trypanosoma cruzi*
   d. *Trypanosoma amazonensis*
2. *Trypanosoma cruzi* is transmitted through the feces of ________:
   a. Sandfly
   b. Cat flea
   c. Tsetse fly
   d. Reduviid bug
3. Megaesophagus is characteristically seen in __________:
   a. Chagas' disease
   b. Sleeping sickness
   c. Mucocutaneous leishmaniasis
   d. Malaria

Chapter 17

Leishmania (Visceral Leishmaniasis)

(*Leishmania donovani* is named after the scientists William Leishman and Charles Donovan)

Case Study and Learning Goals

A 34-year-old male labourer from Bihar presents with low-grade fever and complaints of weight loss and generalised fatigue for the last six months. On examination, he is found to have hepatosplenomegaly and severe anemia. What are the parasitic causes of hepatosplenomegaly? How would you approach the laboratory diagnosis in this case? How would you treat this patient? Detail the elimination programme for this disease.

INTRODUCTION

The protozoa of the genus *Leishmania* are **obligatory intracellular parasites of the reticuloendothelial system** and are responsible for causing a spectrum of diseases called **leishmaniasis**. They are transmitted to the mammal host by the bite of the infected **sandfly, a tiny hopping insect**.

The geographical distribution of *Leishmania* is limited by the distribution of sandfly vectors. The genus has been divided into three subgenera—*Leishmania*, *Viannia* and *Mundinia*. One way to classify leishmaniasis is based on the **geographical distribution** of the parasites, whereby the disease can be classified as 'Old World' and 'New World' leishmaniasis.

The taxonomy of *Leishmania* is controversial and still evolving. In the past, these organisms were classified based on the clinical diseases they caused and the geographic locations in which they were found (Table 17.1). In recent times, however, with the availability of more genetic data, the taxonomic groupings no longer coincide with the recognised disease entities. Around 20 species of the genus *Leishmania* are known to cause the disease.

Subgenera of genus *Leishmania*

- Subgenus *Leishmania*: Development of organisms restricted to the anterior portion of the alimentary tract of the sandfly (*L. donovani*)
- Subgenus *Viannia*: Develop in the midgut and hindgut of the sandfly (*L. braziliensis* complex, *L. guyanensis*)
- Subgenus *Mundinia*: A newly discovered species from the Caribbeans and Thailand (*L. martinique*)

Important species complexes of genus *Leishmania*

- *L. donovani* complex: *L. donovani*, *L. infantum*
- *L. major* complex
- *L. tropica* complex
- *L. aethiopica complex*
- *L. mexicana* complex: *L. mexicana*, *L. venezuelensis*, *L. garnhami*, *L. amazonensis*, *L. pifanoi*
- *L. braziliensis* complex: *L. braziliensis*, *L. peruviana*, *L. colombiensis*
- *L. guyanensis* complex: *L. guyanensis*, *L. panamensis*

Classification based on geographical distribution

- Old World leishmaniasis: Prevalent in Asia, Africa and Europe and transmitted by sandflies of the genera *Phlebotomus* and *Sergentomyia*
- New World leishmaniasis: Prevalent in Central and South America and transmitted by sandfly vectors of the genus *Lutzomyia*

CLINICAL SYNDROMES

Leishmania species produce wide-ranging clinical syndromes—localised or widespread self-healing cutaneous ulcers, destructive mucocutaneous lesions, or fatal systemic disease. These syndromes fall into three broad categories:

- **Visceral leishmaniasis** (also known as **VL, kala-azar, black fever and Dum Dum fever**) is a systemic disease which affects internal organs such as the liver and spleen and typically presents with fever, weight loss, hepatosplenomegaly and pancytopenia. VL is fatal in over 95% of cases if not treated.
    - **Post-kala-azar dermal leishmaniasis (PKDL)** is a clinical condition that presents with skin lesions which manifest after six months or more of apparent cure from VL. It occurs mainly in East Africa and the Indian subcontinent.
- **Cutaneous leishmaniasis (CL)** causes localised or widespread skin lesions. It is the most common form of the disease.
- **Mucocutaneous leishmaniasis (MCL)** affects the mucosal lining of the nose, mouth and throat. It can result in disfigurement, which is linked to social stigma.

Table 17.1 Clinical syndromes and geographical distribution of leishmaniasis

Clinical syndromes	*Leishmania* spp.	Host	Geographical distribution
Visceral leishmaniasis (VL)			
(a) Old World VL	*L. donovani* *L. tropica* (rare)	Humans	Asia East Africa
	L. infantum	Dogs, hares and humans	Mediterranean region and central and western Asia
(b) New World VL	*L. infantum**	Dogs and humans	Latin America
Post-kala-azar dermal leishmaniasis (PKDL)	*L. donovani*	Humans	Indian subcontinent and East Africa
Cutaneous and mucocutaneous leishmaniasis (CL and MCL)			
(a) Old World CL	*L. tropica* *L. major* *L. aethiopica* *L. infantum* (rare)	Humans Hyraxes Rodents	Asia East Africa Central and South America Central Asia, Mediterranean region and the Middle East
(b) New World CL	*L. mexicana* complex *L. braziliensis* complex *L. guyanensis* complex *L. infantum**	Dogs, humans, rodents, hyraxes and opossums	Central and South America
Mucocutaneous leishmaniasis (espundia)	*L. braziliensis* complex *L. mexicana* complex *L. guyanensis* complex	Dogs, humans, rodents, hyraxes and opossums	Central and South America

* In the past, *L. infantum* was designated as *L. chagasi* in the New World; however, with the help of molecular studies, it has now become clear that *L. chagasi* is a sub-population of *L. infantum* and not a separate species.

EPIDEMIOLOGY

Leishmaniasis is largely a zoonosis, although, in certain parts of the world, transmission predominantly follows the human ⟶ vector ⟶ human route. The disease is found in 98 countries in the tropical and temperate belts of the world; this includes developing countries of Asia, Africa, South America and the Mediterranean region of Europe. Of these, 68 countries are endemic for both VL and CL, 9 countries are endemic for only VL and 21 countries are endemic for only CL.

More than 350 million people are at risk of contracting leishmaniasis, and the disease has an overall prevalence of 12 million. More than 1.5 million cases are reported annually, of which 0.7–1.2 million are CL and its variations, and 200,000–400,000 are VL. Human leishmaniasis is on the rise worldwide except in the Indian subcontinent, where a VL elimination programme has been implemented effectively.

MORPHOLOGY

Leishmania exists in two forms—the **amastigote form** (Fig. 17.1a) **in the mammalian host and the promastigote form** (Fig. 17.1b) **in the sandfly vector.**

Amastigote

It is ovoid, measures **2–5 μm in size** and is non-motile. It has a prominent nucleus and a **rod-shaped kinetoplast tangential to the nucleus** which contains thousands of maxicircles and minicircles of mitochondrial DNA. A short axoneme extends from the kinetoplast to the margin of the cell. The amastigote form resides **intracellularly** in the mononuclear phagocytic cells.

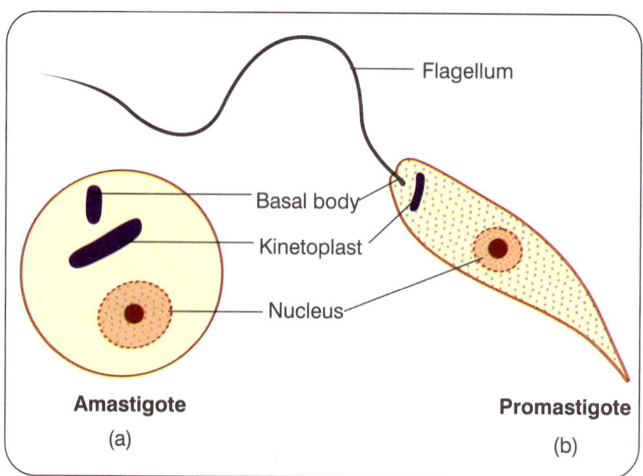

Fig. 17.1 Line diagrams of the two life stages of *Leishmania:* (a) amastigote form and (b) promastigote form

Promastigote

This form is elongated, and measures 15 µm in length. It is **extracellular** and motile with the help of a single long **flagellum,** which lies anteriorly.

LIFE CYCLE (Fig. 17.2a and b)

Vertebrate hosts: Humans and other animals
Insect vector: Sandfly

The various stages in the life cycle of *Leishmania* are as follows:

Human cycle: Humans acquire the infection through the **bite of a sandfly.** The sandfly is a pool feeder, i.e., the appendages in its mouth cut into the skin and create a small blood pool for it to feed. The **infective metacyclic promastigote stages** present in the sandfly's hypostome are thus deposited in the wound. The metacyclic promastigotes are phagocytosed by the **reticuloendothelial cells** and metamorphosed into amastigotes in about 12–24 hours. The amastigotes multiply by binary fission until the cells fill up and rupture. The amastigotes released on cell rupture are phagocytosed by other cells of the body and are infective to the sandfly. It is the macrophages that spread the amastigotes in the body. In cutaneous lesions, the amastigotes remain restricted to the skin.

Vector cycle: When a female sandfly bites an infected person for a blood meal, it ingests free amastigotes and parasitised macrophages. These macrophages disintegrate in a few hours while the amastigotes transform into procyclic promastigotes in the **foregut in 1–2 days (in the hindgut in *L. braziliensis*)** through various intermediate forms. These promastigotes amass in the anterior part of the gut and hypostome of the sandfly as infective metacyclic promastigotes in 1–3 weeks. Thus, transmission continues when the sandfly bites another host. Once infected, a sandfly remains infected for life.

VISCERAL LEISHMANIASIS

The DNA of *L. donovani* has been extracted from Egyptian mummies dating back to about 2000 BC. The disease called kala-azar was first reported in Jessore, India (now Bangladesh), in 1824. However, at the time, it was thought to be a severe form of malaria. In 1903, the parasite was discovered in the spleen of a soldier who succumbed to the disease at Dum Dum in India. The Scottish army doctor, William Leishman, who made the discovery thought of it as a degenerated trypanosome. Around the same time, Charles Donovan, a professor at the University of Madras, independently observed the parasite in a spleen sample collected from a patient suffering from kala-azar. He sought the opinion of Alphonse Laveran, who suggested that it may be a new parasite belonging to the genus *Piroplasma*. Ronald Ross also studied the parasite and concluded that it was a novel parasite and proposed the name *Leishmania donovani*. The intracellular amastigote stage of the parasite was named **Leishman–Donovan (L–D) body** after the scientists who discovered the parasite. The role of *Phlebotomus* in the transmission of kala-azar was demonstrated in 1921 by the Sergent brothers, Edouard and Etienne.

EPIDEMIOLOGY

Visceral leishmaniasis (VL) is caused by the ***L. donovani* complex**, which includes *L. donovani* and *L. infantum* (earlier designated *L. chagasi* in the New World). The causative species of VL in Asia and Eastern Africa is *L. donovani*, whereas *L. infantum* is the causative agent of VL in Central and South America, Central Asia and the Mediterranean region (Table 17.2). Over 95% of the global VL cases are reported from ten countries: India, Brazil, Sudan, South Sudan, Ethiopia, Kenya, Somalia, Nepal, China and Bangladesh.

In the Indian subcontinent and the Horn of Africa, VL affects all age groups. In endemic areas of the Americas and the Mediterranean region, immunocompetent infants and children and immunocompromised adults are affected more commonly than others.

In India, human beings are the only source hosts, and post-kala-azar dermal leishmaniasis (PKDL) patients serve as reservoirs of the infection. In the Mediterranean region, China and Brazil, domestic dogs are considered to be the primary reservoirs of the parasite. In Sudan and Africa, rodents are the main reservoirs of the parasite Thus, **VL is anthroponotic in India but zoonotic in other parts of the world.**

India: In India, VL is most prevalent in the alluvial plains of the river Ganges, a region with temperatures ranging between 15 and 38°C and high humidity. It is most common in economically disadvantaged populations in rural areas where people live in mud houses and keep their livestock under the same roof or in close proximity. Such conditions create a favourable ecological niche for the sandfly vector. Bihar is the most affected state in India, followed by Jharkhand, West Bengal and Uttar Pradesh. The disease has a high incidence in around

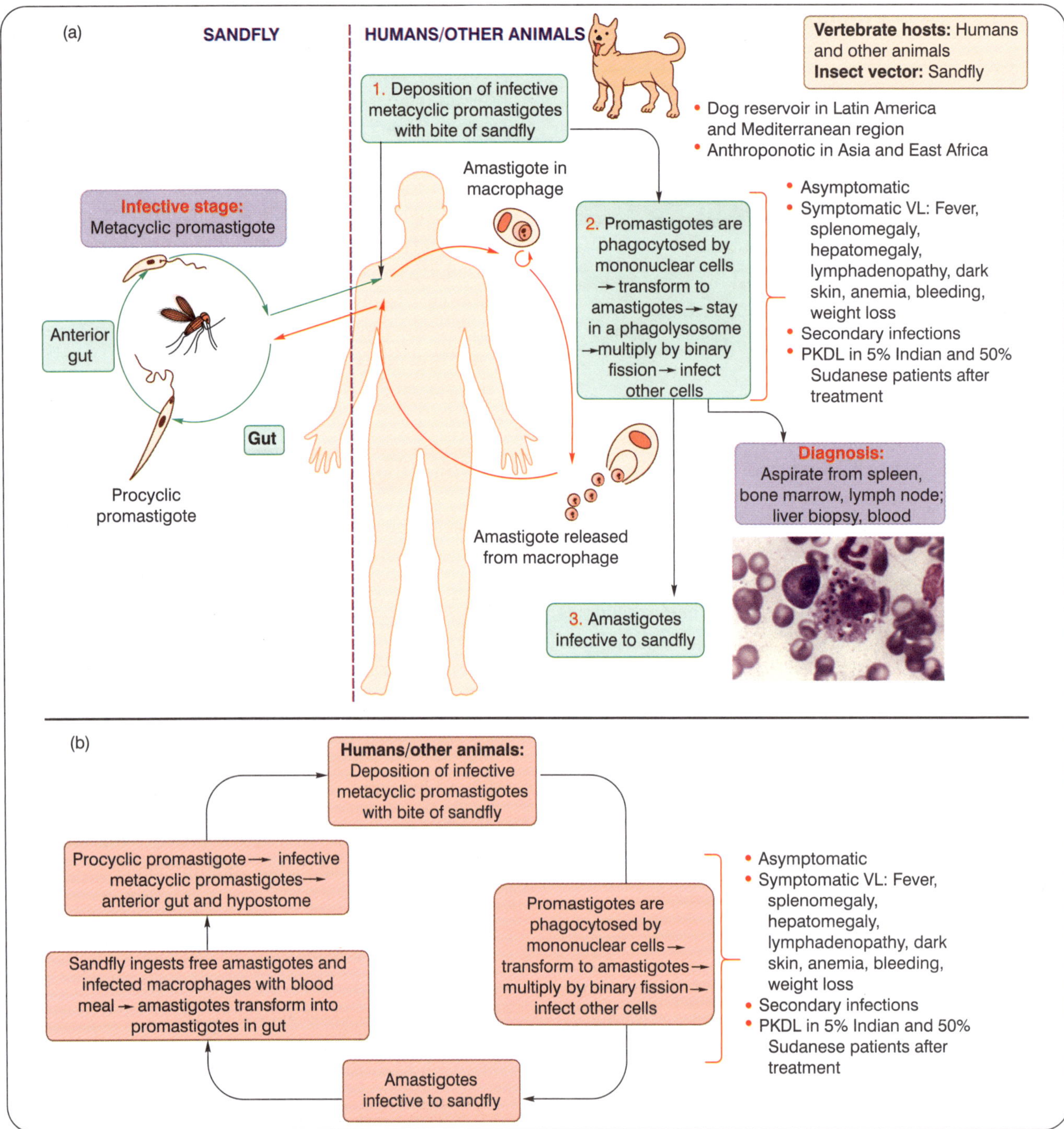

Fig. 17.2 Life cycle of *Leishmania*: (a) detailed and (b) schematic (*Source [inset]:* Centers for Disease Control and Prevention [CDC], Public Health Image Library [PHIL], Image ID 30)

Table 17.2 Infections caused by the *Leishmania donovani* complex

Endemic region	Clinical syndrome	Species	Vector	Transmission
Asia	VL, PKDL	*L. donovani*	*Phlebotomus*	Anthroponotic
East Africa	VL, PKDL	*L. donovani*	*Phlebotomus*	Anthroponotic or zoonotic
Central and South America	VL, CL	*L. infantum*	*Lutzomyia*	Zoonotic
Central Asia, the Mediterranean region and the Middle East	VL, CL	*L. infantum*	*Phlebotomus*	Zoonotic

48 districts with more than 165 million people at risk of contracting the disease. A new focus of the infection has been reported in the sub-alpine valley of the Sutlej river in Himachal Pradesh. The major sandfly vector of kala-azar in India is *Phlebotomus argentipes*. In Himachal Pradesh, *P. chinensis longiductus* has been implicated in the transmission of the disease.

PATHOGENESIS

Leishmaniasis presents with a wide spectrum of clinical manifestations ranging from asymptomatic infection to fatal visceral disease. The mechanisms of the pathogenesis of *Leishmania* infection are as follows:

- **Internalisation:** The intracellular location of amastigotes protects them from the soluble factors of immunity. The promastigotes have GP63 and lipophosphoglycans on their surfaces, which bind to the host receptors on the macrophages and stimulate their opsonization by complement, thus facilitating phagocytosis and spread to other parts of the body.
- **Survival in phagocytes:** A parasitophorous vacuole is formed around the amastigotes which fuses with a lysosome to form a phagolysosome. The amastigote is a very robust structure. It resists the low pH of 5.0 and lytic enzymes of the lysosome and successfully survives them.
- **Pancytopenia:** The accumulation of parasitised reticuloendothelial cells in the organs causes hyperplasia of the spleen, liver, bone marrow, epithelium of the small intestine and lymph nodes. Hematopoiesis is stimulated initially but is eventually depressed. Bone marrow dysfunction, along with the decreased life span of RBCs and WBCs, causes anemia and granulocytopenia.
- **Liver enlargement:** The proliferation of reticuloendothelial cells leads to hepatomegaly. Decreased prothrombin production along with thrombocytopenia leads to mucosal hemorrhage.
- **Spleen enlargement:** Splenomegaly occurs due to the proliferation of reticuloendothelial cells.
- **Hyperpigmentation:** There is an increased level of cortisol and melanocyte production due to the stimulation of adrenocorticotropic hormone (ACTH).
- Concomitant diseases, genetic factors of the host and nutritional status also contribute to the outcome.

IMMUNOLOGY

- The extent of disease progression is determined by the magnitude of the T_{h1} type of immune response early in the disease course. The adequate production of pro-inflammatory cytokines such as IL-2, IL-12, IFNγ and TNFα leads to asymptomatic or self-limiting infection due to the activation of macrophages and reactive oxygen intermediates and nitric oxide-mediated killing.
- Progressive infections show an increase in the T_{h2} type of immune response with increased levels of IL-4, IL-10 and TGFβ and suppression of the T_{h1} response. This suppression allows the parasite to survive, multiply and disseminate. In full-blown VL, there is cellular anergy and suppression of the antigen presentation function of dendritic cells and macrophages. Patients with symptomatic VL have increased non-protective antibody production due to polyclonal activation of B cells; this results in hypergammaglobulinemia.

CLINICAL FEATURES

The **incubation period** of VL ranges from 2–8 months.

Asymptomatic Infection

The majority of the infections remain asymptomatic.

Symptomatic Infection

Only a small fraction of infected individuals in endemic areas eventually develop the disease. However, once it develops, the disease is fatal in >95% of cases if left untreated.

- **Fever:** The most common presentation of VL is an abrupt onset of moderate to high-grade fever associated with chills and rigors. The fever may continue for several weeks and may be of variable patterns—intermittent, remittent with bimodal peaks, or continuous and associated with a loss of appetite, weakness and abdominal protrusion due to hepatosplenomegaly.
- **Splenomegaly:** Soft, non-tender splenomegaly is the most consistent sign of VL. The spleen may become massively enlarged.
- **Hepatomegaly:** Liver enlargement follows soon after splenomegaly with elevated liver enzymes.
- **Lymphadenopathy:** It is commonly seen in most endemic areas of the world except India.
- **Skin changes:** Hyperpigmentation is mostly seen in India and Bangladesh and gives the disease its name—**kala-azar**. The skin of infected individuals becomes dark, dry, thin and scaly with hair loss in the affected areas.
- **Peripheral edema and ascites:** In advanced illness, hypoalbuminemia may manifest with pedal edema and ascites.

- **Hematological abnormalities:**
  - **Anemia** is an early feature and may be severe enough to cause congestive heart failure.
  - A **bleeding tendency** may manifest as epistaxis, gingival bleeding, retinal hemorrhages and gastrointestinal bleed associated with thrombocytopenia and increased prothrombin time.
  - **Hypergammaglobulinemia** occurs due to the polyclonal activation of B cells.
- **Weight loss (cachexia):** Loss of weight and wasting are also seen.
- **Secondary infections:** Other infections such as measles, pneumonia, septicemia, tuberculosis and dysentery may develop in VL patients.

DIAGNOSIS

The approach to the diagnosis of VL is based on the demonstration of the parasite, its antigen or nucleic acid along with a specific serological response.

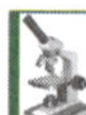

Lab diagnosis

- **Microscopy:** By visualising L–D bodies in mononuclear cells or tissue macrophages
  - Direct microscopy
  - Histopathology: Of biopsy
- **Culture:** NNN medium and modified Tobie's medium
- **Antigen detection:** Immunochromatographic tests and KAtex in urine
- **Serology:**
  - Direct agglutination test (DAT)
  - rK39 (recombinant kinesin) antibody detection
- **DNA detection:** PCR and real-time PCR
- **Skin test:** Montenegro test
- **Other diagnostic parameters:**
  - Hypergammaglobulinemia (aldehyde test)
  - Leukopenia, anemia and thrombocytopenia

Microscopy

It is considered the **gold standard** for the diagnosis of VL. A confirmed diagnosis is achieved by the demonstration of the amastigote form of the parasite (**L-D bodies**) in mononuclear cells in the tissues or macrophages. These forms are best visualised in Giemsa- or Leishman-stained smears (Fig. 17.3a).

The sensitivity of microscopy depends on the sample used. The following can be used for microscopic examination:

- **Splenic aspiration:** It has the most sensitivity (93–99%). However, splenic aspiration is associated with fatal hemorrhage in about 0.1% of the patients.

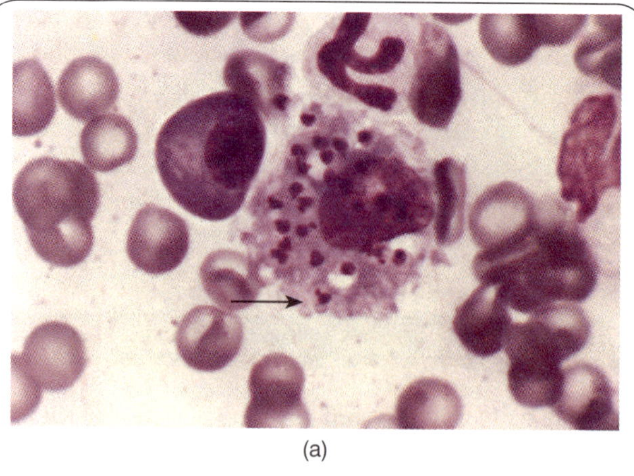

(a)

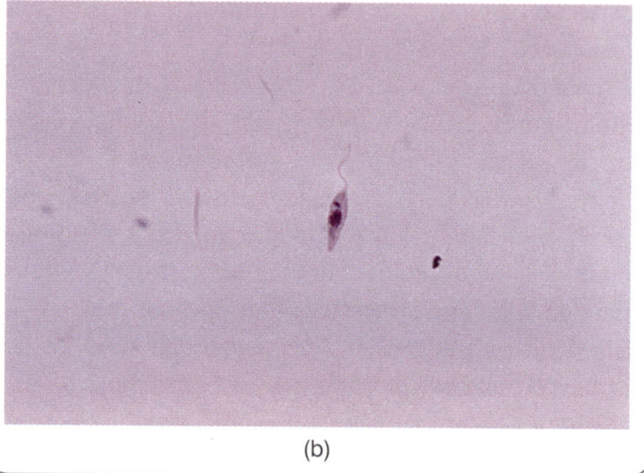

(b)

Fig. 17.3 Features of *Leishmania donovani:* (a) bone marrow smear showing amastigotes (L–D bodies) in a histiocyte and (b) flagellated promastigote form (*Source:* CDC, PHIL, Image IDs 30 and 11073)

- **Bone marrow aspiration:** It has a sensitivity of 65–85% and is safer than splenic aspiration.
- **Lymph node aspiration:** It has a sensitivity of 50–60%.
- **Liver biopsy:** It is about 50% sensitive.
- **Buffy coat from peripheral blood:** It has <50% sensitivity.

Histopathology

L–D bodies may be demonstrated in biopsy specimens after Giemsa staining.

Culture

Clinical samples may be inoculated in biphasic or monophasic culture media, incubated at ambient temperature (22–28°C) and examined weekly for up to four weeks to look for the presence of promastigotes (Fig. 17.3b). Culture is less commonly used as it is tedious and time-consuming and requires expertise. The **sensitivity of culture is**

approximately 70%. The media most suitable for the culture of *L. donovani* are as follows:

- **Biphasic culture media:** Novy-MacNeal-Nicolle medium (NNN) and modified Tobie's medium
- **Monophasic media:** Schneider's insect medium and M199 medium

Serodiagnosis

Numerous serological tests using different antigens have been used for the detection of specific anti-*Leishmania* antibodies. These tests vary in sensitivity and specificity. Some of the commonly used serological tests are the direct agglutination test (DAT), indirect fluorescent antibody test (IFAT), enzyme-linked immunosorbent assay (ELISA) and immunochromatographic tests (ICT).

- **DAT is considered the gold standard for serological tests** for VL diagnosis. The sensitivity and specificity of DAT range from 70–100% and 55–100%, respectively.
- Several recombinant antigens have been used for the diagnosis of VL in ICT and ELISA formats.
- Antibody detection against **recombinant kinesin antigen (rK39)** is the most useful test with a sensitivity of 70–100% and a specificity of 95–100%. ICT (dipstick) using rk39 antigen is the most common **point-of-care** test used in clinical practice in India. Anti-rK39 antibodies have also been detected in urine and sputum.
- Other antigens like rk28 and rk16 have been reported to have better sensitivity in Sudan (92–100%).

Drawbacks:

- Anti-*Leishmania* antibodies remain detectable for months or even years after the patient has been treated. Therefore, they cannot be used to assess recovery or to detect relapse.
- In cases of *Leishmania*–HIV coinfection, serology is less sensitive for the detection of antibodies due to the immunodeficiency produced by HIV.
- In endemic areas, healthy individuals may test positive due to asymptomatic infection.

Leishmanin Skin Test (Montenegro Test)

This test detects delayed hypersensitivity to the purified parasite antigens inoculated intradermally. It is negative in patients with active kala-azar but becomes positive within two months of successful treatment. The test is slowly becoming obsolete.

Antigen Detection

The detection of the 15–20 kDa glycoprotein antigen of *Leishmania* in urine **(KAtex)** is a simple and rapid point-of-care test. It is shown to have a moderate sensitivity (48–87%) and good specificity (89–100%), especially in Nepal.

Advantages:

- It may be useful for the diagnosis of primary VL, for monitoring the efficacy of treatment, and for the detection of subclinical infections.
- It has better sensitivity and specificity in immunocompromised patients.

Drawbacks:

- It has poor sensitivity (48–87%).
- The antigen may be detectable up to six months after treatment, so it cannot be used to assess recovery/cure.

Nucleic Acid-Based Detection

Molecular techniques like PCR, qPCR, NASBA and LAMP are gaining popularity due to their remarkable sensitivity and specificity and because these tests can be performed on any sample. Many genetic targets, especially the transcribed internal spacer (*ITS1*) region and kinetoplast DNA (*kDNA*) have been targeted with these tests.

Advantage:

- These tests enable species and subspecies identification for diagnostic and epidemiological studies.
- They can distinguish between relapse and reinfection.
- They have better sensitivity than other methods.

Animal Inoculation

Specimens can also be inoculated into laboratory animals such as hamsters, mice, guinea pigs or rodents to look for signs of pathology, but it takes months to obtain a positive result.

Other Diagnostic Parameters

- **Aldehyde/antimony test:** Patients with kala-azar have hypergammaglobulinemia which can be detected using a number of tests. However, this method has poor sensitivity and specificity. The following two tests are generally used for this purpose:
  - **Formol-gel (Napier's aldehyde) test:** When the patient's serum is mixed with concentrated 40% formalin solution, it whitens and becomes gelatinous in 20 minutes to 2 hours. This test is usually negative in the first three months of infection. False positivity may be seen in conditions such as chronic liver disease, malaria, chronic myeloid leukemia or other conditions associated with hypergammaglobulinemia.

- **Chopra's antimony test:** The patient's serum is mixed with 4% urea stibamine solution. A positive test is indicated by the appearance of profuse flocculation.

- **Hematological indicators:**
  - Normocytic and normochromic anemia
  - Leukopenia and thrombocytopenia
  - Hypergammaglobulinemia; high globulin levels, even up to 9 g/dl and a high ratio of globulin to albumin
  - Elevated ESR
  - Raised serum hepatic aminotransferases

TREATMENT

Drugs of choice

- *Amphotericin:* Liposomal amphotericin B, 10 mg/kg in a single dose by infusion or 3 mg/kg daily on days 1 to 5, 14 and 21 (total dose 10–15 mg/kg)
  OR
- *Amphotericin B deoxycholate*: 0.5–1 mg/kg per day by infusion, daily or on alternate days × 15–20 doses
  (This is currently the recommended first-line treatment in Bihar, India.)
- *Miltefosine:* For adults, 100 mg/day orally; for children, 2.5 mg/kg/day orally × 28 days
- *Pentavalent antimonial sodium stibogluconate (Sb^V):* 20 mg/kg/day IM or IV × 20–28 days; cure rates are >90% in Africa, the Americas and most of the Old World but are <50% in India due to drug resistance
- *Combination (co-administered) therapy:* Miltefosine 2.5 mg/kg/day orally plus paromomycin 11 mg/kg/day IM, both daily for 10 days

Alternate drug

- *Pentamidine:* 2–4 mg/kg/day IV or IM, up to 15 doses

Adjuvant immunotherapy

- IFNγ in combination with pentavalent antimony has been used with success

Miltefosine is the first oral drug approved for leishmaniasis. Currently, due to the threat of the emergence of drug resistance, monotherapy with miltefosine is discouraged.

Drug Resistance

Since the 1920s, antimonial compounds (sodium stibogluconate [SSG]) were the primary drugs employed against leishmaniasis. However, resistance to SSG has now become widespread, especially in the **Indian subcontinent**. Despite this, these drugs are still in use in other regions of the world, including Latin America and East Africa, where they are still effective. The most important reason for the development of drug resistance is inadequate or improper use of antimonials. In areas where resistance to SSG is reported, liposomal amphotericin or miltefosine are used instead. In recent times, resistance to miltefosine has also been reported, especially from Nepal.

- **Mechanism of resistance to SSG:** Resistance occurs due to the failure of reduction of SbV, the prodrug, to its active form SbIII inside the resistant *L. donovani* amastigotes.
- **Rescue treatment in case of non-response:** Conventional amphotericin B deoxycholate infusions or liposomal amphotericin B at higher doses can be used for longer durations.

VL IN IMMUNOSUPPRESSED PATIENTS

HIV and *Leishmania* co-localise and interact in the same host cells (macrophages and dendritic cells), mutually reinforcing each other's pathogenic effects. VL in immunosuppressed patients who have HIV, those who have had solid organ transplant and those who are malnourished is challenging with respect to diagnosis, treatment and outcome of the disease.

AIDS PATIENTS

HIV and *Leishmania* affect each other's pathogenesis. Individuals who have *Leishmania*–HIV coinfections are more likely to develop the full-blown clinical disease. Patients may have typical or atypical manifestations, some of which may even involve the respiratory or gastrointestinal organs. Splenomegaly may be absent. The relapse and mortality rates are reported to be higher in cases of such coinfections. VL usually manifests when the CD4 T cell count falls below <200/µl in a patient with HIV. PKDL is reported to be more frequent in immunosuppressed individuals.

Effect of *Leishmania* on HIV

Leishmania appears to cause the activation of latent HIV. An increased expression of chemokine receptors (CCR5) is seen on the macrophages, which facilitates the entry of HIV into the cells.

Effect of HIV infection on *Leishmania*

HIV causes the activation of T_{h2} cell response, which results in disease progression. *Leishmania* uptake is enhanced by HIV-infected macrophages.

Diagnosis

A combined approach of microscopy, culture and nucleic acid-based tests is the most sensitive in an immunocompromised host. Serodiagnostic tests may be negative in up to 50% of patients.

Treatment

Ten doses of liposomal amphotericin B, administered as 4 mg/kg on weekly intervals (a total dose of 40 mg/kg) produce good results. VL is an AIDS-defining condition, requiring HAART irrespective of CD4 counts. Antiretroviral treatment arrests the disease development, delays relapses and increases the chances of the patient's survival.

POST-KALA-AZAR DERMAL LEISHMANIASIS (PKDL)

The shift in parasite tropism from visceral organs to the skin after an apparent cure from VL makes PKDL a peculiar phenomenon (Table 17.3). It is chiefly associated with *L. donovani* and rarely with *L. infantum*. Sometimes, PKDL is reported without a prior history of VL. Its pathogenesis is probably immunologically mediated.

PKDL is seen in 5–10% of patients in the Indian subcontinent (predominantly in Bangladesh and India) and 50% of cases in Sudan. It is rarely reported from other parts of the world.

CLINICAL FEATURES

It chiefly presents as hyper- or hypo-pigmented macules and papules resembling those of leprosy. The lesions do not ulcerate. PKDL may also present as nodular lesions in HIV patients. The lesions are chiefly found on the face, but may also be found on the extremities, trunk, oral mucous membranes, etc. The preservation of sensation in the lesions of PKDL differentiates it from leprosy. These **lesions serve as reservoirs for the continued transmission** of the parasite.

DIAGNOSIS

Microscopy

L–D bodies can be detected in skin smears in about 80% of the cases. The sensitivity of this modality can be increased by using *Leishmania*-specific monoclonal antibodies in an immunohistochemistry (IHC) assay.

Culture

This is considered the **gold standard** for the diagnosis of PKDL.

Serological Tests

DAT and antibodies to rK39 antigen are positive in many cases; however, these tests may be negative in immunocompromised patients.

Nucleic Acid-Based Detection

DNA detection yields good sensitivity and specificity.

TREATMENT

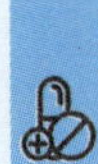

- *Miltefosine:* 150 mg/day orally × 12 weeks
- *Amphotericin B deoxycholate:* 1 mg/kg/day by infusion, up to 60–80 doses over 4 months
- *Liposomal amphotericin B:* 2.5 mg/kg/day IV × 20 days

Table 17.3 Features of post-kala-azar dermal leishmaniasis

Features	Indian subcontinent PKDL	East African PKDL
Incidence among VL patients	5–10%	About 50%
Interval between VL and PKDL	6 months to 10 years after VL treatment	Within 6 months
Persistence of lesions	Long, even for up to 20 years	Few months
Treatment	Required	Generally not required
Disease course	Resolves slowly	Usually gets cured spontaneously

PKDL requires treatment for a longer duration than VL.

PREVENTION AND CONTROL

- The **treatment of VL and PKDL patients** is the mainstay of controlling the spread of these infections.
- The **treatment of animal reservoirs** like dogs and rodents is not practically feasible and has the risk of resulting in the emergence of drug resistance. Dog collars treated with deltamethrin can reduce the risk of infection by sandflies.
- **Personal prophylaxis** includes insect repellents, bed nets and curtains or wire meshes on doors and windows.
- **Indoor residual spraying** of insecticides in the house is effective.
- Habitats of animal reservoirs should be avoided.
- *Phlebotomus* flies do not fly very high above the ground (rather, they hop from one point to another) and are nocturnal in their habits. For this reason, sleeping above ground level helps in avoiding the insect's bites.
- No vaccine is currently available for leishmaniasis but clinical trials on the same are ongoing.
- The Government of India launched the Kala-azar Elimination Programme in 1990–91 (also see **Chapter 57**, *Control Programmes for Parasitic Diseases*) to eliminate the disease from the country.

QUESTIONS

1. Discuss the pathogenesis of visceral leishmaniasis.
2. Discuss the diagnosis and management of visceral leishmaniasis.
3. Discuss post-kala-azar dermal leishmaniasis.

MULTIPLE CHOICE QUESTIONS

1. The vector of kala-azar (visceral leishmaniasis) is ___________:
   a. Tsetse fly b. Reduviid bug
   c. Sandfly d. Mansonoides
2. The diagnosis of visceral leishmaniasis is made by all the following EXCEPT ___________:
   a. Microscopy of splenic/bone marrow aspirates
   b. Culture in non-nutrient agar (NNA) medium
   c. Antibody detection by rk39 antibodies
   d. Polymerase chain reaction
3. Visceral leishmaniasis is caused by the following species ___________:
   a. *L. donovani* b. *L. braziliensis*
   c. *L. aethiopica* d. *L. major*
4. Which of the following statements is NOT TRUE about post-kala-azar dermal leishmaniasis?
   a. It is more common in patients with untreated visceral leishmaniasis
   b. It appears 6 months to 10 years after VL treatment in the Indian subcontinent
   c. Lesions may persist for long periods, sometimes even up to 20 years
   d. It requires treatment, especially in the Indian subcontinent
5. Miltefosine is a drug approved for the treatment of ___________:
   a. Toxoplasmosis b. Visceral leishmaniasis
   c. Malaria d. Syphilis
6. The first line of treatment for kala-azar in India is ___________:
   a. Antimonial stibogluconate b. Miltefosine
   c. Amphotericin B d. Paromomycin
7. Which of the following statements is NOT TRUE about visceral leishmaniasis in India?
   a. It is an anthroponotic disease.
   b. It is endemic in Bihar and a few adjoining regions and has a focus in Himachal Pradesh.
   c. Post-kala-azar dermal leishmaniasis is reported in about 5–10% of patients in India.
   d. Antimonial stibogluconate is the treatment of choice.
8. Montenegro skin test is used for the diagnosis of ___________:
   a. Toxoplasmosis
   b. Visceral leishmaniasis
   c. Malaria
   d. Syphilis
9. Demonstration of L–D bodies in ___________ sample is most sensitive for the diagnosis of visceral leishmaniasis.
   a. Liver aspirate
   b. Lymph node aspirate
   c. Splenic aspirate
   d. Bone marrow aspirate
10. Which of the following statements is NOT TRUE about the serodiagnosis of visceral leishmaniasis?
    a. Rk39 is the most commonly used point-of-care test.
    b. Direct agglutination test is considered the gold standard for VL diagnosis.
    c. Anti-leishmanial antibodies are the most useful to assess cure or to detect relapse.
    d. In HIV patients, *Leishmania* serology is less sensitive due to immunodeficiency.

Chapter 18

Leishmania (Cutaneous and Mucocutaneous Leishmaniasis)

Case Study and Learning Goals

A 28-year-old male from Bikaner, Rajasthan, presents with a painless ulcerative lesion on his face. What are the parasitic causes of ulcerating lesions? How would you approach the laboratory diagnosis in this case? How would you treat this patient?

INTRODUCTION

Cutaneous leishmaniasis (CL), which affects the skin, is a **disfiguring disease** in which the parasites invade mononuclear cells in the skin but not the viscera. The parasite's morphology and life cycle are similar to those of *Leishmania donovani* with slight variations in sizes and vectors according to the causative species. Another difference is that in CL, the **amastigotes remain confined to the skin**.

The cutaneous forms of leishmaniasis are as follows:

- **Localised cutaneous leishmaniasis (LCL):** It is characterised by localised ulcers and lesions on the exposed parts of the body that leave permanent scars.
- **Diffuse cutaneous leishmaniasis (DCL):** This is characterised by multiple nodules all over the body without ulceration. It is a rare disease.
- **Mucocutaneous leishmaniasis (MCL):** In this disease, the lesions spread to the mucosa of the nose, mouth and pharynx.

CUTANEOUS LEISHMANIASIS

CL is the most common form of leishmaniasis. The typical skin lesions associated with this disease have been known by different names across the world. Arab physicians of the 10th century were the first to describe these classical lesions, which they called **Balkh sores.** Over the years, depending on where they were recorded, these lesions have been called **Oriental sores, Baghdad boils, Jericho boils, Delhi boils** and **Aleppo boils** in different parts of the **Old World.** In the **New World**, these lesions were known as **chiclero ulcers (or bay sores).**

Cutaneous lesions resembling those of leishmaniasis have been described in ancient Assyrian literature from the 7th century BC; it is believed likely that these descriptions were derived from even more ancient texts, possibly dating as far back as 1500 to 2500 BC. In the New World, the lesions are evident in sculptures from the 5th century. The parasite that causes this disease was probably first seen in 1885 by D. D. Cunningham in a Delhi boil and in 1898 by Peter Borovsky, but neither of them recognised it. It is J. H. Wright who is credited with discovering the parasite in 1903 and describing it in detail. The different species and vectors of the Old and New World parasites were subsequently discovered.

EPIDEMIOLOGY

About 95% of CL cases occur in the Central and South Americas, the Mediterranean region, the Middle East and Central Asia—chiefly, Afghanistan, Algeria, Brazil, Columbia, Iran, Iraq and Syria. CL is classified into Old World CL and New World CL (Table 18.1) as follows:

- **Old World CL:** It is usually a sporadic disease in areas endemic to it, but epidemics have also been known to occur. The sandfly ***Phlebotomus*** acts as a vector for the parasite. The disease is usually anthroponotic or

Table 18.1 Agents of cutaneous leishmaniasis (CL)

Type of CL	Etiological agents	Vector	Reservoirs	Geographical distribution
Old World CL	*L. tropica* *L. major* *L. aethiopica* *L. infantum*	*Phlebotomus*	Anthroponotic or zoonotic (rodents, dogs and hyrax)	Asia, East Africa, Central and South America, Central Asia, the Mediterranean region and the Middle East
New World CL	*L. mexicana* complex *L. braziliensis* complex *L. guyanensis* complex *L. infantum*	*Lutzomyia*	Zoonotic (forest rodents)	Central and South America

zoonotic. In the 1990s, there was a major outbreak of anthroponotic CL in war-ridden Kabul, Afghanistan; the epidemic affected thousands. The entity also took a viscerotropic form affecting the spleen and lymph nodes in a small group of American military personnel who were infected in the Persian Gulf War in 1991.

India: CL in India is mainly caused by *L. tropica* and *L. major* and is reported chiefly from Rajasthan. Some cases have also been reported from states in the dry north-western half of the Indo-Gangetic plain, including Punjab, Himachal Pradesh, Delhi, Uttar Pradesh and even Jammu and Kashmir.

- **New World CL:** It is a zoonotic disease seen in persons working around the forest fringes or in travellers or military personnel returning from endemic areas. The sandfly vector of this disease belongs to the genus ***Lutzomyia***.

PATHOGENESIS

Malnourished and immunosuppressed persons are at a higher risk of developing lesions of CL; however, genetic factors of the host may also play a role in the pathogenesis of the disease. Different types of cutaneous lesions may develop as follows:

- **'Wet' lesions:** These are caused by *L. major*. This type of disease is characterised by numerous lesions. A 'wet' lesion has a necrotic and exudative centre over a granulomatous base.
- **'Dry' lesions:** These are caused by *L. tropica*. These lesions are less necrotic with lesser exudate. Unlike the 'wet' type, only a few lesions are formed in the 'dry' type.
- **Diffuse cutaneous leishmaniasis (DCL):** It is characterised by the lack of both cell-mediated and humoral immune responses, which results in the uncontrolled multiplication and spread of the parasites over a wide area.
- **Leishmania recidivans (LR):** It is associated with a strong cell-mediated immune response.

Typically, there are no systemic manifestations of CL, but there may be regional lymphadenopathy of the affected site. The ulcers may be superinfected by bacteria.

CLINICAL FEATURES

The incubation period ranges from a few days to weeks. The skin lesions (Fig. 18.1) may be few and localised or diffuse. The following are the typical clinical features of the CL:

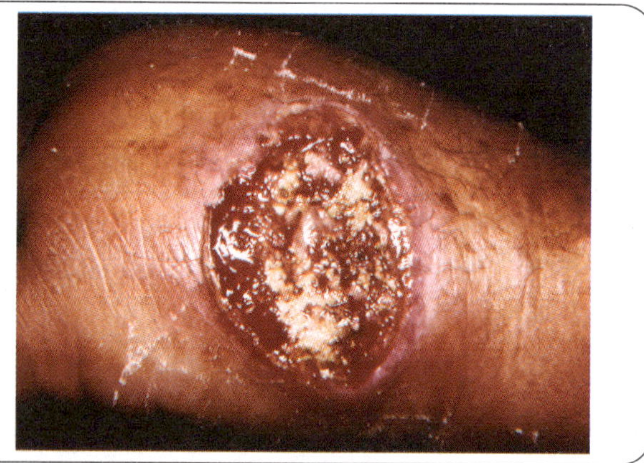

Fig. 18.1 Cutaneous leishmanial lesion (*Source:* Centers for Disease Control and Prevention [CDC], Public Health Image Library [PHIL], Image ID 17625)

- A few days or weeks after the bite of a sandfly, a **painless papule** develops, which enlarges over a period of several days to weeks to form a nodule that commonly ulcerates. The development of lesions is commonly preceded by lymphatic spread and involvement of the lymph nodes. Most patients have one or two lesions varying in size from 0.5–3 cm in diameter, usually on the exposed parts of the body such as the face, arms or legs. Pain is typically absent despite significant destruction of tissue.
- The lesions usually heal spontaneously after 2–15 months but may cause significant disfigurement before healing. However, once healed, it leads to lifelong immunity. CL lesions on the exposed body parts may lead to permanent scar formation which causes social stigmatisation, anxiety and depression. This, in turn, may affect the quality of life of CL patients.
- The lesions caused by *L. major* are multiple, exudative and associated with severe inflammation; these lesions are slow to heal. They are associated with severe scarring if left untreated.
- The lesions of *L. tropica* are usually multiple, dry and painless, and usually self-heal in less than a year.
- In *L. braziliensis* and *L. guyanensis* infections, single or multiple ulcerating lesions are seen. These heal by themselves. Diffuse or disseminated cutaneous lesions may also be seen. Lymphadenopathy may precede the development of cutaneous lesions. Healing is usually followed by immunity to reinfection with that particular species of the parasite. About 2.5% of these cases may progress to involve the mucosa, which results in the development of MCL.
- **Chiclero ulcers**, seen in Central America, are caused by *L. mexicana*. The lesions are characterised by persistent ulcerations on the pinna. These lesions are

usually seen in individuals who live in forests to collect chewing gum latex (by harvesting **chicle** plants).

Leishmaniasis recidivans (LR): In this form of CL, which is caused by *L. tropica*, small, non-ulcerating lesions develop in the periphery of a healed sore. These may extend to cause gross disfiguration.

Diffuse cutaneous leishmaniasis (DCL): It is a rare form of leishmaniasis caused by *L. amazonensis* and *L. mexicana* in South and Central America (New World) and by *L. aethiopica* in Ethiopia and Kenya (Old World). It presents as multiple non-tender, non-ulcerating papules and nodules resembling those of lepromatous leprosy. The lesions are usually widespread and located in two or more parts of the body. They may also involve the mucosa. The leishmanin skin test (LST) is usually negative in DCL, which reflects the absence of a cellular immune response. A large number of parasites are found in the lesions, making it is difficult to treat the disease; the lesions do not self-heal. Immunosuppression is a risk factor for both diffuse and disseminated cutaneous leishmaniases.

DIAGNOSIS

The approach to the diagnosis of CL is based on the demonstration of the parasite in material obtained from slit skin smears, aspirates or biopsies from a lesion (papule or ulcer) or on the documentation of a serological response to the infection.

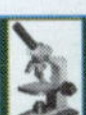

Lab diagnosis

- **Microscopy/histopathology:** By visualising amastigotes in slit skin smears, aspirates or biopsies from lesions
- **Culture:** NNN medium
- **Skin hypersensitivity:** Montenegro test
- **Serodiagnosis:** Not very useful
- **DNA detection:** PCR and real-time PCR

Microscopy/Histopathology

The demonstration of amastigotes is the diagnostic **gold standard**. Amastigote stages within macrophages or close to disrupted cells can usually be visualised in tissue imprints, biopsies or smears stained with Giemsa stain.

Culture

Aspirates or biopsy samples from the ulcers can be cultured in NNN medium to isolate the promastigote forms of the parasite.

Leishmanin Skin Test (LST/Montenegro Test)

A positive leishmanin skin test indicates delayed hypersensitivity reaction to the parasite. It is occasionally used for the diagnosis of CL, especially in epidemiological surveys, because it is simple to use and has high sensitivity and specificity.

Antigen Detection Test

A rapid immunochromatographic test targeting the peroxidoxin antigen of the parasite has become commercially available and may be useful.

Serodiagnosis

This is not very useful in the diagnosis of cutaneous leishmaniasis because of variable sensitivity and specificity.

Nucleic Acid-Based Detection

PCR is more sensitive than microscopy and culture and allows species differentiation which may have bearing on therapy decisions.

TREATMENT

Topical
- Intralesional injection of a pentavalent antimonial
- Ointment containing 15% paromomycin sulfate
- Adjuvant immunotherapy with topical imiquimod (5–7.5%) plus parenteral antimonials
- Heat therapy with an FDA-approved radiofrequency generator
- Cryotherapy with liquid nitrogen

Systemic
- *Pentavalent antimonial:* 20 mg/kg IM/IV × 20 days
- *Fluconazole:* 200 mg/day orally × 4–6 weeks
- *Ketoconazole:* 600 mg/day orally × 4–6 weeks
- *Miltefosine:* 2.5 mg/kg orally × 4–6 weeks
- *Amphotericin B deoxycholate:* 1 mg/kg IV on alternate days (a total of 25–45 mg/kg max.)
- *Liposomal amphotericin B:* 2–3 mg/kg/day IV (a total of 6–10 doses)

Although lesions heal spontaneously in the majority of cases, their spread or persistence is an indication for treatment. **Relapses** usually respond to a second course of treatment. DCL does not heal spontaneously and is difficult to treat. For this reason, treatment for DCL should be continued for some time after the lesions have healed and parasites can no longer be isolated.

One or more small lesions can be treated with topical agents, whereas lesions over the face, hands or joints, multiple lesions, large ulcers, New World CL with the potential to develop into MCL and CL in HIV-co-infected patients require **systemic treatment**.

MUCOCUTANEOUS LEISHMANIASIS (ESPUNDIA)

Mucocutaneous leishmaniasis (MCL) causes the partial or total destruction of the mucosa of the nose, mouth and throat. Over 90% of MCL cases occur in Bolivia, Brazil, Ethiopia and Peru (Table 18.2). In Central and South America, where infections caused by the subgenus *Viannia* (*L.* [*V.*] *braziliensis* complex) are widespread, cutaneous lesions may be accompanied by the spread of the disease to the mucosa, or they may be followed by the involvement of the mucosa years later. It is seen in 1–3% of patients infected with *L. braziliensis*. *L. amazonensis* may also cause MCL in rare cases. Young men with chronic lesions of CL are at particular risk of developing MCL.

PATHOGENESIS

The parasite spreads via the lymphatics or the bloodstream to the mucosal tissues of the upper respiratory tract with lesions in or around the nose, mouth or ear (**espundia**). The parasitised cells stimulate necrosis with inflammatory infiltrates.

MCL predominantly elicits a T_{h1} type of immune response with an increase in IFNγ and TNFα levels and varying levels of T_{h2} cytokines, IL-10 and TGFβ. This is associated with deep erosion locally and massive destruction due to intense inflammation and reactive fibrosis. Patients have a stronger delayed hypersensitivity response with MCL than with CL.

CLINICAL FEATURES

Patients usually provide a history of spontaneously healed cutaneous lesions about 1–5 years before presenting with MCL. However, MCL may also present without a prior history of CL. Typically, patients present with stuffiness of the nose and bleeding followed by nasal cartilage destruction, perforation of the nasal septum and collapse of the nasal bridge, resulting in a **'Tapir nose'**. The involvement of the upper respiratory tract leads to difficulty in swallowing and speech. There may be involvement of the lips, cheeks and soft palate. Superadded bacterial infections are common and may lead to fatal aspiration pneumonia.

DIAGNOSIS

This is the same as that for cutaneous leishmaniasis.

TREATMENT

First-line
- *Pentavalent antimonial (SbV):* 20 mg/kg IV or IM × 4 weeks

Second-line
- *Amphotericin B:* 0.5–1mg/kg IV daily (a total of 25–45 mg/kg max.)
- *Liposomal amphotericin B:* 2–3 mg/kg/day IV × 20 days
- *Miltefosine:* 2.5 mg/kg orally × 4 weeks
- With the failure of therapy or relapse, patients may require repeated courses of an antimonial or second-line drugs.

PREVENTION AND CONTROL

The methods of preventing and controlling CL and MCL follow those prescribed for visceral leishmaniasis (**Chapter 17**, *Leishmania [Visceral Leishmaniasis]*).

Table 18.2 Agents of mucocutaneous leishmaniasis (MCL)

Disease	Etiological agent	Vector	Reservoir	Geographical distribution
Mucocutaneous leishmaniasis (espundia)	*L. braziliensis* complex *L. mexicana* complex *L. guyanensis* complex	*Lutzomyia*	Zoonotic (wild rodents, sloths and opossums)	Central and South America

QUESTIONS

1. Discuss the diagnosis and management of cutaneous leishmaniasis.
2. Discuss the diagnosis and management of mucocutaneous leishmaniasis.

MULTIPLE CHOICE QUESTIONS

1. Chiclero ulcer is caused by which of the following?
   a. *Leishmania donovani*
   b. *Mycobacterium tuberculosis*
   c. *Calymmatobacterium donovanosis*
   d. *Leishmania mexicana*
2. The amastigote form of *Leishmania* resides in the ____________:
   a. Red blood cells
   b. Cells of the reticuloendothelial system
   c. Neuroglial cells
   d. Hepatocytes
3. Which of the following statements is NOT TRUE about espundia (mucocutaneous lesions)?
   a. It is caused by the *Viannia* (*L.* [*V.*] *braziliensis*) complex.
   b. It is commonly seen in Central and South Africa.
   c. The first line of treatment is pentavalent antimonial compounds.
   d. Tapir nose is a common finding.
4. All the following statements are true about cutaneous leishmaniasis in the Old World EXCEPT ___________:
   a. It is caused mainly by the *Leishmania donovani* complex.
   b. In India, it is predominantly seen in Rajasthan and a few other foci.
   c. Diagnosis is made mainly by the demonstration of parasites by microscopy, culture or DNA detection.
   d. Lesions may be self-resolving.
5. Which of the following statements about leishmaniasis recidivans (LR) is NOT TRUE?
   a. It is caused by *Leishmania donovani*.
   b. New small, non-ulcerating lesions develop in the periphery of a healed sore.
   c. Gross disfiguration may occur.
   d. It is caused by *Leishmania tropica*.

CHAPTER 19

Toxoplasma

([From Greek] *toxon* = crescent-shaped + *plasma* = formed structure)

Case Study and Learning Goals

A 25-year-old male patient who has AIDS presents with headache, low-grade fever, altered mental status, confusion and lethargy for the last two weeks. His CD4 cell counts are <100/µl, and his CT scan reveals multiple cerebral lesions with ring enhancement on contrast. What are the parasitic causes of encephalitis? How would you approach the laboratory diagnosis in this case? How would you treat this patient? What secondary prophylaxis would you recommend for him?

INTRODUCTION

Toxoplasma gondii is an obligate intracellular coccidian protozoan that is estimated to infect about a third of the world's population. Though it lies **dormant** in most infected individuals, it is associated with two significant human health concerns. They are as follows:

- **Reactivation** of the dormant parasite in immune-deficient conditions, particularly HIV/AIDS, which results in **encephalitis or systemic disease**
- **Transplacental transmission** of the parasite from a freshly infected pregnant woman to the fetus, which results in **congenital toxoplasmosis**

The parasite is ubiquitous in its presence, infecting several species of warm-blooded animals. It is one of the most common **zoonoses** and a significant veterinary pathogen.

T. gondii was discovered independently in 1908 by C. Nicolle and L. Manceaux in the rodent *Ctenodactylus gondi* at the Pasteur Institute, France, and A. Splendore in rabbits in Brazil. The first congenitally acquired infection in an infant was reported by Josef Janků in 1923; its association with encephalitis in neonates was recognised by A. Wolf and D. Cowen in 1937. The passage of the oocyst of this parasite in cat's feces was first observed in 1965 by W. M. Hutchison, who suggested that the organism may be *T. gondii*. This was later confirmed by other scientists, and by 1970, the complete life cycle of the parasite had been elucidated. Its importance as a pathogen in immunocompromised hosts came to be recognised in due course, especially after its association with CNS disease in AIDS patients became apparent in the mid-1980s.

EPIDEMIOLOGY

T. gondii infects more than 350 host species including mammals, birds, reptiles and marine animals. Environmental contamination occurs due to the shedding of the oocysts by the definitive hosts, felids, especially cats. Though it is a cosmopolitan parasite, its incidence is higher in tropical areas and found to decrease with increasing latitude. Globally, about around 25–30% of the human population is infected by *T. gondii*, with a higher prevalence in Latin America and tropical African countries.

Risk Factors

The following are factors that increase an individual's risk of developing disease:

- Having three or more cats at home as pets
- Immunocompromised conditions like HIV/AIDS and malignancies (due to the reactivation of latent cysts in such conditions)
- Receiving a blood transfusion or organ transplantation

MORPHOLOGY

There are various stages in the life cycle of *T. gondii*, namely, oocysts, sporozoites, tachyzoites and bradyzoites in tissue cysts (Fig. 19.1a, b and c).

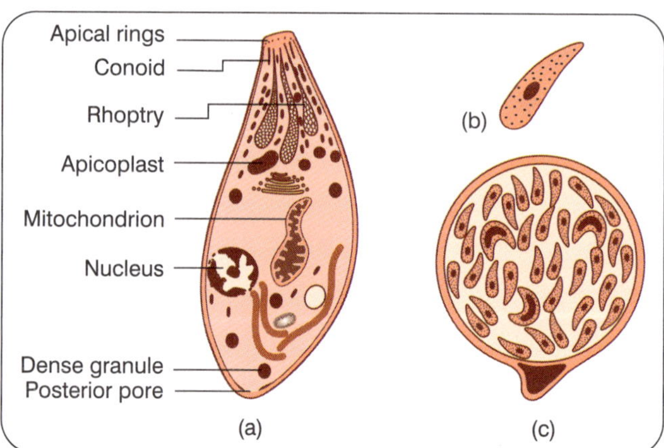

Fig. 19.1 Line diagram of *Toxoplasma gondii*: (a) internal structures of a tachyzoite, (b) a single tachyzoite and (c) tissue cyst with several bradyzoites

Tachyzoites

These are crescent-shaped and **3–7** µm in size. They are motile and **rapidly dividing** invasive forms that are easily destroyed by digestive enzymes. A tachyzoite has a pointy anterior end and a round posterior end. It contains a well-defined nucleus and organelles such as apical rings, conoid rhoptries, micronemes, dense granules and other structures that help in the active penetration of the host cell by the tachyzoite.

Bradyzoites (in Tissue Cysts)

These are slender and 4–6 µm in size. Bradyzoites are **slowly dividing** forms contained in **tissue cysts measuring 5–100** µm in size. They are found in the neural tissues, eyes, muscles, liver, kidney, etc.

Oocysts

These are found in cat feces. They vary in shape from ellipsoidal to sub-spherical, measure **10 × 12** **µm** in size and are environmentally resistant. The mature oocyst contains two sporocysts, each with four slender fusiform **sporozoites** measuring 6–8 µm in size.

LIFE CYCLE (Fig. 19.2a and b)

> **Definitive hosts:** Felids
> **Intermediate hosts:** Rodents, birds, humans and other animals

Felids are the **definitive hosts (mainly cats)** of *T. gondii*, and mice and other animals including humans are its **intermediate hosts**. The various stages in the life cycle of this parasite are as follows:

Definitive host cycle: Cats are infected when they ingest tissue cysts present in rodents or birds or tachyzoites or sporozoites in oocysts.

- Once ingested, the cyst wall of the tissue cyst dissolves in the cat's stomach and small intestine to liberate numerous bradyzoites which penetrate the intestinal epithelium.
- Some forms multiply **asexually by endodyogeny or schizogony**, while others initiate the **sexual cycle** by forming gamonts, which, in turn, produce gametes.
- The fertilisation of the micro- and macrogametes results in the formation of the **oocyst**. On sporulation of the oocyst, which takes 1–5 days, the epithelial cell ruptures, releasing oocysts into the intestinal lumen, from where they are released into the environment through the cat's feces.

Intermediate host cycle: Mice and human beings get infected by either **ingesting tissue cysts in infected meat** or **oocysts** in food or water contaminated with cat feces. **Transplacental transmission, blood transfusion** and **organ transplantation** are also important modes of infection among human beings.

- After infection, the parasite actively penetrates the host cells and produces a **parasitophorous vacuole** around itself. The parasite then multiplies **asexually by endodyogeny** and continues to divide until it fills up the host cell.
- The infected host cells rupture to free the parasites which further infect new cells. Two types of progeny emerge, the rapidly multiplying tachyzoites, which further spread the infection in the body, and the slowly developing bradyzoites, which form tissue cysts.
- The **tissue cysts containing bradyzoites remain latent** in various organs but have a predilection for neural and muscle tissue. The cysts persist for life unless they are reactivated during an immunosuppressed state. The tissue cysts in rodents or birds are ingested by the definitive feline host to continue the life cycle.

> Modes of infection
> - Ingestion of water or unwashed raw vegetables or fruits contaminated with oocysts excreted in cat's feces
> - Ingestion of uncooked or undercooked animal meat from warm-blooded animals and birds containing tissue cysts
> - Infection acquired during pregnancy resulting in congenital infection, i.e., transmission from mother to fetus
> - Blood transfusion
> - Organ transplantation

PATHOGENESIS

Human beings are infected by **tissue cysts** (in infected meat or in transplanted organs), **oocysts** (through food, water and soil contaminated with cat feces) or **tachyzoites** (in transfused blood or through vertical transplacental transmission). The mechanisms of pathogenesis of toxoplasmosis are as follows:

- *T. gondii* enters the host cells by **active invasion** and **lives intracellularly** in almost any tissue of the body. It disseminates in the body via the bloodstream and is capable of infecting all nucleated cells of the body, but not RBCs, which do not have a nucleus. The **parasitophorous vacuole formed around the parasite**

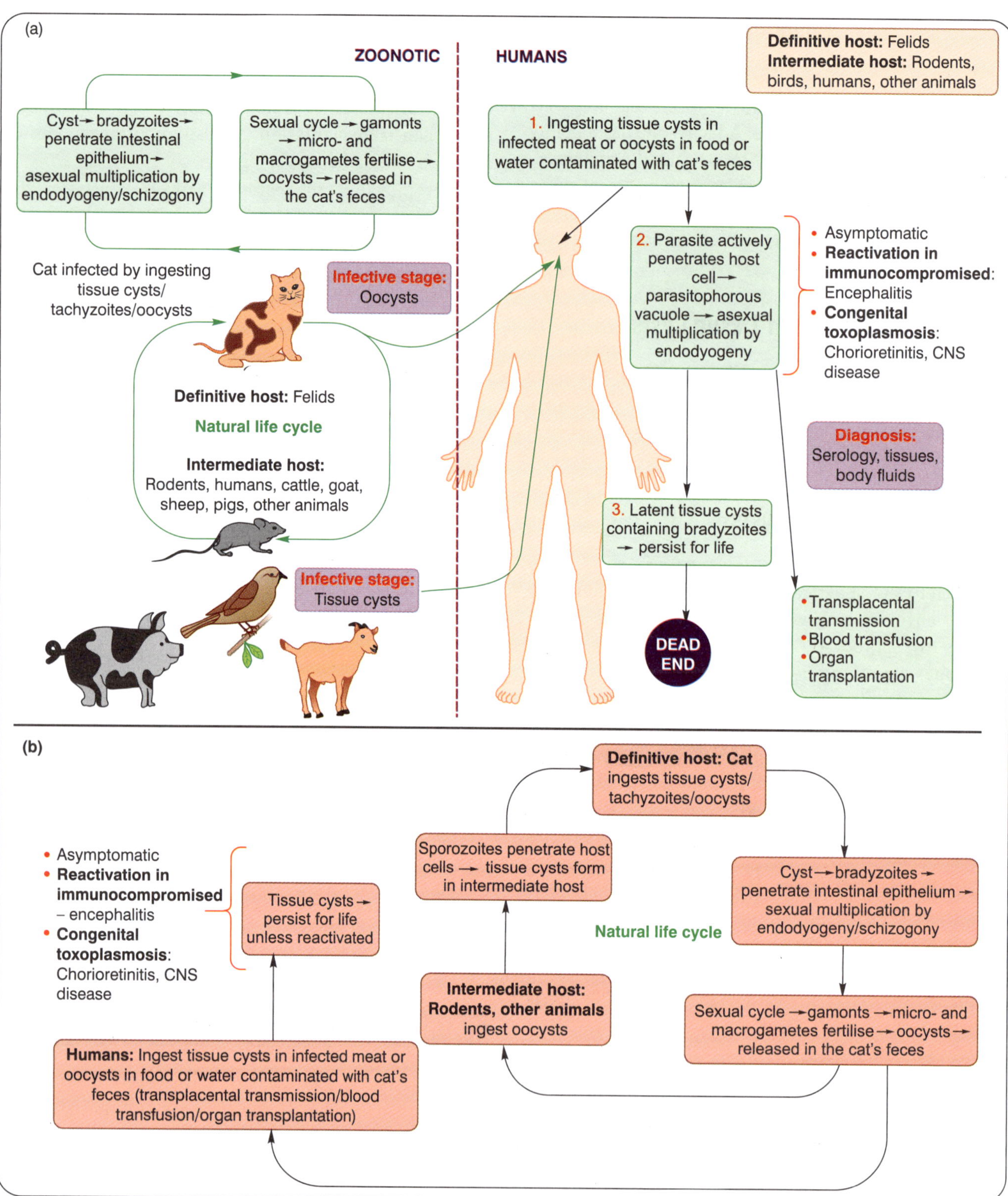

Fig. 19.2 Life cycle of *Toxoplasma gondii*: (a) detailed and (b) schematic

does not fuse with the lysosome. This allows the parasite to survive its intracellular residence.

- Both cell-mediated and humoral immunity are activated in *T. gondii* infections. The extracellular tachyzoites are well-amenable to destruction by the host immunity, chiefly by specific antibodies, macrophage-mediated reactive oxygen intermediates, IFNγ, IL-12, TNFα and cytotoxic T cell lymphocyte-mediated killing. Only the intracellular forms in the tissue cysts survive the host's immune response. Although these **tissue cysts**

persist for life, there are no overt manifestations of the infection in a healthy host.

- Individuals who have fully functional immune systems acquire lifelong immunity against the parasite and are capable of keeping the latent tissue cysts in check. However, **in an immunocompromised host, the latent cysts can get reactivated**. In such cases, there is uncontrolled proliferation of the cyst, dissemination in the body and destruction of the affected tissues by progressively enlarging necrotic lesions surrounded by inflammatory infiltrates.

CLINICAL FEATURES

Asymptomatic Infections

Human infections are asymptomatic in >80% of people infected with *T. gondii*. The parasite persists for life in various organs as latent tissue cysts. However, specific groups of patients including congenitally infected fetuses and immunocompromised persons are at a high risk of acquiring severe disease.

Symptomatic Infections

Approximately 10–20% of patients may present with self-limiting cervical or occipital lymphadenopathy with or without headache, malaise and fever that usually resolves in a few weeks.

Congenital toxoplasmosis

It occurs when a female acquires infection during pregnancy. Such an infection, which is usually asymptomatic or has non-specific features in the woman, gets transmitted to the fetus. The following are features of congenital toxoplasmosis:

- If a woman acquires a *T. gondii* **infection before she gets pregnant**, the infection is not transmitted to the fetus.
- In an **infection is acquired during pregnancy**, the gestational age at the time of infection is the most crucial determining factor of fetal outcome. In general, the chances of transmission increase with the progression of the gestation—from 25% when the woman acquires the infection in the first trimester to 65% when she acquires the infection in the third trimester. The severity of the infection, on the other hand, decreases with increasing gestation, i.e., infections acquired in the early period of organogenesis are the most severe for the fetus.
- Congenital infection may present as follows:
  - **Neonatal or early disease:** In more than 80% of cases of infection during the third trimester of gestation, the neonates are asymptomatic. On the other hand, infections acquired during the first trimester lead to severe abnormalities or abortion. The infection in newborns is marked by fever, pneumonitis and hepatosplenomegaly. Convulsions are also common. The classic triad of chorioretinitis, hydrocephalus and cerebral calcifications is rather rare. Children may show a failure to thrive.
  - **Cerebral lesions:** These may appear as calcifications, and serve as retrospective signs of congenital infection.
  - **Retinochoroiditis:** This leads to profound visual impairment and is a common manifestation, regardless of the time of maternal infection. Retinochoroiditis may not be evident at birth, but develops during subsequent years.
  - **Sequelae or relapse:** The congenital infection may present with mental retardation, seizures, hydrocephalus or microcephaly, deafness, or abnormal muscle tone at a later point in childhood.

Toxoplasma is one of the causative agents of **'TORCH' infections** in developing fetuses and newborns. A battery of investigations are conducted to screen neonates and pregnant women for these transplacentally or congenitally transmitted infections (see box).

TORCH Infections

- T: *Toxoplasma gondii*
- O: Others like *Treponema pallidum* (which causes syphilis)
- R: Rubella virus
- C: Cytomegalovirus
- H: Herpes simplex virus (HSV)

Ocular toxoplasmosis

Chorioretinitis in immunocompetent patients is generally a result of congenital infections acquired during pregnancy. However, some cases of ocular toxoplasmosis have also been reported in recently acquired infections, especially in Brazil.

- The typical findings of *Toxoplasma* **chorioretinitis** include evidently whitish focal lesions with an overlying and intense vitreal inflammation, which has a classic '**headlight in a fog**' appearance.
- It usually develops in the second or third decade of life, after the rupture of intraocular cysts.
- Chorioretinitis is usually bilateral in patients with congenitally acquired infection and is generally unilateral in patients with recently acquired infection.

Toxoplasmosis in immunocompromised patients

Toxoplasma infection in immunocompromised patients is always life-threatening. These patients are usually more at risk of reactivation of latent cysts than a fresh infection, but the risk may differ depending on the underlying condition which causes the immunosuppression.

- In **organ transplant recipients**, severe toxoplasmosis can result from either the reactivation of a latent infection in the recipient or infection from a transplanted organ containing cysts. The highest risk is in heart/heart–lung transplants, followed by liver, kidney and pancreas transplants. Toxoplasmosis should be considered in the differential diagnosis of transplant recipients with multiple organ failure.
- In **HIV-infected patients**, the incidence of toxoplasmosis is closely related to the CD4+ T cell counts, with the risk being highest when the count falls <100 cells/µl. *Toxoplasma* encephalitis (TE) is the most predominant manifestation occurring in 10–50% of these patients. The course of TE varies from a subacute process evolving over weeks to an acute disease evolving over days. The disease may or may not be associated with focal neurological deficits. The clinical features include altered mental status, seizures, cranial nerve defects, sensory and motor abnormalities and neuropsychiatric features. Signs of meningeal involvement are rare. After the brain, the most frequently involved organs are the lungs, eyes and heart.
- All potential transplant recipients and donors should be screened for *Toxoplasma*-specific IgG antibodies to determine their serostatus.

DIAGNOSIS

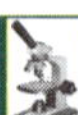

Lab diagnosis

- **Serology:** Detection of IgG, IgM, IgA, IgE antibodies, IgG avidity (*Toxoplasma* serologic profile), Sabin–Feldman dye test, AC/HS test, immunochromatographic test (ICT), indirect immunofluorescent antibody test (IFAT), ELISA and immunosorbent agglutination assay (ISAGA)
- **Microscopy:** Visualisation of tachyzoites in tissue sections or smears of body fluids (CSF, amniotic fluid or bronchoalveolar lavage [BAL])
- **Antigen detection:** Not very sensitive
- **Animal inoculation:** Intraperitoneal inoculation into mice
- **Tissue culture:** Murine alveolar and peripheral macrophage cell lines
- **DNA detection:** PCR and real-time PCR
- **Radioimaging:** Ultrasonography, CT scan and MRI

The diagnosis of toxoplasmosis is usually made by serologic tests. Other tests include DNA detection, microscopic examination of biopsy specimens, buffy coat cells or cerebrospinal fluid and the isolation of the organism in tissue cultures or laboratory animals.

Serodiagnosis

Since the infection is often asymptomatic, serology is useful, especially for the following:

1. Pregnant women, preferably at an early stage of pregnancy
2. Patients with uveitis or retinochoroiditis
3. Organ donors or transplant recipients
4. Congenital toxoplasmosis

- **Detection of IgG antibodies:** IgG antibodies appear as early as 2–3 weeks after the infection, peak at 6–8 weeks, and then decline slowly to a baseline level that persists for life. Due to the lifelong persistence of IgG, this method cannot distinguish recent from past infection. Since IgG antibodies cross the placenta, they are not useful in the diagnosis of congenital infections either.

  IgG avidity test: In an infection, the strength with which the formed IgG antibodies bind to the specific antigenic epitopes after the primary antigenic challenge is initially low, and increases during the subsequent weeks and months. This property can be exploited to differentiate between recent and past infections by using protein-denaturing reagents such as urea to dissociate the weak antibody–antigen complex. This method is known as avidity testing. Avidity is determined from the ratio of antibody titres of urea-treated and untreated serum. Avidity index (AI) values of <0.2 are considered as low, those of 0.2–0.3 as intermediate, and those >0.3 as high. **Low IgG avidity indicates recent infection** acquired during the last three months, whereas high avidity indicates a past infection acquired at least three months ago.
- **Detection of IgM antibodies:** IgM antibodies are produced during the first week of infection and reach a plateau within one month. The levels of specific IgM antibodies usually decrease after 1–6 months of infection, but these antibodies may remain detectable for a year or longer. Thus, IgM cannot be used as a stand-alone test for the diagnosis of acute infection; it is often used in conjunction with other tests.
- **Detection of IgE antibodies:** IgE antibodies may be detected in the sera of acutely infected adults, congenitally infected infants and children

with congenital *Toxoplasma* chorioretinitis. The duration of IgE seropositivity is less than that of IgM or IgA antibodies, which makes the detection of IgE a useful method for identifying recently acquired infections.

Different serological tests measure the levels of different antibodies, each having a unique pattern of rise and fall with time in relation to the infection. A combination of serological tests called ***Toxoplasma* serologic profile (TSP)** is often required to ascertain whether an infection is **recent or of the distant past**.

Several methods like the Sabin–Feldman dye test, differential agglutination (AC/HS) test, immunochromatographic test (ICT), indirect fluorescence antibody test (IFAT), enzyme-linked immunosorbent assay (ELISA), μ-capture ELISA and immunosorbent agglutination assay (ISAGA) are available for IgG, IgM, IgA and IgE detection.

Sabin–Feldman dye test: For many years now, this test has been the **gold standard for serology** in terms of sensitivity and specificity. However, it is currently performed by very few laboratories. In this test, live tachyzoites are incubated with the patient's serum and complement. If anti-*Toxoplasma* antibodies are present in the patient's serum, they bind to the antigens present on the live tachyzoites and kill the latter by complement-mediated lysis. Subsequently, alkaline methylene blue dye is added to differentiate between live and dead tachyzoites—the killed tachyzoites remain unstained and distorted. The dilution of the test serum at which 50% of the tachyzoites are killed is reported as the antibody titre of the test serum.

Drawbacks:

- It requires the maintenance of live tachyzoites.
- It detects IgG antibodies, hence cannot differentiate between recent and past infections.

Differential agglutination test (AC/HS test): The AC/HS test uses two *Toxoplasma* tachyzoite antigens preparations, one treated with acetone (AC) and the other with formalin (HS). The antibodies formed in a recent infection agglutinate both AC and HS suspensions, whereas those formed in past infections agglutinate only HS-treated antigens in higher titres. This helps to differentiate acute from past infection.

Rapid immunochromatographic test (ICT): Lately, rapid ICT-based point-of-care tests have become commercially available for the detection of *Toxoplasma*-specific IgG and IgM antibodies. These have the potential to identify acute infection and are chiefly being used as screening tests.

Microscopy

The demonstration of pseudocysts or tachyzoites in tissue sections or body fluids such as CSF, amniotic fluid or BAL establishes the diagnosis of the infection (Fig. 19.3a–d). The samples may be stained with Giemsa, periodic acid–Schiff, immunoperoxidase or silver stains. The sensitivity of microscopy, however, is quite low. The **direct fluorescent antibody test (DFA)** uses fluorescein-conjugated antibodies against *T. gondii* surface antigens to improve the sensitivity and specificity of microscopy.

Antigen Detection

Antigen detection lacks sensitivity when used on human samples. However, it may be useful in diagnosing toxoplasmosis in an immunocompromised individual in whom antibodies are usually few or absent.

Nucleic Acid-Based Detection

Toxoplasma DNA may be detected by PCR, real-time PCR, LAMP, etc. These methods have been successfully used to diagnose congenital, ocular, cerebral and disseminated toxoplasmosis. Various clinical samples such as CSF (for the diagnosis of TE), vitreous and aqueous fluid (for ocular toxoplasmosis) and other samples such as blood, body fluids, amniotic fluid or placenta can be tested.

PCR on amniotic fluid is considered the gold standard for the diagnosis of congenital toxoplasmosis.

Animal Inoculation

Mice can be inoculated intraperitoneally with clinical samples to isolate *T. gondii*. The inoculated mice usually die in 7–10 days, and peritoneal fluid and spleen aspirates are harvested to demonstrate the tachyzoites (Fig. 19.3b). If the mice do not die, they are observed weekly, and blood from their tails is screened for *Toxoplasma* antibodies. Alternatively, they are sacrificed at 6 weeks to detect encysted parasites or *Toxoplasma* antigens in their tissues (especially those of the brain) by histopathological or immunofluorescent antibody tests.

Tissue Culture

Clinical samples can be inoculated into murine alveolar or peripheral macrophage cell lines. In a positive test, cytopathic effects are observed in 4–12 days. This method is less sensitive than mouse inoculation.

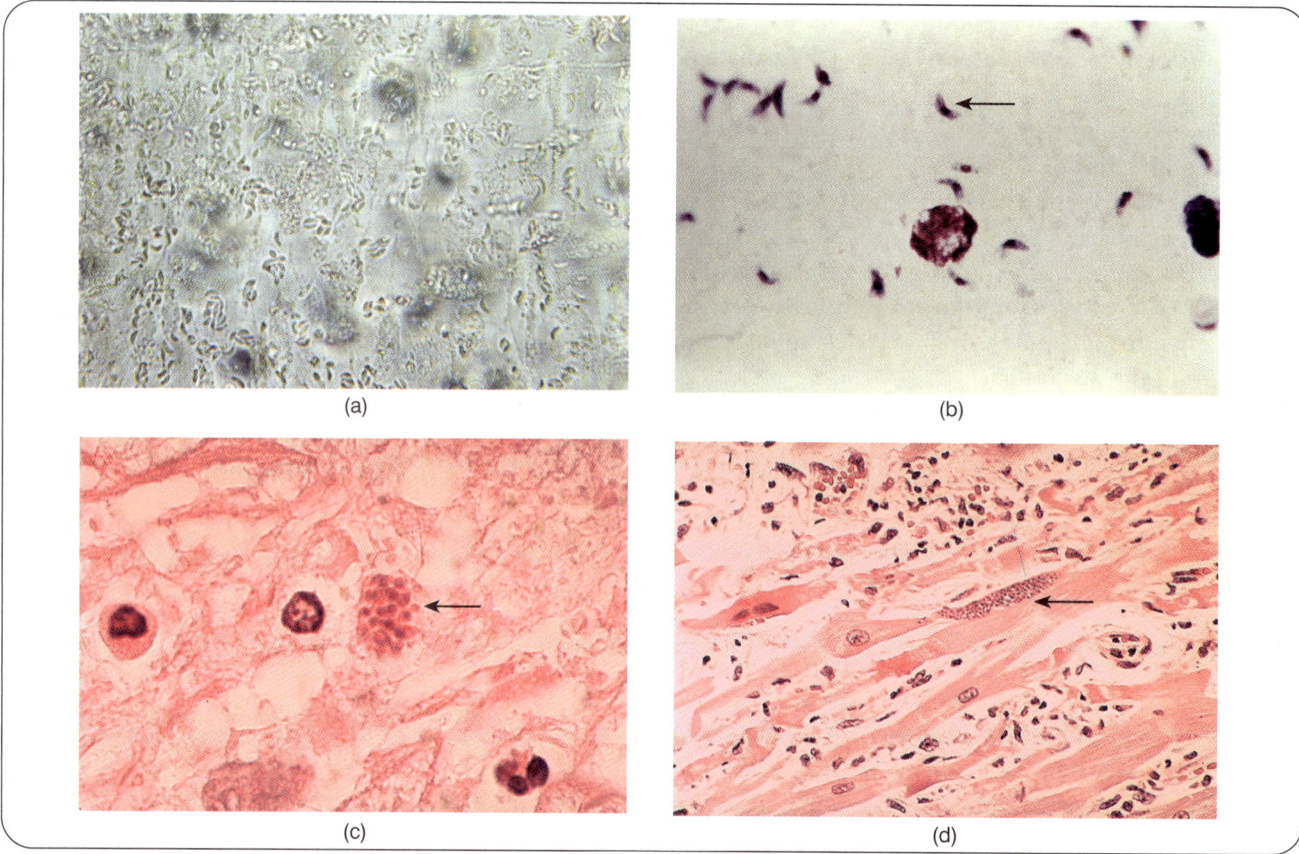

Fig. 19.3 Microscopic features of *Toxoplasma gondii*: (a) numerous unstained, crescent-shaped tachyzoites in human embryonic lung fibroblast cell culture, (b) stained tachyzoites in murine ascitic fluid, (c) a pseudocyst containing numerous bradyzoites in the brain tissue in a case of neurotoxoplasmosis and (d) a pseudocyst in the heart muscle in a case of cardiac toxoplasmosis (*Source:* Centers for Disease Control and Prevention [CDC], Public Health Image Library [PHIL]; Image IDs 20816, 16546, 575 and 572)

Other Diagnostic Parameters

Radioimaging: Serial ultrasonographic (USG) examinations may be performed to monitor congenital defects in the developing fetus. Computed tomography (CT) scan or magnetic resonance imaging (MRI) of the brain can be done to demonstrate multiple ring-enhancing lesions to diagnose TE in HIV patients.

Diagnosis in Special Settings

Diagnosis of congenital toxoplasmosis

Prenatal diagnosis and follow-up during pregnancy: Prenatal diagnosis of congenital toxoplasmosis in utero is necessary for early anti-parasitic treatment. This is done by one of the following methods:

- **Serology:** A low-avidity IgG antibody-positive ELISA, coupled with high IgM or IgE antibody titre is suggestive of acute infection.
- **Nucleic acid-based detection:** An amniotic fluid puncture is performed after 16 weeks of gestation or at least four weeks after maternal infection for the detection of *Toxoplasma* DNA by PCR.
- **Animal inoculation/tissue culture:** Amniotic fluid may be inoculated into mice or tissue culture.
- **Radioimaging:** Monthly USG surveillance to monitor fetal development is recommended.

Postnatal diagnosis of congenital toxoplasmosis:

- **Radioimaging:** At birth, a complete clinical and neurological workup of the neonate should be undertaken. A transfontanellar USG examination may be performed to detect cerebral calcification. A CT scan may subsequently be performed if there are abnormal findings.
- **Animal inoculation or tissue culture:** Parasite detection may be attempted in the placenta or cord blood.
- **Serology:** The testing of neonates is done at birth, after a month of life, and subsequently, every 2 or 3 months to monitor the decrease in maternally transmitted antibodies, which usually disappear within 5–8 months.

- The detection of specific IgM or IgA antibodies, which cannot cross the placental barrier, is a key marker of fetal infection.
- As maternal IgG is passively transferred to the fetus in utero, a positive IgG serology may only reflect maternally transferred antibodies. Therefore, a qualitative analysis is required to differentiate between maternal antibodies and antibodies synthesised by the infected neonate. A comparative analysis of IgGs specific to the mother and the neonate (by Western blot, for example) may help provide serologic evidence of fetal infection.

- **Nucleic acid-based detection:** Placenta or cord blood may be tested for *Toxoplasma* DNA.

Diagnosis of ocular toxoplasmosis (retinochoroiditis)

This depends on the presence of typical lesions (white focal lesions and vitreal inflammation) along with the following tests:

- **Serology:** *Toxoplasma*-specific antibodies can be detected in ocular fluids either quantitatively or qualitatively and compared to serum IgG titres.
  - The **Goldmann–Witmer coefficient** (GWC cut-off = 2) may be used as evidence of local antibody production against *T. gondii*, i.e., antibody production in the eye compared to systemic production.

GWC = [anti-*Toxoplasma* IgG in aqueous humor/total IgG in aqueous humor]/[anti-*Toxoplasma* IgG in serum/total IgG in serum]

- **Nucleic acid-based detection:** The detection of parasite DNA in aqueous or vitreous fluid is diagnostic for ocular toxoplasmosis.

Diagnosis in immunocompromised patients

- **Demonstration of parasite:** This can be done in a tissue sample obtained by biopsy, BAL or autopsy.
- **Isolation:** The parasite can be inoculated into culture systems or animals to isolate the parasite.
- **Nucleic acid-based detection:** *Toxoplasma* DNA can be amplified from blood, CSF and/or BAL.
- **Serology:** It may be useful in the differentiation of graft-transmitted and reactivation toxoplasmosis. The disadvantage of serology is the absence of seroconversion in some cases because of profound immunosuppression.

TREATMENT

Treatment regimes are based on the type of toxoplasmosis and the specific target group, as described in Table 19.1.

Pregnant Women

- Spiramycin is indicated for pregnant women suspected of having acquired the infection at <18 weeks of gestation with low suspicion of fetal infection (documented negative results of amniotic fluid PCR and negative findings on USG at follow-ups). It

Table 19.1 Treatment regimes for toxoplasmosis

Pregnant women	Congenital toxoplasmosis	Ocular toxoplasmosis	AIDS
Infection at <18 weeks of gestation *Spiramycin:* 1 g TDS until delivery **Infection at >18 weeks of gestation** *Pyrimethamine:* 50 mg BDS × 2 days followed by 50 mg daily PLUS *Sulfadiazine:* 75 mg/kg initial dose, followed by 50 mg/kg BDS (maximum 4 g/day) PLUS *Folinic acid (leucovorin):* 10–20 mg daily (during and one week after the completion of pyrimethamine therapy)	*Pyrimethamine:* 1 mg/kg PLUS *Sulfadiazine:* 100 mg/kg PLUS Folinic acid (Continued for at least a year)	*Pyrimethamine:* 100 mg OD for 1 or 2 days and then 25–50 mg OD PLUS *Sulfadiazine:* 1 g QID (OR *Clindamycin:* 1 mg intravitreal) PLUS *Folinic acid:* 10–20 mg OD +/– *Prednisolone:* 1 mg QID may be administered for a short time (Continued for at least 1–2 weeks after the resolution of symptoms)	*Pyrimethamine:* 200 mg loading dose, then 50–75 mg oral OD PLUS *Sulfadiazine:* 1 g QID PLUS *Folinic acid:* 10–25 mg OD (Continued for at least 4–6 weeks after the resolution of signs and symptoms followed by secondary prophylaxis) **Secondary prophylaxis** *Trimethoprim-sulfamethoxazole (Cotrimoxazole):* 160/800 mg daily

prevents the vertical transmission of infection but does not treat the fetal infection.

- Pyrimethamine is teratogenic and should **not be used before 18 weeks of gestation**. It is indicated for women suspected of having acquired infection at >18 weeks of gestation and those with documented fetal infection (positive amniotic fluid PCR or abnormal USG findings).
- Folinic acid is administered to prevent bone marrow suppression associated with pyrimethamine.

AIDS Patients

- Untreated toxoplasmosis is rapidly fatal in immunocompromised patients. **Secondary prophylaxis**, i.e., long-term maintenance therapy, is required for HIV-positive patients treated for toxoplasmosis. It should be started if the $CD4^+$ T lymphocyte count decreases to <100/µl. However, it can be discontinued if the patient is asymptomatic and has a $CD4^+$ T lymphocyte count of >200/µl for at least three months.

PREVENTION AND CONTROL

- **People who have cats for pets should follow certain hygiene practices** like wearing gloves while changing cat litter, changing litter boxes regularly, washing hands frequently, especially after petting or stroking cats, etc.
- Hands should also be washed thoroughly after outdoor activities that involve contact with soil. Ideally, gloves should be worn for gardening.
- Raw fruits and vegetables should be thoroughly washed before consumption, especially if they grow close to the ground.
- Meat should be cooked fully or frozen at –20°C for 15 days. Hands, knives and containers used for manipulating meat should be washed thoroughly.
- **Prenatal and antenatal screening** should be performed routinely to detect *Toxoplasma* infection in women of childbearing age.
- **Primary prophylaxis for HIV patients:**
  - AIDS patients with $CD4^+$ T lymphocyte cell counts <100/µl should receive prophylaxis against TE, which can be discontinued when $CD4^+$ T cell count stays above 200/µl for at least three months.
  - Trimethoprim-sulfamethoxazole (cotrimoxazole) is the drug of choice; sulphadiazine-pyrimethamine can be given as an alternative to sulpha drugs.
- In transplant recipients, **pre-transplant evaluation** should be done (by serological screening of both donor and recipient) to eradicate the infection or to start suitable chemoprophylaxis in high-risk patients.

Questions

1. Elaborate on the morphology and life cycle of *Toxoplasma gondii*.
2. Discuss the diagnosis and management of congenital toxoplasmosis.
3. Discuss the diagnosis and management of toxoplasmosis in pregnant women.
4. Discuss the diagnosis and management of ocular toxoplasmosis.
5. Discuss immunodeficiency and toxoplasmosis.
6. Describe the Sabin–Feldman dye test.

Multiple Choice Questions

1. All the following statements about toxoplasmosis in humans are true EXCEPT ___________:
   a. Most infections are asymptomatic.
   b. It causes encephalitis in AIDS patients.
   c. The chances of transmission from a pregnant woman to the fetus decrease with the progression of gestation.
   d. The involvement of the eye in the case of congenitally transmitted disease is bilateral.
2. The Sabin–Feldman dye test is used for the diagnosis of _______:
   a. Syphilis
   b. Toxoplasmosis
   c. Gonorrhea
   d. Kala-azar
3. *Toxoplasma gondii* infection can be transmitted to the fetus ___________:
   a. If the infection is acquired during pregnancy

b. If the infection is acquired before pregnancy
c. By blood transfusion
d. During delivery only

4. The definitive hosts for *Toxoplasma gondii* are ___________:
   a. Humans
   b. Felines
   c. Canines
   d. All warm-blooded mammals

5. AIDS patients with CD4$^+$ T lymphocyte count of _________ should receive prophylaxis against *Toxoplasma* encephalitis.
   a. <500/µl b. <100/µl
   c. <300/µl d. <400/µl

6. The drugs chiefly used for the treatment of toxoplasmosis are ___________:
   a. Pyrimethamine, sulphadiazine and folinic acid
   b. Albendazole and DEC
   c. Ivermectin and DEC
   d. Nitazoxanide and metronidazole

7. A low-avidity ELISA titre for anti-*Toxoplasma* antibodies signifies ___________:
   a. Past infection
   b. Recent infection
   c. Maternally transmitted antibodies
   d. Congenital infection

8. What is the most predominant manifestation of the disease in AIDS patients?
   a. Uveitis b. Encephalitis
   c. Myocarditis d. Megacolon

9. The 'headlight in a fog' appearance is a characteristic ocular finding in ___________ .
   a. Syphilis b. Gonorrhea
   c. Rubella d. Toxoplasmosis

10. The classical triad of chorioretinitis, hydrocephalus and cerebral calcifications is described in ___________ :
   a. Syphilis
   b. Gonorrhea
   c. Rubella
   d. Toxoplasmosis

Chapter 20

Naegleria

(Named after scientists Mathieu Naegler and Malcolm Fowler)

Case Study and Learning Goals

A 16-year-old male presents to the emergency with a severe headache and high fever, which he has had for the last five days. Signs of meningeal irritation are noted at presentation. The patient has a history of going swimming in a lake ten days ago. The CSF examination shows pus cells but fails to reveal any apparent bacterial cause. What are the parasitic causes of meningoencephalitis? How would you approach the laboratory diagnosis in this case?

FREE-LIVING AMOEBAE

Amoebae that exist as free-living organisms in nature and only occasionally invade a host to live as parasites are termed **amphizoic** or **free-living amoebae**. Pathogenic and opportunistic free-living amoebae such as ***Acanthamoeba, Balamuthia*** and ***Naegleria*** are worldwide in their distribution and can potentially cause infections in humans and other animals. They can be isolated from a wide variety of samples including soil and fresh and brackish water. All these amoebae can cause **central nervous system (CNS) infections, especially in immunocompromised individuals**, and are associated with high mortality. Apart from CNS infections, *Acanthamoeba* is also associated with vision-threatening **corneal infections in immunocompetent individuals and contact lens users**. Besides causing disease themselves, free-living amoebae may also harbour and transmit a number of other pathogens like *Legionella, Pseudomonas*, mycobacteria and viruses such as adenoviruses and echoviruses (playing the role of a **trojan horse**). Another free-living amoeba, ***Sappinia diploidea*** (two nuclei), has recently been identified as a cause of CNS disease in humans.

NAEGLERIA

INTRODUCTION

Naegleria fowleri is a **thermophilic** free-living amoeba which is typically found in warm freshwaters such as ponds, lakes, rivers, hot springs, swimming pools, sewage and discharges of industrial plants. In 1970, R. F. Carter identified *N. fowleri* as the causative agent of a CNS infection—a **rapidly fatal primary meningoencephalitis (PAM)**—in humans. *N. fowleri* is the only species of *Naegleria* known to cause infection in humans. It is also referred to as the **'brain-eating amoeba'**.

EPIDEMIOLOGY

Since the time *N. fowleri* was recognised as a human pathogen, more than 200 cases of PAM have been reported worldwide. The infection is more common in otherwise healthy children or young adults with a history of swimming in lakes or heated swimming pools.

There is no specific reservoir host for *N. fowleri* as it is ubiquitous and free-living in the environment. However, infections have been documented in a variety of animal species.

MORPHOLOGY

N. fowleri exists as a trophozoite, a transitory flagellated trophozoite and as a dormant cyst. It is also known as an amoeboflagellate.

Trophozoite

The trophozoite is **amoeboid, elongated** and **measures 10–30 µm** in size when active (it is **rounded** and **measures 9–15 µm when inactive**). It has a single nucleus with a prominent, centrally-placed nucleolus and a conspicuous contractile vacuole. It feeds on gram-negative bacteria through phagocytic structures called amoebostomes, reproduces by simple binary fission and exhibits rapid motion produced by a single, blunt pseudopodium called lobopodium (Fig. 20.1a).

Flagellate Form

The trophozoite transforms into a transient, pear-shaped, non-feeding and non-dividing flagellated stage with two flagella at its anterior end. The flagellated form can swim rapidly with the help of its flagella. It ranges in length from 10 to16 µm and possesses a single nucleus with a prominent nucleolus (Fig. 20.1b).

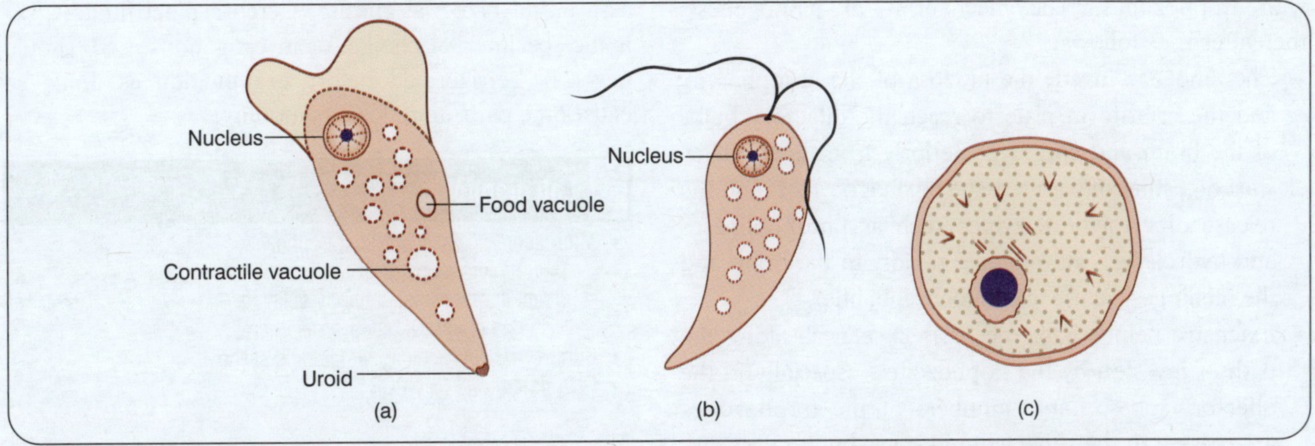

Fig. 20.1 Line diagrams of the various stages of *Naegleria fowleri*: (a) trophozoite, (b) flagellate stage and (c) cyst

Cyst

The cyst is usually **spherical** and measures **7–15 μm** in size. It has a single nucleus with a large nucleolus and a relatively thin cyst wall with mucoid plugs or ostioles. Cysts are often clumped together (Fig. 20.1c).

LIFE CYCLE (Fig. 20.2)

Habitat: Free-living in moist soil and freshwater bodies

Amoebae of the genus *Naegleria* exist in a free-living state in moist soil and freshwater bodies. The different stages in their life cycles, namely trophozoite, flagellate and cyst, rapidly transform from one form to another. Encystation occurs in harsh conditions, whereas excystation takes place when the conditions are favourable. The cyst stage is not found in the human body. The flagellate stage seems to form quickly and spontaneously. Humans acquire *N. fowleri* infections on exposure to freshwater.

PATHOGENESIS

Human beings acquire *Naegleria* infections through the nasal passage by the aspiration of water contaminated

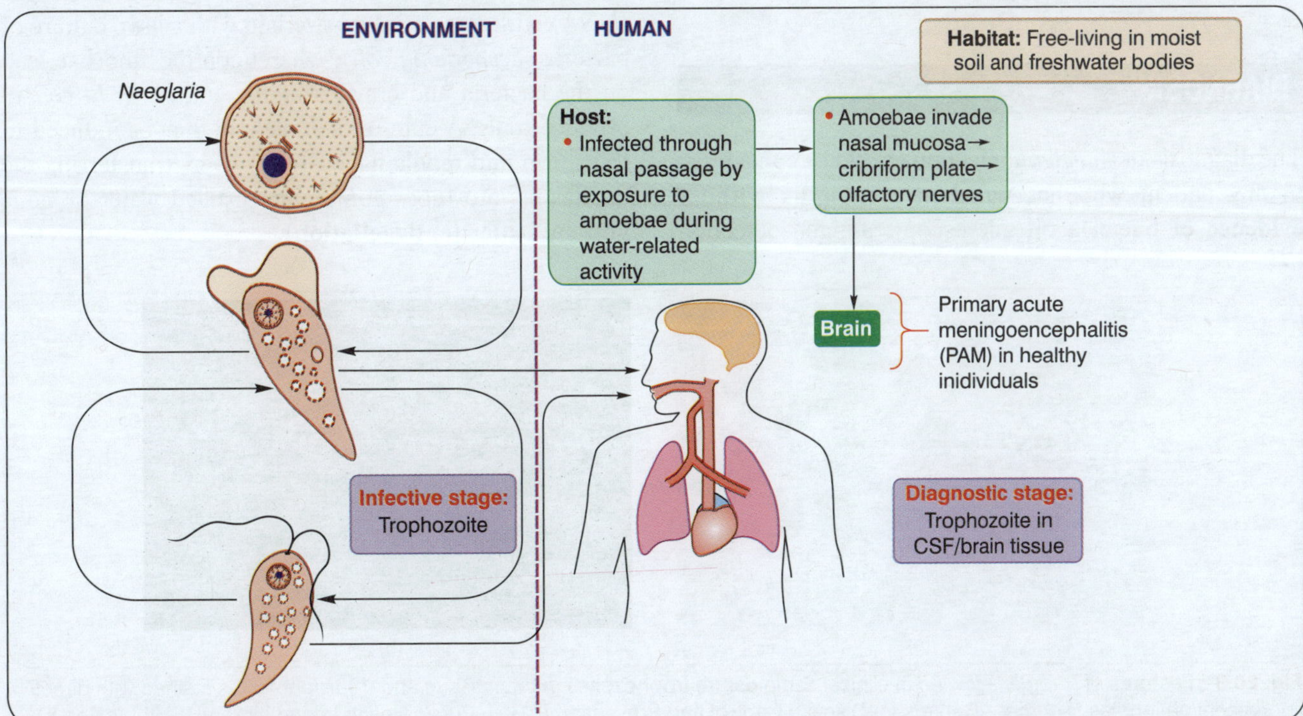

Fig. 20.2 Life cycle of *Naegleria*

with trophozoites. The mechanism of pathogenesis thereafter is as follows:

- The amoebae invade the mucosa of the nasopharynx and the cribriform plate to reach the olfactory bulbs of the brain and spread posteriorly from there. They start digesting the brain tissue by phagocytosis and the release of cytolytic enzymes such as phospholipases and hydrolases, and multiply rapidly in the brain and the meninges (acute meningoencephalitis).
- Extensive hemorrhagic necrosis is seen all along the path of invasion by the trophozoites, especially in the olfactory lobes. Large numbers of the trophozoites are present in the subarachnoid space but no cysts are found. Death occurs in a few days.

CLINICAL FEATURES

The incubation period ranges from two days to two weeks. *N. fowleri* causes acute and fulminant suppuration in the CNS and closely mimics pyogenic meningitis.

- The initial symptoms include alternations in taste and smell due to olfactory nerve involvement.
- In the later stages, severe headache, high fever, nausea, vomiting, signs of meningeal irritation, photophobia and cranial nerve palsies are common.
- Rapid progression to seizures and coma may follow.
- The disease is **almost always fatal**, and death occurs within 7–14 days of exposure.

DIAGNOSIS

The diagnosis of *Naegleria* infection should be considered in any patient who has **purulent meningitis without evidence of bacteria** on microscopy, antigen detection assays and bacterial culture. Cerebrospinal fluid (CSF) is the specimen of choice for investigations. CSF should never be refrigerated before examination as doing so causes the parasite to lose its motility.

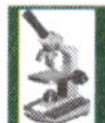

Lab diagnosis

- **Microscopy:** By visualising trophozoites
  - Direct microscopy of CSF
  - Direct fluorescence antibody staining
  - Histopathology: Of biopsy specimen
- **Culture:** NNA medium with Page's saline
- **DNA detection:** By PCR

Microscopy

- **Wet mount:** Motile amoeboid trophozoites can be demonstrated in wet mount preparations of the CSF. Care should be taken to differentiate trophozoites from leukocytes.
- **Giemsa or trichrome staining:** Stained smears are better suited for discerning the trophozoite morphology (Fig. 20.3a).
- **Direct fluorescence antibody staining:** Specific monoclonal antibodies may be used on centrifuged CSF or biopsy tissue to demonstrate trophozoites (Fig. 20.3b).

Culture

CSF samples may be inoculated on **non-nutrient agar (NNA) with Page's saline** overlaid with a lawn culture of bacteria (*Escherichia coli*), whereupon the amoebae feed on the bacteria and crawl over the culture of *E. coli* to produce trails. A culture of *Naegleria* may be induced to transform into motile flagellate forms by transferring the organisms into tubes containing distilled water or non-nutrient buffer **(enflagellation)**.

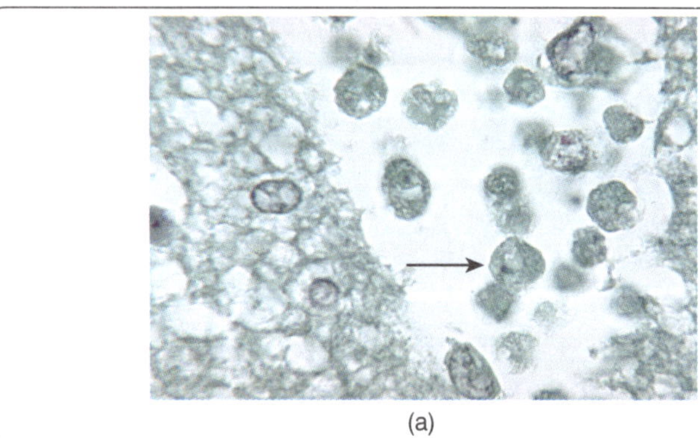

(a)

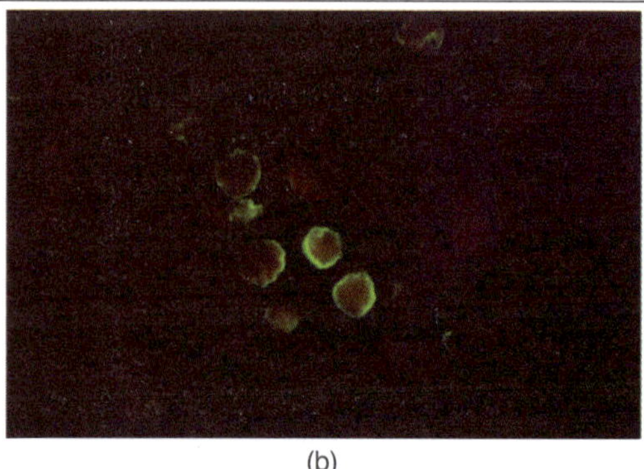

(b)

Fig. 20.3 Features of *Naegleria fowleri* in clinical samples: (a) trophozoites in brain tissue and (b) trophozoites stained with direct fluorescent antibodies (*Source:* Centers for Disease Control and Prevention [CDC], Public Health Image Library, [PHIL] Image IDs 614 and 17617)

Serodiagnosis

Antibodies to *Naegleria* species have been detected in healthy adults. However, in acute infections, the rapid progression of the disease does not allow time for antibodies to be produced. For this reason, serologic testing is not useful in the diagnosis of acute infection.

Nucleic Acid-Based Detection

PCR on CSF or biopsied tissue samples may be used for diagnosis with good sensitivity and specificity.

Histopathology

Biopsy samples from the brain may be examined after staining to demonstrate characteristic trophozoites and the absence of cysts.

Other Diagnostic Parameters

- **CSF examination:** As in pyogenic meningitis, predominantly polymorphonuclear leukocytosis, increased proteins and decreased sugars are found in the CSF.
- **Radioimaging:** Computed tomography (CT) scan and magnetic resonance imaging (MRI) show obliteration of the cisterns and diffuse enhancement around the midbrain, subarachnoid space and cerebrum.

TREATMENT

Drug of choice
- *Amphotericin B (AmB):* 1–15 mg/kg/day IV × 3 days, followed by 1 mg/kg/day × 6 days
- Intrathecal AmB should also be considered

Aggressive therapy should be considered with a combination of AmB and rifampicin, miltefosine or azoles like voriconazole and miconazole. Despite such treatment, only a few patients survive, probably because of delayed diagnosis.

PREVENTION AND CONTROL

- **Education and awareness** are key to the prevention of disease.
- Bathing in unsafe waters and hot springs should be avoided.
- Public water supplies should be adequately **chlorinated**, maintaining 0.5 mg residual chlorine per litre of water.

QUESTIONS

1. Discuss the diagnosis and management of primary meningoencephalitis.

MULTIPLE CHOICE QUESTIONS

1. A young man with a history of swimming in a pond recently developed high-grade fever with headache, vomiting and signs of meningeal irritation. His condition deteriorates rapidly. Which parasitic infection could lead to such a presentation?
   a. *Acanthamoeba*
   b. *Naegleria*
   c. *Echinococcus*
   d. *Toxocara*
2. *Naegleria* causes which of the following?
   a. Granulomatous amoebic encephalitis
   b. Contact lens-associated keratitis
   c. Primary amoebic meningoencephalitis
   d. All of these
3. Which free-living amoeba shows a flagellate stage?
   a. *Acanthamoeba* b. *Balamuthia*
   c. *Naegleria* d. *Entamoeba*

Chapter 21

Acanthamoeba and Balamuthia

(*Acanthamoeba* from *Acantha* [Greek] = thorn + amoeba; *Balamuthia* named after parasitologist William Balamuth)

Case Study and Learning Goals

A 20-year-old female presents to the OPD with complaints of pain in her right eye along with photophobia and watering. She has a history of using contact lenses regularly. On examination, a ring-like corneal infiltrate is seen in her eye. What are the parasitic causes of keratitis? How would you approach the laboratory diagnosis in this case? How would you treat this patient?

ACANTHAMOEBA

INTRODUCTION

Acanthamoeba spp. are among the most prevalent protozoans in the environment. They have been isolated from freshwater as well as brackish water, dust, air and soil.

Free-living amoebae were first isolated from dust in 1931 by B. M. Puschkarew, who named them *Amoeba polyphagus*. The first suggestion that *Acanthamoeba* could act as a human pathogen was made in 1958 during the polio vaccine trials. These organisms were described as the causative agents of **granulomatous amoebic meningoencephalitis (GAE)** and **keratitis** in humans in the 1960s and 1970s respectively. The name *Acanthamoeba* was proposed by T. K. Griffin and J. L. Sawyer based on the presence of spine-like pseudopodia (called acanthopodia) in the trophozoite form.

So far, more than 24 species of *Acanthamoeba* have been documented to be the causative agents of infections in humans, e.g., *A. castellani, A. polyphaga, A. hatchetti, A. lenticulata, A. healyi, A. griffini, A. rhysodes, A. divionensis* and *A. culbertsoni*. The members of the genus *Acanthamoeba* have been classified into 20 genotypes (T1 to T20).

Reservoir for Microorganisms

Acanthamoeba harbours a number of microorganisms such as *Listeria monocytogenes, Legionella* spp., *Chlamydia, Vibrio cholerae, Mycobacterium, Burkholderia, Yersinia,* mimivirus, coxsackievirus and adenovirus (**the trojan horse of the microbial world**). Residing inside *Acanthamoeba* protects these organisms from unfavourable conditions and allows them to evade the host defence, resist antibiotics and enhance their virulence.

EPIDEMIOLOGY

Though human diseases caused by *Acanthamoeba* were initially considered a rarity, they are now recognised as a significant human health concern. *Acanthamoeba* is implicated in the causation of encephalitis and keratitis.

- **Granulomatous amoebic meningoencephalitis (GAE)** most often develops in immunocompromised individuals such as patients who have AIDS and those on immunosuppressants or chemotherapy. However, a few cases are also reported in malnourished children.
- ***Acanthamoeba* keratitis (AK)** varies markedly in its incidence across the globe. Approximately 85% of documented AK cases in the developed countries are associated with contact lens usage. On the other hand, in developing countries including India, AK is mainly associated with corneal trauma.

MORPHOLOGY

Acanthamoeba exists in two forms—trophozoites and cysts (Fig. 21.1a and b). Both these forms can be found in the human body.

Trophozoite

It is amoeboid in shape, is **25–40 μm in size**, has a nucleus with large karyosome and moves slowly with the help of thorn-/spine-like pseudopodia called **acanthopodia**.

Cyst

Cysts are usually round but vary in shape. They are **10–25 μm** in size and are **double-walled with a wrinkled ectocyst** on the outside and an endocyst on the inside.

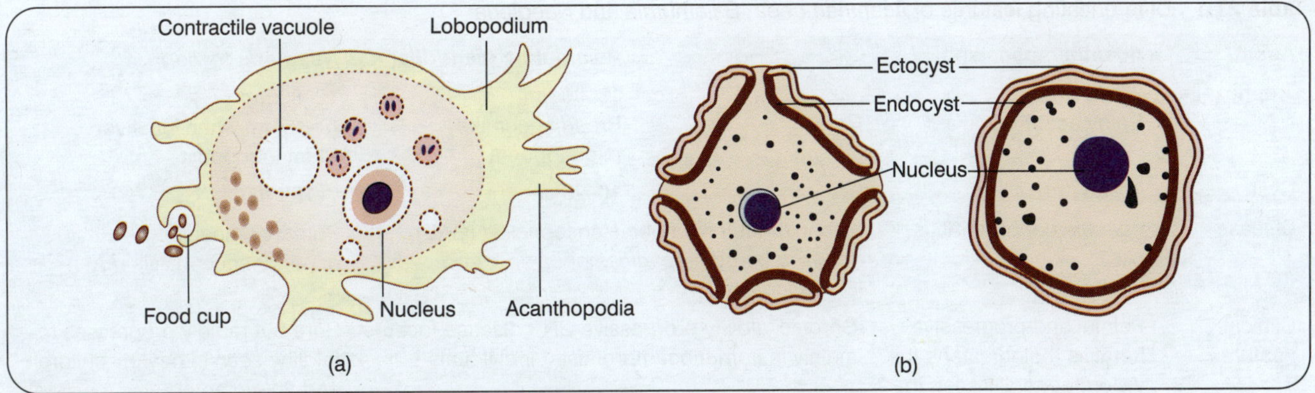

Fig. 21.1 Line diagrams of the two forms of *Acanthamoeba*: (a) trophozoite and (b) cyst

LIFE CYCLE (Fig. 21.2)

> **Habitat:** Free-living in moist soil and freshwater bodies

Like *Naegleria*, *Acanthamoeba* and *Balamuthia* exist in moist soil and freshwater bodies either in the feeding trophozoite stage or the resting cyst stage; no flagellate stages have been documented. These organisms alternate between stages depending on the environment. On encountering harsh conditions such as starvation and dryness, they become encysted. Upon the return of favourable conditions, excystation takes place. *Acanthamoeba* and *Balamuthia* infect humans through the respiratory tract or a breach in the integument. Table 21.1 presents the differentiating features of *Naegleria*, *Acanthamoeba* and *Balamuthia*.

PATHOGENESIS

Human infection is acquired when aerosols contaminated with cysts or trophozoites gain entry into the body **through the respiratory tract or a skin breach**. Further invasion of the central nervous system (CNS) possibly occurs through the **hematogenous route**. The following are the mechanisms of pathogenesis of the infection:

- **Parenchymal necrosis and focal granulomas** with foreign body giant cells are seen in the brain (usually not

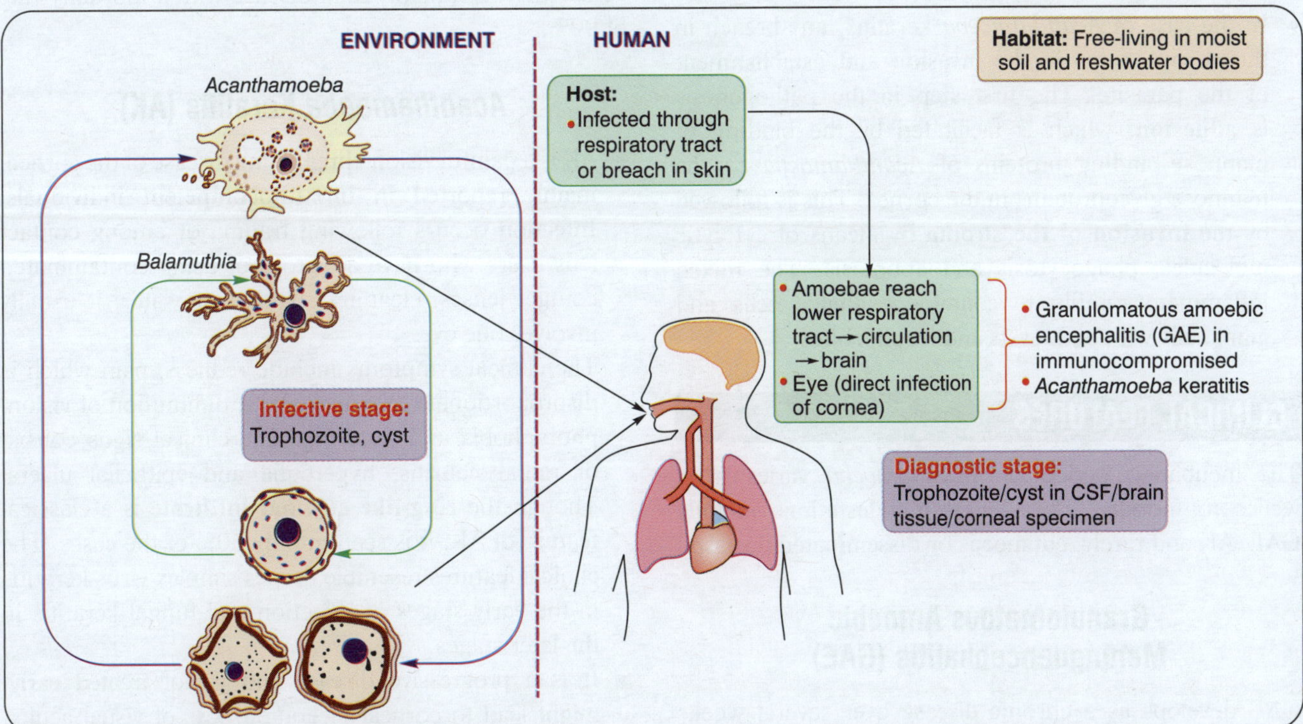

Fig. 21.2 Life cycles of *Acanthamoeba and Balamuthia*

Table 21.1 Differentiating features of *Acanthamoeba*, *Balamuthia* and *Naegleria*

<table>
<tr><th>Agent</th><th colspan="2">Acanthamoeba spp.</th><th>Balamuthia mandrillaris</th><th>Naegleria fowleri</th></tr>
<tr><td>Trophozoite</td><td colspan="2">25–40 μm
Spiny acanthopodia</td><td>15–60 μm
Broad/finger-like pseudopodia</td><td>10–30 μm
(9–15 μm when inactive)
Blunt lobopodia</td></tr>
<tr><td>Cyst</td><td colspan="2">10–25 μm</td><td>10–25 μm</td><td>7–15 μm</td></tr>
<tr><td>Disease</td><td>Acanthamoeba keratitis (AK)</td><td colspan="2">Granulomatous amoebic encephalitis (GAE) (caused by both Acanthamoeba spp. and B. mandrillaris)</td><td>Primary amoebic meningoencephalitis (PAM)</td></tr>
<tr><td>Clinical Features</td><td>Painful and progressive keratitis that threatens the vision; generally seen in immunocompetent lens wearers or those with corneal trauma</td><td colspan="2">Chronic, slowly progressive CNS disease; occurs mainly in immunocompromised individuals</td><td>Rare but rapidly progresses to fatality; seen in healthy children and young adults with a history of exposure to freshwater bodies</td></tr>
<tr><td>Entry</td><td>Corneal abrasion</td><td colspan="2">Respiratory tract, skin (hematogenous spread)</td><td>Olfactory epithelium (direct neural spread)</td></tr>
<tr><td>Incubation</td><td>Days</td><td colspan="2">Weeks to months</td><td>Days</td></tr>
<tr><td>Diagnostic methods</td><td>Corneal scrapings or biopsy, calcofluor white staining, non-nutrient agar (NNA) culture, confocal microscopy</td><td>For Acanthamoeba: Brain biopsy, CSF smear, wet preparation, NNA culture, indirect immunofluorescence of tissue, PCR</td><td>For Balamuthia: Brain biopsy, CSF wet preparation, culture on mammalian cells, indirect immunofluorescence of tissue, PCR</td><td>Brain biopsy, CSF wet preparation, NNA culture with Page's saline, indirect immunofluorescence of tissue, PCR</td></tr>
</table>

seen in the immunocompromised host) with trophozoites and cysts. Usually, the posterior regions of the brain are involved without the involvement of the olfactory bulbs. Amoebic phagocytosis and the production of toxins and enzymes result in the death of the host cell.

- In the case of *Acanthamoeba* keratitis, any breach in the cornea helps in the invasion and establishment of the parasite. The first step in the pathogenesis is **adhesion**, which is facilitated by the binding of mannose-binding proteins of *Acanthamoeba* to the mannose glycoproteins in the cornea. This is followed by the **invasion of the stroma** by means of cytolytic molecules, phagocytosis and apoptosis. The mixed inflammatory infiltrate contains epithelial cells and giant cells with both cysts and trophozoites.

CLINICAL FEATURES

The incubation period of *Acanthamoeba* varies from weeks to months. The clinical manifestations include GAE, AK and rarely, cutaneous or disseminated disease.

Granulomatous Amoebic Meningoencephalitis (GAE)

GAE develops as a chronic disease over several weeks or months. It typically occurs in **immunocompromised** individuals and often mimics a space-occupying lesion. It is characterised by headache, nausea, low-grade fever, vomiting, stiff neck, lethargy, visual disturbances, mental abnormalities, cerebellar ataxia, hemiparesis, seizures and coma. GAE is a highly fatal disease with a mortality rate of 90%.

Acanthamoeba Keratitis (AK)

- AK is a painful vision-threatening disease of the cornea, mainly reported in **immunocompetent** individuals. Infection occurs following trauma or among contact lens users who have a history of using contaminated contact lenses, cleaning solution or water; it usually involves one eye.
- The clinical symptoms include redness, pain which is disproportionate to ocular signs, diminution of vision, photophobia and watering. The clinical signs consist of radial neuritis, hyperemia and epithelial ulcers. Though the **ring-like stromal infiltrate** is a classical feature of AK, it is seen in only 50% of the cases. The clinical features resemble herpes simplex virus keratitis in the early stages of infection and fungal keratitis in the later stages.
- It is a progressive disease and if not treated early, might lead to corneal ulceration, loss of visual acuity, perforation of the cornea and ultimately, loss of the eye.

Cutaneous Acanthamoebiasis (CA)

- CA is a rare opportunistic disease caused by *Acanthamoeba* spp. and is mostly seen in **immunocompromised** individuals. It may or may not be associated with GAE.
- The characteristic feature of CA is the presence of hard erythematous nodules or papulonodules which develop into non-healing indurated ulcers.

DIAGNOSIS

The diagnosis of *Acanthamoeba* infection largely depends on the demonstration of trophozoites and cysts or DNA in CSF, brain tissue, corneal scrapings or biopsy and skin lesions, depending on the clinical disease.

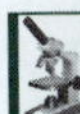

Lab diagnosis

- **Microscopy**: Visualising trophozoites and cysts
  - Direct microscopy of CSF
  - Staining: Giemsa, H&E
  - Calcofluor white
  - Histopathology of biopsy samples
- **Culture:** Non-nutrient agar (NNA)
- **Serology**: Not helpful
- **DNA detection**: PCR, real-time PCR
- **Other diagnostic parameters**:
  - Radioimaging
  - Confocal microscopy

Microscopy (Fig. 21.3a–d)

- **Wet mount:** Direct examination of CSF for trophozoites and cysts in unstained wet mount. The sensitivity of microscopic examination is quite low—reportedly only about 33%.
- **Staining:** Both trophozoites and cysts may be observed on Giemsa or hematoxylin and eosin (H&E) staining.
- **Fluorescent brightener – calcofluor white:** It stains the cyst walls but not the trophozoites.

Culture

The isolation and cultivation of *Acanthamoeba* can be done by direct inoculation of clinical samples onto 1.5% non-nutrient agar (NNA) plates overlaid with *Escherichia coli*. The NNA plates are incubated at 28–37°C for one week. The presence of the *Acanthamoeba* can be determined using an inverted light microscope.

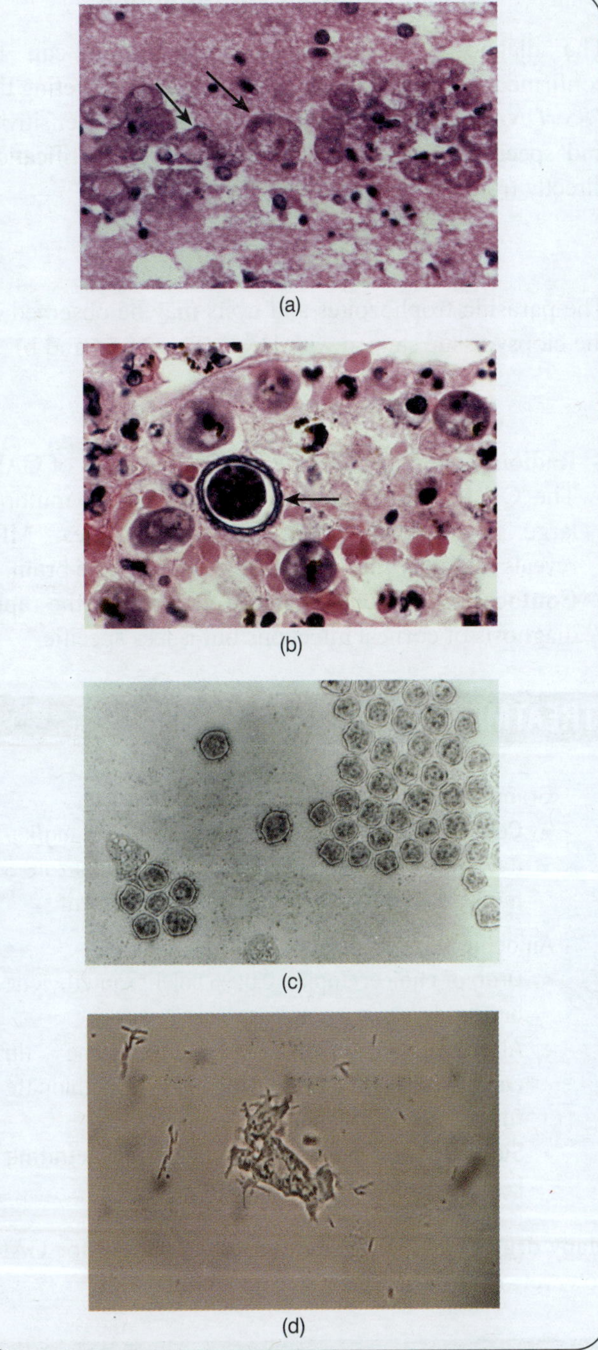

Fig. 21.3 Features of *Acanthamoeba* spp. in clinical samples: (a) trophozoite in brain tissue stained with hematoxylin and eosin (H&E) stain, (b) cyst in brain tissue stained with H&E, (c) cysts seen in an eye swab from a patient with keratitis and (d) trophozoite from a culture showing slender acanthopodia (*Source (a–c):* Centers for Disease Control and Prevention [CDC], Public Health Image Library [PHIL], Image IDs 18941, 9927 and 18944)

Serodiagnosis

Though patients have a higher titre of antibodies than healthy controls, this method is not very useful for diagnosis.

Nucleic Acid-Based Detection

The diagnosis of *Acanthamoeba* infection can be confirmed by conventional or real-time PCR targeting the *18S rDNA* gene. These methods have a higher sensitivity and specificity and also allow for species identification directly from the sample.

Histopathology

The parasitic trophozoites and cysts may be observed in the biopsy tissue stained with H&E (Fig. 21.3a and b).

Other Diagnostic Parameters

- **Radioimaging:** It is helpful for the diagnosis of GAE. The CT scan of the brain shows single or multiple large, low-density, space-occupying masses. MRI reveals multiple, ring-enhancing lesions in the brain.
- **Confocal microscopy:** It is a useful tool for the rapid diagnosis of corneal infections but is less specific.

TREATMENT

Granulomatous amoebic encephalitis

- **Combination therapy:** Cotrimoxazole 20 mg/kg/day, rifampicin 10 mg/kg/day and ketoconazole 5 mg/kg/day until there is clinical improvement

Amoebic keratitis

- **Drug of choice:** Topical 0.02% polyhexamethylene biguanide
- **Alternate drug:** 0.02% Chlorhexidine in combination with 0.1% propamidine isethionate for 3–4 weeks or longer
- **Surgery:** In severe cases, therapeutic penetrating keratoplasty may be required.

Many drug combinations have been attempted for GAE; however, no specific regimen is recommended.

PREVENTION AND CONTROL

Contact Lens Hygiene

- Contact lenses should be removed before swimming.
- Lenses should **not** be cleaned with water or home-made saline.
- Lens cases should be throughly cleaned on a regular basis.
- Contact lenses should not be used for periods longer than that recommended by the manufacturers.

BALAMUTHIA

Balamuthia mandrillaris is a free-living amoeba that was first isolated from the brain of a mandrill baboon that died of meningoencephalitis. In rare cases, it causes a disease of the CNS resembling **granulomatous amoebic encephalitis** with a sub-acute to chronic course; it is usually fatal. *B. mandrillaris* is the only species known to cause disease in humans. The life cycle of *Balamuthia* is similar to that of *Acanthamoeba*, consisting of both the trophozoite and the cystic stages. The size of the trophozoite ranges from **15–60 µm.** It generally moves with the help of broad pseudopodia, although it can also form finger-like pseudopods and display spider-like 'walking' in Vero cell cultures (Fig. 21.4a). The cysts of *Balamuthia* are similar in size and morphology to *Acanthamoeba* cysts except that they have triple-layered cyst walls (Fig. 21.4b). In contrast to *Acanthamoeba*, *Balamuthia* does not grow on NNA culture (Table 21.1). It can, however, be cultured on cell lines like Vero, monkey kidney cell line, HEp2, etc.

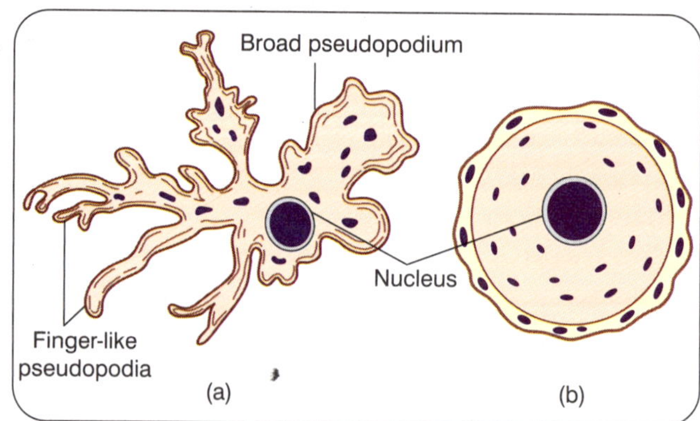

Fig. 21.4 Line diagram of *Balamuthia mandrillaris:* (a) trophozoite and (b) cyst

QUESTIONS

1. Discuss the diagnosis and management of granulomatous amoebic encephalitis.
2. Discuss the diagnosis and management of amoebic keratitis.
3. Differentiate between *Acanthamoeba*, *Balamuthia* and *Naegleria*.

Multiple Choice Questions

1. The culture medium used for growing *Acanthamoeba* is ______:
   a. Novy-Neal-Nicolle medium
   b. Non-nutrient agar medium
   c. Nelson's medium
   d. Nougot medium
2. Which of the following parasites causes contact lens-associated keratitis?
   a. *Entamoeba*
   b. *Acanthamoeba*
   c. *Naegleria*
   d. *Giardia*
3. Which of the following is NOT a feature of granulomatous amoebic encephalitis?
   a. It is sub-acute or chronic.
   b. Both trophozoites and cysts can be demonstrated in CSF.
   c. It responds very well to metronidazole treatment.
   d. It usually presents in immunocompromised patients.

CHAPTER 22

Helminths – Introduction and Classification

([From Greek] *helmins* = intestinal worm)

INTRODUCTION

Helminth is a general term that means 'worm'. These organisms are categorised under the **kingdom Animalia.** Worm infections are among the most prevalent infections, with about one-fourth of the global population of human beings infected with at least one type of worm. Helminths are multicellular eukaryotic organisms which exhibit bilateral symmetry with collagenous connective tissue between two dissimilar epithelia. They feed on organic material and digest it internally, i.e., they have heterotrophic nutrition.

In general, helminths exist in three morphological forms—**adult worm, larva and egg.** The knowledge of the different stages in relation to their growth and development is the basis for understanding the epidemiology and pathogenesis of helminthic diseases, as well as for the diagnosis and treatment of patients harbouring these parasites. Helminth parasites can be broadly differentiated on the basis of their morphology (Table 22.1). The systemic classification of the helminths of human importance is as follows (Fig. 22.1, 22.4 and 22.7):

I. Phylum Platyhelminthes (flatworms)
   1. Cestoidea (tapeworms)
   2. Trematoda (flukes)

II. Phylum Nematoda (roundworms)

III. Phylum Acanthocephala (spiny- or thorny-headed worms)

PLATYHELMINTHES (FLATWORMS)

These are dorsoventrally flattened worms with either a tape-like (cestodes) or leaf-like appearance (trematodes/flukes). The phylum Platyhelminthes is divided into three classes:

1. Cestoidea (tapeworms)
   a. Order Pseudophyllidea (e.g., *Diphyllobothrium*)
   b. Order Cyclophyllidea (e.g., *Taenia, Echinococcus, Hymenolepis*)
2. Trematoda (flukes)
   a. Order Strigeida (e.g., *Schistosomes*)
   b. Order Echinostomida (e.g., *Fasciola*)
   c. Order Plagiorchiida (e.g., *Opisthorchis*)
3. Monogenea (mainly ectoparasites of fishes)

Table 22.1 General morphological features of helminths of human importance

Phylum	Nematoda	Platyhelminthes (Flatworms)	
Adult worm	**Nematodes (Roundworms)**	**Cestodes (Tapeworms)**	**Trematodes (Flukes)**
	Bilaterally symmetrical Elongated Cylindrical with tapering end Unsegmented	Bilaterally symmetrical Flattened Tape-like Segmented	Bilaterally symmetrical Flattened Leaf-like Unsegmented
Head end	No suckers No hooklets Well-developed buccal capsule in some	Suckers present Some have hooklets	Suckers present No hooklets
Alimentary canal	Complete from mouth to anus	Absent	Present but incomplete
Body cavity	Present	Absent	Absent
Sexes	Separate male and female, i.e., dioecious	Not separate, i.e., hermaphrodite or monoecious	Monoecious (except schistosomes)
Larval forms	Rhabditiform Filariform Microfilaria	Coracidium Procercoid Plerocercoid Oncosphere Cysticercus Cysticercoid Coenurus Hydatid	Miracidium Sporocyst Redia Cercaria Metacercaria
Stages responsible for pathology in humans	Larva and adult	Larva and adult	Eggs, larva and adult

CESTODES (TAPEWORMS)

The classification of the members of the class Cestoidea is presented in Fig. 22.1.

General Characteristics

- The adult worms are long, **segmented and flattened** dorsoventrally, hence the name, 'tapeworm'.
- The worms vary in size from a few millimetres (*Echinococcus* spp.) to several meters (*Taenia* spp.) and may have as few as three or as many as several thousand segments.
- There are three regions in the body of an adult worm: a 'head' (scolex), a 'neck' and a strobila (body or trunk) consisting of a series of segments (proglottids).
- The head usually possesses one or more suckers (slit-like or cup-like; Fig. 22.2a and b) and sometimes hooks, which serve as organs of attachment.
- The sexes are not separate, i.e., each worm is **monoecious**.
- These worms do not have a body cavity or an alimentary canal.
- They have both excretory and nervous systems.
- Their reproductive systems are highly developed and complete in each segment (Fig. 22.2c). According to the maturity of the reproductive organs, three types of proglottids can be recognised from the head end to the body:
  a. **Immature proglottids:** Male and female organs are not differentiated in the immature segments.
  b. **Mature proglottids:** Male and female organs are differentiated (the male organs appear first).
  c. **Gravid proglottids:** The uteri in these segments are filled with eggs.
- The eggs of pseudophyllidean tapeworms are operculated, i.e., they have a lid, whereas those of cyclophyllidean species are not. The eggs of all tapeworms, however, contain an **embryo or oncosphere** at some stage of development.

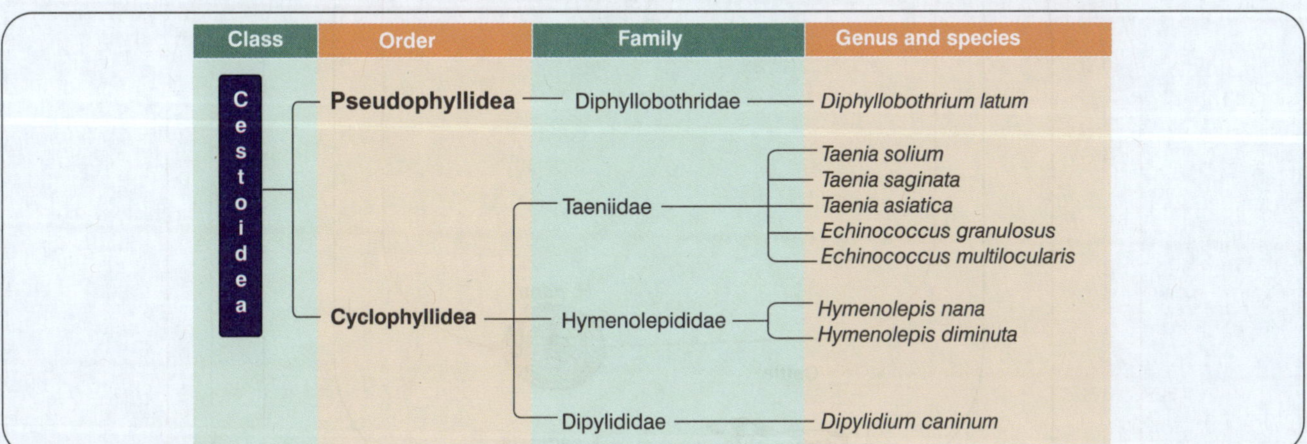

Fig. 22.1 Classification of Cestoidea

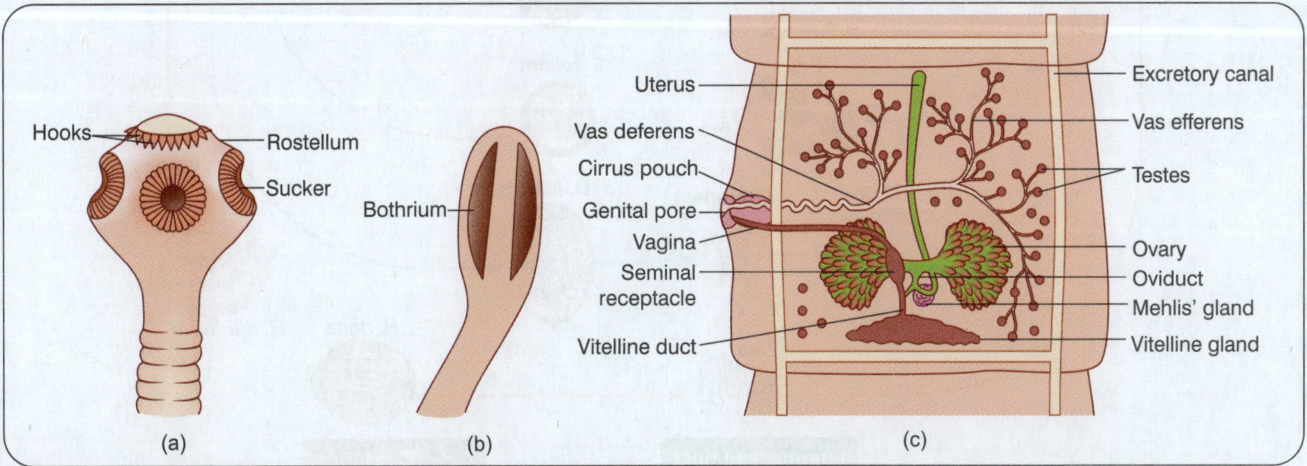

Fig. 22.2 Line diagrams of the morphology of cestodes: (a) head with cup-like suckers and hooks, (b) head with slit-like suckers and (c) a segment

LIFE CYCLE (Fig. 22.3)

Cestodes require two different hosts to complete their life cycle. The exception is *H. nana*, which is capable of autoinfection in humans without involving any intermediate host.

Definitive host: Humans are the definitive hosts for most cestodes, i.e., they **harbour the adult worm**, which usually resides in the intestine and generates progeny.

Intermediate host: The larval form of the worm is harboured by the intermediate host. Cattle, pig, fish, insects, etc., are the **natural** intermediate hosts of cestodes. Sometimes, humans act as the **accidental** intermediate hosts for some worms. In such cases, the larval forms of the worms are present in the tissues and may lead to serious disease (e.g., *Echinococcus* causes hydatid cyst and *Taenia solium* causes neurocysticercosis).

Development in Pseudophyllidea: The larval development takes place first in water and then in two intermediate hosts (e.g., *Diphyllobothrium*) as follows:

- The first larval stage develops from the egg in water and is called '**coracidium**'. The second-stage larva is called '**procercoid**' and develops in the cyclops (first intermediate host). The third larval stage is called '**plerocercoid**' and develops inside fish (second intermediate host).

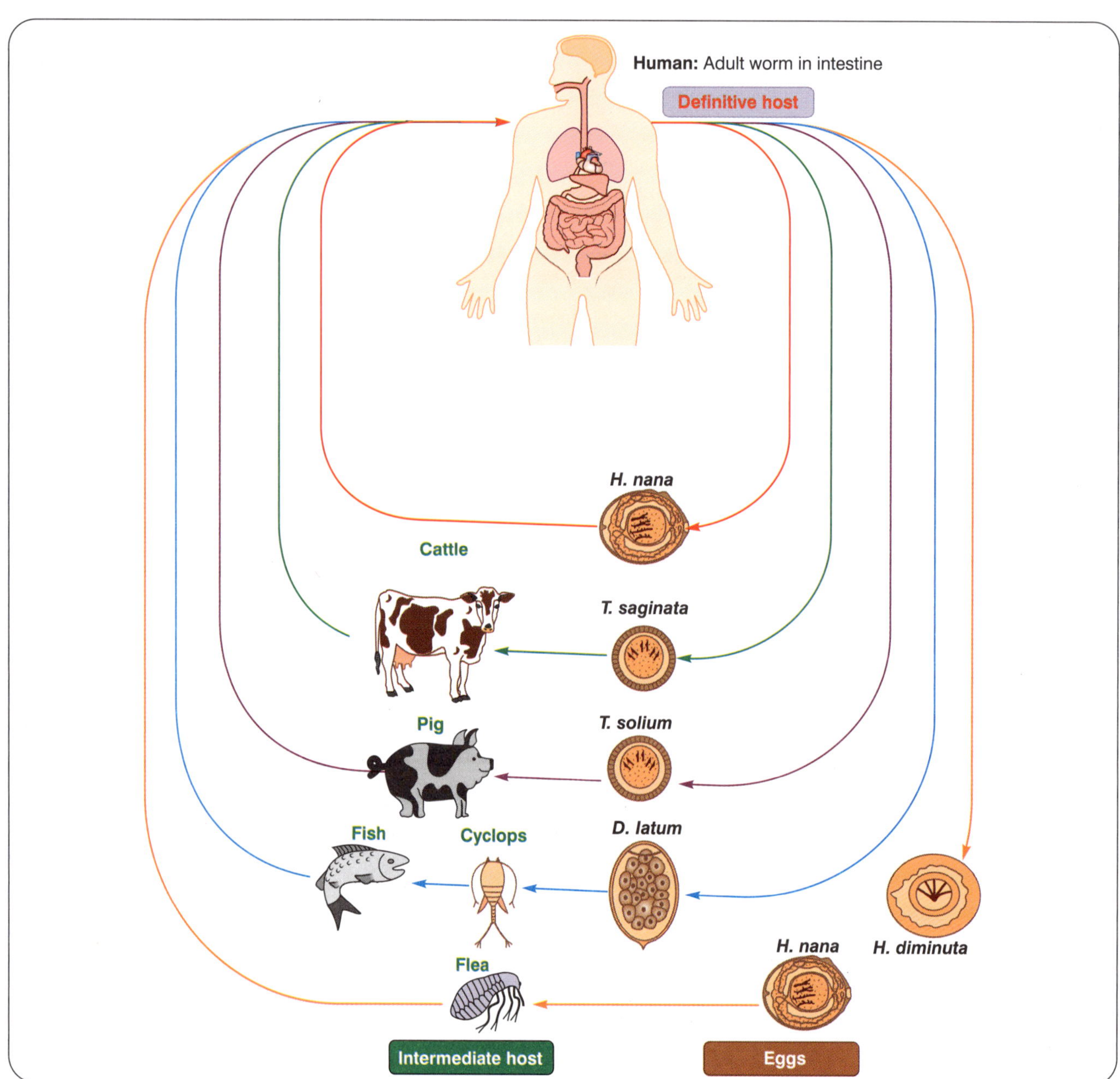

Fig. 22.3 Life cycle of cestodes

- Humans acquire the infection by ingesting plerocercoid larva in inadequately cooked fish. These larvae develop into adult worms in the human intestine and release eggs on reaching maturity.

Development in Cyclophyllidea: The natural larval development takes place in only one intermediate host as follows:

- The larvae (oncosphere) are transformed into sac-like structures resembling bladders. These **bladder worms** (called cysticercus in *Taenia* or hydatid cyst in *Echinococcus*) develop in animals like cattle, goat, sheep, pigs, etc., depending upon the worm species.
- When humans acquire the infection by the ingestion of cysticerci in meat, the adult worm develops in their intestines. However, when humans acquire the infection by the ingestion of eggs, they become the intermediate hosts, and the larval stage develops in their tissues. Such an event is a dead end for the larva.

TREMATODES (FLUKES)

The classification of medically important trematodes is presented in Fig. 22.4.

GENERAL CHARACTERISTICS (Fig. 22.5)

- While most adult worms are **unsegmented and flattened** dorsoventrally (leaf-like), some have thick, fleshy bodies (schistosomes).
- They range in size from less than 1 mm to a few centimetres (<10 cm).
- They have two suckers—an anterior oral sucker through which the digestive tract opens and a ventral sucker (acetabulum) for attachment to the host.
- They lack a body cavity, and their organs are embedded in specialised connective tissue.
- The digestive system is incomplete and consists of an anterior mouth continuing into an esophagus which bifurcates in front of the ventral sucker into a pair of blind intestinal pouches called caeca. These worms do not have an anus.
- The excretory system is bilaterally symmetrical and consists of flame cells and collecting tubules which lead to an excretory pore at the posterior end of the body, usually on the dorsal aspect.
- The nervous system consists of a group of paired ganglion cells at the anterior end from which nerves extend anteriorly and posteriorly.
- Most trematodes are hermaphrodites (**monoecious**), i.e., they have both male and female reproductive organs. The exception to this are schistosomes which have separate sexes (dioecious).
- These worms have highly developed reproductive systems. The male reproductive system consists of two testes and two vasa efferentia joining to form one vas deferens, which opens into the common genital pore. The female reproductive system consists of an ovary, vitelline glands surrounding the ovary, an oviduct, an ootype and the egg-containing uterus which opens near the ventral sucker and into the common genital pore.

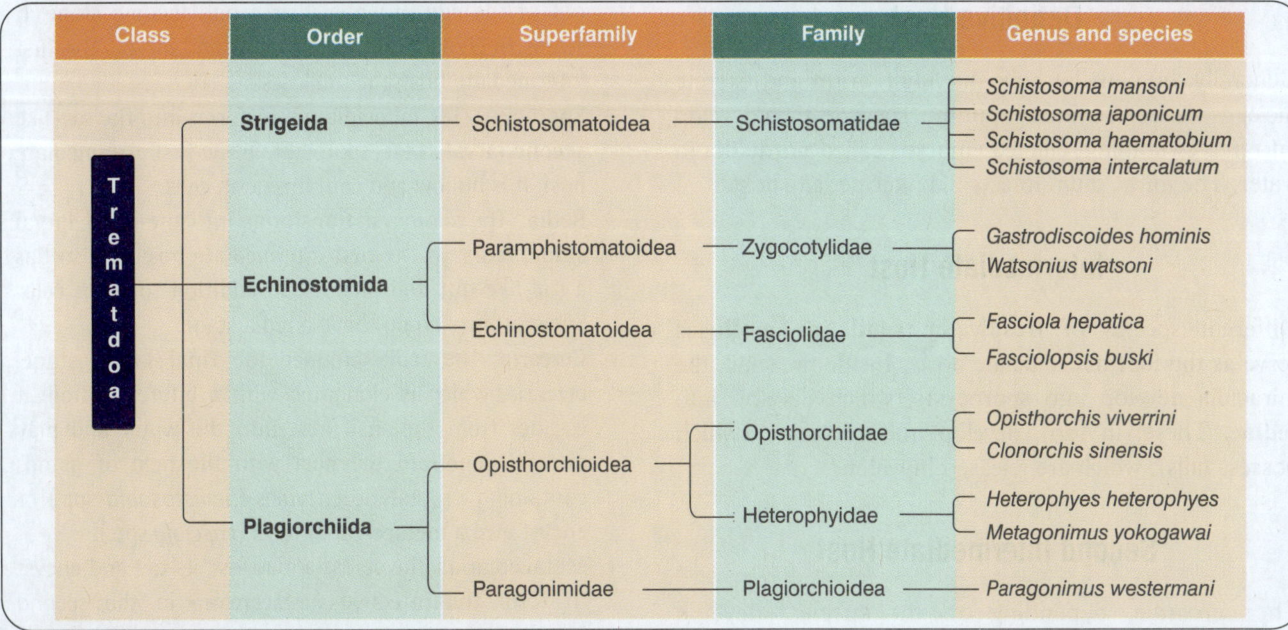

Fig. 22.4 Classification of medically important trematodes

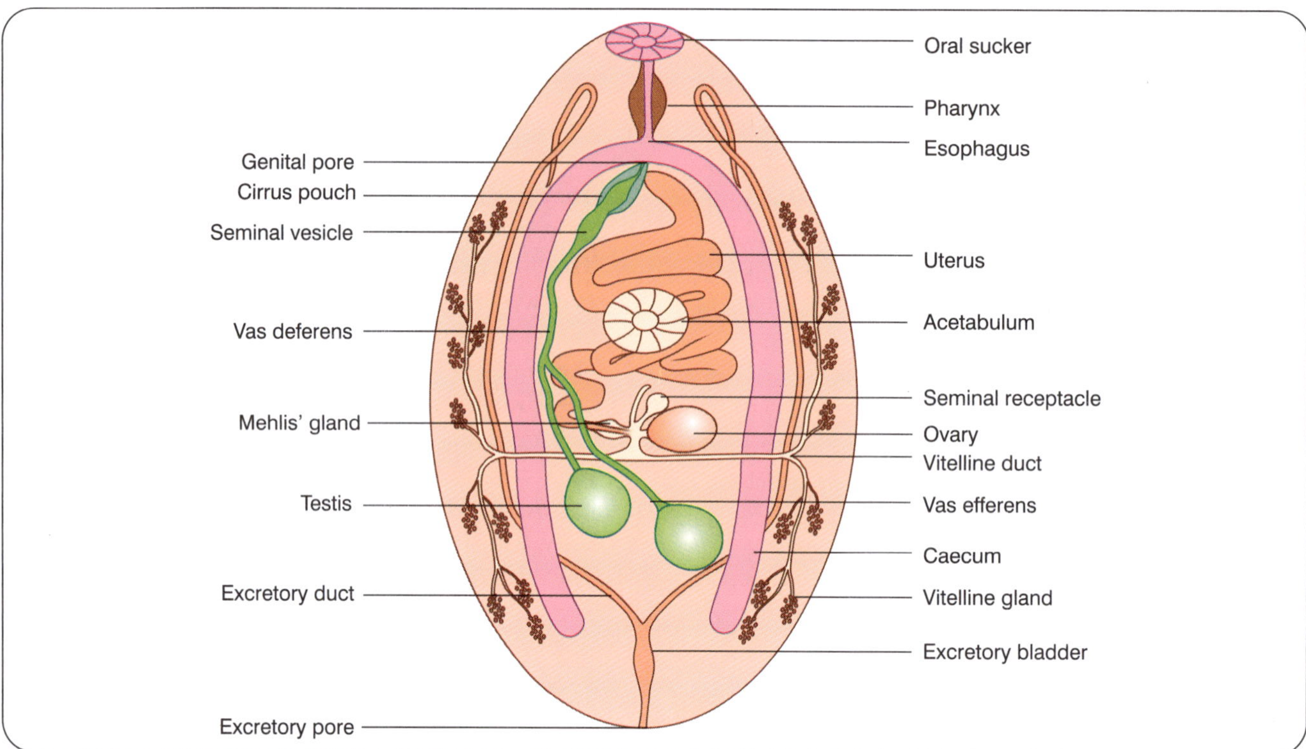

Fig. 22.5 Line diagram of the morphology of trematodes

- Fluke eggs, except for those of schistosomes, are operculated.

LIFE CYCLE (Fig. 22.6)

Trematodes complete their life cycle in two or more different hosts.

Definitive Host

Generally, humans harbour the adult worm and excrete the eggs via feces, urine or sputum. The eggs then develop into free-swimming, ciliated embryos called **miracidia** in water. The miracidium infects the intermediate host.

Intermediate Host

Different species of **freshwater snails** or **molluscs** serve as the first intermediate hosts. Inside the snail, the miracidia develop into **sporocysts**, which develop into **rediae.** These, in turn, develop into **cercariae** (which possess tails), which are released in water.

Second Intermediate Host

The cercariae, depending on the species, develop further in one of three ways—(a) they penetrate the definitive host and transform directly into adults, (b) they penetrate a **second intermediate host (fish or crab** in some trematodes) and develop into encysted **metacercariae** or (c) they latch on to aquatic vegetation and develop into metacercariae. When a metacercarial

> **Larval stages of trematodes**
>
> - **Miracidium:** It is the **first larval stage** which hatches out of the egg in water. It is a non-feeding stage. It swims freely with the help of cilia and infects the first intermediate host, the molluscs.
> - **Sporocyst:** The miracidium transforms into the sac-like **second larval stage**, sporocyst, in the first intermediate host. It is hollow and contains germ cells.
> - **Redia:** The sporocyst transforms into the **third larval stage**, redia, in the first intermediate host. It also has a sac-like gut and pharynx in addition to germ cells. Schistosomes do not have a redia stage.
> - **Cercaria:** The redia produce the **final larval stage**, cercaria, which is elongated with a bifurcated tail. It escapes from the snail host into the water and may directly penetrate the host with the help of glands containing proteolytic enzymes (*Schistosoma* spp.) or encyst into a metacercarial form (*Fasciola* spp.).
> - **Metacercaria:** The cercaria may lose its tail and encyst to form the infective metacercaria in the second intermediate host or on an aquatic plant.

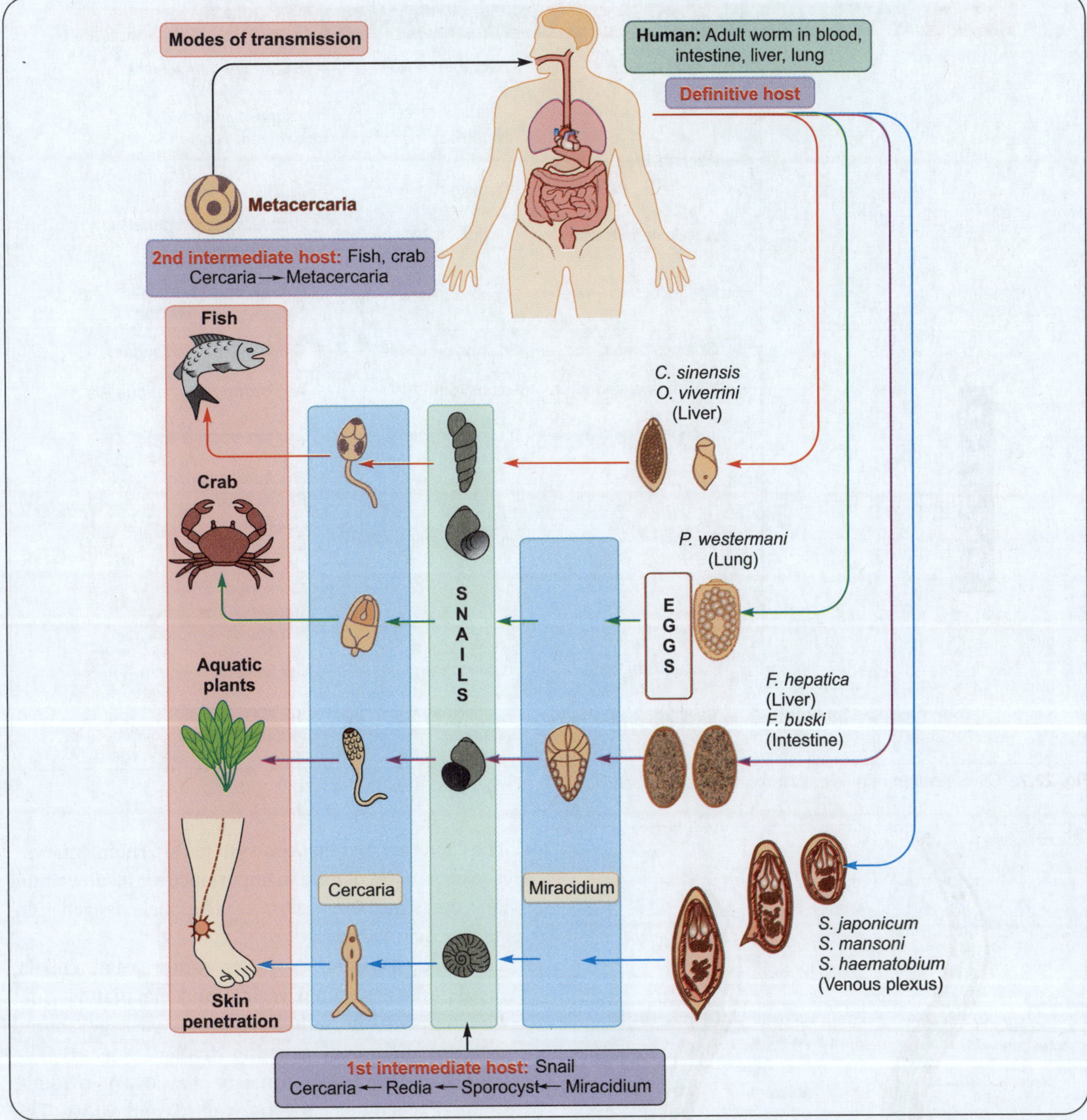

Fig. 22.6 Life cycle of trematodes

cyst is ingested, it is digested to liberate an immature fluke which migrates to a specific organ site and develops into its adult worm.

NEMATODA (ROUNDWORMS)

The nematodes are the most abundant animal groups in the environment. The classification of nematodes is presented in Fig. 22.7.

GENERAL CHARACTERISTICS (Fig. 22.8)

- Nematodes are elongated, **cylindrical** worms. Their bodies are **unsegmented**, do not have any appendages and taper at the ends. The nematode's body is covered with a tough cuticle.
- They range in size range from 5 mm (*S. stercoralis*) to 1 metre (*D. medinensis*).
- They possess a body cavity in which various organs such as the digestive and genital organs are present.

Phylum	Class	Superfamily	Family	Genus and species
Nematoda	Secernentea	Oxyuroidea	Oxyuridae	*Enterobius vermicularis*
		Ascaridoidea	Ascarididae	*Ascaris lumbricoides*
				Toxocara canis
				Toxocara cati
			Anisakidae	*Anisakis simplex*
		Ancylostomatoidea	Ancylostomatidae	*Ancylostoma duodenale*
				Necator americanus
		Rhabditoidea	Strongyloididae	*Strongyloides stercoralis*
				Strongyloides fulleborni
		Gnathostomatoidea	Gnathostomatidae	*Gnathostoma spinigerum*
		Metastrongyloidea	Angiostrongylidae	*Angiostrongylus cantonensis*
		Trichostrongyloidea	Trichostrongylidae	*Trichostrongylus* spp.
		Filarioidea	Onchocercidae	*Wuchereria bancrofti*
				Brugia malayi
				Brugia timori
				Loa loa
				Onchocerca volvulus
				Mansonella ozzardi
				Mansonella perstans
				Mansonella streptocerca
		Dracunculoidea	Dracunculidae	*Dracunculus medinensis*
	Adenophorea	Trichinelloidea	Trichinellidae	*Trichinella spiralis*
			Trichuridae	*Trichuris trichiura*

Fig. 22.7 Classification of medically important nematodes

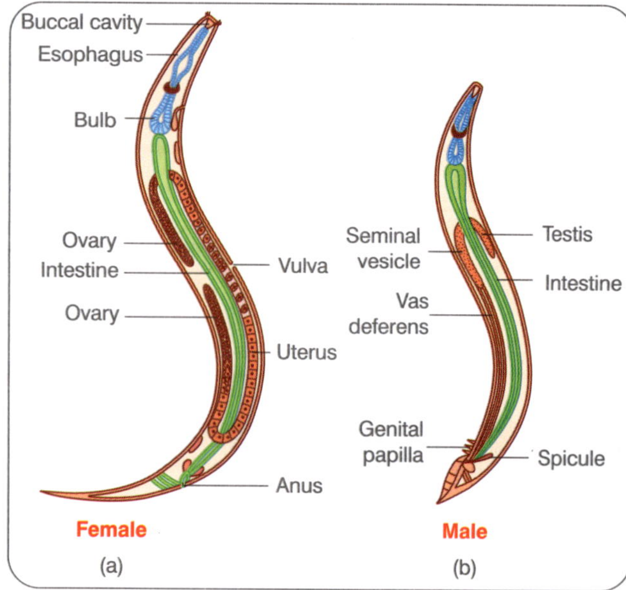

Fig. 22.8 Line diagram of representative morphology of nematodes: (a) female and (b) male

- The alimentary canal is complete, from an oral aperture to an anus. The mouth cavity, when present, may have teeth or cutting plates.
- The excretory and nervous systems are rudimentary.
- The nematodes of human importance are all **dioecious**, i.e., the sexes are separate. The male is generally smaller than the female.
- The male reproductive system comprises of a testis, vas deferens, seminal vesicle and ejaculatory duct which opens through a common passage shared with the intestinal opening (called cloaca). The female genital system consists of an ovary, oviduct, seminal receptacle, uterus, vagina and vulva. The genital pore lies in the middle of the nematode's body.
- The female nematodes are categorised as follows:
  a. **Viviparous:** Give birth to larvae, e.g., *Dracunculus medinensis* and filarial worms
  b. **Oviparous:** Lay eggs, e.g., *Enterobius* and *Ascaris*
  c. **Ovoviviparous:** Lay eggs which immediately hatch to release larvae, e.g., *Strongyloides*
- Nematodes are usually long-living—the roundworm usually lives for one year, the pinworm for several months to years, the hookworm for 5–7 years and *Strongyloides stercoralis* for >30 years.

LIFE CYCLE (Fig. 22.9)

Most nematodes complete their life cycle in **one host**. Humans are the optimal hosts, and the adult worm usually lives in the human intestine. An insect vector is the second host for filarial worms, whereas members of the genus *Cyclops* serve as the second host for *Dracunculus*. After hatching from the egg, the first-stage larva (L1)

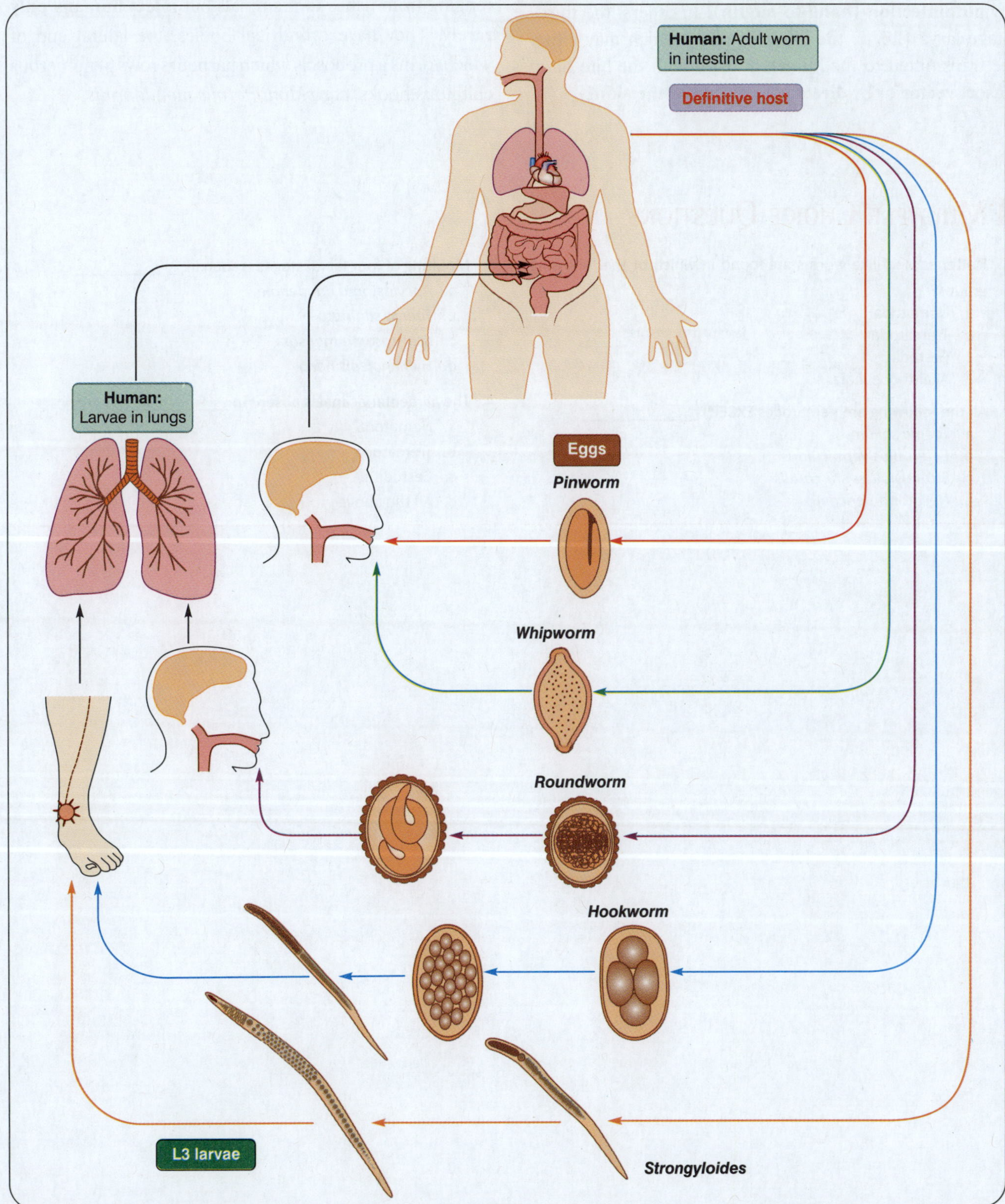

Fig. 22.9 Life cycle of nematodes

undergoes four sequential moultings of the cuticle to form L2, L3 and L4 larvae and finally, the adult stage. For some species, the embryonated egg is the infective stage. The host acquires the infection by ingesting the egg, usually through the **fecal-oral route or fomites or by autoinfection (hand-to-mouth)**. In others, the third-stage larva (L3) is the infective stage, which may either be transmitted to the human host through the bite of an **insect vector** or by **direct penetration of the skin**.

ACANTHOCEPHALA (SPINY- OR THORNY-HEADED WORMS)

These parasites live in the intestine of different vertebrates ranging from fishes to mammals but **infect humans only rarely.** They have cylindrical bodies, the lateral end of which forms a proboscis which harbours rows of numerous chitinous hooks, e.g., *Moniliformis moniliformis.*

Multiple Choice Questions

1. Flattened, leaf-like worms are found in which of the following groups?
   a. Nematoda
   b. Trematoda
   c. Cestoda
   d. Acanthocephala
2. All the following are nematodes EXCEPT ____________ :
   a. *Taenia solium*
   b. *Enterobius vermicularis*
   c. *Strongyloides stercoralis*
   d. *Necator americanus*
3. Moulting of four larval stages is seen in ____________ :
   a. *Ancylostoma duodenale*
   b. *Taenia saginata*
   c. *Schistosoma mansoni*
   d. *Hymenolepis nana*
4. The alimentary canal is absent in ____________ :
   a. Nematoda
   b. Trematoda
   c. Cestoda
   d. All the above

Chapter 23

Soil-Transmitted Helminths

Learning Goals

- What are soil-transmitted helminths (STH)?
- What are the strategies used for the control of STH?

INTRODUCTION

The term **soil-transmitted helminths (STH)** or **'geohelminths'** applies to a group of nematode worms consisting of **roundworms, whipworms and hookworms**. These nematodes are transmitted to humans through **fecally contaminated soil** without any intermediate hosts or vectors. STH infections are highly prevalent but are preventable by public health measures. These worms have many similarities in their epidemiology and population biology; the approach to their diagnosis, treatment and prevention strategies is also similar. For this reason, members of this group are dealt with under one umbrella to optimise public health resources. Other helminths such as *Strongyloides stercoralis*, which are also transmitted after development in soil, are not covered under STH programmes due to differences in their epidemiology, diagnosis, treatment modalities, etc.

The specific differences between the individual species of the STH group are detailed in the chapters ahead and summarised in Table 23.1.

EPIDEMIOLOGY

- The communities affected by different STH are similar or overlap due to the common environmental conditions needed for the transmission of these worms. The most favourable environmental conditions are warm weather (25–35°C), a minimum rainfall of 50–60 inches, and loose and moist soil—conditions prevalent in many **tropical and subtropical regions** of the world.
- More than a billion individuals are infected with STHs, mostly in the tropical and subtropical regions of the world with **poor sanitary conditions and open defecation**. Almost 70% of the STH infections occur in Asia; India contributes to a major portion of this percentage.
- Generally, children are the most affected group; however, adults are not entirely spared. For hookworms, the prevalence rises with age; other population groups such as females of childbearing age are also commonly affected.
- Many infected individuals harbour mixed infections.

CLINICAL FEATURES

The clinical features depend on the intensity of infection, i.e., the worm load in an individual (Table 23.2).

- Individuals who have light infections usually remain asymptomatic.
- In chronic or heavy-intensity infections, STH are implicated in significant growth and cognitive malfunctions due to nutrient deficiency.

DIAGNOSIS

The diagnosis of STH infections is important in many aspects. **Clinically**, it is essential to confirm the infection and treat the patient; **epidemiologically**, it is crucial to determine the environmental hotspots of transmission with the ultimate aim of planning focused interventions by control programmes and lastly, it is vital to **assess the impact** of **mass drug administration (MDA)** in various deworming programmes.

The diagnosis of STH infections is generally made by direct microscopic examination of fecal samples to demonstrate the **characteristic eggs or the worm**. In field surveys, it is important to estimate the intensity of infections.

- **Intensity of the infection** can be measured indirectly by counting the number of eggs per gram (epg) of feces or directly by counting the number of worms expelled in the feces after anti-helminthic treatment. WHO-approved **Kato-Katz and Mini-FLOTAC** techniques can be used to measure the intensity of the infection. However, epg is not an accurate measure of infection since the number of eggs produced by different female worms in the gut is variable.

Table 23.1 Differences between soil-transmitted helminths

Feature	Roundworm	Whipworm	Hookworm
Species	*Ascaris lumbricoides*	*Trichuris trichiura*	*Necator americanus* *Ancylostoma duodenale*
Size of adult	15–35 cm	3–5 cm	0.7–1.1 cm
Shape of adult	Cylindrical, pink	Whip-like, white–grey	Cylindrical, anterior end hook-like, grey–white
Location	Small intestine	Large intestine	Small intestine
Eggs/day/female	2,40,000	3,000–5,000	9,000–10,000 (*Necator*) 25,000–30,000 (*Ancylostoma*)
Egg morphology	Unfertilised egg: long and narrow, 85–95 × 43–47 mm; fertilised egg: round to oval, 45–75 × 35–50 mm; both are bile-stained (brown)	Barrel-/lemon-shaped, 55 × 25 μm, bile-stained (brown) with bipolar mucus plugs	Oval, 60 × 40 μm, thin hyaline shell, 4–32 celled, non-bile-stained (colourless)
Infective stage	Egg	Egg	L3 larva
Route of transmission	Fecal–oral	Fecal–oral	Skin penetration
Extra-intestinal migration	Yes	No	Yes
Complications of heavy intensity infections	Malnutrition, growth retardation, poor cognitive development, intestinal obstruction, extra-intestinal ascariasis, allergic reactions	Malnutrition, growth retardation, poor cognitive development, rectal prolapse, chronic dysentery, anemia	Malnutrition, growth retardation, poor cognitive development, severe anemia
Treatment (first-line)	Albendazole, 400 mg, single dose	Albendazole, 400 mg OD × 3 days	Albendazole, 400 mg, single dose

Table 23.2 Intensity of STH infections

Organism	Light intensity	Moderate intensity	Heavy intensity
Roundworm	1–4,999 epg*	5,000–49,999 epg	>50,000 epg
Whipworm	1–999 epg	1,000–9,999 epg	>10,000 epg
Hookworm	1–1,999 epg	2,000–3,999 epg	>4,000 epg

*epg denotes eggs per gram

- Real-time PCR-based molecular methods are more sensitive for the quantitative estimation of infection and are particularly useful for low-intensity infections. These can also be used for epidemiological studies to assess the impact of deworming post-MDA.

TREATMENT

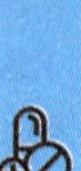

- *Albendazole:* For adults and children >2 years, 400 mg oral or 10 ml 4% suspension as a single dose; for children aged 1–2 years, 200 mg oral or 5 ml 4% suspension as a single dose
- *Mebendazole:* 500 mg BDS × 3 days
- *Supportive treatment:* Iron and nutritional supplements

Albendazole and mebendazole can be used for **preventive chemotherapy in MDA programmes.** A single dose of albendazole has a good safety and efficacy profile and better compliance than other drugs. These factors, when coupled with its ease of administration, make albendazole the preferred drug for MDA. These drugs are **not recommended in the first trimester of pregnancy and in children below one year** due to possible embryotoxic and teratogenic effects.

PREVENTION AND CONTROL

- **STH control programmes:** The goal of STH control programmes is to reduce morbidity from STH in school-age children (SAC, 5–14 years) and pre-SAC (1–4 years) to a level where it is no longer considered a public health problem. MDA programmes are implemented by governments for the control of STH based on infection prevalence in particular areas (Table 23.3).

- Target populations for STH control programmes:
  - **School-age children (SAC) and pre-SAC** have the highest worm burden and can be mass-treated at school.
  - **Women of the reproductive age** including pregnant women in the second and third trimesters and lactating mothers should receive treatment.
  - **Adults at high risk** such as individuals who work at tea plantations and those employed in mining are also targeted.
- Albendazole (more common) or mebendazole are used and have been shown to reduce morbidity due to STH among children.
- In India, **February 10 is the National Deworming Day**. Deworming is also done as a part of many other national programmes such as the Lymphatic Filariasis Elimination Programme, the Weekly Iron and Folic Acid Supplementation Programme of the Reproductive and Child Health (RCH) Division, the School Health Programme, the Integrated Child Development Scheme, etc., which are also aimed at reducing the burden of STH.

Table 23.3 Frequency of deworming for STH infections

Category of risk	Prevalence	Frequency of deworming
Low-risk areas	<20%	Case-to-case basis treatment
Moderate-risk areas	≥20–<50%	Annual MDA
High-risk areas	≥50%	Biannual MDA

- **Education, hygiene and sanitation** play a significant role in the prevention and control of STH. This includes the following:
  - Health education
  - **WASH** programme, i.e., safe **wa**ter, **s**anitation and **h**ygiene with measures like hand washing and discouraging open defecation is an important strategy for the prevention of diarrheal diseases including STH as it reduces environmental transmission of the parasite
  - Composting of human feces before it is disposed
  - **Use of footwear** serves as a primary preventive measure against hookworms
- Reinfection is quite common post-deworming and should be guarded against.
- There are no vaccines for STH at present.

Questions

1. Describe STH control programmes.
2. Discuss the laboratory diagnosis of soil-transmitted helminthic infections.

Multiple Choice Questions

1. The parasites commonly referred to as soil-transmitted helminths are ______:
   a. Roundworm
   b. Hookworm
   c. Whipworm
   d. All these
2. Which technique is used to quantify the intensity of infection by soil-transmitted infection in an individual?
   a. Kato-Katz method
   b. Baerman's technique
   c. NNN culture method
   d. Immunofluorescence microscopy
3. In STH control programmes, which population is targeted for mass drug administration?
   a. Preschool-age and school-age children
   b. Women of reproductive age
   c. High-risk adults
   d. All these

Chapter 24

Ascaris (Roundworm)

(*Ascaris lumbricoides* from *ascaris* [Greek] = worm; *lumbricus* [Latin] = earthworm)

Case Study and Learning Goals

A 5-year-old boy from a rural area presents with generalised abdominal pain, vomiting and mild distension. He has a history of worm expulsion from the anus. What is the parasitic cause of abdominal distension? How would you approach the laboratory diagnosis in this case? What preventive measures would you advise?

INTRODUCTION

Ascariasis is caused by the common **'roundworm'** ***Ascaris lumbricoides*** (named by Carl Linnaeus in 1758), which is **categorised under soil-transmitted helminths (STH)**. It is one of the earliest documented worms—it is mentioned in Egyptian medical papyri dating back as far as 1500 BC, and in several other ancient medical literature including Hippocratic texts and records of Chinese, Roman and Arabian physicians. The eggs of *Ascaris* have been found in fossilised human feces from Peru (dating back to 2277 BC) and Brazil (dating back to 1660–1420 BC), and in Egyptian and Chinese mummies. Its anatomy was described much later by Edward Tyson (1683) and Francesco Redi (1684). The development of human infection following the ingestion of eggs was described by Giovanni Grassi (1881) and Casimir Davaine (1862), and the complete life cycle of *Ascaris* was described by Shimesu Koino as recently as in 1922.

Ascaris suum, another species which rarely causes human infections, is transmitted through contact with domestic pigs infected with this parasite. Though it is prevalent worldwide, the exact burden and harmful effects of this zoonosis in humans is not clear.

EPIDEMIOLOGY

Across the world, more than **800 million** people are estimated to be infected with *A. lumbricoides*, with about 100,000 deaths annually. However, these could be underestimations as the true prevalence is quite difficult to calculate. It is estimated that 20–25% of infected individuals are from India. The heaviest infections occur in parts of the world where human feces are used as manure. The **most commonly affected are children**, who ingest the eggs while playing in soil contaminated with eggs or acquire the infection after eating contaminated raw vegetables. Adults acquire the infection while farming or by eating contaminated raw vegetables, generally from crops fertilised with untreated sewage. *Ascaris* exhibits a highly variable frequency distribution, which means that the worms are **aggregated or over-dispersed heavily in a few individuals** who harbour a disproportionately large number of worms.

MORPHOLOGY

Adult Worm

A. lumbricoides is the **largest intestinal nematode** parasite of humans (Fig. 24.1) (refer to Chapter 22 for the general morphological features of nematodes). The following are the morphological characteristics of *Ascaris*:

- Its body is pink, cylindrical and tapers gradually at the anterior end and less so at the posterior end.
- The mouth opens at the anterior end and possesses three finely-toothed, well-developed lips (one dorsal and two ventral).
- The digestive and respiratory organs float inside the body cavity, which contains a toxic fluid called 'ascaron' or 'ascarase'. This fluid is responsible for allergic manifestations.

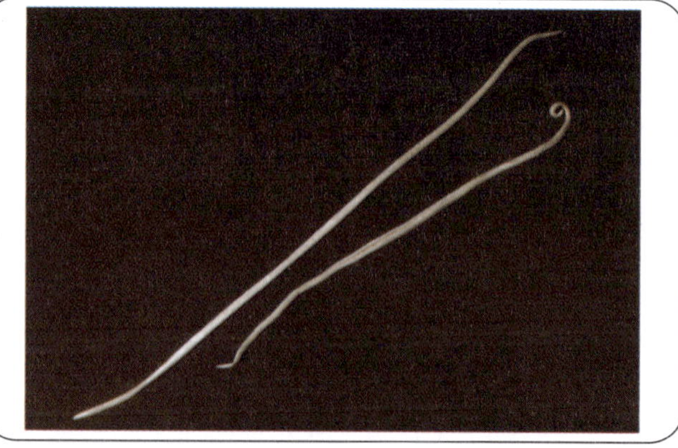

Fig. 24.1 Adults of *Ascaris lumbricoides:* female (left) and male (right) (*Source:* Centers for Disease Control and Prevention [CDC], Public Health Image Library [PHIL], Image ID 10176)

- The male worm measures 15–30 cm in length × 3–4 mm in diameter. Its posterior end is curved ventrally. The ejaculatory duct and anus open into the cloaca, from which arise a pair of copulatory spicules.
- The female worm is longer and stouter than the male and measures 20–35 cm in length × 2–6 mm in diameter. A minute vulva opens at the junction between the anterior and middle third of the body—the narrowest part of the worm's body (vulvar waist). The anus is situated in the subterminal part and opens like a transverse slit on the ventral surface.

Eggs

The female lays eggs after maturation and is capable of laying **as many as 240,000 eggs per day** (Fig. 24.2).

The following are characteristics of *Ascaris* eggs:

- The inner eggshell consists of a lipid layer and a chitin–protein layer. It contains ascaroside, a very hardy lipoprotein, which helps the eggs to survive harsh conditions.
- The outer surface of the egg has an irregular or mammillated mucopolysaccharide (cortical layer) coat which is formed as the egg passes out through the uterus. This mucopolysaccharide layer helps the egg to adhere to its surrounding objects. Sometimes, this layer is lost, and the egg becomes decorticated.
- Both fertilised and unfertilised eggs can be found in stool. However, if only female worms are present in the intestine, fertilised eggs will not be produced.
- The fertilised eggs characteristically float in a saturated salt solution, whereas the unfertilised eggs, being the heaviest of all the helminths eggs, do not float. There are many other features that differentiate fertilised eggs from unfertilised ones (Table 24.1, Fig. 24.2).

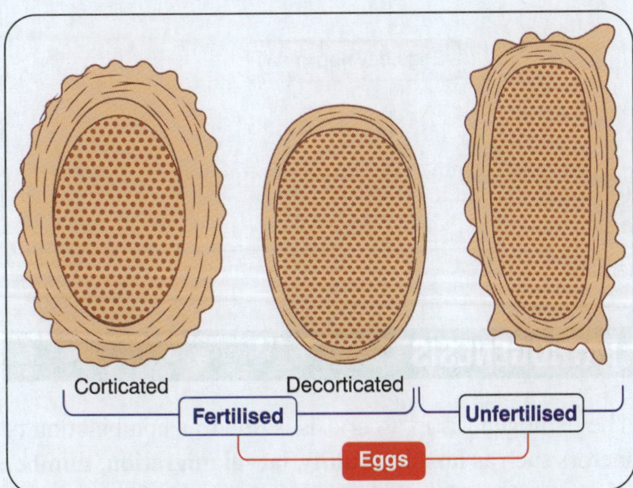

Fig. 24.2 Line diagram of the eggs of *Ascaris lumbricoides*

Larva

Ascaris has four larval stages, L1 to L4.

LIFE CYCLE (Fig. 24.3a and b)

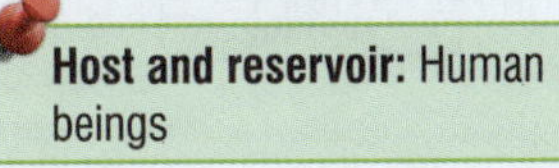

Humans are the **only hosts and reservoirs** of *A. lumbricoides*. No intermediate host is required by this parasite. The normal life span of the worm is about 1–2 years. The various stages in the life cycle of *A. lumbricoides* are as follows:

- The infection is acquired by ingesting embryonated eggs containing second-stage larvae (L2) via contaminated food, water or raw vegetables. The eggs hatch in the **stomach and duodenum** and release larvae which penetrate the intestinal wall and enter the mesenteric vessels and lymphatics. The larvae then pass through hepatic veins and enter the right side of the heart.
- From the heart, the larvae spread through the pulmonary circulation to the **lungs**, where they undergo two moultings (to form L3 and L4 stages). They then penetrate the alveoli to finally ascend into the bronchioles, bronchi and trachea and are coughed into the hypopharynx.
- Upon swallowing, these larvae (L4) pass down into the **small intestine** where they undergo the fourth moulting to become young adults, which then grow

Table 24.1 Differences between fertilised and unfertilised eggs of *A. lumbricoides*

Feature	Unfertilised egg	Fertilised egg
Size and shape	85–95 mm × 43–47 mm Long and narrow	45–75 mm × 35–50 mm Round to oval
Ovum	Small, disorganised and refractile	Large, unsegmented, with clear crescentic area towards both poles; initial stages of cleavage may be seen
Bile-stained/colour	Yes, brown	Yes, brown
Saturated salt solution	Do not float	Float

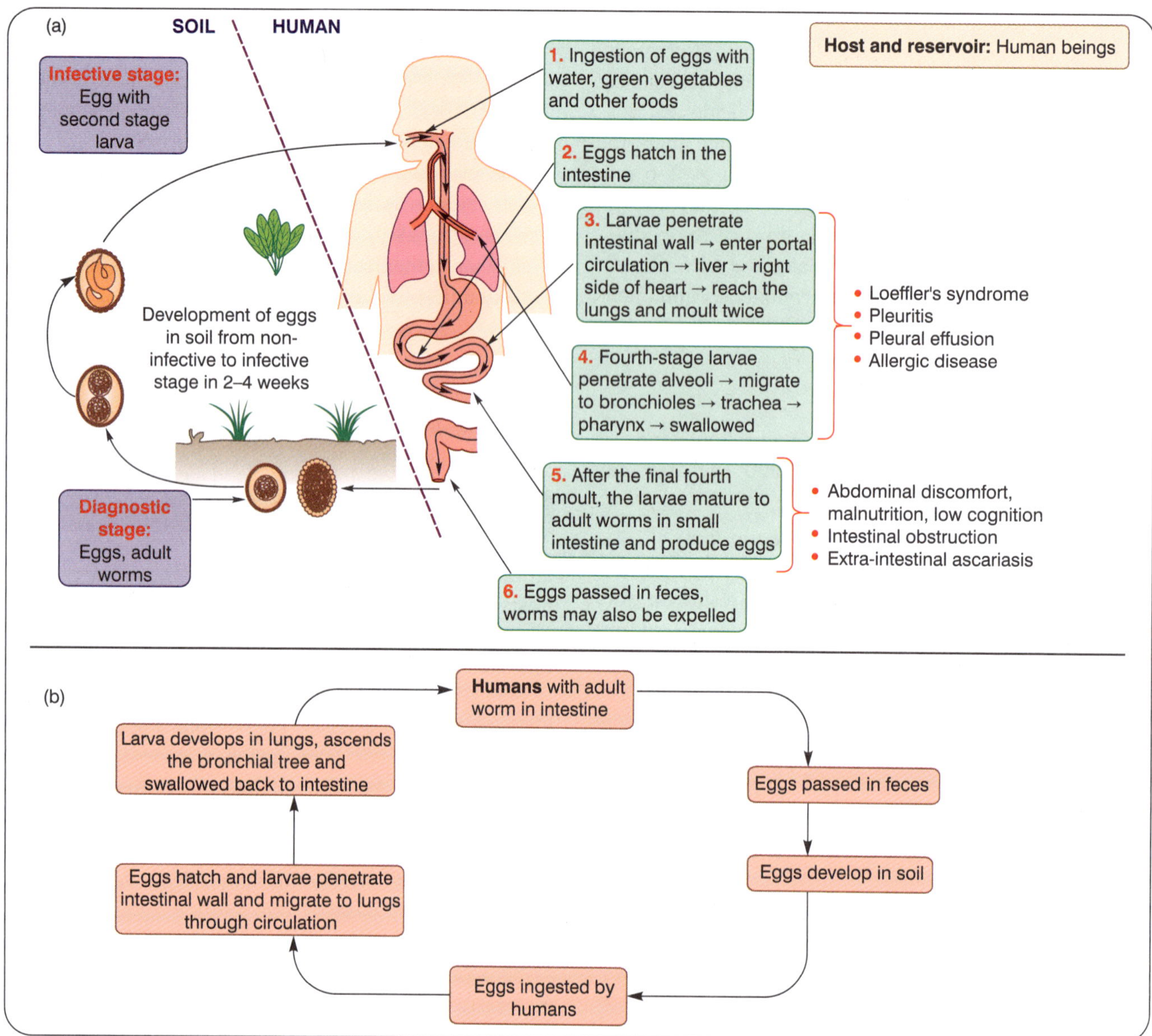

Fig. 24.3 Life cycle of *Ascaris lumbricoides:* (a) detailed and (b) schematic

into mature adult worms. The adults are ready to lay eggs after a period of 6–12 weeks (pre-patent period).

The freshly laid eggs are not infective to humans. In the soil (ideally, temperature 20–40°C and humidity >40%), first-stage **(L1)** rhabditiform larvae develop inside the eggs within 10–15 days. The L1 larvae then moult to the L2 larval stage and render the eggs infective. These **embryonated eggs containing L2 larvae** are now ready to infect another host. A large proportion of the eggs are known to survive and remain infective in the environment for as long as ten years and possibly longer. *Ascaris* eggs can also remain suspended in the air along with dust, whereby they may be inhaled and swallowed.

PATHOGENESIS

The pathogenesis in ascariasis is due to a combination of factors such as **host immunity, larval migration, number of worms, mechanical effects of the adult worm and malnutrition-related** consequences. A host predisposition to infection is indicated with respect to susceptibility to *Ascaris* infection as well as the tendency to harbour heavy infection. The various mechanisms of pathogenesis of the *A. lumbricoides* infection are as follows:

- The worms polarise the host cellular response to the T_{h2} type, as a result of which, eosinophils and mast cells are produced, and there is increased mucus secretion. The parasite antigens also elicit a humoral immune response, whereby the levels of IgG4, IgA and

IgE antibodies are elevated. Helminthic infections are also known to suppress the immunity by modulating the host immune mediators and immunoregulation. The toxic fluid of the worm elicits IgE production, leading to hypersensitivity and histamine release. This produces allergic manifestations such as urticarial and facial edema.

- A large number of larvae migrating through the lung tissue may elicit an inflammatory reaction, which may produce signs of pneumonitis with cellular infiltration of eosinophils and macrophages along with allergic reactions.
- The adult worm is well-tolerated in the intestine unless there is a heavy worm load, in which case, there may be intestinal symptoms. The adult worms are restless wanderers and can enter the ampulla of Vater and thereby, any small space of the hepatobiliary-pancreatic duct system and the gallbladder to cause obstructive symptoms and biliary or pancreatic strictures. In addition, the worm may carry gut bacteria along with it, which may cause secondary abscesses in the liver.
- Nutritional impairment is a common feature of ascariasis, especially in children, due to maldigestion and malabsorption. This results in growth and development problems.

CLINICAL FEATURES

In humans, the infection has an **incubation period of about 60–75 days** from the time of the ingestion of the eggs to the development of clinical features produced by the adult worm. The majority of infections occur in childhood. While the majority of the low-intensity infections remain asymptomatic, an estimated 8–15% of infected individuals develop symptoms. The symptoms depend on the stage of the parasite's life cycle and the intensity of the infection.

Acute Infection

These are manifestations of the early stages of worm migration or are produced by the migratory tendency of the adult worm at a later stage.

- During the **larval migration**, which is about 10–14 days after infection, the patient may develop eosinophilic pneumonia with cough, dyspnea and blood-tinged sputum (hemoptysis). In rare cases, pleuritis or pleural effusion might occur. Radiographic consolidation and widening of the pulmonary hilum may be seen, and the eosinophil count increases significantly (**Loeffler's pneumonia**). This pneumonia is usually self-limiting but can become life-threatening as well. The clinical picture of transient pulmonary infiltrates that clear within a few weeks and are associated with peripheral eosinophilia is referred to as **Loeffler's syndrome**. The patient's sputum or gastric washings may show eosinophils and Charcot–Leyden crystals along with the migrating filariform larvae of *Ascaris*.
- **Allergic manifestations** like fever, urticaria, angioneurotic edema or conjunctivitis may develop due to the release of toxic fluid (ascaron) by the adult worm. Ascariasis may also be a risk factor for asthma and atopy.
- A heavy burden of worms may produce **mechanical effects** such as acute abdomen, which includes intestinal obstruction (the most common complication), upper gastrointestinal bleeding, volvulus (twisting of the intestine), intussusception (inversion of one segment of the intestine within an adjacent segment), peritonitis and even perforation.
- The worms may crawl out of the mouth or enter the nasal meatus via the nasopharynx and then pass out of the nares. They may also enter the trachea and produce respiratory obstruction.
- **Extra-intestinal or ectopic ascariasis** develops when the worms migrate to the hepatobiliary and pancreatic systems. In such cases, patients may present with biliary pain, obstructive jaundice, ascending cholangitis, acalculous cholecystitis and acute pancreatitis. Other organs such as the lungs, eyes, kidneys and brain may also be involved.

Chronic Infection

A long-standing *Ascaris* infection **interferes with growth and development** during childhood.

- Intestinal ascariasis may present as abdominal discomfort, distension, nausea or vomiting, asthenia, lack of appetite, diarrhea or other altered bowel habits.
- Weight loss, protein-energy malnutrition, growth stunting and cognitive disabilities are attributed to ascariasis, especially in children.

DIAGNOSIS

Microscopy

The diagnosis of ascariasis is generally made by the direct demonstration of the **eggs or adult stage of the worm** (Fig. 22.1, 22.2 and 22.4a–d).

Lab diagnosis

- **Microscopy:** By visualising eggs and adult worms
  - Direct microscopy of stool samples
  - Microscopy after concentration of sample with formol ether, Mini-FLOTAC and FLOTAC
  - Egg quantification: Kato-Katz and McMaster
- **Serology:**
  - ELISA: IgG4 antibodies against excretory/secretory (ES) antigens
  - IHA and IFA
- **DNA detection:** PCR and real-time PCR
- **Other diagnostic parameters:**
  - Eosinophilia, ↑ IgE
  - Skin test (scratch test): Type-I hypersensitivity reaction
  - Radiology: Linear filling defects

Usually, the microscopic examination of stool samples on a direct wet mount readily reveals the **eggs** of the worm. However, it may be necessary to concentrate the specimen by salt floatation or formol ether to detect low-intensity infection. Microscopy of stool is not useful in the detection of extra-intestinal infection or during the pre-patent period since no eggs are found in stool in such scenarios.

Often, both fertilised and unfertilised eggs are found in the same specimen. The **unfertilised eggs are easily differentiated as they do not float in the salt solution.** The eggs may appear as debris in a darkly stained smear, which could result in them being missed on microscopy.

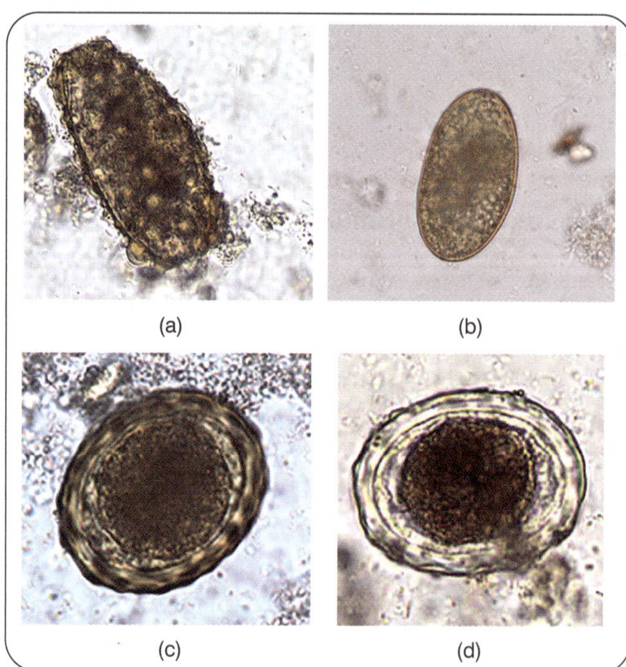

Fig. 24.4 Features of eggs of *A. lumbricoides:* (a) unfertilised corticated egg in an unstained wet mount, (b) unfertilised decorticated (lacking the mammillated layer) egg in an unstained wet mount, (c) fertilised corticated egg in an unstained wet mount and (d) fertilised de-corticated egg in an unstained wet mount (*Source:* CDC, DPDx)

For this reason, stool samples should also be examined in saline wet mounts.

- In field-based surveys, the World Health Organization recommends the use of Kato-Katz and Mini-FLOTAC techniques for concentration and estimation of eggs per gram (epg), and thus help to indirectly assess the intensity of infection. The WHO defines heavy-intensity infection of *Ascaris* as more than 50,000 epg of feces. *A. lumbricoides* and *Trichuris trichiura* eggs remain recognisable for many months but hookworm eggs disintegrate in a Kato-Katz preparation.
- Other techniques such as McMaster and FLOTAC also concentrate the eggs and may be more sensitive than the Kato-Katz technique.

When the patient has pulmonary symptoms, the migrating filariform larvae of *Ascaris* may be detected in sputum or gastric washings along with eosinophils and Charcot–Leyden crystals.

The **adult worm** often passes out through the anus, mouth, nose, and rarely through the ear, and can be identified based on its morphological features. Often, only the female worms are recovered from the intestine.

Serodiagnosis

Serological tests are used for the diagnosis of extra-intestinal ascariasis such as Loeffler's syndrome or for seroepidemiological surveys.

- ELISA can be used for the detection of serum IgG4 antibodies against the excretory/secretory (ES) antigens of *A. lumbricoides* excellent sensitivity and specificity.
- Indirect hemagglutination (IHA) and immunofluorescence (IFA) assays can also be used.

Nucleic Acid-Based Detection

The detection of the parasite's DNA by PCR or its modifications may be used in epidemiological studies to monitor response to mass drug programmes.

Other Diagnostic Parameters

- **Indirect tests:** Eosinophilia and increased IgE titres are chiefly seen during the larval invasion stage. Endoscopy may be useful in identifying duodenal ascariasis.
- **Skin test (scratch test):** This test is based on immediate hypersensitivity reaction to a purified crude extract of *Ascaris* inoculated intradermally. It presents as erythema and edema within a few minutes at the site of inoculation of the antigen. This test is, however, no longer used for diagnosis.

- **Radiology:** Elongated adult worms can be seen in the gas-filled intestine in plain radiographs. On barium meal, linear filling defects are quite conspicuous when two worms are lying parallel in a manner resembling **trolley car lines**. In Loeffler's syndrome, chest X-ray may show infiltrates, and bronchoscopy may show evidence of bronchitis.

TREATMENT

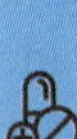

- *Albendazole:* For adults and children >2 years, 400 mg oral or 10 ml 4% suspension in a single dose; for children aged 1–2 years, 200 mg oral or 5 ml 4% suspension in a single dose
- *Mebendazole:* 500 mg in a single dose or 100 mg BDS × 3 days
- *Pyrantel pamoate:* 11 mg/kg (maximum 1 g) in a single dose

Albendazole and mebendazole act on the adult worms by **inhibiting microtubule polymerisation**. Since the worms can potentially migrate to numerous body sites and cause complications, all infections should be treated.

Surgery is required for intestinal obstruction, volvulus, intussusception, biliary strictures and peritonitis. Endoscopic retrograde cholangiopancreatography (ERCP) can be performed to remove worms from hepatobiliary ducts and the duodenum.

PREVENTION AND CONTROL

The prescribed measures for the prevention and control of ascariasis broadly follow those prescribed for STH infections and include the following:

- Safe water, sanitation and hygiene (WASH) programmes
- Preventive chemotherapy by mass drug administration (MDA) programmes
- Health education

ZOONOTIC SPECIES

BAYLISASCARIS PROCYONIS

It is a parasite of **raccoons** in North America. Humans may be accidentally infected, and the larvae of the worm may wander in the body and invade various body organs. The infection may be fatal at times.

Questions

1. Describe in detail the life cycle and pathogenesis of *Ascaris*.
2. Discuss the clinical features, management and prevention of ascariasis.
3. Write a short note on Loeffler's syndrome.

Multiple Choice Questions

1. The drug of choice for ascariasis is ________:
   a. Nitazoxanide b. Albendazole
   c. Metronidazole d. Praziquantel
2. The parasite responsible for causing Loeffler's syndrome is ___:
   a. *Enterobius vermicularis* b. *Ascaris lumbricoides*
   c. *Strongyloides stercoralis* d. *Entamoeba histolytica*
3. Which of the following statements about *Ascaris lumbricoides* is INCORRECT?
   a. It is the largest intestinal nematode.
   b. The female worm is larger than the male.
   c. Female worms may lay eggs without mating with male worms.
   d. The eggs are immediately infectious when excreted in feces.
4. Which of the following statements about *Ascaris lumbricoides* is NOT TRUE?
   a. It is a soil-transmitted helminth.
   b. Infection is acquired by the oral route.
   c. Larvae migrate through the lungs during their life cycle.
   d. The diagnosis of *A. lumbricoides* infection is made by the demonstration of bile-stained eggs in stool samples.
5. The diagnosis of Loeffler's syndrome is made by the demonstration of ________:
   a. Eggs in sputum or gastric washings
   b. Filariform larvae in sputum or gastric washings
   c. Eosinophils and Charcot–Leyden crystals
   d. Eggs in stool samples
6. All the following may be clinical features of ascariasis EXCEPT ______:
   a. Loeffler's syndrome
   b. Intestinal obstruction
   c. Protein-energy malnutrition
   d. Pernicious anemia

Chapter 25

Trichuris (Whipworm)

([From Greek] *trichos* = fine hair + *ura* = tail)

Case Study and Learning Goals

A 4-year-old boy presents with rectal prolapse. Several small, white worms are visible on his rectal mucosa. He also has features of iron deficiency anemia and growth retardation. On examining his stool sample, barrel-shaped eggs with bipolar mucus plugs are seen. What are the parasitic causes of anemia? How would you treat this patient? How can this infection be prevented?

INTRODUCTION

Trichuris trichiura, along with the other **soil-transmitted helminths (STH)**, is among the commonest agents of infections on earth. The characteristic *Trichuris* eggs have been recovered from a glacier mummy thought to be more than 5,000 years old and also from a human colon dating back as far as 3200 BC, establishing a long history of association between the parasite and human beings. In 1771, Carl Linnaeus became the first to describe this worm.

Trichuris suis, the pig whipworm, has also been known to infect humans on rare occasions.

EPIDEMIOLOGY

T. trichiura, which is commonly known as **whipworm,** infects an estimated **500 million** individuals, with the highest prevalence being among children. It is known to co-infect individuals who are infected with *Ascaris lumbricoides*. The infection is cosmopolitan, but like other STHs, it is far more common in the warm and moist regions of the world. It is even more common in rural communities with poor sanitary conditions. In most tropical and subtropical areas, the infection is almost universally acquired in childhood.

MORPHOLOGY

Adult Worm

The adult worm is white–grey with a characteristic **long and slender anterior end** and a **thick posterior end, which gives it the shape of a 'whip with a handle'** (hence the name whipworm) (Fig. 25.1a and 25.2).

- The females are longer (35–50 mm) than the males (30–45 mm).
- The long, slender anterior end makes up 3/5th of the worm's body. This part of the worm burrows into the mucosa of the host's intestine. It contains an esophagus which makes up 2/3rd of the body length. The esophagus is lined with a characteristic single layer of glandular cells called stichocytes.
- The thick posterior end makes up 2/5th of the worm's body and extends into the lumen of the host's gut. This part of the worm's body contains the intestine and the reproductive organs. In female worms, the posterior end is comma-shaped, whereas in males, the posterior end is entirely coiled and equipped with a single spicule (Fig. 25.1a).

Eggs

These are **barrel-/lemon-shaped, measure 55 × 25 µm in size** and are **brown and bile-stained with characteristic bipolar, chitin-rich mucus plugs** (Fig. 25.1b). The embryo hatches out of the mucus plugs with the help of chitinases. The eggs float in a saturated solution of common salt. The female lays about 14,000–20,000 eggs per day.

Trichuris suis ova (pig species of *Trichuris*) are being investigated for a possible role in therapy of inflammatory bowel disease.

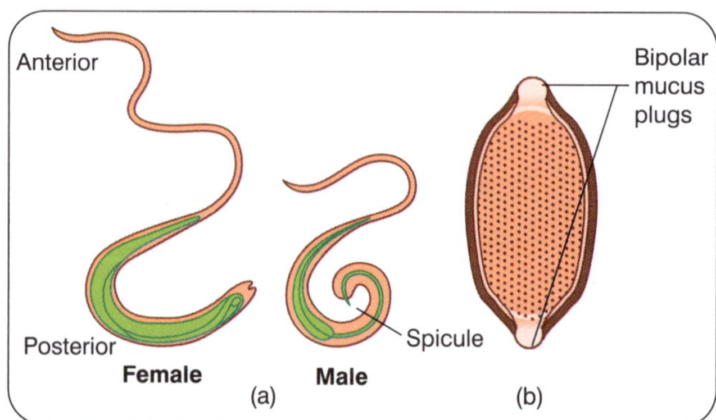

Fig. 25.1 Line diagrams of *Trichuris trichiura:* (a) female and male adults and (b) egg

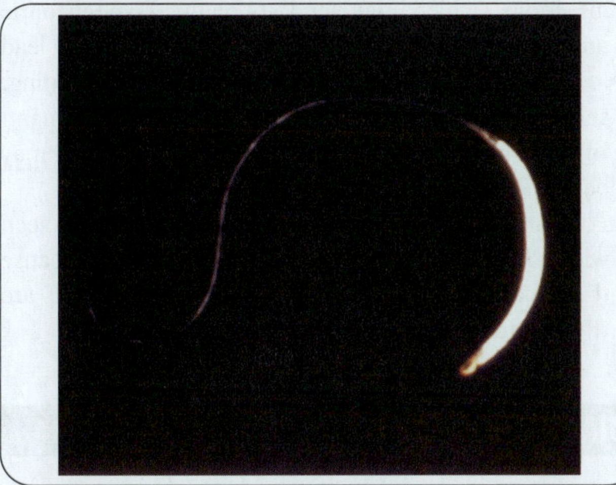

Fig. 25.2 An adult female of *Trichuris trichiura* with the characteristic 'whip with a handle' appreance (*Source:* Centers for Disease Control and Prevention [CDC], Public Health Image Library [PHIL], Image ID 414)

LIFE CYCLE (Fig. 25.3a and b)

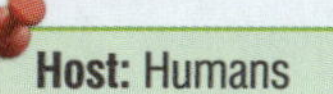

Humans are the **only definitive hosts** of *Trichuris*; no intermediate hosts are required. Whipworm **infection is acquired by the fecal–oral route** through soil, food or hands contaminated with embryonated ova. Geophagia (pica) is commonly implicated in trichuriasis. The eggs hatch in the small intestine and undergo four moultings to mature into the adult stage in about three months. The adults live in the **large intestine (caecum and ascending colon)** with their anterior ends embedded in the mucosa (they are often considered as tissue parasites). After mating, the adult females produce unembryonated eggs which are subsequently passed in stool. In favourable conditions like warm and moist soil, the eggs mature in 2–4 weeks and

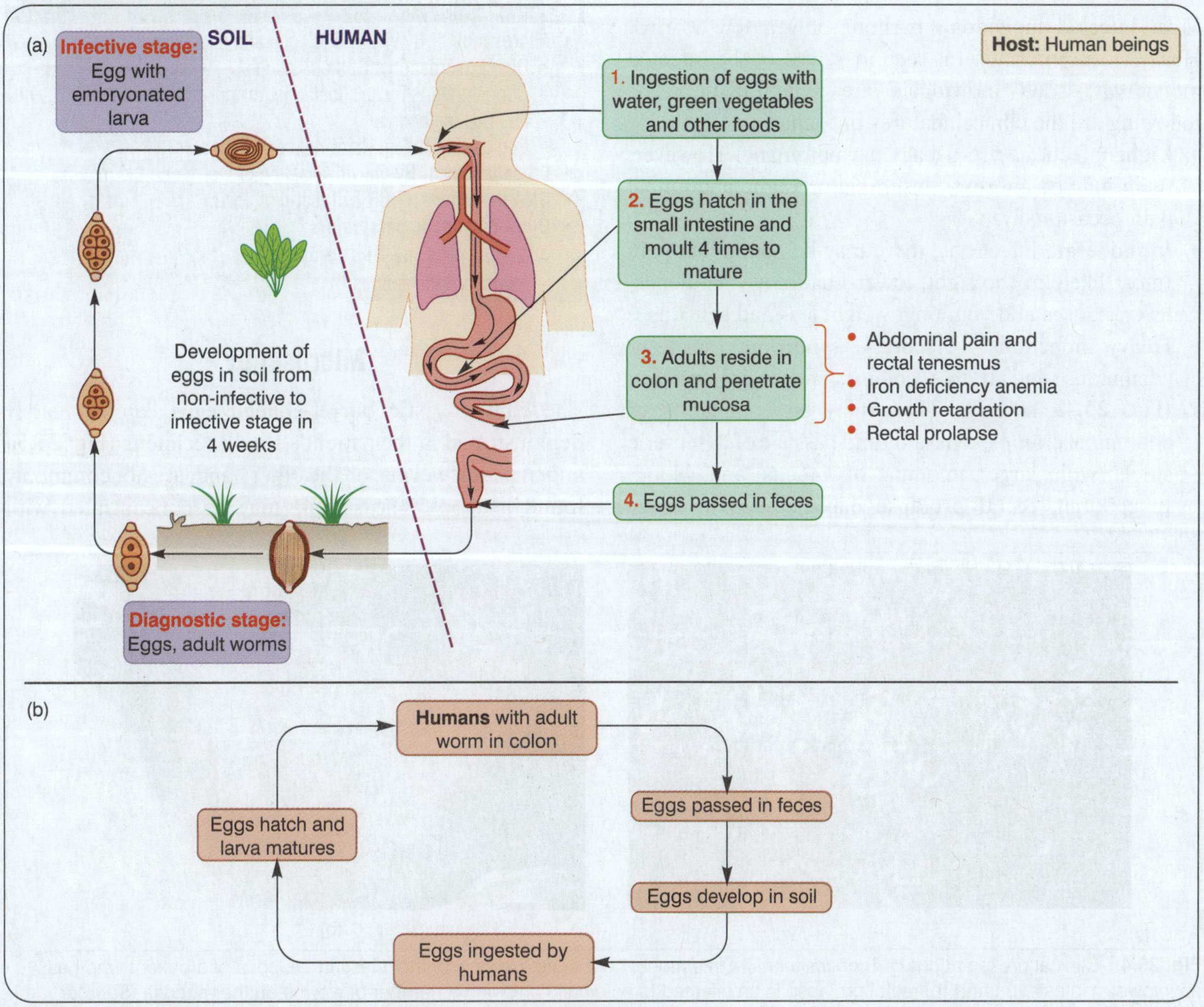

(a) Infective stage: Egg with embryonated larva

SOIL

HUMAN

Host: Human beings

1. Ingestion of eggs with water, green vegetables and other foods

2. Eggs hatch in the small intestine and moult 4 times to mature

3. Adults reside in colon and penetrate mucosa

- Abdominal pain and rectal tenesmus
- Iron deficiency anemia
- Growth retardation
- Rectal prolapse

4. Eggs passed in feces

Development of eggs in soil from non-infective to infective stage in 4 weeks

Diagnostic stage: Eggs, adult worms

(b)

Humans with adult worm in colon

Eggs passed in feces

Eggs develop in soil

Eggs ingested by humans

Eggs hatch and larva matures

Fig. 25.3 Life cycle of *Trichuris trichiura:* (a) detailed and (b) schematic

become infective. The eggs can survive outside the human body for many months. The life span of the worm is 1–3 years.

PATHOGENESIS

The morbidity of trichuriasis is associated with a **heavy worm burden, which causes chronic inflammation of the intestinal mucosa.**

- The intestinal mucosa is inflamed, edematous and friable, and is affected from the distal part of the small intestine to the rectum. The chronically edematous state of the rectal mucosa may lead to a prolapse on straining during defecation.
- Blood loss due to the mucosal damage leads to anemia.

CLINICAL FEATURES

Most infected individuals harbour only a few worms. Heavy worm infestation is seen in <10% of the infected individuals; such individuals are symptomatic. The following are the clinical features of trichuriasis:

- **Light** infections are usually asymptomatic. However, there may be anorexia, insomnia or vague abdominal pain occasionally.
- In **moderate** infections, there may be abdominal pain (most likely in the right, lower quadrant), flatulence, fever, nausea and vomiting, weight loss and pruritus.
- **Heavy** infections (**dysentery syndrome**) lead to edematous and friable colonic and rectal mucosa (Fig. 25.4a and b). There may be complaints of abdominal cramps, tenesmus and passage of dysenteric stools with large amounts of mucus and blood. In children, **rectal prolapse** may be seen in heavy infections, which may tend to recur. **Hypochromic anemia** seen in prolonged massive infections may lead to the clubbing of fingers, growth retardation, stunting, severe weight loss, cachexia and cognitive impairment.
- In some individuals, allergic reactions or urticaria may be seen.
- Polyparasitic co-infections are commonly seen with *Trichuris*, *Ascaris* and hookworms because these parasites live in similar environments and are transmitted through soil.

DIAGNOSIS

Given the large number of eggs produced by the worm, a simple stool examination may be sufficient to establish a diagnosis of trichuriasis.

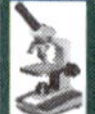

Lab diagnosis

- **Microscopy:** By visualising eggs and adult worms
  - Direct microscopy: Of stool sample
  - Concentration: By salt floatation, formol ether, Mini-FLOTAC, and FLOTAC methods
  - Egg quantification: Kato–Katz and McMaster
- **Colonoscopy:** By the visualisation of worms on the mucosa
- **DNA detection:** PCR and real-time PCR
- **Other diagnostic parameters:**
  - Eosinophilia and ↑ IgE
  - Hypochromic anemia

Microscopy

The **characteristic barrel-shaped eggs** can be readily demonstrated in the patient's stool specimens (Fig. 25.5a and b). Adult worms, on the other hand, are not commonly found in stool. The sample may be concentrated with

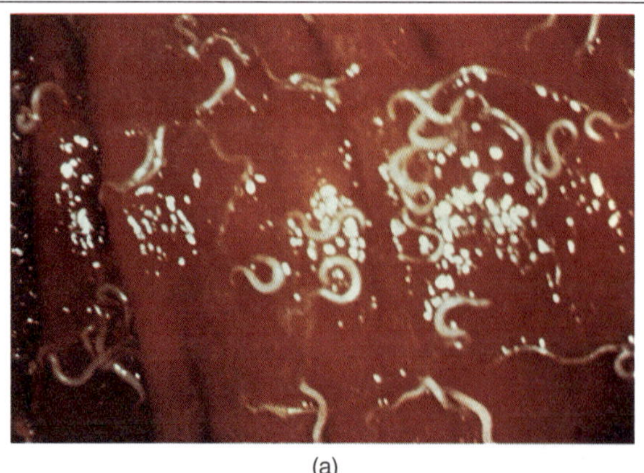

(a)

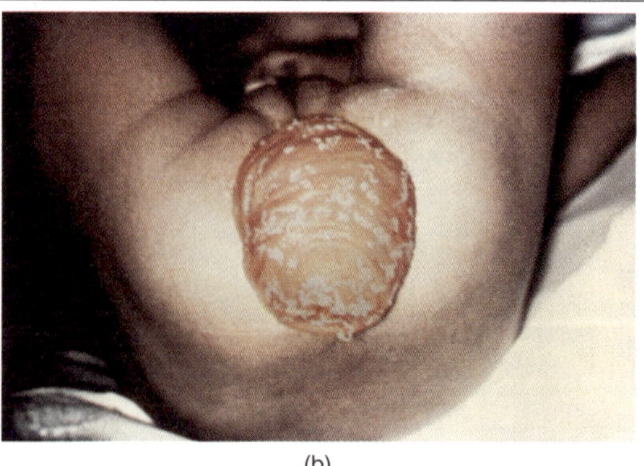

(b)

Fig. 25.4 Clinical presentations of *Trichuris trichiura* infections: (a) a close-up view of the intestinal mucosa of a patient who has a whipworm infestation and (b) rectal prolapse in an infected female child showing a number of worms on the mucosa (*Source:* CDC, PHIL, Image IDs 14778 and 13370)

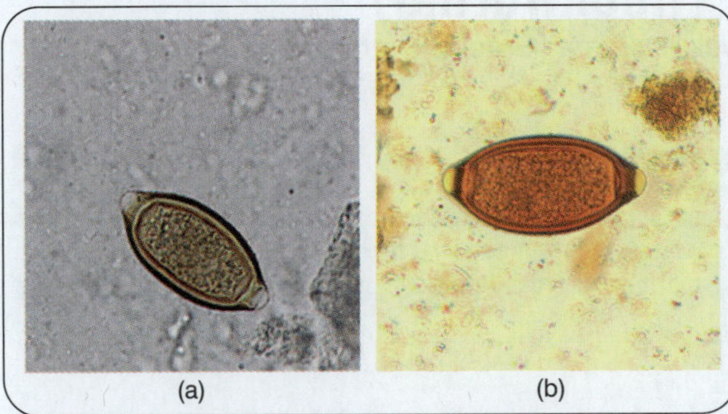

Fig. 25.5 Features of the eggs of *Trichuris trichiura:* (a) an egg in an unstained wet mount and (b) an egg in an iodine-stained wet mount (*Source:* CDC, DPDx)

formol ether or by floatation techniques for better visualisation.

Kato–Katz and Mini-FLOTAC techniques are recommended by the World Health Organization (WHO) for field studies to concentrate the stool samples and quantify the intensity of infection by indirectly counting the eggs per gram (epg) of feces. The WHO definition of heavy-intensity infection of *Trichuris* is more than 10,000 epg of feces.

Colonoscopy

Adult worms may be visualised on the intestinal mucosa.

Nucleic Acid-Based Detection

The detection of parasite DNA by PCR may be employed in epidemiological studies to monitor response to mass drug programmes.

Other Diagnostic Parameters

Other parameters indicative of trichuriasis are as follows:

- Mild to moderate peripheral blood eosinophilia is seen in about 75% cases
- Increased serum IgE level
- Hypochromic anemia

TREATMENT

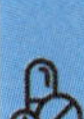

- *Albendazole:* 400 mg oral daily × 3 days for light/moderate infections and 5–7 days for heavy infections
- *Mebendazole:* 100 mg BDS × 3 days for light/moderate infections and 5–7 days for heavy infections
- *Supportive treatment:* Iron and nutritional supplements

In cases of rectal prolapse, the prolapsed intestine should be replaced gently and the buttocks should be held together. The tendency to prolapse usually subsides within 5 to 7 days.

PREVENTION AND CONTROL

The prescribed measures for the prevention and control of trichuriasis broadly follow those prescribed for STH infections and include the following:

- Safe water, sanitation and hygiene (WASH) programmes
- Preventive chemotherapy by mass drug administration (MDA) programmes
- Health education

Questions

1. Discuss the pathogenesis and clinical features of trichuriasis.
2. Discuss the laboratory diagnosis and treatment of trichuriasis.

Multiple Choice Questions

1. The characteristic barrel-shaped eggs are produced by ______:
   a. Pinworm b. Hookworm
   c. Whipworm d. Roundworm

2. The drug of choice for *Trichuris trichiura* is ________:
   a. Ivermectin b. Albendazole
   c. Nitazoxanide d. Metronidazole

3. The common name of *Trichuris trichiura* is ________:
   a. Pinworm b. Hookworm
   c. Whipworm d. Roundworm

4. Abdominal pain, chronic dysentery and rectal prolapse in children are associated with infection caused by ________:
   a. *Giardia lamblia* b. *Ascaris lumbricoides*
   c. *Trichuris trichiura* d. *Enterobius vermicularis*

5. Unsegmented eggs in stool samples are seen in ________:
   a. *Ancylostoma duodenale*
   b. *Trichuris trichiura*
   c. *Enterobius vermicularis*
   d. *Strongyloides stercoralis*

Chapter 26

Necator and Ancylostoma (Hookworms)

(*necator* [Latin] = killer; *ancylos* [Greek] = hook + *stoma* [Greek] = mouth)

Case Study and Learning Goals

A 15-year-old girl from a rural area complains of on-and-off mild abdominal pain, weakness and fatigue for the last 4–5 years. On examination, she is found to have severe anemia and protein malnutrition. She has a history of walking barefoot and has been missing school notably over the last few years. What are the parasitic causes of anemia? How would you approach the laboratory diagnosis in this case? How would you treat this patient? What precautions would you advise her to take in the future?

INTRODUCTION

Hookworm infections in humans are caused by two nematode species–***Necator americanus,* the 'New World' hookworm** and ***Ancylostoma duodenale,* the 'Old World' hookworm.** These two species are grouped under **soil-transmitted helminths (STH)**.

The first description of hookworm disease has been traced back to as early as 1500 BC in documents from ancient Egyptian civilizations. The complete life cycle of hookworms was documented in 1898 by Arthur Looss who accidentally infected himself and made the discovery that hookworms can penetrate skin.

The early association of hookworms with **'miner's anemia'** and other occupations which involve contact with soil, e.g., farming and working in tea and coffee plantations, emphasised the importance of the infection. Consequently, several public health bodies emerged in the late 19th and early 20th centuries to address the problem of hookworms and other communicable diseases. The early 'sanitary commissions' of the Rockefeller Foundation initiated in the United States of America were among the first of these bodies. Eventually, the crusade for the control of hookworm diseases gained momentum globally, and numerous other governments and agencies succeeded the responsibility, including the World Health Organization (WHO).

A few non-human Ancylostoma species, viz. *A. braziliense, A. caninum* and *A. ceylanicum* may accidentally infect humans and cause skin manifestations known as cutaneous larva migrans (refer to **Chapter 30**, *Toxocara and Other Larva Migrans*).

EPIDEMIOLOGY

Hookworms affect approximately **500 million** people globally and account for **3.2 million** disability-adjusted life years (DALYs) lost; these numbers are likely to be underestimations. While the prevalence of most protozoan and helminth parasitic infections peaks in childhood, the prevalence of hookworm infection, though **high among children**, increases with age and repeated infections and **peaks in adulthood.**

The highest incidence of hookworm infections is seen in South-East Asia followed by sub-Saharan Africa. The infection is concentrated in **rural** areas with **poor sanitation**, where the practices of **open defecation** and habits such as walking **barefoot** are common. The infections are also common in certain occupational groups such as **tea plantation workers** and **miners**.

- *N. americanus* is the globally more prevalent human hookworm species, and is especially common in the Americas (in fact, it was once known as the 'American murderer'), central and south Africa, southern India, South Asia, southern China, South-East Asia and Australia.
- *A. duodenale* is geographically limited to the northern regions of Africa, the Mediterranean region, North India, and the northern parts of China and Japan.
- Overlapping geographical distribution and mixed human infections with *N. americanus* and *A. duodenale* are also common.
- A third species, *A. ceylanicum*, which is primarily a canine parasite, has recently been reported as a highly prevalent species in humans in some regions in Malaysia and Indonesia where it is often co-endemic with *N. americanus*.

India contributes significantly to the global burden of hookworm disease. *A. duodenale* is reported mainly from the northern regions of the country while *N. americanus* predominates in South India. Both species are also commonly known to co-exist. *A. ceylanicum* has recently been reported from a tribal community in Tamil Nadu.

MORPHOLOGY

Adult Worm

Hookworms are **pinkish to grey-white cylindrical** worms measuring 7–11 mm in length and 0.4–0.5 mm in breadth. The males are shorter than the females. The name **'hookworm'** comes from the worm's characteristic **dorsal curve anteriorly,** which gives it a hook-like appearance (Fig. 26.1a and b).

- The subglobular head of the worm is equipped with well-developed mouth parts and **teeth** *(Ancylostoma)* **or cutting plates** *(Necator)* and a large buccal cavity lined with a cuticle; these evolutionary developments are suited for its blood-feeding parasitic life (Fig. 26.2).
- The club-shaped esophagus is undivided and helps the worm to pump blood to its intestine, which opens into the anus.
- The posterior end is cone-shaped in females, whereas in the males, it radiates with the support of rays and forms an expanded bell-shaped caudal bursa. The ray pattern is distinctive and helps in species differentiation.

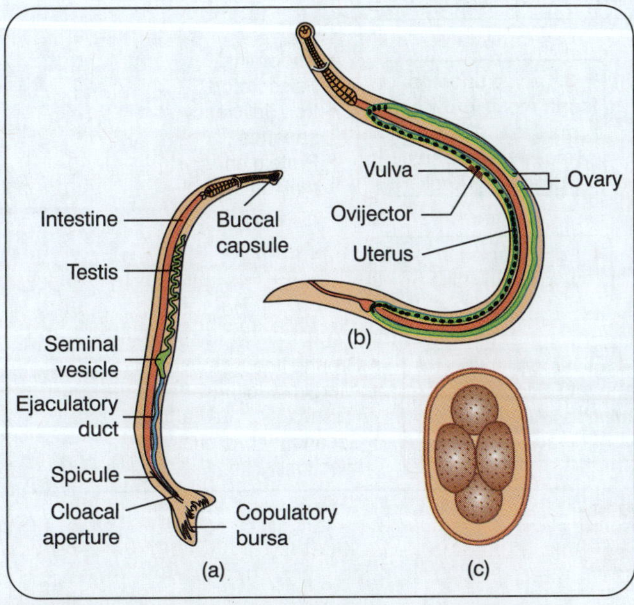

Fig. 26.1 Line diagrams of hookworms: (a) adult male, (b) adult female and (c) 4-celled egg

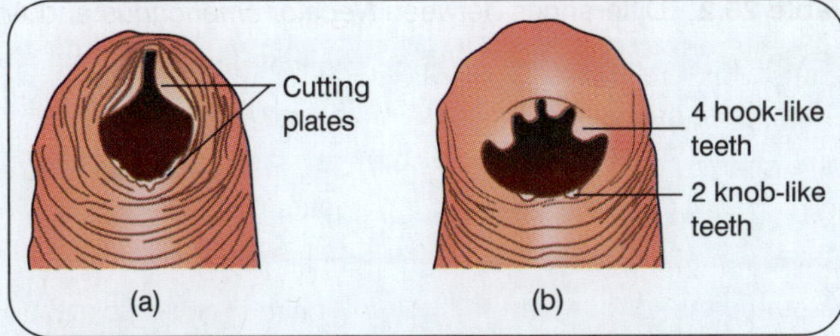

Fig. 26.2 Differences in the mouth parts of hookworms: (a) cutting plates *(Necator americanus)* and (b) teeth *(Ancylostoma duodenale)*

- The genital apparatus of the males opens into the cloaca at its posterior end. In females, the vulva is located at one-third the distance from the posterior. The male copulatory apparatus attaches to this vulva during mating. This accounts for the characteristic Y-shaped arrangement of males and females when they are recovered in pairs.
- The males and females can be easily differentiated based on their size, the shape of their posterior ends and the positions of their genital and anal openings (Table 26.1).

Eggs

These are oval, measure **60 μm** × **40** μm in size and are covered with a **thin, colourless hyaline shell.** There is a **clear space** between the shell and the developing embryo (Fig. 26.1c). Other features of hookworm eggs are as follows:

- They contain a segmented ovum with four blastomeres.
- They float in a saturated salt solution.
- The eggs of *Necator* and *Ancylostoma* are indistinguishable morphologically.

The differentiating features of *N. americanus* and *A. duodenale* are presented in Table 26.2.

LIFE CYCLE (Fig. 26.3a and b)

Humans are the **only definitive hosts** of hookworms; no intermediate hosts are required

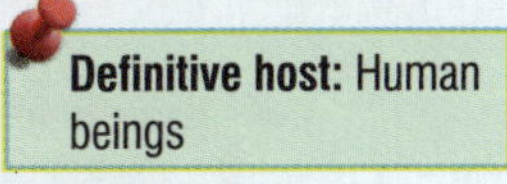

Table 26.1 Differences between male and female hookworms

Feature	Male	Female
Size	Shorter than the female	Longer than the male
Posterior end	Bell-shaped (due to copulatory bursa)	Cone-shaped (no copulatory bursa)
Anus	Opens into the cloaca	Subterminal
Genital apparatus	Opens into the cloaca	1/3rd the distance from the posterior end

Table 26.2 Differences between *Necator americanus* and *Ancylostoma duodenale*

Feature	*N. americanus*	*A. duodenale*
Vernacular name	'New World' hookworm	'Old World' hookworm
Life span	3–5 years; may even live as long as 18 years	1–5 years
Size	Relatively short	Relatively long
Mouth parts	2 pairs of cutting plates	2 pairs of hook-like and 1 pair of knob-like teeth
Dorsal curve	Opposite to body curve	Same as body curve
Position of the vulva in the female	Middle or slightly anterior to midpoint	One-third the distance from the posterior tip
Eggs/day/female	5,000–10,000	10,000–25,000
Egg morphology	No perceptible difference	No perceptible difference
Route of transmission	Skin	Skin/Oral
Tissue maturation	In the lungs	In the lungs (but not essential)
Blood loss/day/worm	0.04 ml	0.2 ml
Anemia	Less severe	More severe
Geographic distribution	Americas, central and south Africa, southern India, southern Asia, southern China, South-East Asia and Australia	Northern regions of Africa, Mediterranean regions, northern India, northern China and Japan

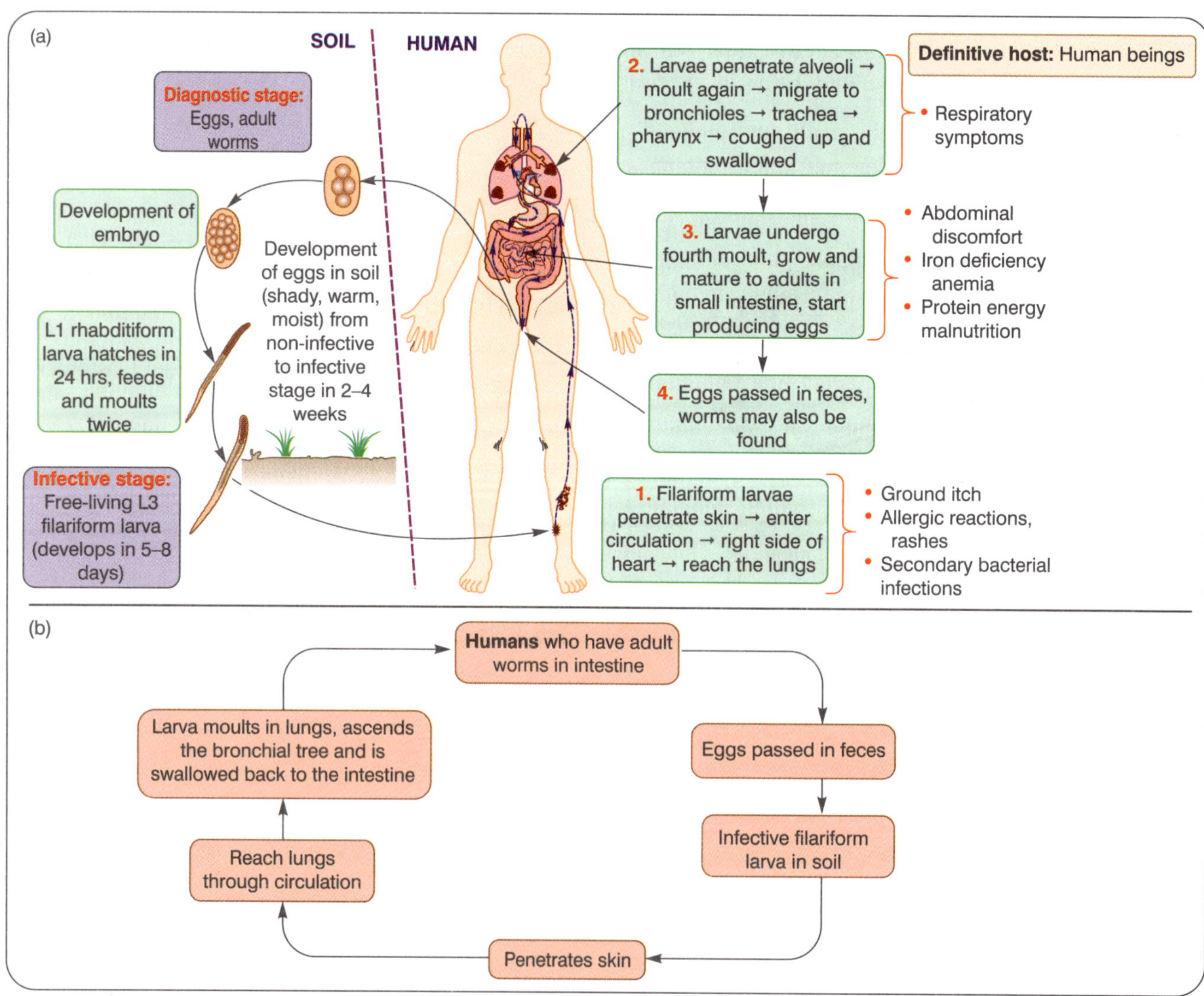

Fig. 26.3 Life cycle of hookworms: (a) detailed and (b) schematic

by these parasites. Infected humans excrete the immature hookworm eggs in their feces. **Loose, shady, warm and moist soil** is the most favourable environment for the development of the further life stages of the parasite.

- Once the egg is liberated, the embryo develops, and the mature rhabditiform larvae (L1) hatch in about 24 hours. These larvae feed on bacteria and organic debris voraciously to accumulate sufficient energy reserves and subsequently moult twice to develop into non-feeding **infective filariform larvae (L3)** within 5–8 days. The L3 larva rests and awaits contact with the skin of another host. It is viable for 3–4 weeks, after which it usually desiccates. The L3 larva is receptive to various stimuli in the environment and initiates **skin penetration** on attraction to the essential fatty acids present on the human skin.

Ancylostoma larvae are also capable of entering the host directly through the fecal-oral route with contaminated food which makes them candidates for food-borne infections in addition to transcutaneous route of transmission. On the other hand, *Necator* larvae strictly penetrate the host only through the skin.

- After skin penetration, the larva migrates through the epidermis and dermis, through the veins to the right side of the **heart** and then the **lungs**, from where it migrates through the alveoli and bronchial tree to reach the trachea and pharynx. Once there, the larva is readily swallowed through the esophagus.
- After reaching the **small intestine**, the larva undergoes maturation. The adult worm holds fast onto the mucosa using its strong buccal apparatus and feeds on the capillary blood and plasma. It keeps moving to new areas for feeding. On sexual maturation and mating, the females start producing thousands of eggs a day. The worms may stay in the intestine for several years.

PATHOGENESIS

The third-stage filariform larva **releases various enzymes** to facilitate skin penetration such as **hyaluronidase and aspartyl protease**. These enzymes digest collagen, elastin and other compounds that maintain skin integrity. The various mechanisms of pathogenesis of the hookworm infection are as follows:

- **Skin:** Allergic reactions, rashes and vesicles may develop at the site of penetration, which may be secondarily infected with bacteria.
- **Pulmonary:** The migration of the larvae through the lungs may result in pulmonary features and hypereosinophilia depending on the intensity of infection.
- **Intestinal:** The intestinal phase is long-lasting and characterised by blood and nutrient loss due to the rupture of mucosal capillaries at the attachment sites. The hookworms release anticoagulants to facilitate smooth blood flow. When a worm moves from one site to another, the residual anticoagulant activity continues at the first site, causing blood and plasma leakage for some time. Thus, there is a two-pronged loss of blood—by direct feeding of the worm and also by hemorrhage from the abandoned feeding site—eventually leading to **iron deficiency anemia (microcytic and hypochromic)**.

The degree of anemia is related to the infecting species. *A. duodenale* **leads to five times more blood loss** than *N. americanus*–0.2 ml/worm per day for the former and 0.04 ml/worm for the latter.

In chronic and repeated infections, the **severity of anemia increases with the worm load**. The clinical manifestations of anemia and nutrient deficiency depend on the physiological needs and underlying nutritional status of the host. Thus, **symptoms are more apparent in growing children, pregnant and menstruating females and labourers** who perform rigorous manual labour. Severe anemia may also lead to cardiomegaly and mental and physical retardation.

CLINICAL FEATURES

The majority of hookworm infections are **light infections**; in such cases, the infected individuals remain **asymptomatic**.

Acute Infection

A small number of individuals with acute infection may develop a pruritic maculopapular rash known as **'ground itch' at the site of entry** of the larva; in other cases, the event may go unnoticed. Once they gain entry into the body, the migrating larvae make their way to the **lungs**, and may produce features of pneumonitis. Such respiratory manifestations are less commonly seen in hookworm infections than in *Ascaris* or *Strongyloides* infections. After about a month of larval entry, the parasite reaches the **intestine**. At such time, patients may experience epigastric pain, diarrhea and nausea, and their eosinophil counts may be raised.

Chronic Infection

In chronic infections, the chief clinical features are **iron deficiency anemia and protein-energy malnutrition**, especially in **children and adolescent girls**. Such individuals may exhibit both physical and mental retardation leading to poor performance and **absenteeism** at the school and workplace. The skin and mucous membranes may show extreme pallor and there may be puffiness of the face, swelling of the feet, bulging of the abdomen, dryness of the skin and hair and koilonychia (spoon-shaped nails) due to profound anemia and malnutrition. In most severe cases, the anemia caused by hookworms may even lead to **congestive heart failure**. On occasion, **severe hematemesis** is also reported.

- **Pica:** This is a disorder characterised by the habitual ingestion of substances like mud, soil and chalk. It is usually a manifestation of iron deficiency anemia and is commonly observed in patients who have hookworm infections. Patients who have this disorder are also exposed to other soil-borne infections.
- **Wakana disease:** This entity is mostly seen in **Japanese** patients due to the ingestion of infective larvae of ***A. duodenale*** along with raw vegetables. The patient presents with gastrointestinal and pulmonary symptoms. The diagnosis is made by demonstrating **larvae in the patient's sputum**. An increase in IgE and eosinophilia are usually seen.

DIAGNOSIS

The diagnosis of hookworm infection is made by the microscopic examination of fecal samples to demonstrate the **eggs** or the **worm**. Several specimens (**at least three**) should be collected over a period of ten days to factor in the **intermittent shedding** of eggs.

Lab diagnosis

- **Microscopy:** By visualising eggs, larvae and adults
  - Direct microscopy of stool
  - Concentration: Salt floatation, formol ether, Mini-FLOTAC and FLOTAC
  - Egg quantification: Kato–Katz and McMaster
- **Culture:** By Harada Mori filter paper method and Baermann's funnel technique (detection of larvae)
- **Coproantigen detection**
- **DNA detection:** PCR and real-time PCR
- **Other diagnostic parameters:**
  - Eosinophilia and ↑ IgE
  - Iron deficiency anemia
  - Occult blood test
  - Radiology: Non-specific

Microscopy

Hookworm eggs are normally passed in stool when they are in the **developing embryo stage** (usually the **4–32 celled** stage). They are thin-shelled and appear hyaline and colourless (non-bile stained) (Fig. 26.4a and b). The eggs of *A. duodenale* and *N. americanus* cannot be differentiated microscopically.

Since the egg wall disintegrates soon after being released from the human body, the samples should be processed **within 3–4 hours of collection.**

Egg quantification:

- The number of eggs per gram (epg) of feces is used to quantify the intensity of infection. Another method that can be used for quantifying worm load is **Chandler's index**, which is also based on epg.
- For field surveys, Kato–Katz and Mini-FLOTAC are the most common methods recommended by the WHO for concentrating and quantifying helminth eggs. The WHO definition of heavy intensity infection of hookworm is more than 4,000 epg of feces. When the Kato–Katz method is used, microscopy should be done within 30 minutes of preparing the slides (because the hookworm egg wall disintegrates quickly). Another commonly used method is Stoll's egg counting technique. McMaster and FLOTAC techniques can also be used.

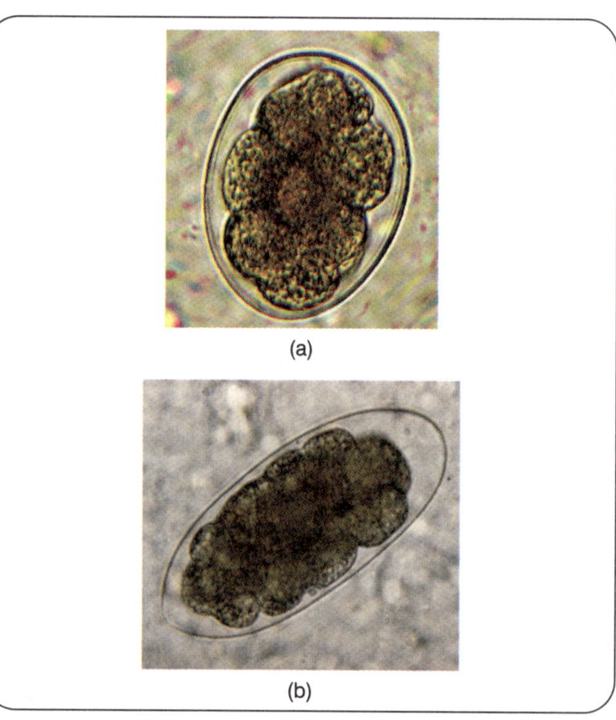

Fig. 26.4 Features of eggs of hookworms: (a) 8-celled stage and (b) 16-celled stage (*Source:* Centers for Disease Control and Prevention [CDC], DPDx)

Table 26.3 Characteristics of the rhabditiform larvae of hookworms and *Strongyloides stercoralis*

Feature	Hookworm larva	*Strongyloides stercoralis* larva
Size	100–150 μm × 15–17 μm	200–300 μm × 15–18 μm
Buccal cavity	15 μm	4 μm
Genital primordium	7 μm	22 μm
Anal pore	80 μm from the posterior tip	50 μm from the posterior tip

Sometimes, the egg may contain a motile larva. In a warm and humid environment, the larvae hatch from the eggs **within 24 hours**, which may lead to them being confused with the larvae of *Strongyloides stercoralis.* The two species need to be differentiated since the treatments for the two species differ (Table 26.3, Fig. 26.5a and b).

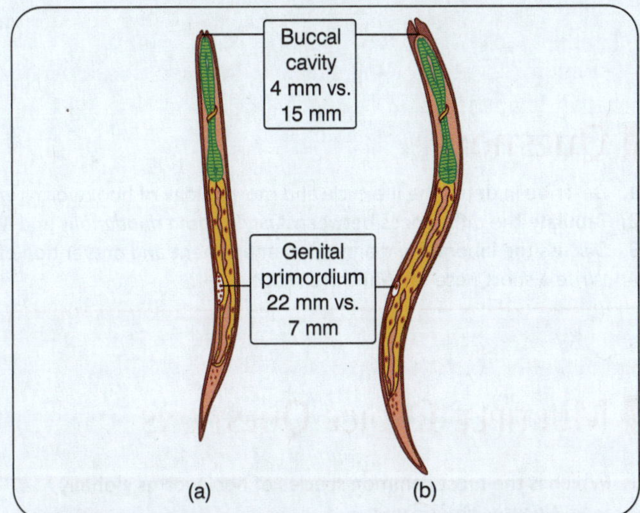

Fig. 26.5 Differences between the larvae of (a) *Strongyloides* and (b) hookworm

Stool Culture

A fresh stool sample may be cultured by various techniques such as Harada-Mori filter paper method, Baermann's funnel technique, charcoal culture or agar plate culture to detect larvae hatching out of hookworm eggs (refer **Annexure 1**, *Approach to the Laboratory Diagnosis of Parasitic Infections*).

Coproantigen Detection

Coproantigens are antigens of the parasite found in the feces (*kopros* [Greek] means dung). To detect hookworm coproantigens, cross-reacting IgG antibodies against the excretory/secretory (ES) antigens of another species, *A. ceylanicum,* are used.

Nucleic Acid-Based Detection

Parasite DNA can be detected in the stool samples by molecular techniques such as PCR and its modifications. These methods are rapid, provide quantification of the infection, and can differentiate the infecting species from similar parasites.

Other Diagnostic Parameters

- **Hemogram:** Eosinophilia (>600 cells/μl or >6% of the total leukocyte count) may be used as a marker of STH infection and may be observed in about 60% of cases of hookworm infection. Low hemoglobin (≤5 g/dl) and ferritin may be noted due to iron deficiency anemia.
- **Occult blood test:** Occult blood in stool in patients with heavy intensity infections has been used as a surrogate marker.
- **Radiology:** Non-specific features such as intestinal hypermotility, proximal jejunal dilatation and coarsening of the mucosal folds are associated with hookworm infections.

TREATMENT

- *Albendazole:* For adults and children >2 years, 400 mg oral or 10 ml of a 4% suspension as a single dose; for children aged 1–2 years, 200 mg oral or 5 ml of a 4% suspension as a single dose
- *Mebendazole:* 500 mg BDS × 3 days
- *Pyrantel pamoate:* 11 mg/kg × 3 days
- *Supportive treatment:* Iron and nutritional supplements

A single 400 mg dose of albendazole has a cure rate of 72%. On the other hand, a single 500 mg dose of mebendazole has a cure rate of only 15%, and three consecutive daily doses are required for efficacy.

PREVENTION AND CONTROL

The prescribed measures for the prevention and control of hookworms broadly follow those prescribed for STH infections and include the following:

- WASH programme
- Preventive chemotherapy by mass drug administration (MDA) programmes
- Health education
- Use of footwear as a primary preventive measure

There is no hookworm vaccine available presently. However, enormous efforts and monetary resources are being invested in developing an effective vaccine with the aim to induce protective immunity to prevent moderate to heavy infections among the most affected population groups.

Hookworm vaccines: Two recombinant vaccines targeting parasite-derived enzymes **APR-I (aspartic protease) and ASP-2 (*Ancylostoma-secreted* protein)** are undergoing clinical trials.

Questions

1. Describe in detail the life cycle and morphology of hookworms with suitable diagrams.
2. Tabulate the differences between *Ancylostoma duodenalis* and *Necator americanus*.
3. Discuss the laboratory diagnosis, management and prevention of hookworm disease.
4. Write a short note on Wakana disease.

Multiple Choice Questions

1. Which is the most common species of hookworms globally?
   a. *Necator americanus*
   b. *Ancylostoma duodenale*
   c. *Ancylostoma caninum*
   d. *Ancylostoma braziliense*
2. Through which route are hookworms transmitted most often?
   a. Oral
   b. Inhalational
   c. Transcutaneous
   d. Congenital
3. The adult worms of *Necator* can be morphologically distinguished from *Ancylostoma* on the basis of _______ :
   a. The route of acquisition of infection
   b. Differences in the eggshell
   c. Presence of cutting plates
   d. They cannot be distinguished
4. *Necator* causes _______ blood loss per worm while *Ancylostoma* causes _______.
   a. 0.2 ml/worm per day; 0.04 ml/worm
   b. 0.04 ml/worm per day; 0.2 ml/worm
   c. 2 ml/worm per day; 0.4 ml/worm
   d. 1 ml/worm per day; 2 ml/worm
5. Which of the is NOT a characteristic of hookworm eggs?
   a. Bile-stained
   b. Thin-shelled
   c. *Necator* eggs cannot be differentiated from *Ancylostoma* eggs
   d. Need to mature in soil before they become infective
6. Which stage of *Ancylostoma duodenale* is infective to human beings?
   a. Filariform larva
   b. Rhabditiform larva
   c. Egg
   d. Adult worm
7. Wakana disease is associated with _______ :
   a. *Gnathostoma spinigerum*
   b. *Toxocara canis*
   c. *Baylisascaris*
   d. *Ancylostoma duodenale*

Chapter 27

Strongyloides

([From Greek] *strongylos* = rounded + *oides* = similar)

Case Study and Learning Goals

A 25-year-old farmer on corticosteroids for an autoimmune disorder presents with complaints of itchy, progressive and linear rashes on his buttocks which subside in a few hours—he says the "rash comes and goes". There is peripheral eosinophilia, and his IgE levels are elevated. What are the parasitic causes of progressing linear rashes? How would you approach the laboratory diagnosis in this case? How would you treat this patient?

INTRODUCTION

While there are over 50 species of the genus *Strongyloides* that are known to infect birds, reptiles, amphibians, livestock and other primates, *Strongyloides stercoralis* is the primary species implicated in human disease. Though the transmission of this parasite chiefly involves humans, zoonotic transmission is also possible through dogs. It was identified as a cause of disease only in 1876 by Louis Alexis Normand who found the parasites while autopsying soldiers who had returned from French colonies in what is now Vietnam. In the same year, A. Bavay named the intestinal and fecal forms *Anguillula intestinalis* and *Anguillula stercoralis* respectively; however, it was later discovered that these were actually different stages of the same parasite. In 1883, Rudolf Leuckart discovered the alternations between the free-living and parasitic generations, and in 1914, Friedrich Fülleborn proposed the parasite's auto-infective cycle while working on dogs.

Strongyloides fuelleborni, a non-human primate species, can also infect humans.

EPIDEMIOLOGY

It is estimated that approximately **100 million** people are infected with *S. stercoralis* globally. The disease is more prevalent in the rural areas of developing countries that lie in the tropical and warm temperate belts of the world where **the exposure of bare skin to fecally contaminated soil** is common. The infection has a prevalence of up to 60% among Aboriginal populations in Australia.

S. stercoralis infections are more common among males than females and the prevalence increases with age. The infection is frequently imported by **travellers, refugees, immigrants** and **military personnel** to areas where it is not endemic. It shows clustering in households and among prisoners of war and institutionalised people.

With the increasing prescriptions of corticosteroids, *S. stercoralis* is likely to become a growing clinical challenge.

Other **predisposing factors** associated with severe or disseminated disease are hematological malignancies, human T cell lymphotropic virus type-1 (HTLV-1) infection, cytotoxic chemotherapy and radiotherapy, immunosuppressive therapy for organ transplants, autoimmune diseases, alcoholism, malnutrition and old age.

MORPHOLOGY

Adult Worm

The adult worms exist in nature as both free-living as well as parasitic stages. The **parasitic females** live in the intestine and are considered parthenogenic (a type of reproduction in which the egg can develop into an embryo without fertilisation by sperm) since parasitic males are not recovered from the human body. The females are **ovoviviparous** and lay eggs inside the intestine; these eggs hatch immediately to release larvae. Other features of the adult females are as follows:

- Parasitic females are 2–3 mm long and 30–50 µm wide.
- The anterior portion contains the esophagus with a distinct esophageal bulb.
- The ovaries are aligned linear to the body and with the eggs arranged longitudinally inside them.

Both males and females exist in the short-lived **free-living stage** (Fig. 27.1a).

- The free-living females are shorter in size than the parasitic females.
- The free-living males live in soil and are smaller and thinner than the female.

Larvae

In its life cycle, *S. stercoralis* goes through larval forms which are as follows:

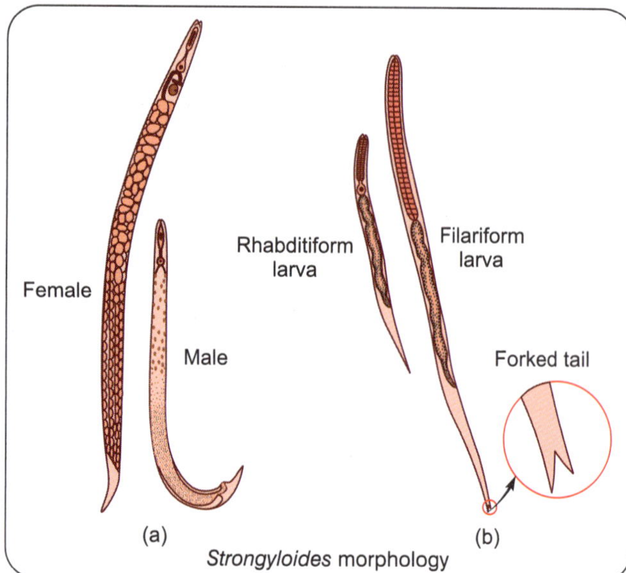

Fig. 27.1 Line diagrams of *Strongyloides stercoralis*: (a) adults and (b) larvae

- **Rhabditiform larva (rod-like esophagus):** It is 250–300 µm long and 15 µm wide. The anterior third of the body contains a muscular esophagus with a short buccal cavity (Fig. 27.1b).
- **Filariform larva (thread-like esophagus):** It is 550–630 µm × 16 µm wide. The esophagus occupies about a third of the total body length. The tail end is **forked** (Fig. 27.1b). This is the **infective and non-feeding stage** of the parasite. The development of the larva is arrested at this stage, and further development is only possible in a host.

LIFE CYCLE (Fig. 27.2a and b)

> **Hosts:** Human beings and other mammals
> **Free-living form:** In soil

Both **free-living and parasitic forms** of *S. stercoralis* exist in nature. **Humans are the definitive hosts** of the parasite; no intermediate host is required. Human beings get infected when the **infective filariform larva penetrates their bare skin** with the help of hydrolytic enzymes. After penetration, the larva finds its way into the **venous circulation** and reaches the **right side of the heart**, and thereafter, the **lungs** through the pulmonary circulation. It gets trapped in the lung capillaries, breaks into the alveoli and ascends the **bronchial tree** to the **trachea and epiglottis** from where it is swallowed and reaches the **small intestine**, where it matures.

The adult parasitic female resides in the intestinal crypts and (most likely **parthenogenetically**) deposits embryonated eggs in the mucosa. These eggs rapidly hatch to release the first-stage rhabditiform larvae which are excreted in the host's feces. It is for this reason that the eggs of the parasite are generally not found in feces. The rhabditiform larvae may develop along one of the following courses of development:

- **Parasitic:** The rhabditiform larvae moult into the filariform stage before passing out through the intestine. The filariform larvae may penetrate the intestinal mucosa or the perianal skin and reach the circulation (**autoinfection**). In this way, the infection is maintained in the host for decades without fresh exposure. In the case of a host with an altered immune status, there is explosive and uncontrolled amplification in the number of larvae known as **hyperinfection**. In such a situation, the parasite is found in increased numbers in the intestine and the lungs. The larvae may also enter the systemic circulation during hyperinfection and may widely disseminate to various organs of the body.
- **Free-living:** The larvae are passed out into the environment along with feces. In suitable conditions such as moist and warm soil, they feed on debris and soil bacteria. In such a setting, the development of the larvae could proceed as follows:
  - The rhabditiform larva may directly grow into an infective filariform larva.
  - The rhabditiform larva may develop into one generation of free-living male and female adults. These adults would then generate progeny which would develop into the infective filariform stage.

The infective filariform larva stands on its tail and 'waits' for stimuli such as heat, odour and chemical signals from the host body, following which, it gets activated and penetrates the host's skin. This stage is very resistant to environmental conditions and can survive for several days in moist soil.

PATHOGENESIS

The disease process starts as soon as the infective larvae of *S. stercoralis* penetrate the host's skin. The nature of the immune response to the infection is not well known; IgE may confer some protection. HTLV-1 co-infection leads to a defect in IgE responses, because of which, the host becomes predisposed to develop a hyperinfection.

- **Skin:** At the site of penetration, there may be petechial hemorrhages, congestion and edema.
- **Lungs:** The larvae, while passing through the lungs, elicit features of bronchopneumonia with lobular consolidation. Alternatively, their passage may be

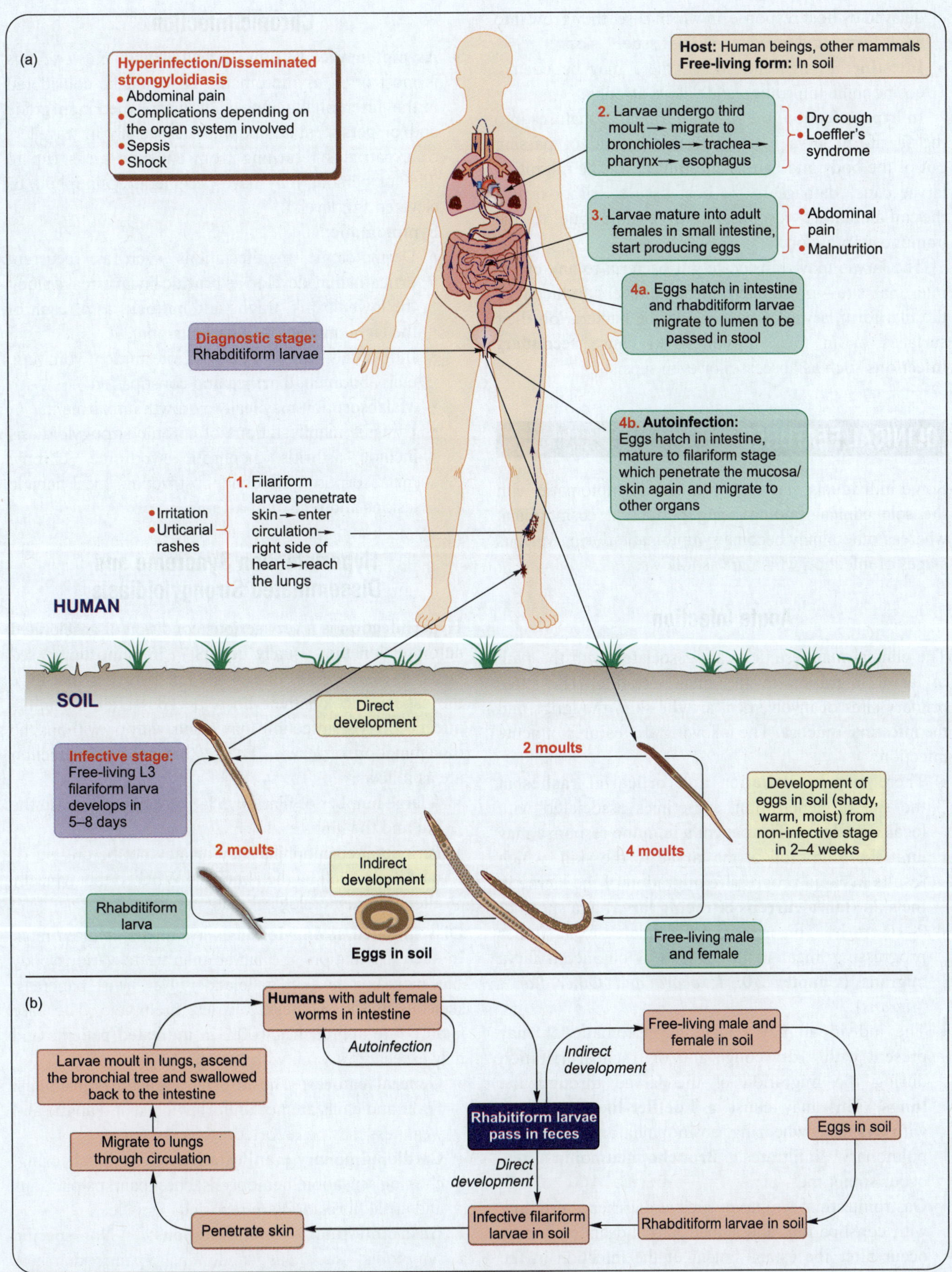

Fig. 27.2 Life cycle of *Strongyloides stercoralis*: (a) detailed and (b) schematic

delayed by host response, in which case, they grow into adult forms and invade the lung tissue.
- **Intestine:** In light infections, there may be edema, eosinophilic infiltration and villous atrophy.

In **hyperinfection**, the rhabditiform larva matures into the filariform larva in the intestine instead of passing out of the body and causes autoinfection. The migrating larvae cause damage to the host tissues. Paradoxically, the inflammatory response may be mild due to the immunosuppression.

The larvae may translocate gut bacteria to any extra-intestinal site—presumably through ulcers induced by the filariform larvae or by carrying the bacteria on their surfaces or in their intestines—to cause **secondary infections** such as abscesses or even sepsis.

CLINICAL FEATURES

Some individuals may remain totally asymptomatic with the sole clinical finding being peripheral eosinophilia, whereas others may become symptomatic during various stages of infection which are as follows.

Acute Infection

The clinical manifestations are associated with the path of larval migration to the small intestine. The three primary sites of involvement are the skin, the lungs and the intestinal mucosa. The following are features of acute infection:
- There may be **irritation and urticarial rashes** at the site of penetration, sometimes associated with localised edema. The patient's immune response may limit the migration of the larvae to the skin, which results in rapid progressive migration of the larvae in the skin (**larva currens or racing larva**) at a speed of 2–10 cm/hr. This is to be differentiated from similar progressing linear rashes caused by cutaneous larva migrans (**Chapter 30**, *Toxocara and Other Larva Migrans*).
- The individual may remain asymptomatic or may present with a dry cough and/or tracheal irritation during the migration of the larvae through the **lungs**. This may cause a **Loeffler-like syndrome** with dyspnea, wheezing, eosinophilia and migratory pulmonary infiltrates. **Bronchopneumonia** may occur sometimes.
- Gastrointestinal symptoms such as diarrhea alternating with constipation, abdominal pain and anorexia may occur after the establishment of the infection in the small intestine.

Chronic Infection

- **Asymptomatic:** Chronic infection with *S. stercoralis* is most often asymptomatic. It should be considered in the differential diagnosis of unexplained high-grade and/or persistent eosinophilia, especially in travellers or expatriates returning from endemic areas (up to 75% of persons may have peripheral eosinophilia or elevated IgE levels).
- **Symptomatic:**
  - Dermatologic manifestations such as recurrent urticaria may develop as pruritic linear streaks along the lower trunk, thighs and buttocks as a result of the larval migration (**larva currens**).
  - Individuals may complain of intermittent vomiting, pain abdomen, diarrhea and constipation.
  - Malabsorption may lead to growth impairment.
  - Unusual manifestations of chronic strongyloidiasis include arthritis, nephrotic syndrome, chronic malabsorption, duodenal obstruction, focal hepatic lesions and recurrent asthma.

Hyperinfection Syndrome and Disseminated Strongyloidiasis

Hyperinfection is a very serious condition of accelerated autoinfection that usually occurs in immunosuppressed hosts. *S. stercoralis* is one of the few parasites that have the capacity to kill their hosts decades after the initial infection. Hyperinfection may occur with or without the dissemination of larvae. The features of hyperinfection are as follows:
- A large number of filariform larvae can be found in the gut and the lungs.
- Peripheral eosinophilia may or may not be present or may be masked by the abnormal WBC counts typically altered in hematological malignancies.

Disseminated strongyloidiasis in humans is often fatal. In such a situation, the larvae migrate to various body sites including the skin, gallbladder, liver, heart, pancreas, skeletal muscle, kidneys, ovaries, brain, etc. The case fatality rate approaches 100% in untreated patients and may exceed 25% even with treatment.
- **General features:** The onset may be acute or insidious. Fever and chills are not uniformly present. Fatigue and weakness may be reported.
- **Cardiopulmonary manifestations:** Cough, wheezing, choking sensation, hemoptysis, chest pain, palpitations and atrial fibrillation are reported.
- **Gastrointestinal manifestations:** Non-specific symptoms such as abdominal pain, diarrhea, constipation, bleeding, anorexia, weight loss, difficulty

in swallowing, vomiting and gastrointestinal bleeding are commonly reported.

- **Central nervous system (CNS) manifestations:** Meningeal signs and symptoms are the most common manifestations of CNS involvement. In patients with meningitis, the spinal fluid may show features of aseptic meningitis (i.e., pleocytosis, elevated protein and normal glucose with sterile bacterial cultures) or demonstrate features of a gram-negative bacterial infection when the bacteria are translocated to the CNS. Larvae may or may not be present.
- **Sepsis and multi-organ failure:** Hyperinfection/dissemination is often complicated by secondary bacterial infections including group D streptococci, *Streptococcus bovis, Escherichia coli, Klebsiella pneumoniae, Proteus mirabilis, Pseudomonas aeruginosa, Enterococcus faecalis,* coagulase-negative staphylococci, *Streptococcus pneumoniae* and *Candida.* Polymicrobial infections may also occur.
- **Dermatologic manifestations:** Pruritic linear streaks on the lower trunk, thighs and buttocks frequently accompany hyperinfection.

DIAGNOSIS

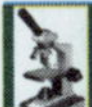

Lab diagnosis

- **Microscopy:** By visualising larvae
  - Direct microscopy of stool, sputum, bronchoalveolar lavage, body fluids and duodenal aspirates
  - Histopathology: Of biopsy specimen of the small intestine or infected extra-intestinal site
- **Culture:** On Koga agar plate or by Harada–Mori filter paper method or Baermann's funnel technique
- **Coproantigen detection:** ELISA
- **Serology:** IgG antibody detection
- **DNA detection:** PCR and real-time PCR
- **Other diagnostic parameters:**
  - Eosinophilia, ↑ IgE, leukocytosis
  - Radiology: Non-specific features

The diagnosis of *Strongyloides* infection is usually made by a combination of serology and microscopic detection of rhabditiform and occasionally filariform larvae in feces, duodenal fluid or biopsy specimens. Sometimes, larvae may be recovered from sputum samples in disseminated infections.

Microscopy

The rate of recovery of larvae in fecal samples is low. A single sample is positive in 20–30% of cases. The sensitivity of microscopy can be improved by examining multiple stool samples. The **rhabditiform larvae** of *S. stercoralis* must be differentiated from those of hookworms that sometimes develop in stool samples at room temperature. This can be done on the basis of the **shorter buccal cavities** of *S. stercoralis* larvae which distinguishes them from hookworm larvae (Fig. 27.3a, b and c) (refer **Chapter 26**, *Necator and Ancylostoma [Hookworms]*).

- The diagnosis of 'hyperinfection syndrome' is based on the recovery of filariform larvae (in addition to rhabditiform larvae) from stool samples examined immediately after the collection of the samples. The presence of larvae or eggs in the **sputum**, bronchoalveolar lavage or other body fluids is also diagnostic. **Biopsies** from the skin, intestine, lymph nodes and other infected organs may show larvae in cases of hyperinfection syndrome/disseminated disease.
- **Duodenal aspirates** may be collected for investigations if stool examination is negative. The parasite can be demonstrated (along with eosinophil infiltration of the lamina propria) in small intestine biopsy specimens taken from the gastric crypts or duodenal glands.

Stool Culture

Only a fresh stool sample should be used for culturing. The L3-stage filariform larvae are formed within two days of inoculation; they should be differentiated from the larvae of hookworm on the basis of their **forked**

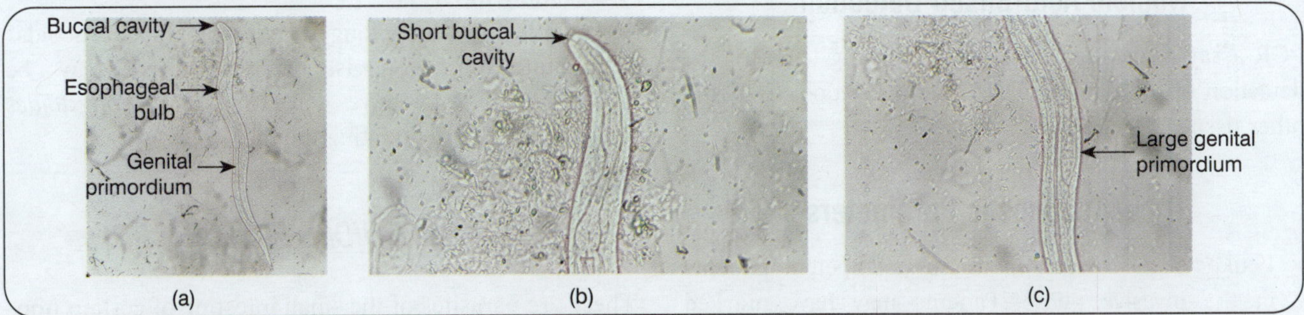

Fig. 27.3 Larvae of *Strongyloides stercoralis*: (a) rhabditiform larva, (b) its short buccal cavity and (c) large genital primordium

tails. Various culture methods can be used, like the Harada–Mori filter paper method, Baermann's funnel technique and the Koga agar plate method (refer **Appendix I**, *Approach to the Laboratory Diagnosis of Parasitic Infections*). These methods have much better sensitivity than microscopy.

> **Note:** Stool samples and larval cultures should be handled carefully to avoid skin exposure to filariform larvae. Personal protective equipment like gloves, gowns, and eyewear should be worn while handling samples. Agar plate cultures should be sealed with parafilm or tape prior to incubation. Lugol's iodine (1% povidone-iodine) or 70% ethanol may be used to kill the infective larvae on exposed skin and surfaces.

Coproantigen Detection

Several assays have been developed for the detection of coproantigens for *S. stercoralis* but they are not yet commercially available in developing countries. Moreover, the efficacy of many of these methods needs to be evaluated.

Serology

Serological tests for the detection of IgG antibodies using crude antigens of *S. stercoralis* (or from closely-related *S. ratti* or *S. venezuelensis*) filariform larvae or recombinant antigens are commercially available. These are increasingly being used for both diagnosis and post-treatment evaluation. Most of these tests possess good sensitivity and specificity, and their high negative predictive value can be particularly useful in excluding *S. stercoralis* infection. However, these tests cannot distinguish between current and past infection even though antibody levels decrease markedly within six months of successful chemotherapy. Another disadvantage is that cross-reactions may occur in patients with ascariasis, filariasis or schistosomiasis, leading to false positivity. A false negative test may occur in immunocompromised patients.

Nucleic Acid-Based Detection

PCR assays, when available, are promising tools for the detection of the parasite DNA in stool, blood, CSF and other tissue specimens.

Other Diagnostic Parameters

- Leukocytosis is seen in immunocompetent patients in the invasive phase. Patients may have **marked peripheral eosinophilia or elevated IgE levels**; these usually vary with the stage of the infection. Eosinophil levels may be high during larval migration and decline with chronicity and are generally higher in patients from non-endemic areas as compared to those from endemic areas. During hyperinfection, patients may or may not show eosinophilia.
- **Radiology** may reveal non-specific features such as patchy infiltrates, interstitial pneumonitis and bronchopneumonia.

TREATMENT

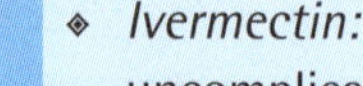

Drug of choice
- *Ivermectin:* 200 µg/kg oral for 2 days in uncomplicated strongyloidiasis and for 7 days or more in hyperinfection syndrome
- *Thiabendazole:* 25 mg/kg twice daily

Alternate drug
- *Albendazole:* 400 mg twice a day for 10–14 days (less effective)

The goal of therapy is the eradication of the infection. To achieve this, follow-up should compulsorily be done at two weeks. If larvae are still found in the patient's specimens, a **repeated course** of the drugs should be administered.

In immunocompromised patients, treatment should be continued for at least 14 days. Response to treatment should be followed up with serial stool examination or antibody titres for 1–2 years. In such patients, reduction of immunosuppressive therapy may be considered and concurrent bacterial infections should be treated.

PREVENTION AND CONTROL

- The **use of footwear** helps as a primary preventive measure.
- WASH programme, i.e., the provision of safe water, sanitation and hygiene including hand washing and discouraging of open defecation is an important strategy for the prevention of diarrheal diseases including the STH.
- Patients for whom long courses of glucocorticoids/ immunosuppression is being planned may be considered for active screening for *Strongyloides* infection before initiating the therapy.

STRONGYLOIDES FUELLEBORNI

These are parasites of the small intestine of certain **non-human primates**. Human infections are reported from some parts of Africa and Papua New Guinea. In addition to skin contact, transmammary transmission is also propounded for this infection. Children are the most affected and present with protein-losing enteropathy, abdominal distension and pulmonary symptoms. Severe hypoproteinemia without proteinuria is classical and leads to peripheral edema and ascites (**'swollen belly syndrome'**). The diagnosis is made by demonstrating eggs (not larvae as in the case of *S. stercoralis*) in stool. The eggs are smaller than those of hookworms (45–55 × 30–35 μm), possess a thin shell and contain larvae which fill the egg. **Thiabendazole** is the treatment of choice. If left untreated, this infection is associated with high mortality.

Questions

1. Describe hyperinfection syndrome in *Strongyloides stercoralis* infection.
2. List the intestinal parasitic infections that are common in immunocompromised individuals.
3. Discuss the laboratory diagnosis and management of strongyloidiasis.
4. Describe the life cycle of *Strongyloides stercoralis*.
5. Discuss *Strongyloides fuelleborni*.

Multiple Choice Questions

1. Larva currens is associated with ________:
   a. *Ancylostoma duodenale*
   b. *Necator americanus*
   c. *Strongyloides stercoralis*
   d. *Toxocara canis*
2. Hyperinfection syndrome is caused by ________:
   a. *Ascaris lumbricoides*
   b. *Toxocara canis*
   c. *Ancylostoma duodenale*
   d. *Strongyloides stercoralis*
3. Swollen belly syndrome is caused by ________:
   a. *Strongyloides fuelleborni*
   b. *Strongyloides stercoralis*
   c. *Ascaris lumbricoides*
   d. *Toxocara canis*
4. The larvae of which of the following parasites can be recovered from stool samples?
   a. *Ascaris lumbricoides*
   b. *Toxocara canis*
   c. *Trichostoma duodenale*
   d. *Strongyloides stercoralis*
5. The route of transmission of *Strongyloides stercoralis* infection is ________:
   a. Transcutaneous b. Fecal-oral
   c. Inhalational d. Vertical
6. The drug of choice for the treatment of *Strongyloides* infection is ________:
   a. Nitazoxanide b. Diethylcarbamazine (DEC)
   c. Ivermectin d. Mebendazole

Chapter 28

Enterobius (Pinworm)

([From Greek] *endon* = inside)

Case Study and Learning Goals

A 12-year-old girl presents to the pediatric OPD with a two-month history of itching in the anal area, especially at night, and occasional abdominal pain. What is the preferred sample for laboratory diagnosis in this case? What is the mode of transmission of the infection? How would you treat this patient? What preventive measures would you recommend?

INTRODUCTION

Enterobiasis is the world's most common helminthic infection in humans. It is caused by *Enterobius vermicularis* (named by Carl Linnaeus who originally called the organism *Ascaris vermicularis*), commonly called **'pinworm'** or **'threadworm'** because of the characteristic needle-/thread-like posterior end of the female. Historically, these parasites have long been known to cause human infections. *E. vermicularis* infections were known to the Roman physician Celsus (25 BC–AD 50). They were also described by Paulus Aegineta (AD 625–690) and by the Arabic physician Avicenna.

Enterobius gregorii is the less common species to infect humans and is quite similar to *E. vermicularis* morphologically except for the smaller posterior spicule in male worms.

EPIDEMIOLOGY

In contrast to the other nematodes, pinworm infections are **not limited** to the tropical and sub-tropical regions of the world and lower socioeconomic groups. The following are epidemiological features of enterobiasis:

- These infections are highly prevalent **across the world** with higher endemicity in cool and temperate zones where bathing and changing of clothes are less frequent. Infections are also common in families of the higher socioeconomic groups.
- Enterobiasis is highly transmissible and often spreads fast in households or institutions due to **direct person-to-person transmission.**
- The prevalence of enterobiasis is maximum among children aged 5–14 years; the infection is also more common in females than in males.
- Reinfection is quite common.
- **Autoinfection** in children due to the habit of nail-biting after scratching the perineum plays an important role in the maintenance of the infection.

MORPHOLOGY

Adult Worm

They are tiny, thread-like white worms (Fig. 28.1a and b and 28.2a–d).

- The **males** are 2–5 mm long and 0.1–0.2 mm wide with their posterior ends curved ventrally. **Females are longer**, 8–14 mm long and 0.3–0.5 mm wide with a sharply **pointed posterior** end (hence the name 'pinworm'). The females are **oviparous** and lay eggs containing larvae. The gravid female lays up to 17,000

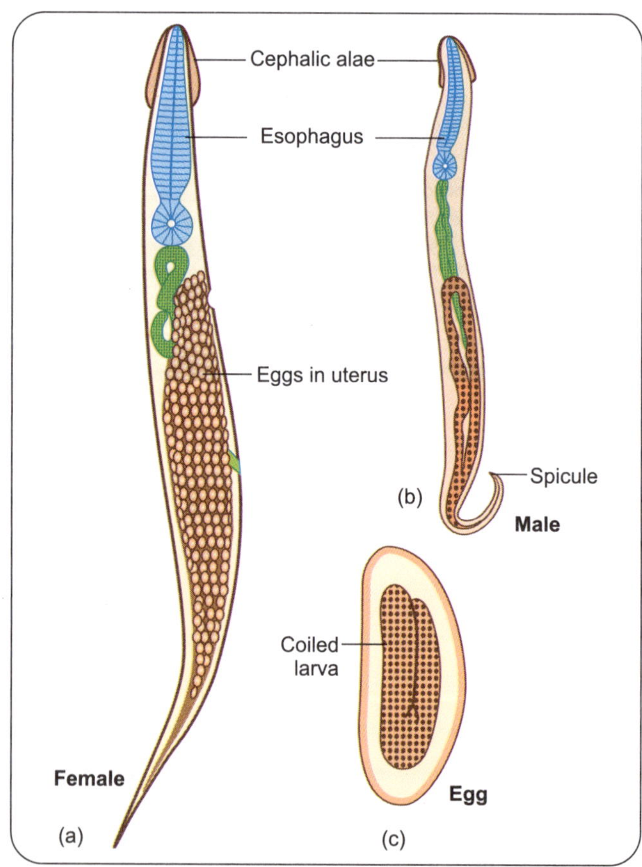

Fig. 28.1 Line diagrams of *Enterobius vermicularis*: (a) adult female, (b) adult male and (c) egg

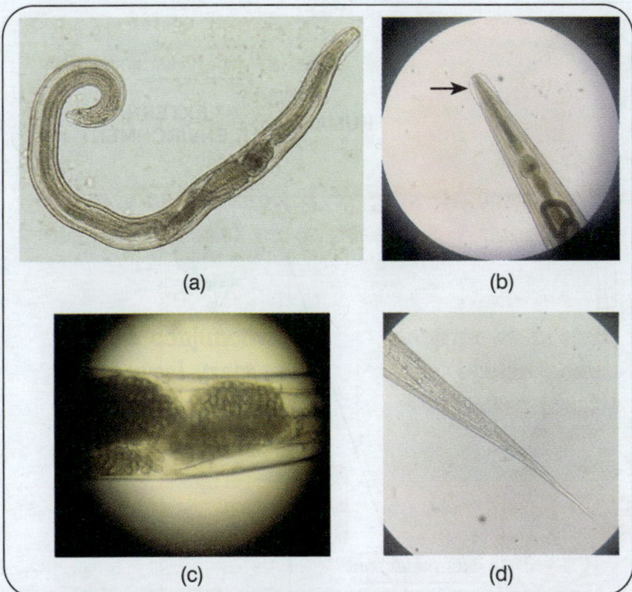

Fig. 28.2 Adults of *Enterobius vermicularis*: (a) adult male (*Source:* Centers for Disease Control and Prevention [CDC], DPDx, image contributed by the Centre for Tropical Medicine and Imported Infectious Diseases, Bergen, Norway), (b) the anterior end of a female worm showing cephalic alae (arrow) and esophagus divided into muscular and bulbous portions, separated by a narrow isthmus, (c) the body of a female worm filled with eggs and (d) the pin-like posterior end of a female worm

eggs and has a distended uterus due to the large number of eggs inside it. It dies within 2–3 weeks of oviposition.
- A characteristic cephalic wing-like prominence called '**alae**' is present in both sexes.
- There is no buccal cavity; the esophagus is divided into muscular and bulbous portions separated by a narrow isthmus.

Eggs

These are oval/**plano-convex** (flattened on one side), **50–60** µm × **20–30** µm in size, and **contain the coiled larva** surrounded by a thin shell membrane (Fig. 28.1c). The eggs are **non-bile stained and float** in a saturated solution of common salt. These mature rapidly and become infective within six hours of being released.

LIFE CYCLE (Fig. 28.3a and b)

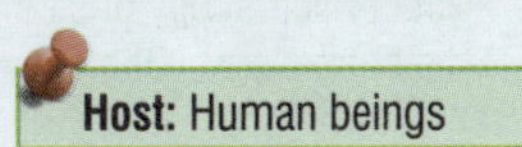

Humans are the only hosts of *Enterobius vermicularis*; no intermediate host is required. The life span of adult male worms is about 7 weeks and that of females is 5–13 weeks.

The **infective form of the parasite is the embryonated egg**. When **ingested**, the infective larvae hatch in the **small intestine** and develop into adults in about 5 weeks without any tissue migration. The adult worms **inhabit the large bowel**, especially the caecal portion and feed on the epithelial cells and bacteria. The male usually dies after fertilising the female. The gravid female worms, which are full of eggs, migrate to the large intestine and **lay eggs around the perianal skin,** especially at night. Once outside the body, the **eggs mature in about six hours** at body temperature and can survive for long periods. The modes of transmission of the infection are as follows:
- **Autoinfection** is the direct transmission of eggs from hand to mouth. This type of transmission occurs when a hand used to scratch the contaminated anal area is subsequently put in the mouth. This mode of transmission is very common.
- Infection is also transmitted by **contact with fomites** carrying viable eggs such as contaminated nightclothes or bed linens. It is also transmitted from the hands of other people and even food.
- Rarely, there may be **sexual transmission** or **inhalation** of dust containing airborne embryonated eggs.
- In **retroinfection**, the eggs hatch on to the anal mucosa and the larvae migrate up the intestine.

PATHOGENESIS

Enterobius vermicularis produces features in the intestine which are usually mild. There may be small ulcers and mild inflammation. The gravid female worm migrating to the perianal area at night is the primary cause of pathology. The mechanisms of pathogenesis of *E. vermicularis* infection are as follows:
- There is perianal/perineal pruritus and excoriation, mostly at night, probably due to the **migration and movement of female worms to the perianal area**. Scratching of the area may lead to secondary infections.
- The female worms may sometimes migrate aberrantly to the female genitourinary tract, fallopian tubes or appendix, causing **inflammation**. Granulomata may form at the ectopic sites and may show polymorphonuclear leukocytes, eosinophils, fibroblasts, macrophages and Charcot-Leyden crystals.

CLINICAL FEATURES

The majority of *E. vermicularis* infections are asymptomatic. When symptomatic, the infection may have the following features:
- **Itching** is the commonest symptom; children may wake up crying because of intense irritation in the perianal area.

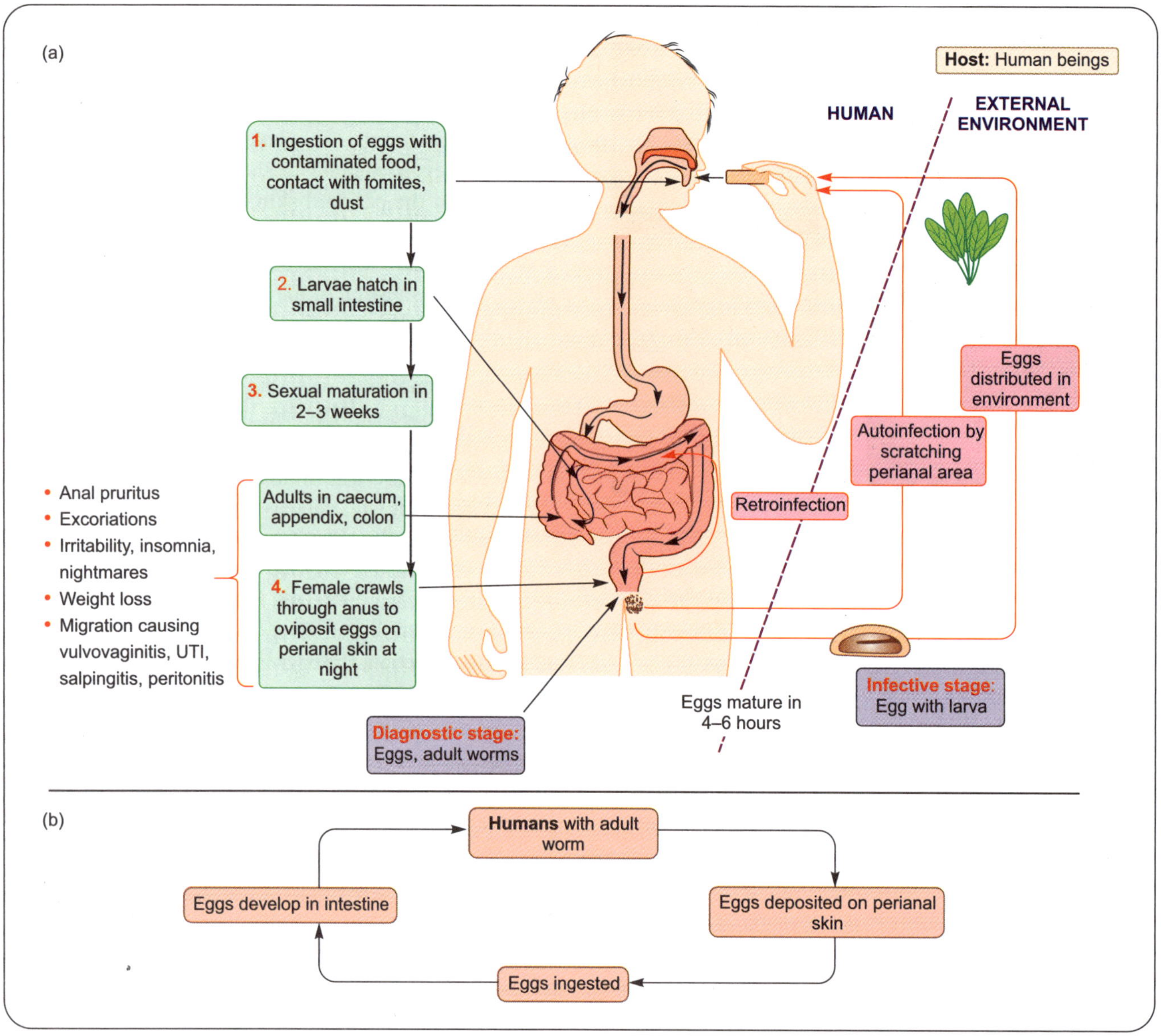

Fig. 28.3 Life cycle of *Enterobius vermicularis*: (a) detailed and (b) schematic

- Insomnia, nightmares and nervousness are recorded in children.
- Enuresis and weight loss may be seen.
- Appendicitis has been linked to enterobiasis.

Ectopic localisation: Sometimes, vulvovaginitis is associated with pinworm infection. Though tissue invasion is not a characteristic of the worm, the parasite has occasionally been recovered from several ectopic sites such as lungs, liver, urinary tract, uterus, fallopian tubes, lymph nodes, eyes and the peritoneal cavity.

DIAGNOSIS

The female pinworms intermittently come out of rectum to the perianal area to lay eggs. They **do not** release their eggs in the intestine. Hence **stool is not the preferred sample** for investigations and is positive in only about 5% of the cases.

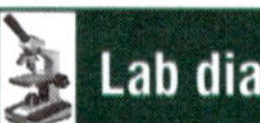

Lab diagnosis

- **Microscopy:** By visualising the eggs and adult worms
  - Specimen: NIH swabs, scotch tape from the perianal area and anal swabs
  - Direct microscopy of stool samples less useful
  - Histopathology: Of biopsy of ectopic sites

Microscopy

The diagnosis is made by demonstrating eggs (Fig. 28.4) or adult worms in a wet mount of a '**scotch tape**' or '**NIH swab**' collected **from the perianal area**

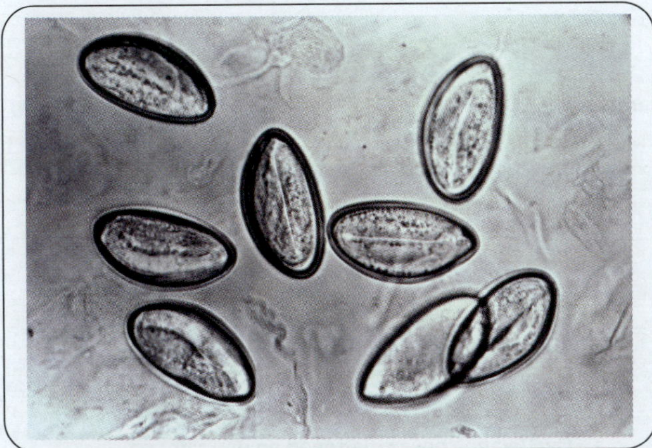

Fig. 28.4 Eggs of *Enterobius vermicularis* mounted on a cellulose tape (*Source:* CDC, Public Health Image Library [PHIL], Image ID 5229)

or an anal swab. The specimen should preferably be collected early in the morning before the patient has had a bath. The sensitivity for a single sample is 50%, which improves to >90% with 3–5 samples collected on different days. The various methods of collecting the specimen are as follows:

- **Scotch tape:** A 6 cm long piece of scotch tape is folded with its sticky side out over the end of a wooden tongue blade or glass rod and then firmly applied against either side of the patient's perianal region (Fig. 28.5). In the lab, the tape is placed with its sticky side down on a glass slide and examined microscopically. The slide with the affixed tape can be stored in a refrigerator for a long time.
- **NIH swab method (from the National Institute of Health, USA):** A square inch transparent cellophane sheet is fastened to a glass rod with a rubber band and used for swabbing the anal region. After swabbing, the rod is placed inside a test tube for transportation. For examination, the cellophane sheet is spread out on a glass slide holding a drop of saline in such a way that the swabbed material lies between the cellophane and the slide (Fig. 28.6).
- **Swube tubes:** Commercially available 'Swube tubes' containing a paddle coated with adhesive material can also be used for sample collection and transportation.

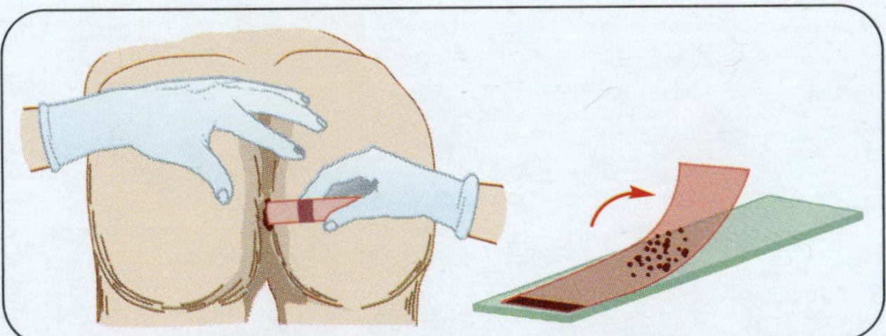

Fig. 28.5 Scotch tape method

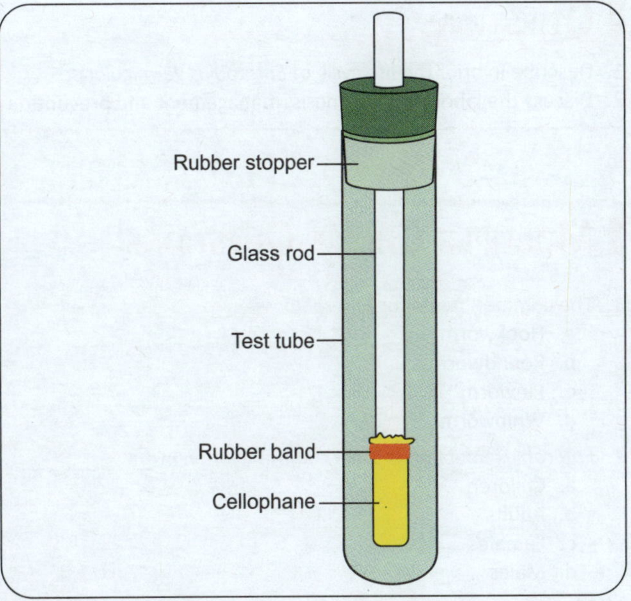

Fig. 28.6 NIH swab

Other Diagnostic Parameters

- For histopathology, biopsy samples should be obtained from ectopic sites.
- Enterobiasis is not usually associated with eosinophilia or elevated IgE.

TREATMENT

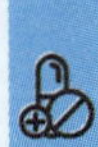

- *Albendazole:* 400 mg as a single dose
- *Mebendazole:* 100 mg as a single dose
- *Pyrantel pamoate:* 11 mg/kg (maximum 1 g) as a single dose

Since reinfection is quite common, all patients should receive a **second course of treatment after two weeks** of the first course. All family members should be treated simultaneously. Parents should be counselled about maintaining proper hygiene.

PREVENTION AND CONTROL

Total prevention is not realistically possible. However, health education for **improving personal hygiene**, thorough washing of clothes and clipping of nails may help.

Questions

1. Describe in brief the life cycle of *Enterobius vermicularis*.
2. Discuss the laboratory diagnosis, management and prevention of enterobiasis.

Multiple Choice Questions

1. The common name for *Enterobius* is ____________ :
   a. Hookworm
   b. Roundworm
   c. Pinworm
   d. Whipworm
2. *Enterobius* infection is most commonly seen in ____________ :
   a. Children
   b. Adults
   c. Females
   d. Males
3. Diagnosis of *Enterobius* infection is best made by __________ :
   a. The detection of eggs in stool samples
   b. The detection of eggs in perianal swabs
   c. Serology
   d. Culture of stool samples
4. All the following are characteristics of *Enterobius* eggs EXCEPT ____________ :
   a. Oval/plano-convex (flattened on one side)
   b. Contain a coiled larva surrounded by a thin shell membrane
   c. Bile-stained
   d. Float in saturated solutions of common salt
5. Pinworm infection is treated by ____________ :
   a. Nitazoxanide
   b. Albendazole
   c. Fluconazole
   d. Cefoxitin

Chapter 29

Trichinella

(*Trichinella* from *thrix/trichos* [Greek] = fine hair + *ella* = small; *spiralis* [Latin] = enrolled)

Case Study and Learning Goals

A 45-year-old hunter presents with complaints of intense muscular pain and swollen eyelids for the last two weeks. He has a history of eating partially-cooked wild boar meat when he visited a forest two months back. Physical examination reveals splinter hemorrhages in his nail bed. A muscle biopsy reveals a coiled helminth larva. What are the parasites acquired by pork consumption? What is the pathogenesis of this disease? How would you treat this patient?

INTRODUCTION

Trichinella species can infect mammals, birds and reptiles. In humans, these parasites cause a systemic illness called trichinellosis (or trichinosis), which is often fatal. While the disease is caused by many of the closely related species of *Trichinella*, ***T. spiralis* is the most important species to cause human disease**. It is a **zoonotic** infection acquired mainly from **pigs or other carnivores**. The parasite was first described in 1835 by James Paget, a medical student who incidentally found calcified nurse cells harbouring the larval form of the parasite in the muscles of a man who had died of tuberculosis.

EPIDEMIOLOGY

Trichinella has a **worldwide** distribution. However, some species are reported predominantly from certain geographical regions (see box). These parasites have distinct **sylvatic** (in bears, walruses, hyenas and other carnivores) and **domestic** life cycles (in pigs and rats) in nature. The infection is acquired by **ingesting raw or undercooked meat, most commonly pork** (sausages), though **horse and polar bear meat** have also been implicated in causing outbreaks. **Hunters** and their friends and relatives are at risk due to the exposure to the raw or improperly cooked meat of game animals. Individuals who maintain a vegetarian diet are not at risk.

- *T. spiralis* and *T. pseudospiralis* – cosmopolitan
- *T. britovi* – Europe, North Africa, the Middle East and Asia
- *T. nelsoni* – Africa
- *T. nativa* – Arctic and Subarctic regions
- *T. papuae* – New Guinea

MORPHOLOGY

Adult Worm

These worms are the **smallest nematode parasites of humans**. They are equipped with characteristic glandular cells called 'stichocytes', which are arranged in a row after the short esophagus.

- The male (Fig. 29.1a) is about 1.5 mm long with conspicuous claspers at its posterior end.
- The female (Fig. 29.1b) is 3.5 mm long with a single uterus in its anterior portion containing the fully developed larvae (**viviparous**).

Larvae

The freshly hatched larva measures around **100 μm in length**. Its esophagus has a spear-like 'stylet' which helps it to penetrate host cells. When fully developed, it reaches a length of **1,000 μm (1 mm)** and is found intracellularly

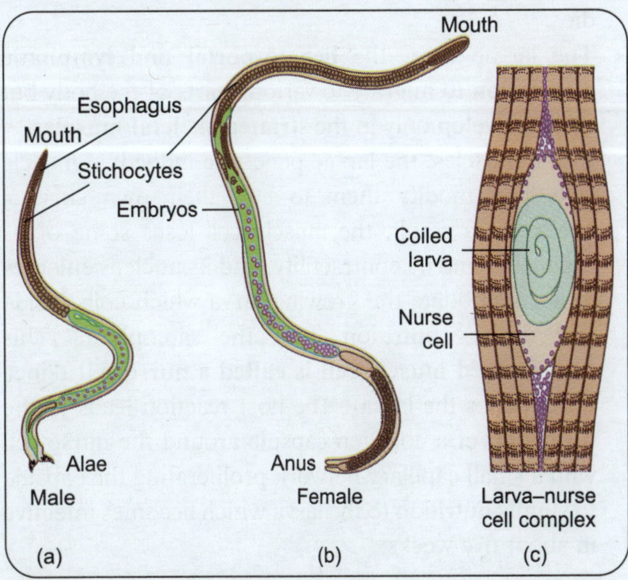

Fig. 29.1 Line diagrams of (a) *Trichinella* male, (b) female and (c) larva–nurse cell complex

in the muscle fibres of the host, enclosed in a pseudocyst (Fig. 29.1c).

LIFE CYCLE (Fig. 29.2a and b)

Definitive and intermediate hosts: Pigs, rats, bears and other carnivores and human beings (**dead-end hosts**)

Trichinella is a peculiar parasite as it uses a **single host as its definitive and as its intermediate host**. Pigs, rats, bears and other carnivores serve as hosts for the parasite, and the adult and larval stages of the life cycle of these parasites occur in different organs of the host. Human beings also serve as hosts and are involved in the transmission of the parasite; however, they are the **dead end** in the parasite's life cycle. Clinical features appear only in the human host. The various stages in the life cycle of *Trichinella* are as follows:

- The infection is acquired by ingesting the encapsulated larva (L1) in nurse cells present in undercooked infected meat or garbage containing pork/rat waste. Once ingested, the nurse cells are broken down by the digestive enzymes to release the larvae, which subsequently reach the **small intestine**. Once there, the larvae invade the intestinal columnar epithelium, rapidly moult four times (L1→L4) and develop into adult males/females within 30 hours.
- The sexually mature male fertilises the female and subsequently dies; it is then excreted in the feces. Meanwhile, the fertilised **viviparous female** burrows deep into the intestinal wall and releases hundreds to thousands of larvae (L1) for several weeks before it dies.
- The larvae enter the **hepato-portal and lymphatic circulation** to migrate to various parts of the body but finally develop only in the **striated skeletal muscles**.
- In the muscles, the larvae penetrate individual muscle cells and modify them to suit their own survival needs. As a result, the muscle cell loses some of its organelles and its contractility, and its nucleus enlarges to accommodate the growing larva which coils inside and derives nutrition from the sarcoplasm. This **transformed muscle cell is called a nurse cell** (since it nourishes the larva). The host reaction leads to the formation of a collagen capsule around the nurse cell with a small capillary network proliferating the capsule to supply nutrition to the larva which becomes infective in about five weeks.

Trichinella is the largest known intracellular parasite.

- After this, the larva enters a stage of developmental arrest and usually calcifies in six months. However, it may remain viable for many years. There may be thousands of larvae per gram of muscle in severe disease.
- When ingested by another host, the parasite continues its life cycle.

PATHOGENESIS

The features of the disease depend on stage of the infection. The various mechanisms of pathogenesis of *Trichinella* infection are as follows:

Intestinal stage: The penetration of the adult worm into the intestinal mucosa causes **traumatic damage and inflammation**. This stage is often asymptomatic.

Parenteral stages: This stage can be further divided into two stages which are as follows:

- **Migratory stage:** During migration, the larvae reach various host tissues and destroy the cells they enter. This results in a marked local and systemic inflammatory reaction in the affected organ. There may be pneumonia, encephalitis, meningitis, nephritis, myocarditis, peritonitis and localised damage. The migration of larvae is associated with concomitant bacterial invasion; heavy infections can lead to bacterial sepsis.
- **Encystment stage:** The larval antigens present in its metabolic products and secretions cause host immune reactions and the associated pathology of the affected body site. There may be localised edema, swelling, decreased blood pressure and reduced muscle contractility. Extreme eosinophilia and elevated IgE levels are common.

CLINICAL FEATURES

Most light *Trichinella* infections are asymptomatic and self-limiting. The **clinical features may appear simultaneously in family members or a group** of individuals who shared a common activity. The clinical presentation depends on the stage of the parasite's life cycle.

Intestinal Stage

This stage develops **1–7 days** after infection. The individual may remain asymptomatic or present with symptoms like those of food poisoning. Abdominal pain, vomiting and diarrhea may be present.

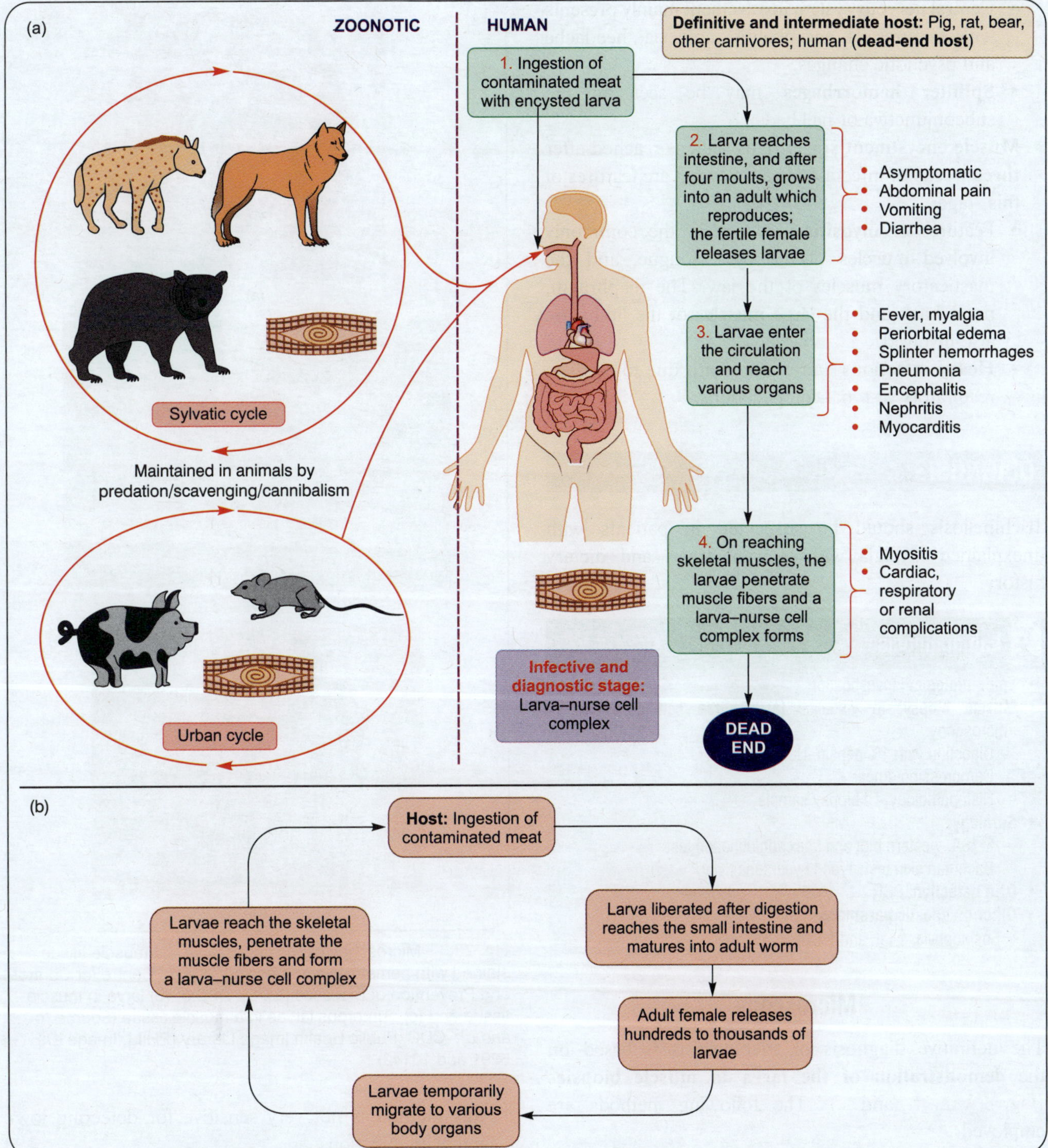

Fig. 29.2 Life cycle of *Trichinella:* (a) detailed and (b) schematic

Parenteral Stage

- **Larval migration stage:** This stage is reached **7–21 days** after infection. The following clinical features may be seen at this stage:
    - There is characteristic **hypereosinophilia**. Urticarial rashes and maculopapular exanthemas may be seen.
    - There may be high-grade fever, myalgia, periorbital or facial edema, dysphagia, headache and paraesthesia.
    - Heart involvement presents as tachycardia, hypotension and elevated venous pressure. **Myocarditis is the most important cause of mortality** in trichinellosis.

- Central nervous system involvement mainly presents with features of encephalitis, amnesia, headache and psychotic changes.
- **Splinter hemorrhages** may be seen in the subconjunctiva or nail beds.

◆ **Muscle encystment stage:** This stage is reached after **three weeks** of infection. The following are features of this stage:
- Features of **myositis** are seen in the commonly involved muscles of the eyes, tongue, and the masticatory muscles of the jaw. The diaphragm, neck, back and the large muscles of the limbs are also involved.
- **Heavy infections can cause death** due to cardiac, respiratory or renal complications.

DIAGNOSIS

Trichinellosis should be suspected in patients with unexplained myalgia with relevant travel and dietary history.

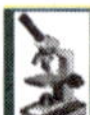

Lab diagnosis

- **Epidemiological** investigation
- **Muscle biopsy:** To visualise **larva–nurse cell** complex by microscopy
  - Digestion with 1% pepsin–HCl
  - Compression smear
  - Histopathology: Of biopsy sample
- **Serology:**
  - ELISA, western blot and latex agglutination test
  - Bachman skin test: Type I hypersensitivity
- **DNA detection:** PCR
- **Other diagnostic parameters:**
  - Eosinophilia, ↑ IgE and ↑ CPK

Microscopy

The definitive diagnosis of trichinellosis is based on the **demonstration of the larva in muscle biopsies** (Fig. 29.3a, b and c). The following methods are employed:

◆ **Digestion:** 1 cm^2 of the muscle biopsy is digested with a mixture of 1% pepsin and 1% HCl at 37°C for several hours and then examined microscopically for larvae. The **preferred muscles for biopsy are the gastrocnemius, deltoid and biceps**. This method can be used for estimating the number of larvae per gram of muscle.

◆ **Trichinoscopy:** In 50% of cases, the larvae can be demonstrated on **compression smears** prepared by pressing the biopsy tissue between two slides. However, this method is not very sensitive for detecting low-intensity infections.

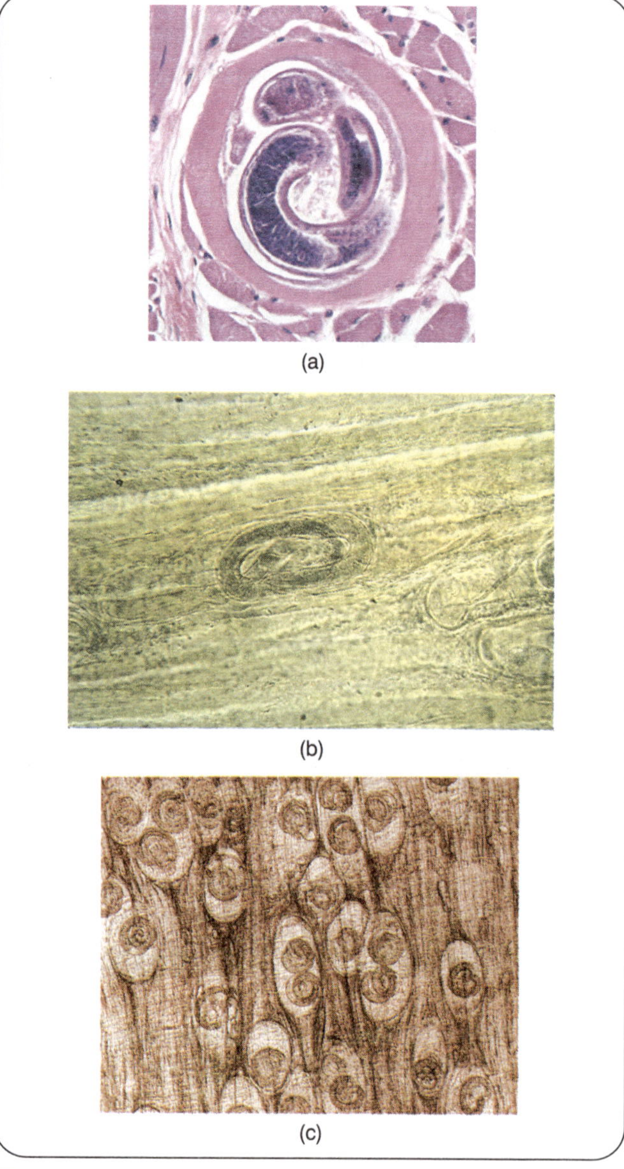

Fig. 29.3 Microscopy of *Trichinella* larva: (a) muscle tissue stained with hematoxylin and eosin (*Source:* Centre for Control and Prevention of Diseases [CDC], DPDx), (b) larva in muscle tissue and (c) numerous larvae in a muscle tissue (*Source [b and c]:* CDC, Public Health Image Library [PHIL], Image IDs 5291 and 10142)

- The pseudocyst containing the tightly coiled larva is oval and has tapering ends.
- It measures 200–350 μm in size with a capsule which is about 15 μm thick.

◆ **Histopathology:** Muscle tissue may be stained with hematoxylin–eosin stain. The larvae may be seen along with features of myositis with abundant eosinophils.

Serology

This is the most commonly employed method for the diagnosis of trichinellosis. However, it is usually negative at the onset of clinical features since the titres tend to peak only in the second or third month after infection and subsequently decline over the next few years.

- ELISA may detect antibodies against the excretory/secretory (ES) antigens of the muscle-stage larvae. Western blot is quite specific but less sensitive. Bentonite flocculation and latex agglutination tests detect antibodies earlier but are non-specific.
- **Skin test (Bachman test)** is an immediate (Type I) hypersensitivity reaction (induration surrounded by erythema in an area measuring about 5 cm diameter in 15–20 minutes) to *Trichinella* antigen injected intradermally. This test is positive after 2–3 weeks of infection. However, it cannot differentiate between recent and past infection as a patient may remain positive for many years after exposure.

Nucleic Acid-Based Detection

The detection of the parasite's DNA by molecular methods like multiplex PCR can be used for species identification.

Stool/Body Fluid Examination

Microscopic examination of stool during the diarrheic stage or of other body fluids such as blood, milk and other secretions during the migratory phase to detect the adult worms and larvae may be helpful, though rarely.

Other Diagnostic Parameters

- **Eosinophilia** of 20–90% (>1,000 cells/µl), especially 2–5 weeks post-infection is very characteristic.
- The total IgE levels are usually raised.
- The levels of muscle enzymes like **creatine phosphokinase** are also raised.
- X-ray may detect calcified cysts.

TREATMENT

Intestinal phase

- *Mebendazole:* 200–400 mg oral TDS × 3 days followed by 400–500 mg oral TDS × 10 days
- *Albendazole:* 400 mg oral BDS × 8–14 days

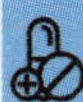

Systemic disease

- There is **no data to support the efficacy of any drug regime** in systemic illness.
- Corticosteroids and anti-inflammatory agents must be administered in conjunction with mebendazole or albendazole in severe disease for 8–14 days.

These drugs may reduce the worm burden but are not effective against larvae in muscle tissues. Despite treatment, the mortality rate stands at about 5%.

PREVENTION AND CONTROL

- **Good animal husbandry practices**, sterilising pig feeds, regular inspection of meat and avoiding the consumption of raw meat can prevent transmission.
- Appropriate garbage management is of immense utility.
- Meat should be thoroughly cooked at about 70°C or above (until there is no pink flesh or fluid left). Meat should be preserved in deep freezers at –15°C × 3 weeks or –30°C × 6 days. Salting, smoking or drying of meat does not destroy the infective larvae.
- Irradiation of sealed packaged meat products destroys the infective larvae.

QUESTIONS

1. List the various tissue nematodes and describe briefly the life cycle of *Trichinella*.
2. Enumerate the parasitic infections caused by the consumption of improperly or uncooked pork.
3. Describe the pathogenesis and clinical features of trichinellosis.
4. Discuss the laboratory diagnosis and management of trichinellosis.

Multiple Choice Questions

1. The muscle fibres that harbour the larvae of *Trichinella spiralis* are called ___________:
   a. Nurse cells
   b. Sleeper cells
   c. Foamy cells
   d. Mother cells
2. *Trichinella* infection is acquired by humans by the ___________:
   a. Ingestion of infected meat
   b. Ingestion of raw vegetables contaminated with *Trichinella* eggs
   c. Penetration of the larva through the skin while swimming
   d. Bite of the tsetse fly
3. The reservoir hosts for *Trichinella* spp. are ___________:
   a. Fish
   b. Humans
   c. Arthropods
   d. Mammals
4. In which of the following parasites does the larval stage reside in muscle cells and cause myositis?
   a. *Taenia solium*
   b. *Strongyloides stercoralis*
   c. *Ascaris lumbricoides*
   d. *Trichinella* spp.
5. Which of the following is the largest intracellular parasite?
   a. *Taenia saginata*
   b. *Trichinella spiralis*
   c. *Strongyloides stercoralis*
   d. *Sarcocystis hominis*

Chapter 30 Toxocara and Other Larva Migrans

([From Greek] *toxon* = crescent-shaped + *kara* = head)

Case Study and Learning Goals

A 7-year-old boy from a rural area presents with a low-grade fever, wheezing cough, myalgia and pain in the right hypochondrium for the past three months. On examination, he is found to have noted hepatomegaly, and investigations reveal high eosinophilia. What are the parasitic causes of eosinophilia? List the animal parasites that can accidentally infect humans?

INTRODUCTION

Eosinophilia is associated with numerous parasitic infections (Table 30.1), and is especially notable in invasive helminthiases. It can also be caused by a number of allergic and immunologic disorders. The degree of eosinophilia is highly variable and is influenced by various factors, which are as follows:

- Helminths whose migration through tissues is limited, such as those localised to the gastrointestinal tract or skin, are generally associated with little or no eosinophilia.
- In contrast, **helminths that migrate extensively through the internal or visceral organs cause profound eosinophilia**.
- Eosinophilia is also higher for those parasites for which humans are aberrant hosts.
- Once the migration of the parasite is complete and the tissues are no longer exposed to it, the eosinophilia usually wanes.

Table 30.1 Parasitic causes of eosinophilia

Nematodes
• *Toxocara canis*/*cati* (larva migrans*)
• *Trichinella spiralis**
• *Wuchereria bancrofti* (Tropical pulmonary eosinophilia*)
• *Brugia malayi* (Tropical pulmonary eosinophilia*)
• *Onchocerca volvulus*
• *Loa loa*
• *Gnathostoma* spp.*
• *Angiostrongylus cantonensis* (Eosinophilic meningoencephalitis)*/*costaricensis*
• *Ascaris lumbricoides* (Loeffler's syndrome*)
• Hookworms
• *Trichuris trichiura*
• *Capillaria* spp.*
• *Strongyloides stercoralis*
• *Anisakis* spp.
• *Dirofilaria* spp.
• *Baylisascaris procyonis**
Trematodes
• *Paragonimus westermani*
• *Fasciola hepatica*
• *Clonorchis sinensis*
• *Opisthorchis viverrini*
• *Schistosoma haematobium**/*mansoni*/*japonicum*
• *Fasciolopsis buski*
• *Heterophyes heterophyes*
• *Echinostoma* spp.
Cestodes
• *Taenia solium* (cysticercosis)
• *Echinococcus granulosus*
• *Hymenolepis nana*
• *Sparganum proliferum*
Protozoa
• *Cystoisospora belli*
• *Dientamoeba fragilis*
• *Sarcocystis* spp.

*Higher degree of eosinophilia

Larva migrans: Larva migrans (LM) is a zoonosis caused by the **migration of larvae of non-human helminth species** to different parts of the human body. It is characterised by **multi-system involvement along with eosinophilia.** When the larvae of animal nematodes accidentally infect humans, they are unable to complete their normal developmental cycle and wander around aimlessly in the human body. LM is of four types depending upon the involvement of body parts. These are as follows:

- Visceral larva migrans (VLM)
- Ocular larva migrans (OLM)
- Neural larva migrans (NLM)
- Cutaneous larva migrans (CLM)

VISCERAL LARVA MIGRANS

INTRODUCTION

Toxocara canis (dog roundworm) and *T. cati* (cat roundworm) are generally associated with VLM in humans. It was Helenor Campbell Wilder who first described the condition (in 1950) when he found a larva of the parasite in a granuloma in a patient's retina.

Causes of VLM
- *Toxocara canis*
- *Toxocara cati*
- *Baylisascaris procyonis*
- *Ascaris suum*

EPIDEMIOLOGY

T. canis and *T. cati* have a cosmopolitan distribution in dogs and cats respectively. Depending on the area, the incidence of *Toxocara* infections in dogs ranges from 2–90%. Puppies and kittens are also heavily infected because of transplacental and lactogenic transmission of the parasite to the fetus. Though the exact prevalence of the infection among humans is unknown, the widespread distribution of *T. canis* and *T. cati* in dogs and cats and other carnivores, and the wide variety of possible transmission routes reported in humans indicate that toxocariasis is a common zoonosis. Children are most susceptible to the disease; other risk factors are geophagia, the habit of eating raw fruits or vegetables and living in rural areas.

MORPHOLOGY

Toxocara are morphologically similar to the human roundworm, *Ascaris lumbricoides.*

Adult Worm

The adult worms are large and pinkish. The males of *Toxocara* species are 4–6 cm in length with a curved posterior end. The females are longer, measuring 6–10 cm. Anteriorly, both males and females possess three lips and large, spear-shaped cervical alae (Fig. 30.1a). The alae are broader in *T. cati* (Fig. 30.1b) than they are in *T. canis*.

Eggs

Toxocara eggs are found in the feces of dogs and cats. They are golden in colour, round to pear-shaped and thick-shelled with a pitted surface. *T. canis* eggs are larger (measuring 80–85 μm) than those of *T. cati* (which measure 65–75 μm). The eggs develop L3 larvae *in ovo* (Fig. 30.1c).

Larvae

When hatched, the L3 larvae are 350–400 μm long and 15–20 μm wide with two large excretory columns and single-pointed lateral alae. These features help in their identification in histopathology sections.

LIFE CYCLE (Fig. 30.2)

> **Definitive hosts:** Dogs and cats
> **Accidental hosts:** Human beings

The various life cycle stages of *Toxocara* spp. are as follows:

Natural life cycle: In dogs and cats, the adult worm lives in the intestine, where it lays non-embryonated eggs which are released in the animal's feces. These eggs embryonate in the soil and transform into the L2 infective larval stage in 2–3 weeks. The eggs are extremely hardy and can survive harsh environmental conditions and

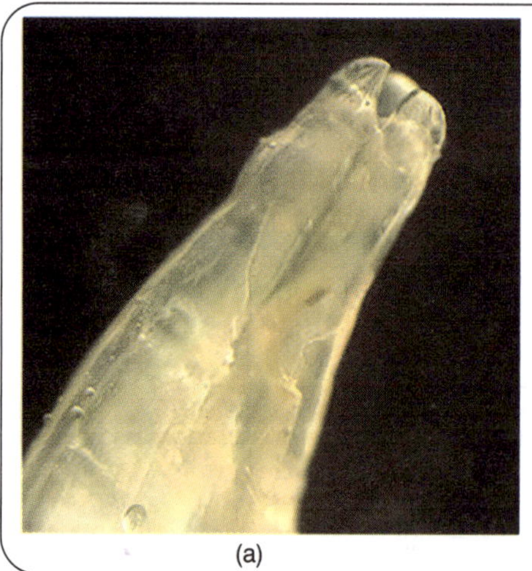
(a)

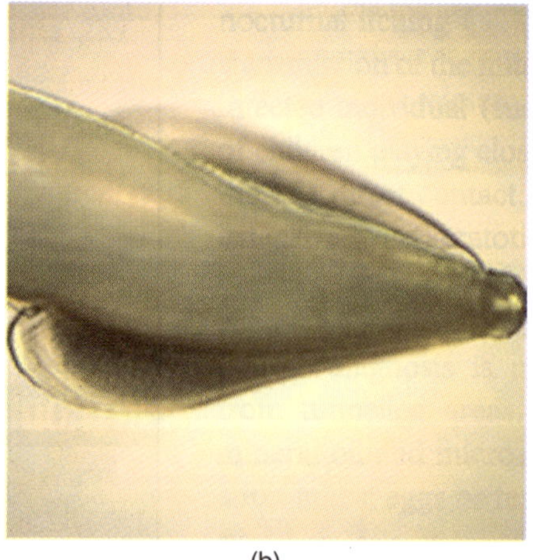
(b)

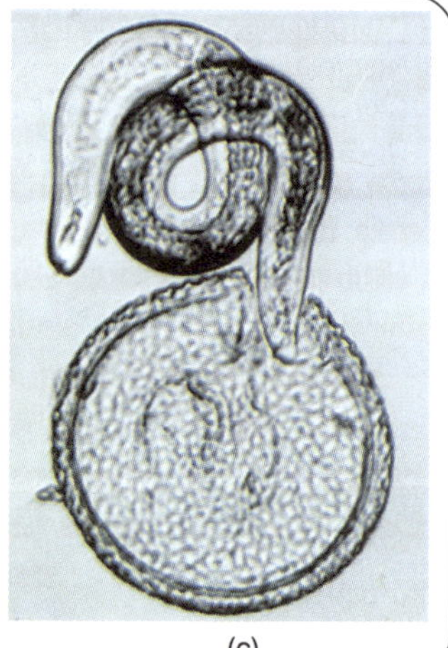
(c)

Fig. 30.1 Features of *Toxocara*: (a) the anterior end of *T. canis* showing three lips, characteristic of ascarid worms, (b) the anterior end of *T. cati* showing broad alae with striations and (c) *T. canis* L3 larva hatching (*Source:* Centers for Disease Control and Prevention [CDC], DPDx)

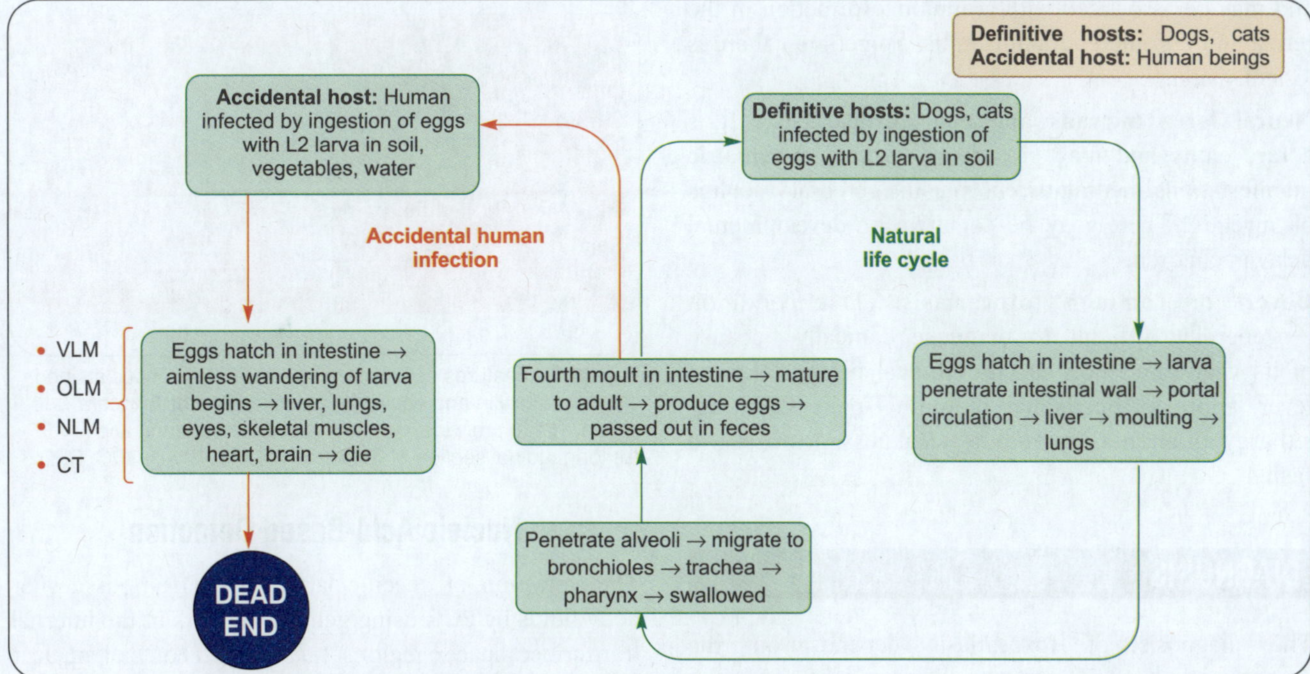

Fig. 30.2 Life cycle of *Toxocara species* (schematic)

survive for months. On ingestion by the natural host, the larvae hatch in the small intestine and reach the liver, where they moult again. These larvae then further migrate to the lungs, penetrate the alveolar space and ascend the trachea to be swallowed into the gastrointestinal tract. Finally, they moult again and mature into adult worms in the intestine, and the life cycle continues.

Human life cycle: Humans acquire toxocariasis by **accidentally ingesting the parasite's eggs** from contaminated soil, water, raw vegetables or fruit or by living in close proximity with dogs or cats that carry the embryonated eggs in their hair. Human beings are not the natural hosts of *Toxocara* species, and are the dead end in the life cycle of the parasite. After hatching in the intestine, the larvae start wandering in the body aimlessly, causing damage in the process until they die. They can survive in the body for periods ranging from months to years.

PATHOGENESIS

In humans, *Toxocara* larvae penetrate the intestinal wall and migrate to various organs by mechanical means and by protease digestion. Various organs can be affected, such as the liver, lungs, skeletal muscles, the heart, the brain and the eyes. Often, the larvae become encapsulated in fibrous tissue in the liver and lungs. The migrating or dead larvae stimulate the host's immune response, resulting in local inflammation. There is eosinophilia and increased production of cytokines and antibodies. This results in the formation of granulomas consisting of lymphocytes, eosinophils, fibroblasts and giant cells.

CLINICAL FEATURES

Asymptomatic Infections

Most *Toxocara* infections are asymptomatic.

Symptomatic Infections

The infection can present as visceral larva migrans (VLM), ocular larva migrans (OLM), neural larva migrans (NLM or neurotoxocariasis) or covert toxocariasis (CT).

Visceral larva migrans: It is the most common LM syndrome and is particularly seen in children. Its clinical features include fever, cough, wheezing, myalgia and cutaneous manifestations like pruritus, rash, eczema and vasculitis. The most involved organ is the liver, with hepatomegaly being a common finding among patients; however, other organs may be involved as well. Less frequently, lymphadenopathy, myocarditis, nephritis and arthritis are observed in some people.

Ocular larva migrans: It is a less common form of LM. Clinically, it is observed more frequently in children. OLM usually occurs unilaterally along with strabismus and may be associated with granuloma formation in the retina and chronic endophthalmitis. Sometimes, there is loss of vision.

Neural larva migrans and neurotoxocariasis: It is a rare entity and may present as seizures, psychiatric manifestations, meningitis, encephalitis, cerebral vasculitis or myelitis. There may be cognitive or developmental delay in children.

Covert or common toxocariasis: This condition is generally difficult to diagnose clinically because of its vague and non-specific clinical presentation as fever, anorexia, headache, abdominal pain, vomiting, lethargy, pulmonary symptoms, weakness, pruritus and rash.

DIAGNOSIS

The diagnosis of toxocariasis depends on the demonstration of *Toxocara*-specific antibodies or the direct visualisation of the worm in a tissue specimen.

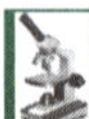

Lab diagnosis

- **Serology:**
  - ELISA: Antibodies against excretory/secretory (ES) antigens
  - Immunoblotting
- **Microscopy:** By visualising characteristic morphology of larvae in tissue biopsies
- **DNA detection:** PCR
- **Other diagnostic parameters:**
  - Eosinophilia
  - Radiology

Serology

ELISA assays have been used to detect excretory or secretory (TES) antigens of the larval stages of *T. canis* or recombinant antigens. Antibodies may also be elevated in asymptomatic patients. The test results may be confirmed by immunoblotting.

OLM is diagnosed on the basis of elevated anti-*T. canis* antibodies in the patient's serum and vitreous or aqueous humour, whereas NLM is diagnosed based on the finding of elevated antibodies in the patient's CSF.

Histopathology

Biopsy of the liver, lungs, brain or the affected part may only rarely reveal the larvae, which may then be identified by their characteristic structures in cross-section (Fig. 30.3a and b).

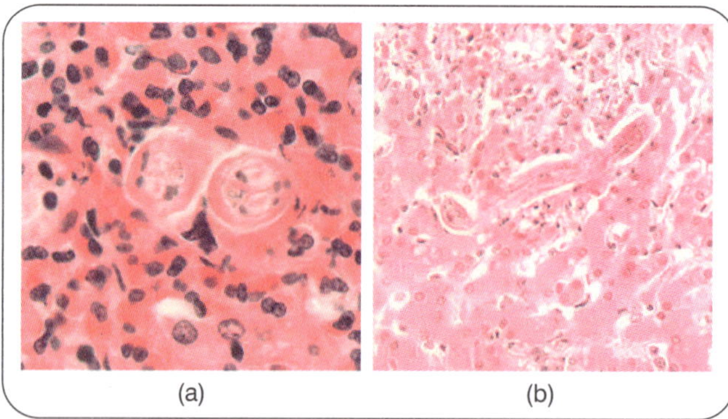

Fig. 30.3 Features of *Toxocara* species in liver tissue stained with hematoxylin and eosin: (a) cross-section of *Toxocara* larvae, 15–20 μm wide, with two excretory columns and (b) longitudinal section of *Toxocara* larva (*Source:* CDC, DPDx)

Nucleic Acid-Based Detection

The detection of specific larval DNA from tissues or body fluids by PCR using genetic markers in the internal transcribed spacer regions (*ITS1* and *ITS2*) of nuclear ribosomal RNA genes is useful in diagnosis.

Other Diagnostic Parameters

- **High eosinophilia** (often reaching up to 90% of the leukocyte count) is a classical feature and is usually accompanied by leukocytosis.
- Radioimaging may be helpful for the diagnosis of OLM or VLM.

TREATMENT

- *Albendazole:* 15 mg/kg × 5 days or mebendazole 20–25 mg/kg × 21 days are commonly used despite their limited efficacy against larvae in tissues.
- *Surgery:* It is required in OLM along with anthelmintic drugs.

In addition to anthelmintic drugs, anti-inflammatory compounds (corticosteroids or NSAIDs) can be prescribed to relieve symptoms caused by allergic responses, specifically for OLM and neurotoxocariasis.

PREVENTION AND CONTROL

- Raw food and vegetables should be thoroughly washed before consumption.
- Hands should be washed well after contact with soil and before eating.

- Dogs and cats, especially puppies and kittens, should be periodically tested and dewormed starting from two weeks of age.
- Cat and dog feces should be removed from areas adjacent to homes and children's playgrounds.
- Health education is also an important control measure.

BAYLISASCARIS PROCYONIS

Baylisascaris procyonis is an ascarid of raccoons. Cases of infections of this parasite are not reported from India since raccoons are not native to the country. The life cycle of *B. procyonis* is similar to that of *Toxocara*. Infection occurs after the ingestion of eggs excreted in raccoon feces, which contaminates soil and the environment. The clinical manifestations are similar to those of *Toxocara* infection and depend on the organs involved, i.e., VLM, OLM and NLM. A more severe and fatal **eosinophilic meningoencephalitis** is reported in more than half of the cases. The diagnosis of *B. procyonis* infection is made by the demonstration of larvae in tissues and is aided by molecular tests. Recombinant antigen-based serodiagnostic assays are being evaluated for their diagnostic value. Albendazole along with corticosteroids are administered for treatment.

CUTANEOUS LARVA MIGRANS (CLM)

As the name suggests, CLM occurs when **nematode larvae of non-human species penetrate the human skin**. Since humans are not their natural hosts, these larvae are not able to complete their life cycle, and do not develop further. Thus, they remain confined to the skin or ectopically migrate deeper into the body. CLM is caused chiefly by the larvae of **non-human hookworm species**, e.g., *Ancylostoma braziliense* and some other zoonotic nematodes.

Causes of CLM
- *Ancylostoma braziliense*
- *Ancylostoma caninum*
- *Ancylostoma ceylanicum*
- *Dirofilaria* species
- *Uncinaria stenocephala*
- *Gnathostoma spinigerum*

Various synonyms such as **creeping eruption, plumber's itch, sandworm, duck hunter's itch** and **epidermatitis linearis migrans** are used to describe CLM.

EPIDEMIOLOGY

The disease is cosmopolitan in distribution but is most commonly reported from tropical and subtropical geographic regions, especially the Caribbean, South America, Africa, South-East Asia and the United States. Due to the increase in international travel in recent decades, however, the entity is no longer restricted to these regions. CLM is the most frequent skin disease among travellers returning from tropical countries. Only a few cases have been reported from India. However, the disease is probably underreported because of the difficulties in its diagnosis.

The factors favouring the disease transmission are tropical climate, overcrowding and poor hygiene and sanitation. Walking barefoot and sleeping in contaminated soil are directly related to the acquisition of CLM.

MORPHOLOGY

Adults worms are typically found in dogs and cats. The males of non-human hookworm species have a bursa with two spicules that do not fuse at their distal ends. Both males and females have a buccal capsule containing either two pairs of teeth as in case of *A. braziliense*, or three pairs as in *A. caninum* (Fig. 30.4). *Uncinaria stenocephala* possesses cutting plates instead of teeth.

LIFE CYCLE

Definitive hosts: Dogs and cats
Accidental hosts: Human beings

Domestic animals such as dogs and cats are the **natural hosts** of these parasites. The adult worms reside in the intestine of

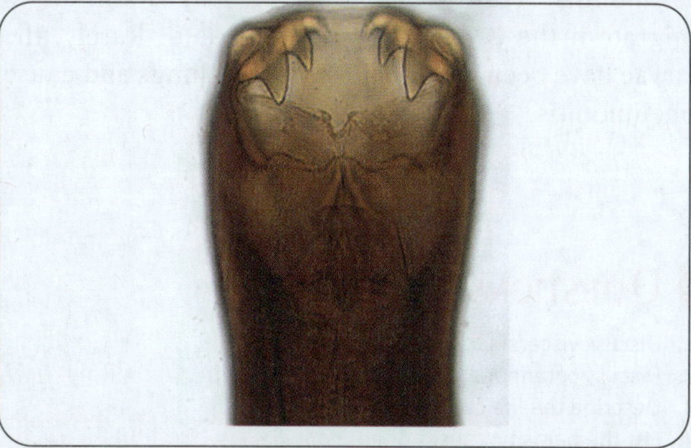

Fig. 30.4 The anterior end of *Ancylostoma caninum* showing three pairs of teeth (*Source:* CDC, DPDx)

the natural host, and their eggs are released into the environment during defecation. The eggs develop into the infective form, the filariform L3 larva, in moist and warm soil. The filariform L3 larva penetrates the skin of its natural host to complete its life cycle in a fashion similar to the human hookworm.

Alternately, it penetrates the skin of the **accidental host human** or gets ingested. The larva gets arrested in the skin instead of migrating along its normal course. It wanders in the superficial layers of the skin at a rate of 2–5 cm per day. It usually dies within 2–6 weeks but may live for many months.

PATHOGENESIS

The larva migrates through the skin by **burrowing a serpiginous tunnel**. The older part of the tunnel turns dry and crusty after the larva advances. As it moves, the larva releases secretions and metabolites which provoke a local inflammatory response and result in the formation of **severely itchy papules. Secondary bacterial infections** may occur because of intense scratching. Deeper ectopic migration to the lungs may cause pneumonitis with eosinophilia.

CLINICAL FEATURES

The clinical features of CLM range from **non-specific dermatitis** to a **creeping eruption**. An erythematous itchy papule (**ground itch**) is observed as the first lesion. It is succeeded by a 2–3 mm thick and raised pink or flesh-coloured swollen lesion. The path of the migrating worm appears as a **linear or serpentine track**, seen most commonly on the feet, legs, thighs, buttocks and the back. The skin eruptions are self-limiting and usually heal spontaneously within weeks or months. However, the larvae may continue to migrate if the condition is left untreated. Rarely, the larvae have been reported to reach the lungs and cause pneumonitis.

***Ancylostoma caninum* eosinophilic enteritis**

This entity is reported from Australia. *A. caninum* larvae migrate to the intestine and cause eosinophilic enteritis. Clinically, *A. caninum* eosinophilic enteritis presents with abdominal pain, diarrhea and small bowel obstruction. Endoscopic findings of mucosal edema, ulceration and inflammation may be noted, and eosinophilic infiltrates are common. However, the worm is usually not demonstrated. Instead, its presence is indicated by serological evidence of exposure to *A. caninum*.

DIAGNOSIS

The diagnosis is mainly based on **clinical presentation and inspection of the lesion** with characteristic history of exposure or recent travel to endemic regions. A biopsy is not useful since the larvae migrate ahead of the visible tract. Patients may have **peripheral eosinophilia,** and Charcot-Leyden crystals may be found in their sputum. In pneumonitis, the larvae may be recovered from the sputum. Epiluminescence microscopy is an effective non-invasive method to detect the larvae and confirm the diagnosis of CLM.

TREATMENT

Drug of choice

- *Ivermectin:* 200 μg/kg once or twice

Alternate drug

- *Albendazole:* 400-800 mg/day × 3–5 days
- Topical application of 10–15% thiabendazole

The associated symptoms may be treated by antihistaminic agents or topical anesthetics.

PREVENTION AND CONTROL

- Walking barefoot should be avoided.
- Health education is an important control measure.

QUESTIONS

1. Discuss visceral larva migrans.
2. Discuss cutaneous larva migrans.
3. Describe the life cycle of *Toxocara canis.*
4. List the parasitic causes of eosinophilia.

Multiple Choice Questions

1. Visceral larva migrans is commonly caused by all the following EXCEPT ____________ :
   a. *Trichinella spiralis*
   b. *Toxocara canis*
   c. *Toxocara cati*
   d. *Baylisascaris procyonis*
2. Cutaneous larva migrans is commonly caused by __________ :
   a. *Ancylostoma duodenale*
   b. *Necator americanus*
   c. *Toxocara canis*
   d. *Ancylostoma braziliense*
3. The natural hosts of *Toxocara canis* are __________ :
   a. Humans
   b. Canines
   c. Felines
   d. All mammals
4. Which of the following infections is NOT associated with moderate to extreme eosinophilia?
   a. *Trichinella spiralis*
   b. *Ascaris lumbricoides*
   c. *Toxocara canis*
   d. *Wuchereria bancrofti*
5. *Toxocara* infection occurs by ___________ :
   a. Penetration of skin by the larvae
   b. Ingestion of food contaminated with larvae
   c. Ingestion of food contaminated with the eggs
   d. Ingestion of meat containing cysts of *Toxocara*

CHAPTER 31

Angiostrongylus

([From Greek] *angeion* = bottle + *strongylos* = round)

Case Study and Learning Goals

A 25-year-old patient from Japan presents with features of meningitis. On CSF examination, he is found to have leukocytosis with a moderately raised eosinophil count. What are the parasitic causes of eosinophilic meningitis? How would you approach the laboratory diagnosis in this case? How would you treat this patient?

INTRODUCTION

Angiostrongylus are nematode parasites of small mammals such as rats which sometimes infect humans. Two members of the genus, *A. cantonensis* and *A. costaricensis,* are especially known to cause pathogenic human infections. However, other species are also reported to cause infections in humans.

A. cantonensis was first discovered in rats in China by T. C. Chen in 1935. The parasite was first isolated from the spinal cord fluid of a patient in Taiwan in the 1940s. However, its importance as a significant human pathogen was only recognised in 1962 by Leon Rosen in Hawaii.

EPIDEMIOLOGY

Rats are the natural reservoirs of these parasites, and snails are the intermediate hosts. Humans are accidentally infected when they ingest snails.

- *A. cantonensis* causes eosinophilic meningitis and is prevalent in South-East Asia and the Pacific regions, where raw snails, slugs or prawns are consumed. In 2000, an outbreak of *A. cantonensis* was reported in a group of 12 American travellers who had recently returned from Jamaica.

Infectious causes of eosinophilic meningitis

- *Angiostrongylus*
- *Gnathostoma*
- *Paragonimus*
- *Schistosoma*
- Neurocysticercosis
- Coccidioidomycosis

- *A. costaricensis* causes abdominal angiostrongyliasis and is prevalent in Central and South America, and is occasionally reported from the Caribbean region and Africa.
- *A. malaysiensis* and *A. mackerrasse,* which are rarely reported in humans, cause eosinophilic meningitis.

MORPHOLOGY

Adult Worm

The adult worms are delicate and slender (Fig. 31.1a and b).

- The adult male is 2.5–3 cm × 0.3–0.4 mm in size with two lateral teeth in the buccal cavity and no lips. It has a well-developed bursa with rays.
- The female worm is 2–3.5 cm × 0.3–0.5 mm in size. Its uterus is spirally intertwined with its intestine, giving it a '**barber's pole**' appearance.

Eggs

The eggs are thin-shelled, measure 30 × 70 µm, and are unembryonated when laid.

LIFE CYCLE (Fig. 31.2)

Definitive hosts: Rats
Intermediate hosts: Molluscs and human beings (accidental)

Natural life cycle: Rats are the natural **definitive hosts** of *A. cantonensis*. They harbour the adult worm in the branches of their pulmonary artery or the right ventricle. **Molluscs are the intermediate hosts**. The following are the stages in the life cycle of *A. cantonensis*:

- In the rat, the mature female worms lay eggs which form emboli in the pulmonary capillaries. There, the

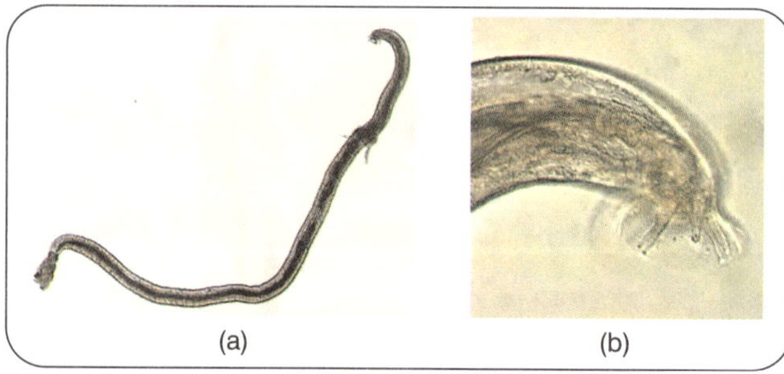

Fig. 31.1 Features of *Angiostrongylus:* (a) an adult worm recovered from a patient's vitreous humour and (b) male copulatory bursa supported by bursal rays (*Source:* Centers for Disease Control and Prevention [CDC], DPDx)

eggs embryonate and form L1 larvae which enter the alveoli and ascend the trachea to be swallowed into the esophagus and thereafter, to be passed out in the animal's feces.

- The L1 larvae are either ingested along with the rodent feces by the intermediate mollusc hosts (**snails, slugs and prawns**) or they penetrate the cuticle and subsequently undergo two moults to become L2- and L3-stage larvae. The L3 larvae can survive in the mollusc host for about a year.
- Rats get infected either by eating the intermediate host (molluscs) or by drinking water contaminated with the L3 larvae. After entering the rat's body, the larvae exsheathe, penetrate the intestinal wall and enter the right side of the heart through hepatic veins. From there, the larvae enter the pulmonary circulation (but do not lodge there at this stage) and reach the left ventricle. Then, they migrate to the brain, either directly or through other tissues. In the brain, they moult twice and form young adults. The adults migrate to the subarachnoid space, penetrate the cranial circulation and reach the pulmonary artery, where they mature sexually to start laying eggs and continue their life cycle.
- Certain hosts (crabs, prawns and pigs) may become infected by ingesting intermediate hosts. However, in such cases, the larvae only survive in the host's tissues without developing further (**paratenic host**).

For *A. costaricensis*, rodents and dogs can be the definitive hosts, from which the L1 larvae enter the intermediate hosts—slugs. In the intermediate hosts, they develop into L3 stage larvae which are shed in the mucus. When rats eat the infected slugs, the larvae penetrate their intestinal walls, enter the lymphatics and moult twice to form young adults. These migrate to the mesenteric arteries and mature to start laying eggs in the intestinal wall. The eggs hatch to release L1 larvae which are released in the feces to be ingested once again by slugs. Transmission to humans occurs by the ingestion of infected slugs or contaminated vegetables.

Human life cycle: Humans are **accidentally** infected by the following modes:

- The ingestion of the intermediate host (mollusc)
- The ingestion of the uncooked meat of infected paratenic hosts
- The ingestion of vegetables or water contaminated with the slime of slugs and snails

Humans are **non-permissive hosts**, i.e., the parasite does not complete its developmental cycle in the human body and dies after reaching the brain, and occasionally, the lungs or eye. It goes no further and does not reach maturity.

PATHOGENESIS

- ***A. cantonensis:*** In human beings, who are non-permissive hosts, the larvae are only permitted to

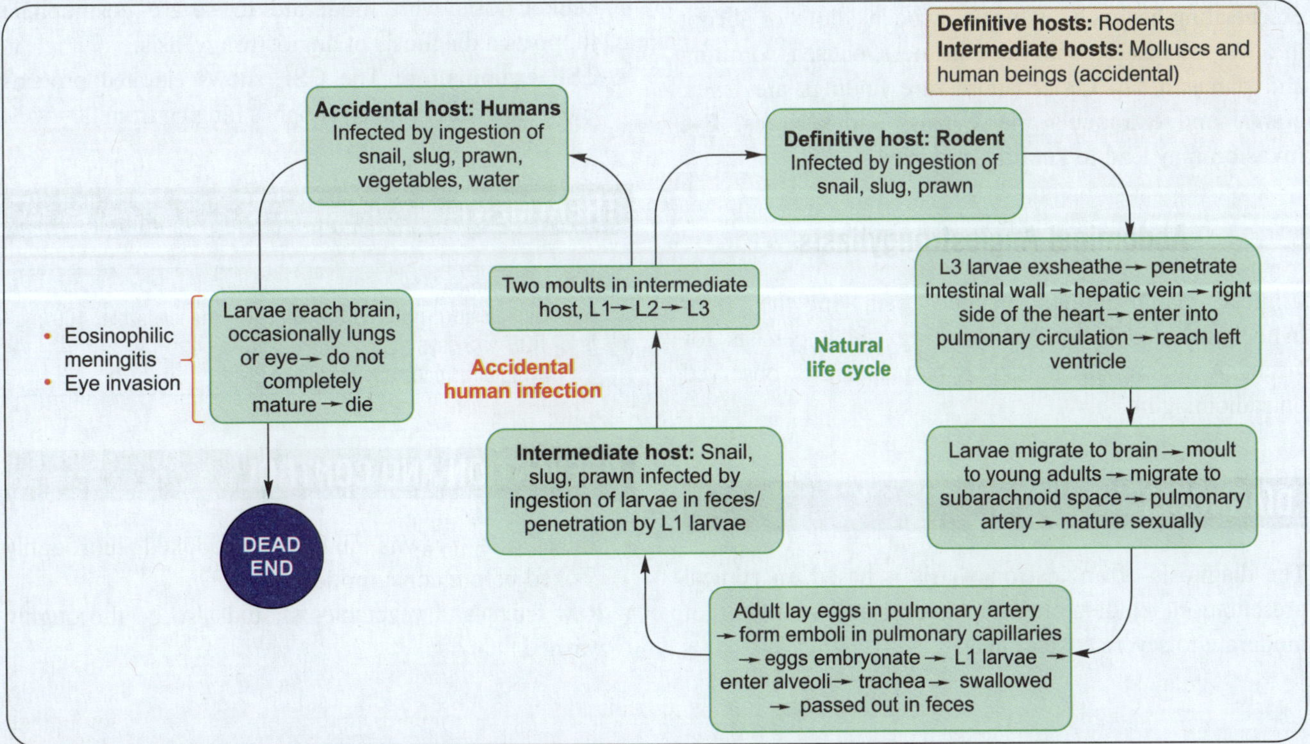

Fig. 31.2 Life cycle of *Angiostrongylus cantonensis* (schematic)

reach as far as the brain but not to develop further. The immature worm dies in the brain, thus eliciting an intense inflammatory reaction with a predominance of eosinophils, monocytes and foreign-body giant cells (eosinophilic meningitis).

- ***A. costaricensis:*** The L3 larva, after infecting a human being, penetrates the intestinal wall and enters the anterior mesenteric artery, where it develops into an adult worm which matures and lays eggs. The worm stimulates an inflammatory reaction that causes thrombosis and necrosis in the vessels along with eosinophilic infiltration and the formation of granuloma around the eggs and adults. The thickening of the intestinal wall may also cause obstruction.

CLINICAL FEATURES

The average incubation period of *Angiostrongylus* is 1–3 weeks, though it may range from one day to six weeks. ***A. cantonensis*** causes **eosinophilic meningitis,** whereas ***A. costaricensis*** causes **abdominal angiostrongyliasis.**

Eosinophilic Meningitis

Clinical symptoms develop 2–35 days after the ingestion of the larvae. Patients usually present clinically with an excruciating headache, which may be insidious or abrupt in onset, associated with neck stiffness, nausea, vomiting and paraesthesia. Other, more rare findings are fever, cranial and extraocular nerve palsy and seizures. **Eye invasion** may lead to keratitis and iritis.

Abdominal Angiostrongyliasis

Clinical manifestations include pain in the right hypochondrium, fever and vomiting which persists for weeks. A tumour-like mass may be palpated or observed on radioimaging.

DIAGNOSIS

The diagnosis of angiostrongyliasis is based on clinical presentation, epidemiological history and a finding of moderate to severe eosinophilia.

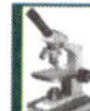

Lab diagnosis

- Clinical suspicion with epidemiological evidence
- Leukocytosis with moderate to severe eosinophilia

Microscopy

The larvae of *A. cantonensis* may sometimes be seen in CSF.

Histopathology

Biopsy of a suspected lesion may demonstrate either the larvae, worms or eggs of the parasite.

Radioimaging

A tumour-like mass and intestinal wall thickening and obstruction may be seen in abdominal disease.

Nucleic Acid-Based Detection

PCR is used to confirm the etiological agent in research laboratories.

Serology

There is currently no approved test available for serodiagnosis.

Other Diagnostic Parameters

- Leukocytosis with moderate to severe eosinophilia supports a diagnosis of angiostrongyliasis.
- **CSF examination:** The CSF shows elevated proteins and leukocytosis with eosinophils ranging from 20–50%.

TREATMENT

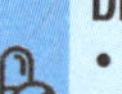

Drug of choice

- Though no drug is 100% effective, mebendazole, 100 mg BDS × 5 days may be attempted
- Symptomatic therapy should be given

PREVENTION AND CONTROL

- Snails and prawns should be cooked thoroughly cooked before consumption.
- Raw fruits and vegetables should also be thoroughly washed.

Questions

1. Write a short note on abdominal angiostrongyliasis.
2. Describe the differential diagnosis of eosinophilic meningitis.
3. Discuss the life cycle of *Angiostrongylus cantonensis* and the diagnosis of its infection.

Multiple Choice Questions

1. Abdominal angiostrongyliasis is caused by ___________ :
   a. *Angiostrongylus costaricensis*
   b. *Angiostrongylus cantonensis*
   c. *Angiostrongylus knowlesi*
   d. *Angiostrongylus stercoralis*
2. *Angiostrongylus cantonensis* causes ___________ :
   a. Tropical pulmonary eosinophilia
   b. Loeffler's syndrome
   c. Eosinophilic meningitis
   d. Burton's disease
3. Infectious parasitic causes of eosinophilic meningitis include all the following EXCEPT ___________ :
   a. *Angiostrongylus*
   b. Malaria
   c. *Paragonimus*
   d. *Schistosoma*

CHAPTER 32

Dracunculus

([From Latin] *draco* = dragon)

Case Study and Learning Goals

A 25-year-old male from South Sudan presents with an intensely itchy blister on his foot. What could be the parasitic etiology in this case based on the patient's geographical location and clinical presentation? How is the etiological agent transmitted? What is the current status of its epidemiology? What are the important features of the control programme for this parasite?

INTRODUCTION

Dracunculus medinensis is known to infect humans since antiquity. Its name, which is derived from Latin, means a 'little dragon from Medina'. It is also known as **Guinea worm, Medina worm, serpent worm or dragon worm**. The disease it causes is called **dracunculiasis, dracontiasis** or the **Guinea worm disease**.

The historical significance of *D. medinensis* in relation with malady, medicine and healing is reflected in the use of the **'Rod of Asclepius'** (Fig. 32.1a and b) in the logos of numerous health organisations. This symbol is most likely to be an ancient Greek representation of the treatment of dracunculiasis by winding the worm on a stick.

The earliest reference of the disease, which dates as far back as 1500 BC, is found in the Ebers Papyrus, which mentions techniques for the treatment of the disease. The worm has also been recovered from ancient Egyptian mummies. The parasite finds mention in ancient Sanskrit literature from the 14th century BC, and is also referred to in the Bible as a 'fiery serpent'. Descriptions of the disease are also noted in Roman, Greek and Arab medical literature of the 10th and 11th centuries. Much later, European travellers to West Africa named the worm 'Guinea worm'. In 1819, Karl Asmund Rudolphi found that the adult female contains larvae and in 1836, D. Forbes found the larvae in water during a visit to India as an officer of the British army. The elucidation of the complete life cycle of the parasite and the knowledge of the involvement of copepods had to wait until they were described by Alekej Pavlovitch Fedchenko in 1870; these findings were later confirmed by Patrick Manson in 1894. The life cycle was further elaborated by an Indian physician, Dnyaneshwar Atmaram Turkhud, who infected human volunteers with *Cyclops*.

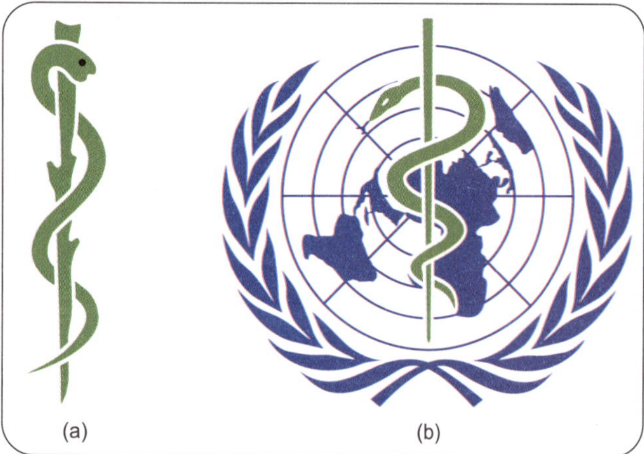

Fig. 32.1 (a) The symbol of healing: the Rod of Asclepius and (b) the logo of the World Health Organization

EPIDEMIOLOGY

In the mid-1980s, dracunculiasis was a major malady with >3.5 million cases globally. It has now been largely eradicated from most parts of the world; only 47 human cases were reported in 2019, mainly from **Chad, South Sudan, Ethiopia and Mali**, and sporadic cases are reported from **Angola**. Increased surveillance has revealed ongoing transmission in dogs, cats and baboons, which presents a challenge to the final stretch of eradication of dracunculiasis.

Dracunculiasis affects economically disadvantaged communities that do not have access to safe drinking water and in which people bathe in or walk through water used for drinking, as was the case with stepwells, which were common in India in the past. The chances of infection increase before the arrival of the monsoon, when the water level in ponds or wells is low. The disease affects all age groups but is more common among young adults, especially males. Infected individuals do not become immune to the disease, and many of them contract the infection repeatedly.

India: The certification of India as a **Guinea worm disease-free country** by the World Health Organization (WHO) in **February 2000** was a major milestone in the history of disease eradication in India. The disease was a significant cause of disability in many states of India before it was eradicated.

MORPHOLOGY

Adult Worm

The adult female is creamy-white, 50–100 cm × 1–2 mm in size (Fig. 32.2a). The male is much smaller, measuring 2–4 cm × 0.4 mm. The coiled uterus of the female is filled with **1–3 million larvae** and entirely occupies its body cavity. The numerous larvae increase the internal pressure on the uterus and body wall, causing it to finally erupt. Alternatively, the uterus is forced out of the worm's mouth to release the larvae. The muscular contractions of the body wall assist the spurts of larval release.

Larvae

The larvae are of the rhabditiform stage and measure 500–750 × 15–25 μm in size (Fig. 32.2b).

LIFE CYCLE (Fig. 32.3a and b)

> **Definitive hosts:** Humans and other mammals
> **Intermediate hosts:** Copepods (*Cyclops*)

Human cycle: The **definitive hosts—humans and other animals—are infected on the ingestion of the intermediate hosts, copepods (*Cyclops*)**. The stages of the parasite's life cycle after ingestion are as follows:

- After ingestion, the copepods are digested and the larvae are released in the duodenum. These penetrate the intestinal wall and traverse the viscera to reach the subcutaneous connective tissue.
- These larvae moult twice in the course of three months and achieve sexual maturation, following which, they begin to mate. The male dies soon after mating.
- The **gravid female migrates to the skin**, preferentially to the parts that frequently come in contact with water, e.g., the feet, legs and arms of washermen and the legs of people who frequently enter stepwells to collect water. Upon reaching the skin surface, the female releases a toxin which leads to the **formation of a blister**. The gravid female takes about a year to reach the skin.
- Contact with cool water is a cue for the worm to expel its uterus through the skin blister and **release hundreds of thousands of larvae in the water**.

Aquatic cycle: The larvae are taken up by copepods within three days, and transmission continues as follows:

- Once ingested by copepods, the larvae enter the hemocoel and undergo two moults over two weeks to become the infective form, which is ready to infect another definitive host.
- The copepods may also be consumed by paratenic hosts such as tadpoles and frogs, which possibly allow alternate transmission cycles in nature.

PATHOGENESIS

The mechanisms of pathogenesis of *Dracunculus* infection are as follows:

- The release of larvae just under the skin stimulates an intense allergic response and the formation of blisters and ulcers on the skin.
- Secondary bacterial infections of the ulcer exacerbate pain and disability and may cause abscesses.
- Worms that fail to emerge get absorbed or calcified in deeper tissues.

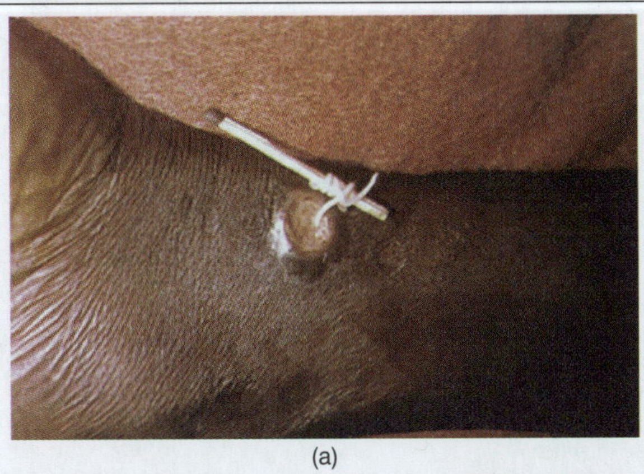

(a)

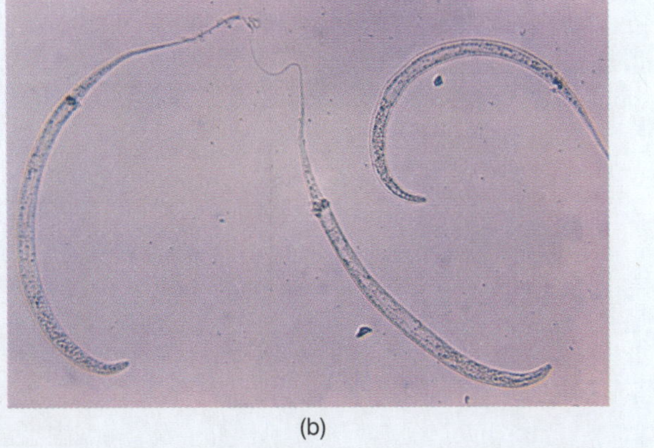

(b)

Fig. 32.2 Adult and larvae of *Dracunculus medinensis*: (a) extraction of a worm and (b) three larvae (*Source:* Centers for Disease Control and Prevention [CDC], Public Health Image Library [PHIL], Image IDs 1342 and 663)

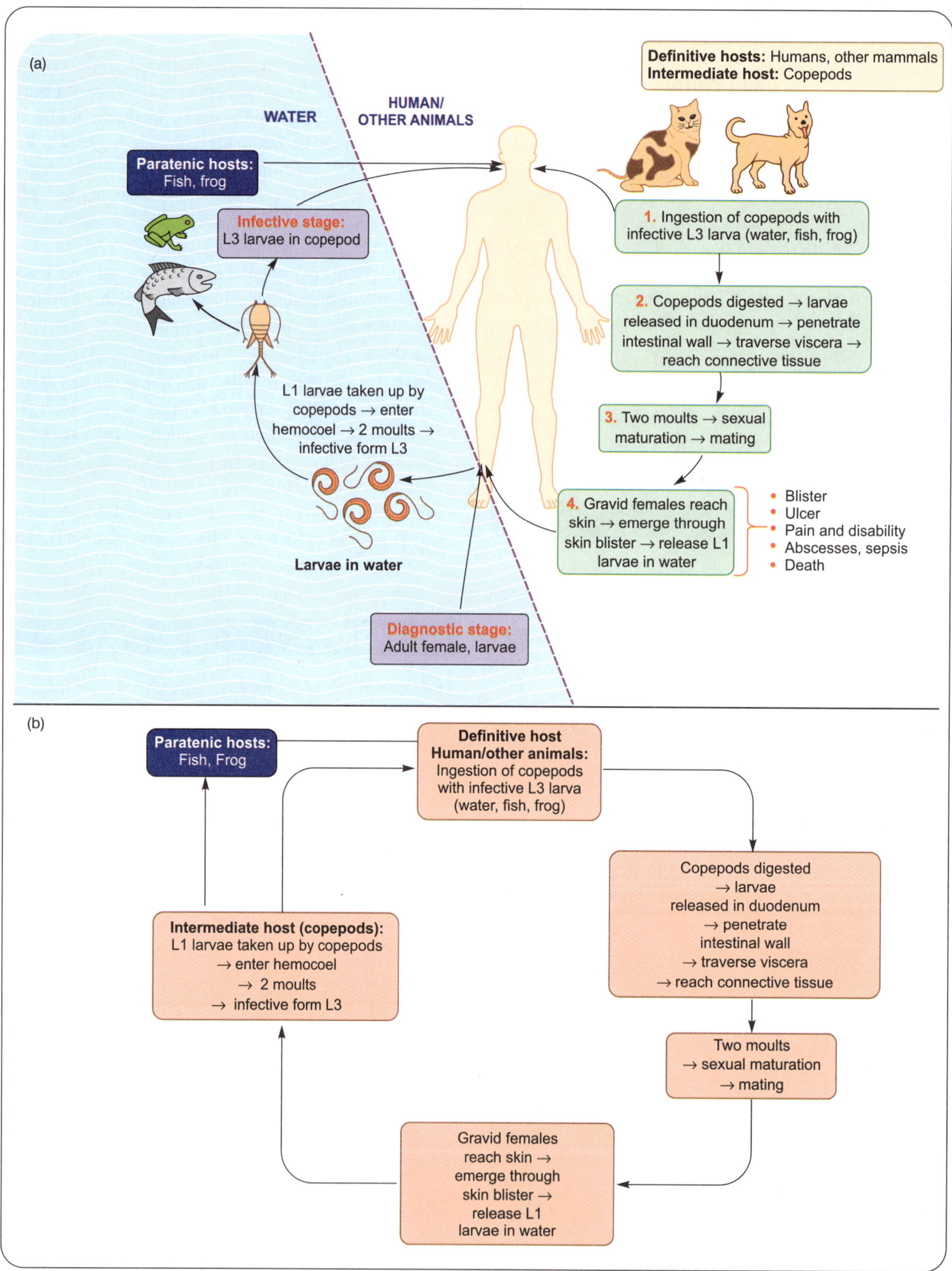

Fig. 32.3 Life cycle of *Dracunculus medinensis*: (a) detailed and (b) schematic

CLINICAL FEATURES

The clinical features of dracunculiasis appear after an **incubation period of about a year** when the gravid adult female worm reaches the subcutaneous tissues, ready to discharge its larvae. The following are the features of the disease:

- A **single or multiple painful papule(s)** appear, commonly on the **lower legs, ankle or foot**. The papule enlarges over the next few days to form a blister, which eventually ruptures to release the larvae. A part of the worm is visible at this stage.
- The blister is accompanied by painful edema and **intense generalised pruritus**; it may ulcerate. There may be fever, nausea and vomiting.
- The ulcers caused by the emergence of the worm invariably develop **secondary bacterial infections**, which exacerbate inflammation and pain and result in temporary disability for a period of weeks to a few months. The disability resulting from clinical disease is of great socioeconomic importance.
- The parasite migrates through the subcutaneous tissues, causing severe pain. Worms near the articular surfaces cause permanent disability.
- Bacterial infections may cause complications such as sepsis, abscesses and pyogenic arthritis.

DIAGNOSIS

The diagnosis is easily made clinically by **visualising the emerging adult worm** through the blister (Fig. 32.2a).

Lab diagnosis

- **Clinical examination:** Blister with emerging adult worm
- **Microscopy:** Visualising larvae in blister fluid
- **Other diagnostic parameter:** Peripheral **eosinophilia**

Microscopy

Examination of the discharged fluid may demonstrate the larvae. The body part with the blister is immersed in cold water. This causes a white fluid containing several **L1 larvae** to be discharged from the blister. This fluid can be examined microscopically (Fig. 32.2b).

Serology

The detection of IgG antibodies is generally reserved for epidemiological purposes.

Other Diagnostic Parameter

Peripheral blood **eosinophilia** is common.

TREATMENT

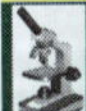

- **Worm removal:** The affected body part is immersed in water every day to encourage more of the worm to come out. The exposed part of the worm is tied with a fine silk thread fastened to a rod or stick. By winding the thread around the rod/stick, the worm is slowly and gently pulled out over a period of 15–20 days (Fig. 32.2a). [**Note:** Heavy traction should be avoided because it could result in the breaking of the worm, which in turn, could result in allergic reaction and secondary bacterial infections.]
- **Anthelmintic drugs:** Drug therapy is not very useful in the treatment of dracunculiasis.
- **Symptomatic treatment:** Wet compresses may be applied to the affected skin, and anti-inflammatory drugs and topical antibiotics may be used to prevent secondary bacterial infections.

PREVENTION AND CONTROL

In the mid-1980s, the World Health Assembly declared the global elimination of dracunculiasis as one of its goals, following which, extensive control programmes were launched across the globe. These programmes have led to a gradual decrease in the number of cases by more than 99% from then to now. This is a striking example of the effectiveness of simple public health measures in controlling infectious diseases even in the absence of a drug or a vaccine.

Global eradication programme: Dracunculiasis is likely to soon become the first parasitic disease to be eradicated across the globe. It is eradicable for the following reasons:

- Its diagnosis is simple and can be made clinically by visualising the emerging worm.
- The disease is geographically restricted.
- The intermediate host, the copepod, can be controlled as it exists only in stagnant water bodies.
- Control interventions are simple, cost-effective and relatively easy to implement, e.g., water filtration with any finely meshed cloth or a filter made of nylon mesh with pores measuring 0.15 mm.
- The political commitment from international agencies and local governments is strong.

Certification of dracunculiasis eradication: The WHO established an independent International Commission for the Certification of Dracunculiasis Eradication (ICCDE) in 1995.

- **Precertification:** An endemic country reporting **zero indigenous cases over one calendar year** is deemed to have prevented disease transmission and is classified in the precertification phase.
- **Eradication:** A country that has reported **zero indigenous cases through active surveillance for at least three consecutive calendar years** is deemed to have stopped the transmission of the disease and is declared free of dracunculiasis.

India's success story: The National Guinea Worm Eradication Programme was launched by the Indian government in 1984 with support from the WHO. India was declared free of dracunculiasis in February 2000. The control measures employed in India included:

1. **Safe drinking water:** This included the filtration of drinking water and the provision of safe drinking water by installing piped supply and boreholes with hand pumps.
2. **Control of *Cyclops*:** Copepods in drinking water were killed with larvicides like abate (temephos).
3. **Health education:** Communities were educated about boiling water or filtering drinking water through four layers of *dhoti* cloth. The contamination of water bodies was averted by preventing people from stepping into the water sources.
4. **Active surveillance:** Infected cases and their treatment regimens were monitored closely.
5. **Treatment of cases:** The detected cases were treated in a timely manner.

Questions

1. Describe the eradication campaign for Guinea worm disease.
2. Discuss the laboratory diagnosis and management of dracunculiasis.

Multiple Choice Questions

1. The only parasitic disease that has been nearly eradicated is ____________:
   a. American trypanosomiasis
   b. Diphyllobothriasis
   c. Dracunculiasis
   d. Schistosomiasis
2. The diagnosis of Guinea worm disease can be easily made by the ____________:
   a. Demonstration of eggs in stool samples
   b. Demonstration of larvae in stool samples
   c. Demonstration of the adult worm coming out of the skin
   d. Demonstration of larvae in sputum samples
3. The only countries still reporting *Dracunculus* cases are in ____________:
   a. South-East Asia
   b. South America
   c. Africa
   d. North America
4. India was certified as a Guinea worm disease-free country by the World Health Organization (WHO) in the year ____________:
   a. 2000
   b. 2002
   c. 2005
   d. 2012
5. Guinea worm is transmitted to humans mostly by ____________:
   a. Ingestion of water contaminated with parasite-infected water fleas
   b. Penetration of larvae through skin during swimming or water-related activities
   c. Ingestion of metacercariae in water
   d. Any of the above
6. Dracunculiasis presents most commonly as all the following EXCEPT ____________:
   a. Severe pain abdomen with fever
   b. A single or multiple painful papules or blisters commonly in the lower legs, ankle or foot
   c. Intense generalised pruritus
   d. Sepsis, abscess and pyogenic arthritis
7. Which of the following is known as dragon worm or serpent worm?
   a. *Trichuris*
   b. *Toxocara*
   c. *Diphyllobothrium*
   d. *Dracunculus*

Chapter 33

Wuchereria and Brugia

(Named after scientists Otto Henry Wucherer, Joseph Bancroft and S. L. Brug)

Case Study and Learning Goals

A 47-year-male from a southern state of India presents with a swelling over his entire lower leg which is non-pitting and not reversible with limb elevation. On palpation, his inguinal lymph nodes are found to be enlarged, firm and tender. A history of recurrent episodes of fever with chills associated with pain in the inguinal region for more than 10 years is elicited. What are the parasitic causes of swelling of the leg? How would you approach the laboratory diagnosis in this case? How would you manage the disease in this patient?

FILARIAL NEMATODES

Filariae (from the Latin word *filum*, meaning thread) are nematode parasites that are transmitted by the bites of infective arthropod vectors. They live in the subcutaneous tissue, deep connective tissue, lymphatic system or the body cavity of humans. Some adult filarial worms can survive in the host for many years.

- The filarial parasites have a complex life cycle requiring two hosts—a human being and a bloodsucking insect.
- The **female worm is viviparous** and produces large numbers of pre-larval stages called microfilariae (mf) which are highly motile, thread-like microscopic structures.
- The released microfilariae can be detected in the peripheral blood or skin, depending on the species. The mf may survive for 1–2 years but do not develop further in the vertebrate host. They show a certain **periodicity of appearing in peripheral circulation** that coincides with the local feeding habits of their insect vectors (see box).

> - **Nocturnal periodicity:** In this type of periodicity, mf appear in peripheral circulation only at night, as seen with *Wuchereria* and *Brugia*.
> - **Diurnal periodicity:** In this type of periodicity, mf circulate only during certain hours of the daytime, as seen with *Loa loa*.
> - **Sub-periodic periodicity:** In this type of periodicity, mf are present throughout the 24-hour period; however, their density increases at certain times. In some geographical regions, *Wuchereria* and *Brugia* are sub-periodic.
> - **Non-periodic:** Certain mf exhibit no periodicity and circulate in the blood at all times in constant numbers, e.g., *Mansonella* and *Onchocerca*.

- The mf are taken up by insect vectors during their blood meal and develop further in such vector hosts to form the infective larvae. Humans are infected by the bite of insect vectors carrying the infective larvae. When not in the peripheral blood, the microfilariae are found primarily in the capillaries and blood vessels of the lungs.
- The pathology is chiefly produced by the adult worms, and the disease may not be evident before significant pathology occurs. The diagnosis of the disease is usually made by the demonstration of microfilariae.
- Adult filariae harbour some obligate intracellular **endosymbiotic bacteria called '*Wolbachia*'**, which are also said to play a role in the pathogenesis.
- There are eight filarial species for which the human being is the definitive host, six of which are pathogenic (Table 33.1).

Table 33.1 Filarial parasites and their various disease manifestations

Parasite	Habitat of the adult worm	Disease manifestation
Wuchereria bancrofti	Lymphatic vessels and lymph nodes	Lymphatic filariasis
Brugia malayi		
B. timori		
Loa loa	Subcutaneous connective tissue, often in the subconjunctival tissue of the eye	Calabar swellings and allergic manifestations
Onchocerca volvulus	Connective tissue	Dermatitis and eye lesions
Mansonella streptocerca	Connective tissue	Skin disease
M. ozzardi and *M. perstans*	Mesentery	They are **non-pathogenic** but can be isolated from blood or skin snips

WUCHERERIA AND BRUGIA

INTRODUCTION

Lymphatic filariasis, commonly known as **elephantiasis (swollen body parts and thickening of skin like that of an elephant)**, is a neglected tropical disease which is caused by three closely related nematode filarial worms—***Wuchereria bancrofti, Brugia malayi*** **and** ***Brugia timori***. The infection occurs when a filarial parasite is transmitted to a human being through a mosquito bite. It is usually acquired in childhood and insidiously causes damage to the lymphatic system. About 40 million people (a third of those infected) have the clinical disease, making lymphatic filariasis the second most common cause of permanent and long-term disability worldwide.

The disease was first described in ancient India by **Sushruta,** who called it ***slipada*** (*sli* meaning elephant and *pada* meaning leg). The gross swellings of the limbs, genitals and other body parts have been represented by the ancient Egyptians, Hindus, Persians, Greeks, Romans and Arabs in various drawings, artefacts, statues and literature. The Dutch explorer Jan Huyghen van Linschoten noticed what was then known as the 'curse of St. Thomas'—lymphatic filariasis—in Goa in the late 16th century. The microfilariae larvae were first visualised in hydrocele fluid by the French surgeon Jean-Nicolas Demarquay in 1863 and in urine by **O. E. H. Wucherer** in 1866. The adult worm was described by Joseph Bancroft in 1876. It was **Patrick Manson, 'the father of tropical medicine'**, who discovered the life cycle of filarial worms in 1877. He also pointed out the involvement of mosquitoes in the disease transmission, a finding which led other workers to implicate mosquitoes in the transmission of malaria and several arboviruses.

The microfilariae of *B. malayi* were described in 1927 by S. L. Brug as a new species in Indonesia; the adults were described in 1940 in India by S. Sundar Rao and P. A. Maplestone who isolated them from the arm of a patient.

EPIDEMIOLOGY

Filarial infections are distributed across the tropics and subtropics, with 886 million people in 52 countries at risk of lymphatic filariasis and requiring preventive chemotherapy to stop its spread and transmission.

- The largest numbers of infected people are present in India and sub-Saharan Africa. The infection is prevalent all over India except in the north-eastern states, Jammu and Kashmir and Punjab.
- ***Wuchereria bancrofti*** is responsible for 90% of the cases of lymphatic filariasis. The major vectors of this disease are ***Culex*** mosquitoes, the most important species being ***C. quinquefasciatus***. In some areas, ***Aedes*** and ***Anopheles*** are responsible for the transmission of the disease.
- ***Brugia malayi*** causes most of the remainder of the cases. ***Mansonia*** mosquitoes are the main vectors for brugian filariasis, though ***Culex*** mosquitos play the role in some areas.
- ***Brugia timori*** is restricted to the Timor island of Indonesia.

MORPHOLOGY

Adult Worm

The adult worms are long, thin and creamy-white. They have tapering ends and a smooth cuticle.

- The adult *W. bancrofti* male is **4 cm × 0.1 mm** in size with a ventrally curved tail end which contains two unequal spicules. The female is **6–10 cm × 0.2–0.3 mm** in size. It has a slightly swollen head with two circles of papillae. The buccal cavity is inconspicuous in both males and females (Fig. 33.1).
- The *B. malayi* male is shorter than the female, measuring **3.5 cm × 0.1 mm** in size, with a ventrally curved tail and two unequal spicules. The female measures **5–6 cm × 0.1 mm**.

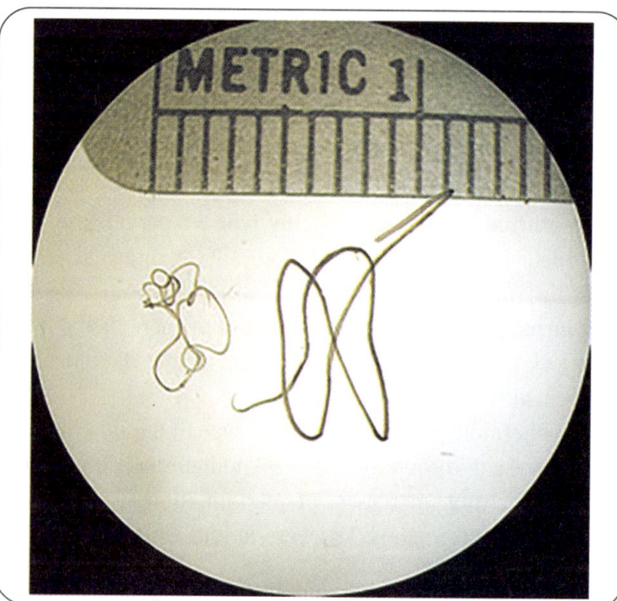

Fig. 33.1 Adults of *Wuchereria bancrofti*: male on the left and female on the right (*Source:* Centers for Disease Control and Prevention [CDC], DPDx)

- The adult filarial worms live in the lymphatic ducts. The male and female worms remain coiled together.

Microfilariae

The females are **viviparous** and give birth to thousands of microfilariae.

- The microfilariae are advanced forms of the embryo or pre-larval stage.
- They have **several internal nuclei** which are visible when stained with suitable dyes. These nuclei appear as granules throughout the length of the body except for the head and tail end and are absent at some definite places (representing rudimentary structures like the excretory system, alimentary canal, etc.).
- The microfilaria retains the egg membrane (**sheath**), which is evident at its head (**cephalic space**) and tail ends. The cephalic space is as long as it is broad in *W. bancrofti*; in *B. malayi*, it is twice as long as it is broad.
- Microfilariae are actively motile and can move against the blood flow. They are capable of living in the peripheral blood without development for few weeks and develop further only when taken up by the insect vector.
- The location of the microfilariae in blood or skin, their size and shape, the arrangement of their internal nuclei, and the presence or absence of the sheath act as markers for the microscopic identification of the various filarial species (Table 33.2 and 33.3 and Fig. 33.2).

Table 33.2 Differentiating features of microfilariae in blood

Species	Sheath	Chief features	Other features
Wuchereria bancrofti (Lymphatic filariasis)	Present	• Large, 250–300 × 8–10 µm • Few and graceful body curves • Sheath stains pink with Giemsa and pale with hematoxylin • Nuclei distinct; there are **no nuclei** in the tail-tip	• Nocturnal periodicity • Differentiated from *Brugia* species and *L. loa* by its tail features • Differentiated from *Mansonella* species by its larger size and sheath
Brugia malayi (Lymphatic filariasis)	Present	• Large, 200–275 × 5–6 µm • Body has many angular curves • Sheath stains dark pink with Giemsa and pale with hematoxylin • Nuclei are dense and stain darkly; there are **2 widely spaced nuclei** in the tail-tip	• Nocturnal periodicity • Differentiated from *W. bancrofti* by its darker stained sheath and nuclei, kinked body and tail features • Differentiated from *B. timori* by its shorter length and darker stained sheath
Brugia timori (Lymphatic filariasis)	Present	Features distinguishing *B. timori* from *B. malayi*: • Longer, 290–325 × 5–6 µm • Sheath does not stain well with Giemsa • Body nuclei are less dense and the space at the head end (cephalic space) is longer • Similar to *B. malayi*, i.e., it has 2 nuclei in the tail-tip	• Nocturnal periodicity • Only found in Indonesia
Loa loa (Loiasis, Calabar swelling)	Present	• Large, 250–300 × 8–10 µm • Body has several curves and kinks • Sheath stains best with hematoxylin • Nuclei not distinct; extend to the tail-tip	• Diurnal • Differentiated from *W. bancrofti* by its tail features • Differentiated from *M. perstans* by its larger size and sheath
Mansonella perstans (Non-pathogenic or of low pathogenicity)	Unsheathed	• Small and thin, 190–240 × 4–5 µm • Body nuclei are irregular • Nuclei extend to the end of the tail, which is rounded • Large nucleus in the tail-tip	• Non-periodic • Differentiated from *L. loa* and *W. bancrofti* by its smaller size, absence of sheath and nuclei in the tail
M. ozzardi (Non-pathogenic or of low pathogenicity)	Unsheathed	• Small and thin, 150–200 × 4.5 µm • Body nuclei not distinct • Anterior nuclei positioned side-by-side • Long tail which is hooked and pointed, tail-tip with no nuclei	• Non-periodic • Differentiated from *W. bancrofti* by its smaller size, absence of sheath and non-periodicity

Table 33.3 Differentiating features of microfilariae in skin

Species	Sheath	Main features in stained preparations
Onchocerca volvulus (Onchocerciasis)	Unsheathed	• Large, 240–360 × 5–9 μm • Head slightly enlarged • Anterior nuclei placed side-by-side • Tail long and pointed, no nuclei in tail-tip • Actively motile in wet preparations
Mansonella streptocerca (Non-pathogenic or of low pathogenicity)	Unsheathed	• Small and thin, 180–240 × 4.5 μm • Anterior nuclei arranged in single file • Tail usually hooked like a 'shepherd's crook', nuclei extend to the tail-tip • Less motile than *O. volvulus*
Mansonella ozzardi (Non-pathogenic or of low pathogenicity)	Unsheathed	• Small and thin, 150–200 × 4.5 μm • Anterior nuclei arranged side-by-side • Tail long and pointed, no nuclei in the tail-tip • Less motile than *O. volvulus*

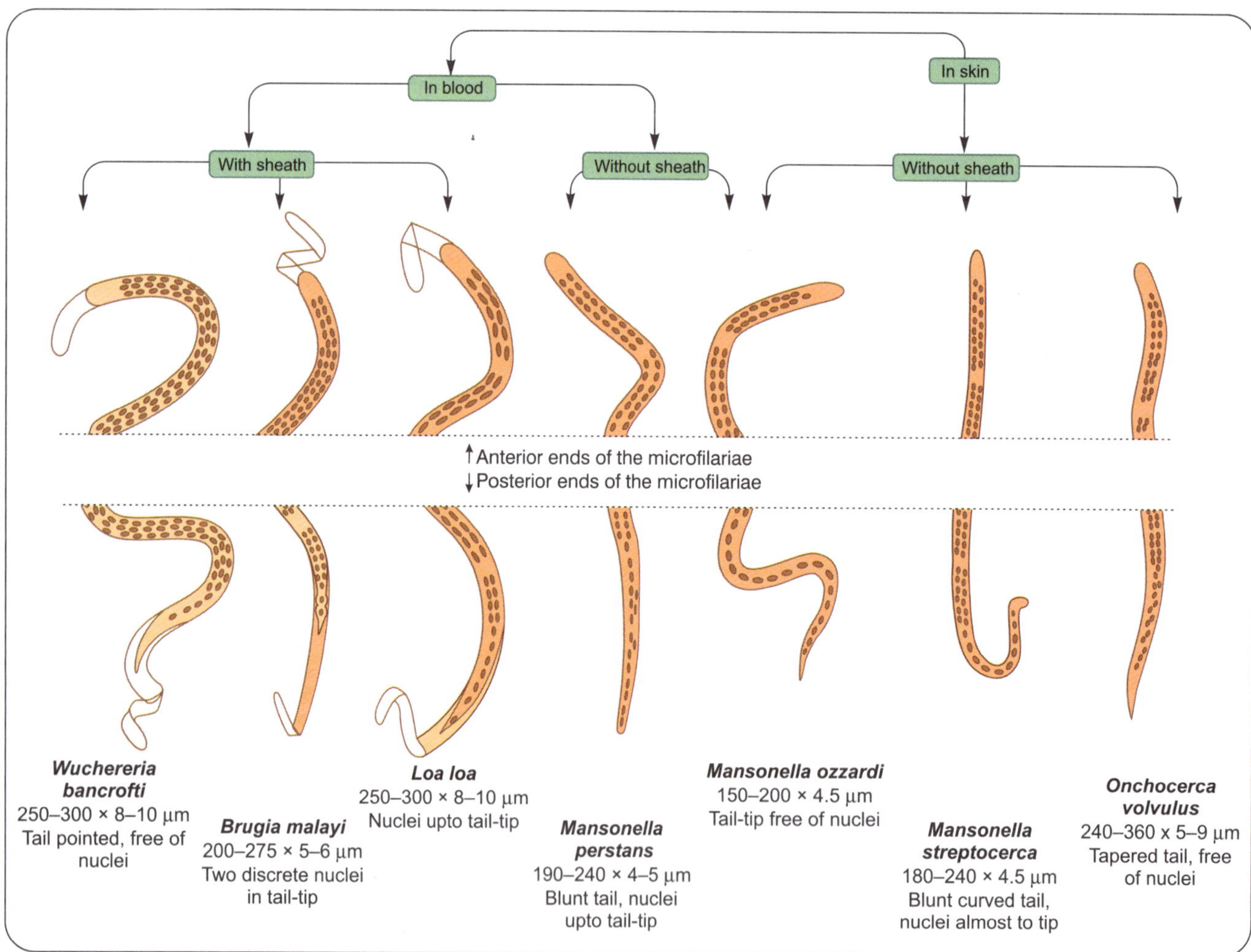

Fig. 33.2 Differentiating features of the anterior and posterior ends of the various microfilariae

Larvae

The L1 to L3 larval stages are seen in the mosquitoes and the L4 stage develops in humans.

LIFE CYCLE (Fig. 33.3a and b)

The various stages in the life cycle of filarial worms are as follows:

Human stage: The **definitive hosts—human beings—get infected by the bite of the intermediate host—mosquito—**which deposits the **L3 larvae** near the site of the bite.

> **Definitive hosts:** Human beings
> **Intermediate hosts:** Mosquitoes

- The L3 larva enters the **skin** wound, traverses the peripheral **lymphatics** and reaches the larger **lymph vessels** and the **lymph nodes** of the inguinal, scrotal or abdominal region. Once there, it settles and matures into an L4 larva in 7–10 days, and subsequently, into the adult in weeks to months. The adult's life span is estimated to be 5–10 years.
- The sexually mature adults fertilise, and the gravid females release several thousand microfilariae in the lymph per day. These mf pass through the lymphatic

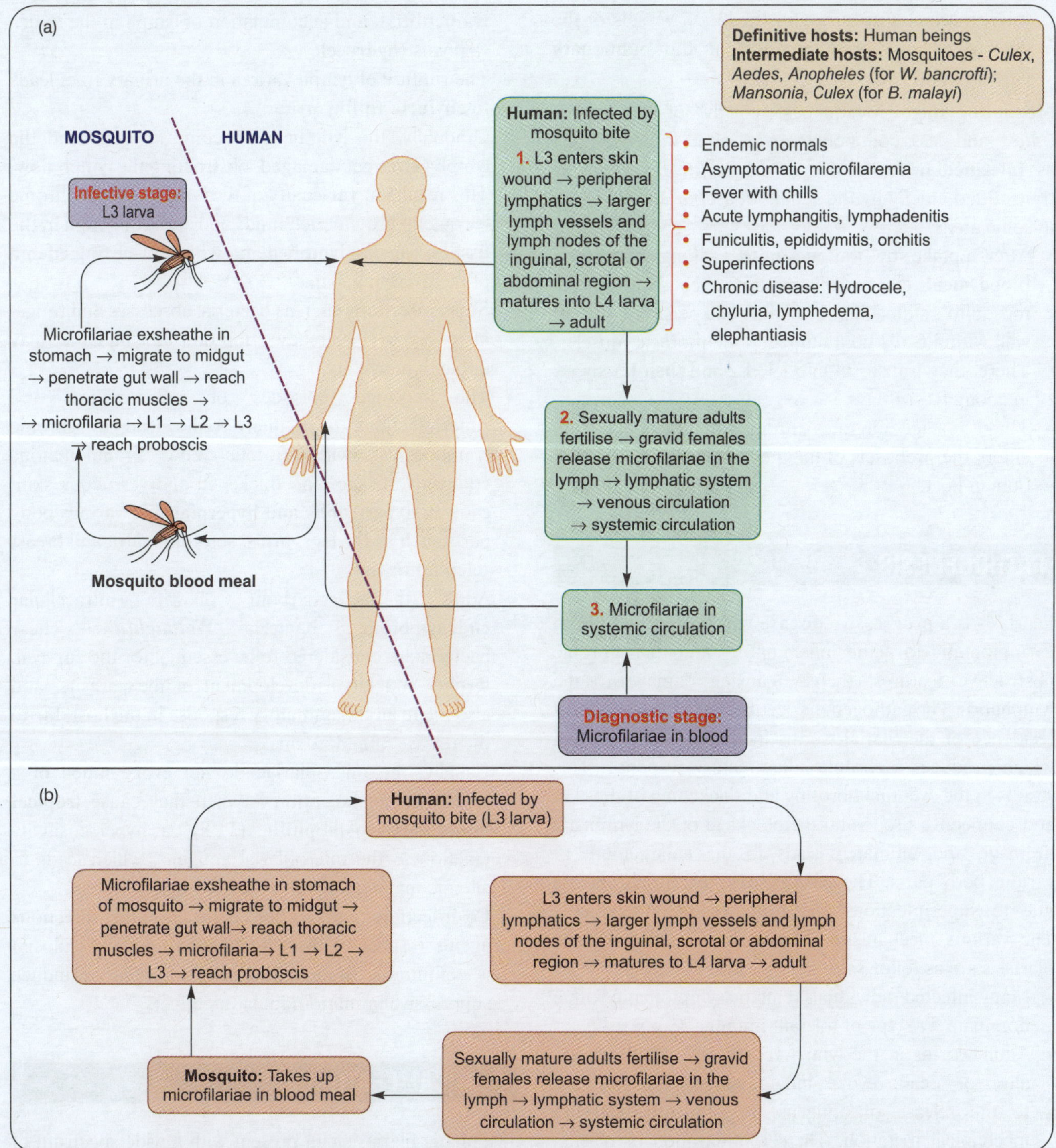

Fig. 33.3 Life cycle of *Wuchereria and Brugia*: (a) detailed and (b) schematic

system to the venous circulation and finally reach the systemic circulation. The period from the inoculation of the L3 larva to the appearance of microfilariae in the blood is called the **pre-patent period**.

- The microfilariae can survive for about two months awaiting uptake by the vector. They show remarkable periodicity in the blood to suit the biting times of their vector hosts. During the daytime, the microfilariae concentrate in the blood vessels of the deeper tissues, predominantly in the pulmonary capillaries.

Mosquito stage: Mosquitoes, chiefly of the genus *Culex*, and less commonly, *Aedes* and *Anopheles*, act as **intermediate hosts** for *W. bancrofti*. *B. malayi* is transmitted chiefly by the genus *Mansonia* and by *Culex* in some areas.

- After uptake by the mosquitoes along with their **blood meal**, the microfilariae lose their sheath in the mosquito's stomach in 1–2 hours and penetrate the gut wall within 6–12 hours to reach the thoracic muscles. There, they transform into L1, L2 and then L3 stages in about 10–14 days.
- The L3 stage migrates through the hemocoel and enters the proboscis of the mosquito to await another human host.

PATHOGENESIS

Filariasis is a **progressive disease** which progresses from asymptomatic to acute inflammatory and then chronic obstructive features, thereby causing damage to the lymphatics. The pathogenesis occurs due to the permanent residence of the filarial worms in the lymphatic system which produces a chronic inflammatory response. This results in the eventual fibrosing and thickening of the skin and connective tissue and the blockage of the lymphatic drainage and ultimately leads to the enlargement of various body parts. The other disease manifestations are due to superinfections and hypersensitivity reactions. The various mechanisms of pathogenesis of lymphatic filariasis are as follows:

- Many infected individuals remain asymptomatic with a dominant T_{h2} type of tolerant immune response.
- Adult worms in the lymph vessels and lymph nodes, alive or dead, evoke inflammatory reactions due to the release of antigens, toxic metabolites and mechanical irritation. There is infiltration of plasma cells, polymorphonuclear cells, eosinophils and macrophages. The dying worms are associated with an even more intense inflammatory response.
- Recurrent inflammation of the lymph vessels (**lymphangitis**) and lymph nodes (**lymphadenitis**) causes proliferation of the endothelial and connective tissues, leading to dilation, thickening and fibrosis of the lymphatic channels.
- There may be inflammation of the testis (**orchitis**), epididymis (**epididymitis**) and spermatic cord (**funiculitis**), and accumulation of lymph in the tunica vaginalis (**hydrocele**).
- The rupture of lymph varices in the urinary tract leads to **chyluria (milky urine)**.
- Gradually, the lymphatics become tortuous and the lymph valves get damaged, obstructing the lymph flow. This results in **varicosity** of the lymph vessels, chronic leakage of protein-rich fluids and stasis of lymph in the tissues, causing **lymphedema with non-pitting edema** of the overlying skin.
- **Superinfections** such as bacterial abscesses and fungal infections in the already compromised lymphatics play a role in morbidity.
- The repeated episodes of inflammation and superinfections over many years lead to chronic lymphedema with fibrous and granulomatous connective tissue, and thickened and verrucous skin, causing **hypertrophy** and **hyperplasia** of various body parts such as the legs, arms, scrotum, vulva and breast (**elephantiasis**).
- Adult filariae harbour obligate intracellular **endosymbiotic bacteria—'*Wolbachia*'**. These bacteria are considered to be essential for the survival, fertility and larval development of the parasite, and also incite an inflammatory response in the host due to the release of endotoxins.
- Usually, the microfilariae do not evoke much of a reaction. The exception is when they cause **tropical pulmonary eosinophilia (TPE)**, a hypersensitivity reaction to the microfilarial antigens, which leads to allergic manifestations of the respiratory system.
- **Co-infection** with other parasites and infectious agents (especially those of malaria and tuberculosis) is common in human filariasis since filariae induce suppressive immunomodulatory effects.

CLINICAL FEATURES

Lymphatic filariasis can present with a wide spectrum of subclinical and clinical conditions.

Endemic Normals

In endemic areas, a proportion of the population seems to remain uninfected and without microfilaremia. It is not clear whether these individuals have low-grade and undetectable or self-limiting infections or if they are immunologically resistant.

Subclinical (Asymptomatic) Microfilaremia

In endemic areas, several individuals demonstrate microfilariae in their blood but none of the symptoms. These individuals serve as carriers of the infection and are known as **asymptomatic microfilaremics**. The parasite burden in these individuals can reach significantly high numbers. Imaging techniques may reveal some degree of subclinical disease pathology in the lymphatics or renal damage.

Acute Clinical Disease

The acute manifestations of lymphatic filariasis are characterised by recurrent episodes of the following:

- **Fever with chills** lasting 1–5 days and associated with **lymphangitis** is a common feature. The lymphatics appear as painful, red, congested streaks on the skin and are cord-like on palpation.
- **Lymphadenitis** is seen, commonly that of the inguinal, axillary and epitrochlear nodes. The nodes are firm and tender.
- In males, the lymphatic system of the genitals is frequently affected, leading to **funiculitis, epididymitis and orchitis**. Early **pitting edema**, which is reversible on limb elevation, may be seen.
- Bacterial and fungal **superinfections** of the affected limbs are common.
- Acute filarial episodes occur in infants too but they are usually more common in older children and continue throughout life.

Chronic Filariasis

It develops over a course of 10–15 years.

- **Lymphedema:** Chronic host immune response against the worms leads to severe lymphatic obstruction and lymphedema (Fig. 33.4a, b and c). The edema may be graded as follows:
  - Grade 1: Pitting edema reversible on limb elevation
  - Grade 2: Pitting/non-pitting edema not reversible on limb elevation with normal overlying skin
  - Grade 3: Non-pitting edema of the limb, not reversible on elevation with thickening of the overlying skin
  - Grade 4: Non-pitting edema with fibrotic and verrucous skin changes **(elephantiasis)**
- **Hydrocele:** In men, scrotal hydrocele is the most common clinical manifestation of chronic filariasis caused by *W. bancrofti*. Chronic epididymitis and funiculitis may also occur (see box). In women, swelling of the vulva and breast may be seen.

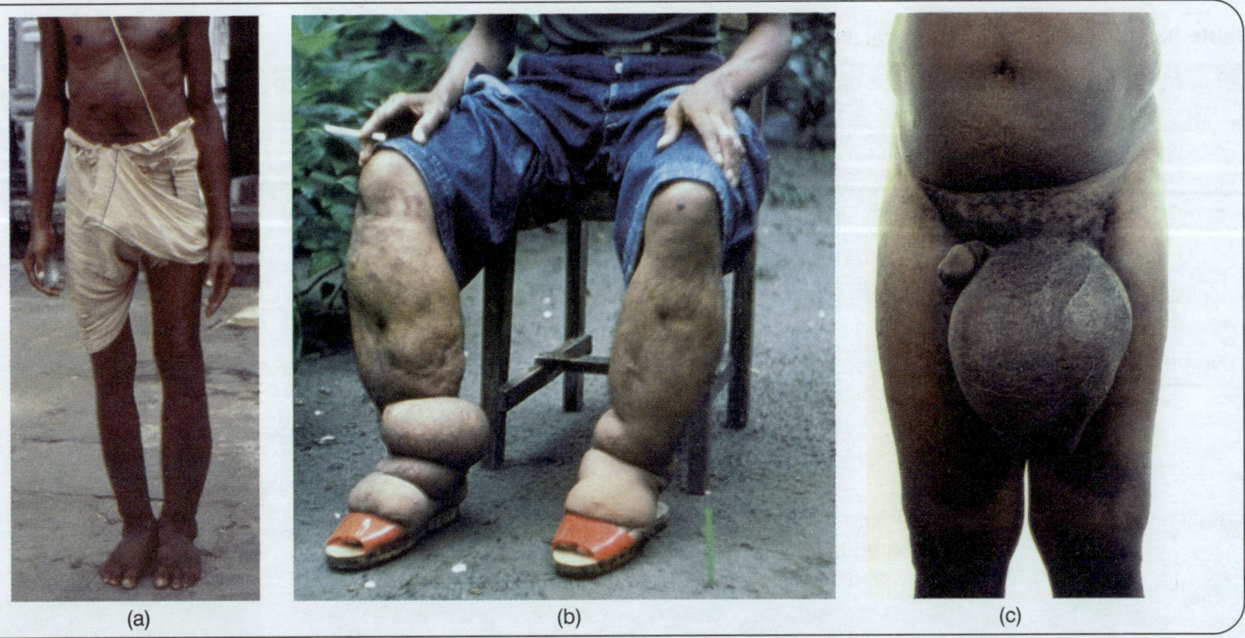

Fig. 33.4 Disease manifestations of lymphatic filariasis: (a) marked swelling of the lower extremities, more pronounced on the left leg, (b) severe edema of the lower legs and (c) hydrocele (*Source:* CDC, Public Health Image Library [PHIL]; Image IDs 17437, 373 and 20246)

- While the genitals are commonly involved in bancroftian filariasis, they are usually spared in brugian filariasis.

- **Chyluria:** The excretion of chyle in the urine (milky urine) is sometimes seen but it is not a very common finding.

Tropical Pulmonary Eosinophilia (TPE)

TPE or **occult filariasis** is a distinct syndrome which develops in some individuals infected with *W. bancrofti* and *B. malayi* (Table 33.4). It is more commonly seen in non-immune individuals living in endemic regions.

- **Epidemiology:** The syndrome affects males more than females (in a ratio of 4:1). The majority of cases have been reported from the Indian subcontinent, South-East Asia, South America and Africa. It is reported in <1% of filarial infections.
- **Pathogenesis:** There is an exaggerated immune response to the microfilarial antigens in which type I, type III and type IV hypersensitivity reactions are elicited with eosinophils playing a pivotal role.
- **Clinical features:** The presentation consists of paroxysmal cough, wheezing, chest pain, weight loss and low-grade fever. The symptoms are usually nocturnal and may be in synchrony with the nocturnal periodicity of microfilariae. Sputum may be viscous, mucoid and scanty, and often contains eosinophils. It is accompanied by pronounced blood eosinophilia (>3,000 cells/µl). Extrapulmonary manifestations include lymphadenopathy and hepatosplenomegaly. Untreated or partially treated TPE may progress to interstitial lung disease.
- **Laboratory diagnosis of TPE:** It is to be noted that **microfilariae cannot be demonstrated in the peripheral blood in TPE**. The following criteria are used for diagnosis:
  - WBC count is raised with peripheral blood eosinophilia (30–80%; absolute eosinophil count >3,000 cells/µl). ESR is always raised.
  - Chest X-ray shows reticulonodular shadows and miliary mottling, which often make differentiation from miliary tuberculosis difficult.
  - Pulmonary function test shows mixed restrictive and obstructive changes in the lungs.
  - Filaria-specific IgG and IgE are elevated in the serum.
  - There is clinical improvement with diethylcarbamazine (DEC).
- **Treatment of TPE:** DEC, 6 mg/kg/day, is given for 2–4 weeks. Steroids may be added with precautions. Relapse may occur in 20% of cases; these patients may require higher doses.

DIAGNOSIS

The demonstration of **microfilariae in blood** was the mainstay of the diagnosis of filariasis until a few years ago. The examination of hydrocele fluid also helps. These

Table 33.4 Comparison of classical and occult filariasis

Feature	Classical lymphatic filariasis	Occult filariasis/tropical pulmonary eosinophilia (TPE)
Etiology	Adult worms of *Wuchereria* and *Brugia*	Microfilariae
Organ involvement	Lymphatics and lymph nodes	Lungs, liver and spleen
Pathogenesis	Recurrent inflammation of the lymphatic vessels and lymph nodes due to adult worms	Hypersensitivity reaction to microfilariae
Clinical manifestations	Varicose lymph vessels and hydrocele, elephantiasis and chyluria	Hepatosplenomegaly and allergic pulmonary manifestations
Diagnosis	• Demonstration of microfilariae in peripheral blood • Antigen detection in serum • Serology not very useful	• Eosinophilia (absolute eosinophil count >3,000 cells/µl) • Elevated serum IgE and filarial-specific IgG and IgE • Microfilariae absent from peripheral blood
Treatment	• Diethylcarbamazine (DEC): 6 mg/kg with or without albendazole 400 mg, single-dose treatment or 6 mg/kg/day × 12 days OR • Doxycycline: 200 mg/day × 4 weeks with ivermectin 400 µg/kg • Management of lymphedema, hydrocele, etc.	• DEC: 6 mg/kg/day for 2–4 weeks

methods have now been superseded by the **antigen detection card test** which is easy to use as a rapid point-of-care test.

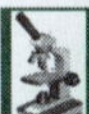

Lab diagnosis

- **Microscopy:** By visualising microfilariae
  - Direct microscopy of night blood smear
  - Blood concentration techniques: Membrane filtration and Knott's centrifugation
  - DEC provocation test
- **Antigen detection:** Rapid immunochromatographic tests
- **Serology:**
  - Subtype IgG4 antibody detection
  - Specific IgG and IgE may help in diagnosis of TPE
- **DNA detection:** PCR and real-time PCR
- **Other diagnostic parameters**
  - Radioimaging: Filarial dance sign
  - Lymphoscintigraphy

Microscopy

Direct wet mount: Blood may be examined as a wet mount on a glass slide to demonstrate the characteristic serpentine movement of the microfilariae. The sample should preferably be collected according to the periodicity of the parasite. Therefore, in India, samples should ideally be collected at night, between **10 p.m.** and **4 a.m.**

Thick or thin smear: Giemsa or hematoxylin and eosin stain of blood films can be performed to observe the morphological features of the microfilariae (Fig. 33.5a–f).

Concentration techniques: Blood can be examined after performing concentration techniques to increase sensitivity. The membrane filtration or Knott's centrifugation technique may be used for this purpose (refer to **Appendix I**, *Approach to the Laboratory Diagnosis of Parasitic Infections*).

Diethylcarbamazine provocation test: The administration of DEC induces the appearance of microfilariae in the peripheral blood. Thus, a blood sample collected within 20–40 minutes of the administration of DEC, 2 mg/kg orally, increases the sensitivity of detection. This test is contraindicated in *Onchocerca volvulus* and *Loa loa* infections.

Quantitative buffy coat (QBC): The use of QBC in microhematocrit tubes coated with acridine orange has been reported to be acceptable for the diagnosis of microfilariae with a sensitivity similar to that of a thick film.

Antigen Detection

Immunochromatographic card tests (ICT) are now the preferred method for the diagnosis of bancroftian filariasis and are now used in the national filaria control programmes. Circulating antigens of *W. bancrofti* can be detected using monoclonal antibodies against Og4C3 and AD12 antigens with excellent sensitivity (96–100%) and

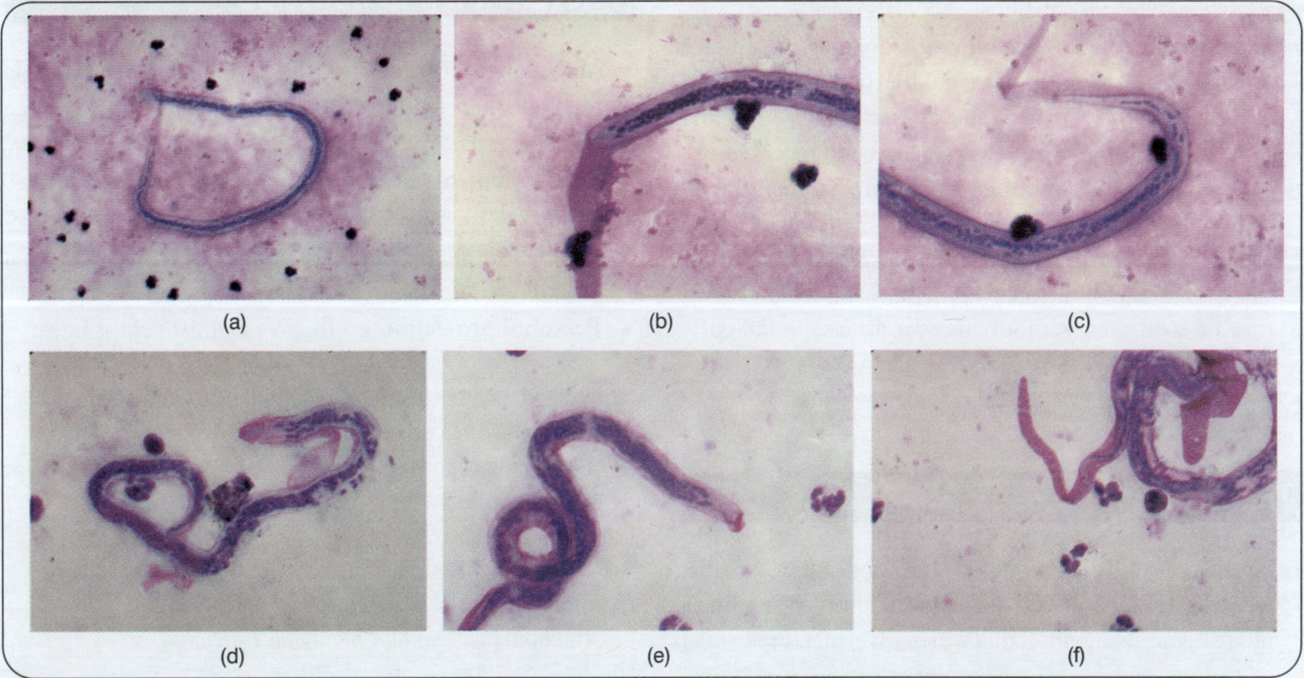

Fig. 33.5 Microfilariae (mf) with conspicuous nuclei and sheath in blood stained with Giemsa stain in a case lymphatic filariasis: (a) *Wuchereria bancrofti* mf, (b) the anterior end of the mf of *W. bancrofti*, (c) the posterior end of the mf of *W. bancrofti*, (d) *Brugia malayi* mf, (e) the anterior end of mf of *B. malayi* and (f) the posterior end of the mf of *B. malayi* (*Source:* CDC, PHIL; Image IDs 3009, 3010, 3007, 3003, 3004 and 3005)

specificity (95–100%). *Brugia malayi* infections can also be diagnosed serologically by ELISA targeting the Bm14 and BmR1 antigens.

Advantages

- It is more sensitive than microscopy.
- It can detect latent infections.
- It can be performed on blood collected at any time.
- It is easy to use.

Serology

Except for epidemiological surveys and monitoring, total IgG antibody detection is not very useful as it cannot differentiate between current and past infections and also because of cross-reactivity to other helminths. The detection of specific **IgG4** subtype is useful as it correlates with the intensity and duration of the infection.

Nucleic Acid-Based Detection

PCR- and real-time PCR-based methods have been developed for the detection of filarial DNA in blood, plasma, paraffin-embedded tissues, urine, sputum and mosquitoes. However, these methods are available only in research centres.

Other Diagnostic Parameters

- **High-frequency ultrasound** with doppler techniques are used to detect changes in the lymphatic vessels as well as adult worms. The characteristic wriggling movement of the worms within the lymphatic vessels, especially in the scrotum, is known as the **filarial dance sign**.
- **Lymphoscintigraphy** of the limbs reliably demonstrates the functional abnormalities of the lymphatics, which may be seen even without an overt disease in the early stages.
- **X-rays** can detect dead and calcified worms.

TREATMENT

- Ivermectin kills microfilaria but not adult worms, whereas DEC is effective against microfilariae and is modestly active against adult worms. Ivermectin can lead to serious and occasionally fatal adverse neurological reactions in people infected with *L. loa*. The severe adverse events occur when the *L. loa* microfilaremia exceeds 20,000–30,000 mf/ml.
- Doxycycline targets *Wolbachia* bacterial endosymbionts but is contraindicated in children and pregnant women.

Individual drug administration	
Diethylcarbamazine (DEC): 6 mg/kg with or without albendazole, 400 mg, single-dose treatment; or 6 mg/kg/day × 12 days OR *Doxycycline:* 200 mg/day × 4 weeks with ivermectin, 400 μg/kg	
Mass drug administration (preventive chemotherapy)	
Across the world except Africa*	**Africa**
Annual DEC and albendazole for at least 5 years to everyone in endemic areas except children <2 years and pregnant women	Annual or biannual ivermectin and albendazole for at least 5 years
*Onchocerciasis (for which DEC is ineffective) is prevalent in Africa along with lymphatic filariasis.	
Morbidity management	
Lymphedema: Hygiene, physiotherapy, doxycycline, 200 mg/day × 6 weeks *Hydrocele:* Surgical hydrocelectomy **Prevention** of secondary bacterial infections	

PREVENTION AND CONTROL

- **Mass chemotherapy** of the population in endemic areas for at least five years is believed to reduce transmission.
- **Vector control measures** such as insecticide sprays, antilarval measures, environmental engineering and public awareness should be employed to abolish larval breeding sites.
- **Personal protection** is effective against vector bites.

Preventive chemotherapy is recommended as a strategy by the WHO for the control of:

- Lymphatic filariasis
- Onchocerciasis
- Schistosomiasis
- Soil-transmitted helminths (hookworm, roundworm and whipworm)
- Trachoma caused by *Chlamydia trachomatis*

Filaria control programme: The **Global Programme to Eliminate Lymphatic Filariasis (GPELF)** was established by WHO with the following aims:

- To stop the spread of infection by vector and adult control measures and mass drug administration (MDA).
- To alleviate suffering among patients by morbidity management and disability prevention (MMDP).

India: The **National Filariasis Control Programme (NFCP)**, which has been in operation in India since 1955, now falls under the ambit of the **National Vector Borne Disease Control Programme (NVBDCP)**, which is an umbrella programme for the prevention and control of vector-borne diseases (refer to **Chapter 57**, *Control Programmes for Parasitic Diseases*).

The National Health Policy (2002) of India envisages the **elimination of lymphatic filariasis (ELF)**. **Elimination** is defined as a scenario where 'lymphatic filariasis ceases to be a public health problem, where the percentage of microfilaria carriers is less than 1 per cent and where the children born after the initiation of ELF are free from circulating antigens or microfilariae'. The elimination strategy includes:

- **Vector control:** This is done by using methods to control the breeding of mosquitoes.
- **Anti-parasitic measures:** This includes the detection of carriers by door-to-door surveys and the treatment of diseased persons in filaria clinics. Annual mass drug administration (MDA) of DEC and albendazole for five years is carried out on National Filaria Day.
- **Morbidity management:** This is done by home-based management of lymphedema cases and hospital-based hydrocele surgery.

Questions

1. Describe the general characteristics of filarial nematodes.
2. Discuss the diagnosis and management of lymphatic filariasis.
3. Differentiate between the microfilariae that appear in peripheral blood.
4. Differentiate between the microfilariae that appear in the skin.

Multiple Choice Questions

1. Which of the following is NOT a characteristic of the microfilariae of *Wuchereria bancrofti*?
   a. Sheathed b. Tail-tip has three nuclei
   c. Nocturnal periodicity d. Nuclei distinct
2. The involvement of genital organs in males is more commonly seen with ____________:
   a. Bancroftian filariasis b. Brugian filariasis
   c. Loiasis d. Onchocerciasis
3. *Brugia timori* is prevalent in ____________:
   a. South America b. South Africa
   c. India d. Indonesia
4. Microfilariae of *Wuchereria* and *Brugia* exhibit ________:
   a. Nocturnal periodicity
   b. Diurnal periodicity
   c. Non-periodic
   d. None of the above
5. Which bacteria are endosymbionts of filarial parasites?
   a. *Vahlkampfia* b. *Wolbachia*
   c. *Campylobacter* d. *Escherichia coli*
6. The drugs administered during mass drug administration in the filaria control programme in India are ____________:
   a. Ivermectin and diethylcarbamazine (DEC)
   b. Diethylcarbamazine (DEC) with or without albendazole
   c. Ivermectin and mebendazole
   d. Any of the above combinations
7. The non-sheathed microfilariae in the blood are ____________:
   a. *Loa loa*
   b. *Mansonella perstans*
   c. *Brugia timori*
   d. *Brugia malayi*
8. The life cycle of filarial worms causing lymphatic filariasis was discovered by ____________:
   a. Antony van Leeuwenhoek
   b. Patrick Manson
   c. Ronald Ross
   d. Charles Laveran
9. The microfilariae of which of the following parasites are detected in skin snips?
   a. *Loa loa*
   b. *Mansonella perstans*
   c. *Mansonella streptocerca*
   d. *Brugia timori*
10. All the following statements are true about tropical pulmonary eosinophilia EXCEPT ____________:
    a. It is associated with filarial nematodes
    b. It is diagnosed by the demonstration of microfilariae in peripheral blood
    c. It is more commonly reported from Asia, South America and South Africa
    d. It is treated with diethylcarbamazine (DEC)

CHAPTER 34

Loa loa

(From an Angolan word *loa* = worm)

Case Study and Learning Goals

A 30-year-old resident of Nigeria complains of a swelling on his arm measuring 10 cm, which changes its location (migratory). His eosinophils and IgE levels are found to be elevated. What are the parasitic causes of migratory swellings? How would you approach the laboratory diagnosis in this case? How would you treat this patient?

INTRODUCTION

Loa loa is often referred to as the **African eye worm** because the adult worm can sometimes be seen moving through the sclera of the eye.

It was first described in medical literature in 1770 by a French surgeon, Mongin, who unsuccessfully attempted the extraction of a worm from the eye of a young girl in Santa Domingo. The migratory swelling of the limbs was described in 1885 by the ophthalmologist Douglas Argyll-Robertson in Old Calabar in Nigeria; thereafter, this feature came to be known as **'Calabar swelling'**. It was Patrick Manson who implicated *L. loa* in these swellings in 1910. Robert Thomson Leiper discovered the role of tabanid flies *Chrysops* in the transmission of the disease in 1912.

EPIDEMIOLOGY

Loa loa has a limited geographic distribution, restricted to tropical rain forest regions of western and central Africa and south of the Sahara Desert, with up to 70% prevalence in areas of Nigeria and the Democratic Republic of the Congo. It is transmitted to humans through the repeated bites of **tabanid flies (also known as deer flies, mango flies or mangrove flies) of the genus *Chrysops*.**

MORPHOLOGY

The morphology of *Loa loa* follows the scheme of filarial worms except for differences in the size of the worms and microfilariae (See Table 33.2 in **Chapter 33**, *Wuchereria and Brugia*).

- The adult female measures 5–7 cm × 0.5 mm and the male measures 3.5 cm × 0.4 mm.
- The microfilariae (mf) are 250–300 × 8–10 μm in size. They are **sheathed, with nuclei extending to the tail-tip** (Fig. 34.1a and b).

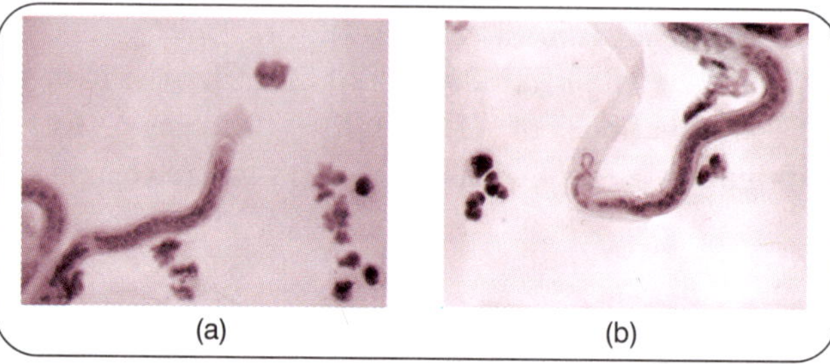

Fig. 34.1 Sheathed microfilaria of *Loa loa*: (a) anterior end and (b) posterior end (*Source:* Centers for Disease Control and Prevention [CDC], Public Health Image Library [PHIL]; Image IDs 21533 and 21534)

LIFE CYCLE (Fig. 34.2)

> **Definitive host:** Human beings
> **Intermediate host:** Female tabanid fly (*Chrysops*)

Human stage: The **definitive hosts—humans**—get infected with the **bite of the female tabanid fly**. The **L3 larva** of the parasite enters through the bite wound and settles in the subcutaneous tissue, where it matures in 6–12 months. The life span of the adult is 1–15 years. The worm migrates subcutaneously or into the deep connective tissue at a rate of 1 cm per minute. After mating, the gravid female releases microfilariae in the blood. The microfilariae show a **diurnal** periodicity peaking at **mid-day** and concentrating, in the pulmonary capillaries at night. The microfilariae can also be found in spinal fluid, urine, sputum and the lungs.

Tabanid fly stage: The female tabanid flies (mango or deer flies) are the **intermediate hosts** for *L. loa*. The **day biting** fly ingests the microfilariae in its blood meal. The life cycle of the parasite in the vector is essentially the same as that of other filarial species.

PATHOGENESIS

The mechanisms of pathogenesis of *L. loa* are as follows:

- The migration of the worm is not painful per se; it is usually inconspicuous unless the worm is moving

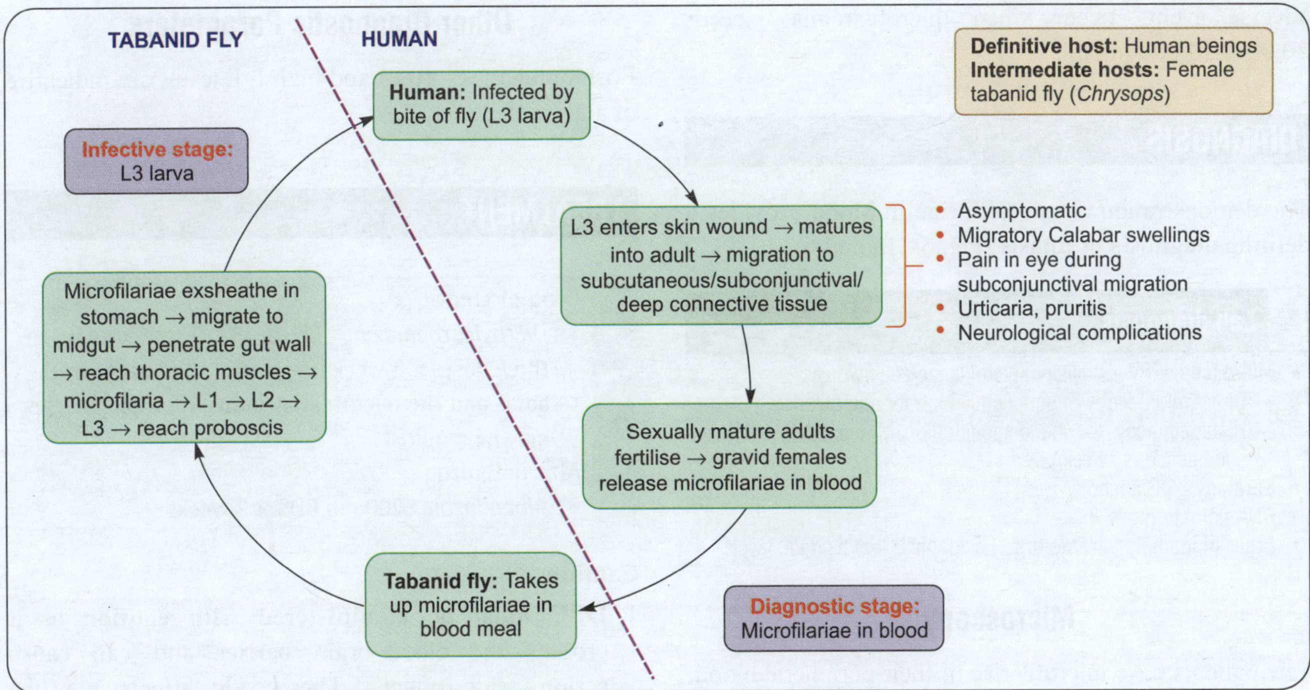

Fig. 34.2 Life cycle of *Loa loa* (schematic)

in the subconjunctival tissue of the eye or across the bridge of the nose.

- Calabar swellings are angio-edematous and represent hypersensitivity responses to the antigens or microfilariae of the migrating adult parasite.
- The complications of the infection are cardiomyopathy due to endomyocardial fibrosis, nephropathy due to immune complex glomerulonephritis and pleural effusions.
- On administration of ivermectin, fatal encephalopathy and encephalitis may result from the microfilariae dying within the vessels of the CNS and stimulating an eosinophil-rich inflammatory response.

CLINICAL FEATURES

Asymptomatic Infections

Most cases of loiasis are asymptomatic, though the bite of the vector may result in redness, swelling and itching.

Symptomatic Infections

The first clinical signs may appear within a few months of infection, but often, they do not appear for more than a decade. The incubation period from the bite of the vector to the appearance of the adult worm in the human host is about 3–4 years.

- **Calabar swellings (fugitive swellings):** This is a characteristic clinical sign of loiasis. These are **evanescent, migratory and angio-edematous swellings**. Such a swelling starts as local pain or itching lasting 1–2 hours, following which, a 10–20 cm wide, non-erythematous and non-pitting swelling develops. The swelling generally resolves in 2–4 days but may last as long as several weeks. Calabar swellings often occur on the limbs, near the joints, which makes movement difficult and painful. Travellers from non-endemic areas tend to have more frequent and debilitating episodes of Calabar swellings with high eosinophilia and IgE antibodies but rarely have microfilaremia.
- **Ocular manifestations:** The migration of the mature worm through the subconjunctiva or sclera of the eye (African eye worm) causes severe eye pain, inflammation and sometimes, blindness. Symptoms may last from minutes to several hours. Adult worms are also occasionally seen in the penis, nipples or across the bridge of the nose.
- **Less specific manifestations:** These include urticaria, pruritus, myalgia and arthralgia.

Complications

L. loa infection can also cause renal, cardiac, pulmonary and neurological diseases. It has gained attention in recent years because of the fatal neurological complications that occur when ivermectin therapy is given as part of mass treatment programmes for onchocerciasis to people co-infected with *Onchocerca volvulus* and *L. loa*. Severe adverse events occur when microfilaremia exceeds 20,000–30,000 mf/ml.

DIAGNOSIS

The demonstration of **microfilariae in blood provides a definite diagnosis of loiasis** (Fig. 34.1a and b).

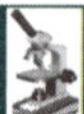

Lab diagnosis

- **Microscopy:** By visualising microfilariae/adult worms
  - Direct microscopy of peripheral blood for microfilariae
  - Histopathology for the demonstration of the adult worm in subcutaneous swellings
- **Serology:** IgG antibody
- **DNA detection:** PCR
- **Other diagnostic parameters:** Eosinophilia and high IgE levels

Microscopy

Few patients have microfilariae in their peripheral blood; the majority of those infected are amicrofilariemic.

- Microfilariae have **diurnal periodicity** and are found circulating in the peripheral blood during the **day**.
- **Delafield's hematoxylin staining** is recommended as Giemsa does not reveal the sheath of the mf.
- Microfilariae of *L. loa* should be differentiated from those of *Wuchereria bancrofti* and *Mansonella perstans* in areas where these parasites are co-endemic.
- Quantification of the *L. loa* microfilariae in peripheral blood may be important for treatment as the drug of choice (diethylcarbamazine) has been associated with severe neurologic manifestations in patients with high filarial burden.

Demonstration of adult worms: *L. loa* adults can be demonstrated in the eye or skin by biopsy of a subcutaneous nodule.

Serology

A lateral flow assay (LFA) to identify subjects with a serological response to Ll-SXP-1, a specific and validated marker of *L. loa*, is commercially available.

Nucleic Acid-Based Detection

PCR assays are available for the detection of *L. loa* DNA in blood in reference laboratories and are highly sensitive and specific.

Other Diagnostic Parameters

Eosinophilia (30–40%) and high IgE levels are indicative of active infection.

TREATMENT

Drug of choice
- *Diethylcarbamazine (DEC):* 8–10 mg/kg/day in three doses × 3 weeks is effective against both the adult and the microfilarial forms; multiple courses may be required

Alternate drug
- *Albendazole:* 200 mg BDS × 3 weeks

Caution:

1. **DEC must be administered with caution** as it crosses the blood–brain barrier and can cause serious side effects. These side effects may be decreased if **adjunctive therapy** with glucocorticoids, anti-inflammatory and anti-histaminic drugs is administered along with DEC to reduce allergic or other inflammatory reactions.
2. **Ivermectin is contraindicated** in loiasis as it can cause serious neurological side effects including coma, encephalitis, retinal hemorrhage and membranous glomerulonephritis.

Surgical extraction of adult worms: A worm visibly migrating through the conjunctiva or the bridge of the nose can be surgically extracted.

PREVENTION AND CONTROL

- Personal protection to reduce fly bites by wearing long, light-coloured clothing, using screens on doors and windows and using insecticides or repellents on exposed skin is recommended.
- Since regions of *L. loa* endemicity in Africa overlap those of *Onchocerca* and lymphatic filariasis, mass drug administration for those diseases takes care of loiasis as well.
- A prophylaxis of DEC, 300 mg, once a week, effectively protects long-term travellers.
- Currently, there are no vaccines available for loiasis.

Questions

1. Describe the morphology, life cycle and clinical manifestations of *Loa loa*.
2. List the causes of subcutaneous filariasis.
3. Describe the diagnosis and management of *Loa loa* infection.

Multiple Choice Questions

1. *Loa loa* is transmitted by __________ :
   a. Tsetse fly
   b. Sandfly
   c. Blackfly
   d. Tabanid fly
2. Calabar swellings are characteristic of __________ infection.
   a. *Chlamydia trachomatis*
   b. *Pseudomonas pseudomallei*
   c. *Loa loa*
   d. *Onchocerca volvulus*
3. Loiasis is chiefly prevalent in __________ :
   a. South-East Asia
   b. The Mediterranean region
   c. Africa
   d. North and Central America
4. The diagnosis of onchocerciasis is made by the __________ :
   a. Demonstration of microfilariae in a blood smear
   b. Mazotti test
   c. DEC patch test
   d. Casoni's test
5. The drug of choice for the treatment of loiasis is __________ :
   a. Praziquantel
   b. Diethylcarbamazine
   c. Ivermectin
   d. Mebendazole

Chapter 35

Onchocerca

(*Onchocerca* [From Greek] *onkos* = nodule + *kerkos* = tail; *volvulus* from *volvere* [Latin] = to roll)

Case Study and Learning Goals

A 25-year-old male from Congo presents with keratitis, generalised pruritus and a rash with hyper- and hypopigmented patches. What are the parasitic causes of keratitis? How would you approach the laboratory diagnosis in this case? How would you treat this patient?

INTRODUCTION

Onchocerca volvulus is a filarial worm that is responsible for causing onchocerciasis or **'river blindness'** in humans. It is one of the leading causes of blindness in the world and also causes significant disfigurement of the skin.

The Irish surgeon John O'Neill first discovered the microfilarial larvae in skin snips of patients in Ghana in 1874. Patrick Manson described the adult worm in 1890. The role of the blackfly in the transmission of this parasite was revealed by D. B. Blacklock in 1926.

EPIDEMIOLOGY

Onchocerciasis occurs predominantly in tropical areas. Around 30 countries are affected in Africa, with more than 90% of the infected people living in the sub-Saharan parts of the continent. In some of the West African communities, around 50% of men over the age of 40 have been blinded by the disease. Six countries in Central and South America are affected—Brazil, Colombia, Venezuela, Ecuador, Guatemala and Mexico. A few cases are reported in Saudi Arabia and Yemen. Onchocerciasis has not been reported in India.

Onchocerciasis is transmitted by repeated bites of **blackflies (*Simulium* spp.)** which breed along fast-flowing rivers and streams. Hence the disease is prevalent along the course of rivers and streams and is called **'river blindness'**.

MORPHOLOGY

Adult Worm

The worm is whitish, long and slender, and lies coiled up in nodules in tissues. The adult male is 3–8 cm × 0.2 mm in size, while the female is longer, measuring 30–80 cm × 0.3 mm. Well-defined transverse ridges and annular and oblique thickenings are seen in the cuticle, especially in the female worm.

Microfilariae

The microfilariae measure 220–360 × 4–5 μm and are **non-sheathed**. The posterior end is angulated, and there are **no nuclei in the tail-tip**.

LIFE CYCLE (Fig. 35.1)

Human stage: The **definitive hosts—human beings—** get infected by the **bite of female blackflies**. The **L3 larva** enters through the bite wound into the subcutaneous tissue and matures there in 6–12 months. The adult resides in the subcutaneous nodules. Its life span is up to 15 years. The gravid female releases microfilariae, which are found in the skin, lymphatics of the connective tissue and eyes. The microfilariae show a **diurnal** periodicity and are taken up by the day biting fly.

> **Definitive host:** Human beings
> **Intermediate host:** Female blackfly (*Simulium*)

Blackfly stage: The **female blackflies are the intermediate hosts** for *O. volvulus*. The life cycle in the vector is essentially the same as that of other filarial species.

PATHOGENESIS

The disease process relates to the immune response of the body to the microfilariae and the adult worms. The adult worms are less pathogenic and simply elicit the **formation of subcutaneous or subconjunctival nodules (onchocercomas)** due to cellular reaction and fibrosis around the worms. The mechanisms of pathogenesis of *Onchocerca* infections are as follows:

- In response to the microfilariae, especially the dead ones, recurrent inflammation occurs, eventually resulting in cutaneous and ocular pathology.
- In the skin, there is permanent **thickening and hypertrophy**. The **loss of elasticity of the skin** causes

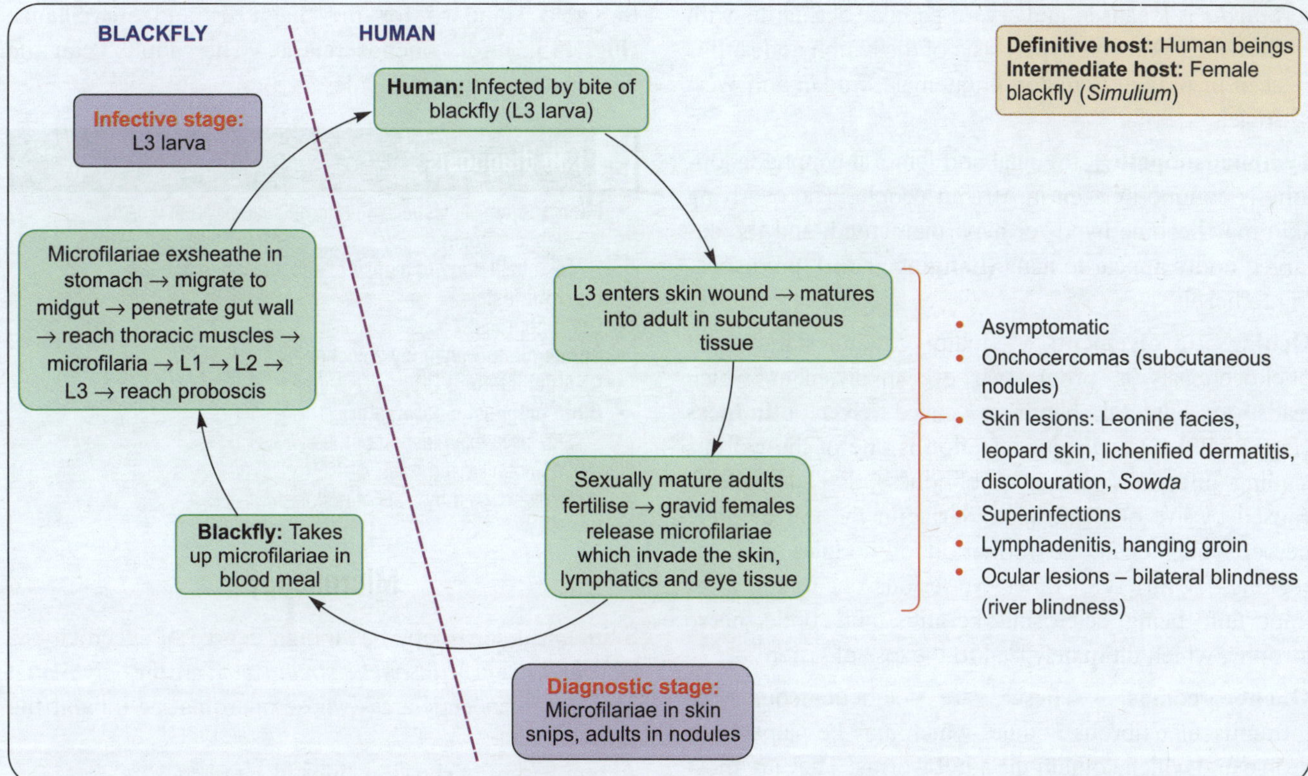

Fig. 35.1 Life cycle of *Onchocerca volvulus* (schematic)

it to hang over the inguinal area. Extensive follicular hyperplasia of the regional lymph nodes is linked to the formation of autoantibodies to defensins and a hyperimmune response. This produces **chronic hyperreactive dermatitis**, which results in the darkening of the skin and the enlargement of lymph nodes.

- A variety of **eye lesions** such as conjunctivitis, corneal opacities, punctate keratitis which progresses to **sclerosing keratitis**, iridocyclitis leading to glaucoma and cataract, chorioretinitis and optic nerve atrophy may be seen, which ultimately lead to **blindness**.

CLINICAL FEATURES

It is chiefly a disease of the **eyes and skin** (Fig. 35.2a and b). The incubation period from the bite of the vector to the development of clinical manifestations in humans is about one year.

Asymptomatic Infections

The infection may be asymptomatic when the worm load is light.

Symptomatic Infections

In heavy infections, the clinical manifestations include dermatitis, subcutaneous nodules, lymphadenitis and ocular manifestations.

Skin lesions: Generalised pruritus and rashes are the most common manifestations of onchocerciasis. The pruritus may be incapacitating. Scratching often leads to ulcers, bleeding, and secondary bacterial and fungal infections. The skin lesions (Fig. 35.2b) resemble those of other skin conditions such as scabies, contact dermatitis, insect bites, dermatomycosis, leprosy, etc., and must be differentiated from these. The following are the skin manifestations of the disease:

- There is recurrent inflammation which eventually results in the permanent loss of elasticity and thickening and premature, exaggerated wrinkling of the skin.
- **Leonine facies** resembling lepromatous leprosy may be seen due to thickened earlobes and facial skin.
- **Leopard or lizard skin** develops, predominantly on the shins, as depigmented spots surrounded by hyperpigmented areas.
- Lichenified dermatitis develops due to thickening, discolouration and cracking of the skin.
- **Mal morado or purplish discolouration** of the skin is a feature seen in Central America.

- ***Sowda*** is localised and severe papular dermatitis with darkened skin and hyperplasia of the lymph nodes. It is seen in Arabia, Ecuador, Guatemala, Sudan and West Africa.

Lymphadenopathy: Inguinal and femoral lymphadenopathy is commonly seen in African people. The overlying skin may become hypo- or hyperpigmented, and the enlarged nodes appear to hang **(hanging groin)**, predisposing to hernia.

Ocular involvement: A major manifestation of onchocerciasis is progressive eye involvement which leads to bilateral blindness called **river blindness** (Fig. 35.2a). *O. volvulus* infection is one of the world's leading infectious causes of blindness. Eye damage is caused by live or dead microfilariae in the eye or optic nerve, which elicit the formation of nodules in these regions. A variety of other eye lesions occur, the most important being sclerosing keratitis and optic nerve atrophy, which ultimately lead to the loss of vision.

Onchocercomas: These are subcutaneous or intramuscular fibrous nodules which may be palpable or visible and which contain the adult worms. They are most common over bony prominences. If the nodules are in the head and neck region, there are more chances of the involvement of the eyes. These nodules may be single or multiple and vary in size from a few millimetres to a few centimetres. They are painless and non-suppurating.

DIAGNOSIS

Traditionally, the microscopic examination of skin biopsies (snips) to demonstrate **microfilariae** has been the gold standard for the diagnosis and surveillance (Fig. 35.3) of onchocerciasis. The adults can be demonstrated in the nodules.

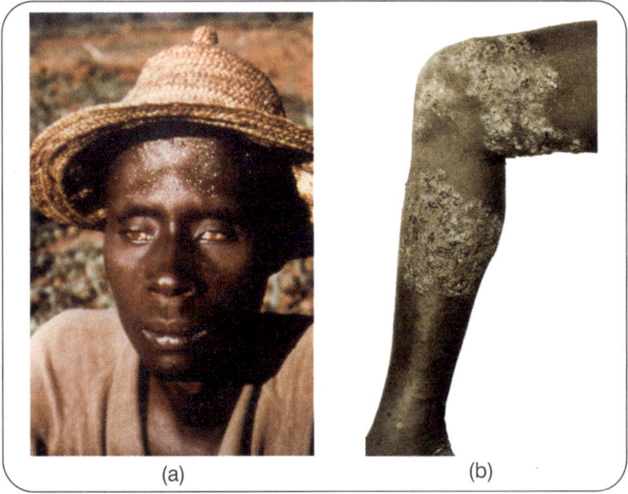

Fig. 35.2 Disease manifestations of *Onchocerca volvulus*: (a) river blindness and (b) cutaneous lesions (*Source:* Centers for Disease Control and Prevention [CDC], Public Health Image Library [PHIL], Image IDs 16634 and 20286)

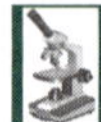

Lab diagnosis

- **Microscopy:** By visualising microfilariae or adult worms
  - Skin snip microscopy
  - Histopathology of biopsy of subcutaneous nodules
- **Mazzotti test**
- **DEC patch test**
- **Serology:** IgG antibody detection by Ov16 ELISA
- **DNA detection:** PCR and real-time PCR
- **Other diagnostic parameters:**
  - Slip lamp examination of the eye
  - Eosinophilia and ↑ IgE
  - Radioimaging by USG of nodules

Microscopy

Skin snip microscopy has a high degree of specificity as *O. volvulus* and *Mansonella streptocerca* are the only filarial parasites in endemic areas whose microfilariae inhabit the skin.

- Incubation of the skin snips in saline at 37°C for a few hours stimulates the microfilariae to emerge.
- The examination of six skin snips has a sensitivity of >90%.
- The sensitivity of skin snip microscopy decreases when mass drug administration programmes are ongoing.

Detection of the adult worm: *O. volvulus* adults can be detected in the biopsy of the subcutaneous nodules but this method is less sensitive.

Mazzotti Test

On administration of DEC, 25–50 mg, orally, acute inflammation occurs, leading to intense pruritis, lymphadenitis and fever. This subsides in a few days.

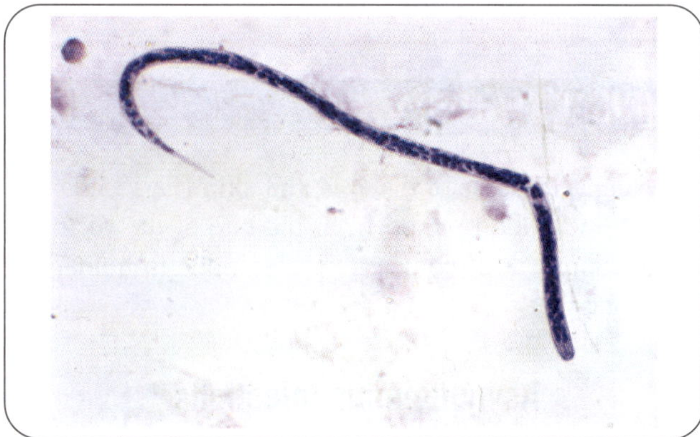

Fig. 35.3 Microfilaria of *Onchocerca volvulus* (*Source:* CDC, PHIL, Image ID 1147)

However, the reaction may be severe in heavily infected individuals.

Diethylcarbamazine (DEC) Patch Test

The problem of severe reactions is eliminated by applying DEC on the skin of individuals infected with *O. volvulus*. This elicits a localised rash with redness and itching within 24–48 hours, indicating a positive test.

Serology

The WHO recommends the use of Ov16 ELISA for the demonstration of IgG antibodies, especially of the IgG4 isotype, to monitor the interruption of transmission of *O. volvulus*. Some rapid immunochromatographic card tests are also being evaluated for use in the field.

Nucleic Acid-Based Detection

PCR, real-time PCR and LAMP assays have been developed for the detection of *Onchocerca* DNA in blood and are highly sensitive and specific.

Other Diagnostic Parameters

- Slit lamp examination of the eye makes it possible to visualise microfilariae.
- Ultrasonography is used to distinguish onchocercomas from other similar-looking lesions.
- Mild to moderate eosinophilia and elevated serum IgE indicate an active infection.

TREATMENT

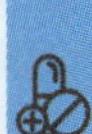

Drug of choice
- *Ivermectin:* 150 µg/kg orally in a single dose, either yearly or semi-annually is active against the microfilariae but not the adult worms; it is contraindicated in those areas of Africa where *Loa loa* infections are co-endemic as it can cause severe neurological reactions in such individuals.

- **Ivermectin** paralyses and kills microfilariae, thus relieving intense skin itching and controlling the ocular damage. Though it does not kill adult worms, it prevents microfilaria production for a few months following treatment, thus helping to reduce transmission.
- Nodules may be removed surgically.

PREVENTION AND CONTROL

- Community-based **mass drug administration (MDA) of ivermectin** every 6–12 months is employed under the African Programme for Onchocerciasis Control (APOC) since 1995 and under Onchocerciasis Elimination Programme in the Americas (OEPA) since 1992.
- Vector control by **aerial dispersion of insecticides** has reduced disease transmission in several African countries.
- Currently, there are no vaccines for onchocerciasis.

Questions

1. Discuss the laboratory diagnosis and management of onchocerciasis.

Multiple Choice Questions

1. *Onchocerca volvulus* is transmitted by ________:
   a. Tsetse fly
   b. Sandfly
   c. Blackfly
   d. Housefly
2. The drug of choice for the treatment of onchocerciasis is ________:
   a. Praziquantel
   b. Albendazole
   c. Ivermectin
   d. Mebendazole
3. River blindness is caused by infection with ________:
   a. *Chlamydia trachomatis*
   b. *Pseudomonas pseudomallei*
   c. *Leishmania donovani*
   d. *Onchocerca volvulus*
4. Onchocerciasis is mainly prevalent in ________:
   a. South-East Asia
   b. The Mediterranean region
   c. Africa
   d. North and Central America

5. *Sowda* and leopard skin are manifestations of _________:
   a. Leishmaniasis
   b. Lymphatic filariasis
   c. Onchocerciasis
   d. Leprosy

6. The diagnosis of onchocerciasis is made by all the following EXCEPT _________:
   a. Demonstration of microfilariae in a blood film
   b. Mazzotti test
   c. DEC patch test
   d. Serology for detection of specific IgG antibodies

Chapter 36

Mansonella and Dirofilaria

(*Mansonella* named after the scientist Patrick Manson; *Dirofilaria* from Latin, *dirus* = fearful + *filum* = thread)

Case Study and Learning Goals

A 15-year-old girl presents with tearing and redness of the eyes and a swelling in her left eye with granulation tissue on the swelling. The swelling is surgically explored, and a whitish worm is extracted from it. What are the parasitic causes of worms in the eye? How is the disease transmitted?

MANSONELLA

INTRODUCTION

Human mansonellosis is caused by *Mansonella perstans, M. ozzardi* and *M. streptocerca,* the three main filarial species of the genus *Mansonella.*

EPIDEMIOLOGY

In endemic areas, mansonellosis is often considered one of the most common human helminthiases. However, it has not been reported from India. *M. perstans* is considered to be most evenly distributed in areas of Africa, South America and the Caribbean, *M. ozzardi* in the tropical regions of Central and South America and the Caribbean and *M. streptocerca* in Western and Central Africa (Table 36.1).

MORPHOLOGY

The morphology of *Mansonella* follows the morphological scheme of filarial worms except for differences in size (see Tables 33.2 and 33.3 and Fig. 33.2 in **Chapter 33**, *Wuchereria and Brugia*).

LIFE CYCLE

Definitive hosts: Human beings
Intermediate hosts: Female midge (also blackfly for *M. ozzardi*)

The life cycle of *Mansonella* is similar to that of other filarial species except for differences in vectors and clinical manifestations depending on the species. Humans, the definitive hosts, get infected by the bite of the insect vector, which transmits the **L3 larvae**. These larvae mature into adults in the subcutaneous tissue and then migrate to the species-specific preferred site (Table 36.1). There, they fertilise and produce microfilariae which show no specific periodicity. These microfilariae are taken up by the vector during its blood meal to continue the cycle of transmission.

CLINICAL FEATURES

Most microfilaremic individuals are asymptomatic, though eosinophilia is a common feature. Non-specific symptoms including pruritus, urticaria, arthralgia, abdominal pain and fatigue have been described.

- In *M. perstans* infections, symptoms are related to the migration of the worms and include transient subcutaneous swellings (similar to Calabar swellings),

Table 36.1 Features of *Mansonella* species that affect humans

Characteristic	*Mansonella perstans*	*Mansonella ozzardi*	*Mansonella streptocerca*
Areas of endemicity	Sub-Saharan and North Africa, South America and the Caribbean	Central and South America and the Caribbean	Western and Central Africa
Arthropod vectors	*Culicoides* spp.	*Culicoides* spp., *Simulium amazonicum* (blackflies)	*Culicoides* spp. (midges)
Adult worm localisation	Serous cavities (pericardium, pleura, peritoneum), mesentery and retroperitoneum	Subcutaneous and connective tissues, lymphatic vessels and peritoneum	Skin of the trunk and upper shoulder
Microfilariae localisation	Blood	Blood and occasionally, skin	Skin

pericarditis, pleuritis and inflammatory granulomatous nodules surrounding dead adult worms.

- Although *M. ozzardi* infection is usually asymptomatic, some patients present with fever, pruritis, urticaria, lymphadenopathy and keratitis.
- The symptoms of *M. streptocerca* infection are similar to those of onchocerciasis, with patients presenting with dermatitis, hypopigmented macules and lymphadenopathy. However, dermatitis and pruritus predominate on the upper parts of the body, and the characteristic nodules of onchocerciasis are absent.

DIAGNOSIS

The diagnosis of mansonellosis is made by demonstrating microfilariae in the skin or peripheral blood depending upon the infecting species.

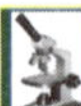

Lab diagnosis

- **Microscopy:** By visualising microfilariae
  - Peripheral blood examined for *M. perstans* and *M. ozzardi* (no periodicity)
  - Skin snips examined for *M. streptocerca* and occasionally, *M. ozzardi*
- **Other diagnostic parameters:**
  - Eosinophilia
  - Raised IgE

Microscopy

The microfilariae of *Mansonella* are unsheathed. They show **no periodicity** and may be demonstrated at any time in peripheral blood (Fig. 36.1a and b).

The microfilariae of *M. streptocerca* and *M. ozzardi* may be demonstrated in skin snips and need to be differentiated from the microfilariae of *Onchocerca volvulus* (see Table 33.3 and Fig. 33.2 in **Chapter 33**, *Wuchereria and Brugia*).

Other Diagnostic Parameters

Eosinophilia and raised IgE are common features in infected individuals.

TREATMENT

***Wolbachia* endosymbionts** are common in some strains of *M. perstans* and *M. ozzardi*. Doxycycline, 200 mg BDS × 6 weeks, which targets the *Wolbachia* has shown efficacy and safety and helps reduce microfilarial load.

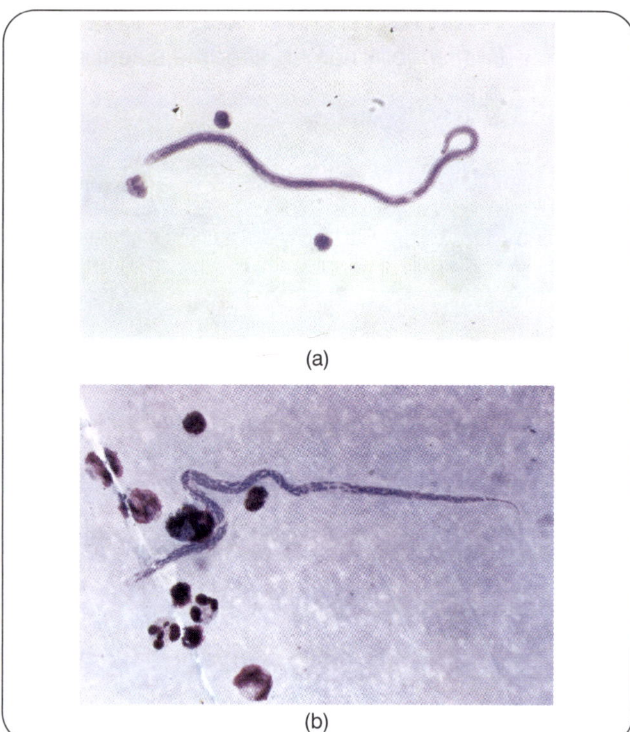

(a)

(b)

Fig. 36.1 Microfilaria of *Mansonella* spp.: (a) *M. perstans* and (b) *M. ozzardi* (*Source:* Centers for Disease Control and Prevention [CDC], Public Health Image Library [PHIL], Image IDs 1144 and 1142)

Drug of choice

- *Mansonella perstans:* Combination therapy of DEC plus mebendazole is preferred; thiabendazole is also effective in reducing microfilaremia; however, there are no definite guidelines.
- *Mansonella ozzardi:* Ivermectin, 150 µg/kg as a single dose has been shown to have good efficacy; optimal treatment not clear.
- *Mansonella streptocerca:* Ivermectin, 150 µg/kg as a single dose is effective; DEC, 6 mg/kg/day, orally in three doses × 12 days has also been used effectively.

PREVENTION AND CONTROL

The prevention and control measures for *Mansonella* are the same as those for *Onchocerca*.

DIROFILARIA

Zoonotic filarial infections are sometimes reported in human beings from across the globe. Among these infections is dirofilariasis, which is considered an emerging zoonotic disease. *Dirofilaria* species are parasites of animals which rarely infect humans. *D. immitis* (dog heartworm), *D. tenuis* (raccoon), *D. repens* (dog and cat), *D. ursi* (bear) and *D. striata* (wild cats) are some of the species known to infect humans. These infections are sometimes also reported in immunocompromised patients.

Humans acquire the infection by the **bite of a mosquito** containing the filariform larvae. Humans are non-permissive hosts, and the parasite undergoes incomplete development in human tissues.

CLINICAL FEATURES

There may be subconjunctival, intraocular, orbital and pulmonary lesions. The most common lesions caused by *D. immitis* are pulmonary nodules. Patients may present with cough, fever, chills, malaise and hemoptysis. When lodged in a pulmonary vessel, it may cause an infarct.

DIAGNOSIS

- The diagnosis of dirofilariasis is made by identifying the adult worms in excised material from the nodules (Fig. 36.2). Careful **histopathologic examination** of biopsies is important because the worm may be present in only a few sections and may be in different stages of disintegration.

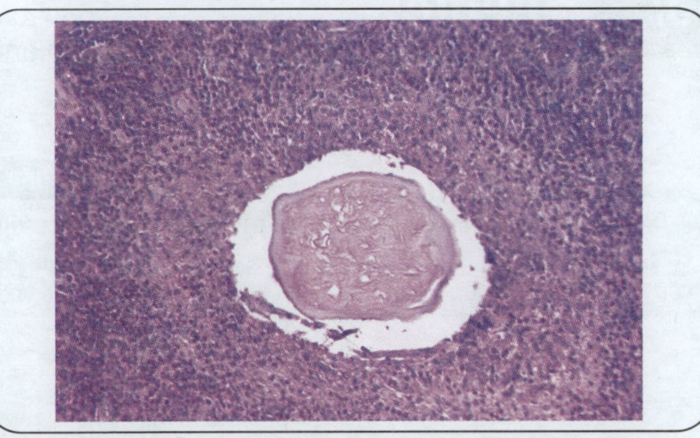

Fig. 36.2 *Dirofilaria* extracted from an eye specimen viewed in an H&E-stained section (*Source:* CDC, PHIL, Image ID 625)

- When the worm can be extracted, its **cuticular ridges** help in its identification.
- Microfilariae of *Dirofilaria* are not found in blood or tissue.
- The pulmonary nodules may appear as **coin lesions** on X-ray examination with sharply defined margins.
- Some patients have moderate eosinophilia.

TREATMENT

- **Surgical removal** of the worm is the only treatment available.
- No chemotherapeutic agents are effective against *Dirofilaria*.

QUESTIONS

1. Describe the clinical manifestations caused by *Mansonella streptocerca* infection.
2. Discuss the morphological differentiation of the different microfilariae seen in skin snips.

MULTIPLE CHOICE QUESTIONS

1. *Dirofilaria immitis* is also known as __________.
   a. African eye worm
   b. Guinea worm
   c. Dog heartworm
   d. Rat tapeworm
2. Which of the following microfilariae CANNOT be isolated from skin snips?
   a. *Mansonella streptocerca*
   b. *Mansonella ozzardi*
   c. *Onchocerca volvulus*
   d. *Mansonella perstans*
3. The ideal sample for the diagnosis of *Mansonella perstans* infection is ____________ :
   a. Blood sample to demonstrate microfilariae
   b. Blood sample to demonstrate adult worms
   c. Skin snip to demonstrate microfilariae
   d. Skin snip to demonstrate adult worms
4. For *Mansonella* infections, humans act as the ___________ :
   a. Definitive host
   b. First intermediate host
   c. Second intermediate host
   d. Paratenic host

CHAPTER 37

Taenia

(*Taenia* from [Latin] *tainia* = belt, band and *saginata* = fed, thick; *solium* from *sosl* [Arabic] = chain)

Case Study and Learning Goals

A 15-year-old male presents with chronic pain abdomen, indigestion and loss of weight over the last two years. His history reveals the occasional consumption of beef and passage of white, motile and rectangular worm-like segments. What would be your differential diagnosis? How would you approach the laboratory diagnosis in this case? How would you treat this patient?

INTRODUCTION

Taenia are tape-like worms of the phylum Platyhelminthes (flatworms), the adults of which live in the intestines of humans (the definitive host), and the larval forms of which are found in intermediate hosts as presented in Table 37.1. The three major species of this genus are *Taenia solium* (**pork tapeworm**), *T. saginata* (**beef tapeworm**) and the recently described species, *T. asiatica* (**Taiwan** ***Taenia*** or **Asian** ***Taenia***).

Knowledge of the pork tapeworm has been traced back to ancient times. The earliest description of the disease was found in the Egyptian Ebers papyrus which dates back to 1550 BC. However, the infection in humans was first observed only in 1558 AD by Gessner. In the later centuries, the two species *T. solium* and *T. saginata* were biologically differentiated, and their two-host life cycle was elucidated. *T. asiatica* was discovered as recently as in 1993 in Taiwan by Keeseon S. Eom and Han-Jong Rim.

The **adults of these worms cause intestinal taeniasis** which may present with mild gastrointestinal and nutritional disturbances in the host. The **larval forms of** ***T. solium*** **cause cysticercosis**, a far more common public health problem than intestinal taeniasis.

T. multiceps and ***T. crassiceps*** are less important species of the genus and may cause occasional infections in humans.

EPIDEMIOLOGY

The *Taenia* spp. are ubiquitous parasites across the globe, with about 100 million people infected with *T. solium* or *T. saginata*.

Table 37.1 Host preferences of human *Taenia* species

Species	Definitive hosts	Intermediate hosts
T. saginata	Humans	Cattle
T. solium	Humans	Pigs, dogs and humans
T. asiatica	Humans	Pigs, cattle and goats

- ***T. saginata*** is the most widely distributed human *Taenia*. It is highly endemic (with a prevalence rate of 10%) in some African countries, the Eastern Mediterranean and parts of the erstwhile USSR.
- ***T. solium*** is endemic in most developing countries including Central and South America, sub-Saharan Africa, South-East Asia, India and the Western Pacific due to poor sanitation and animal husbandry practices. In the United States of America and Europe, *T. solium* cysticercosis is considered an emerging disease due to increased immigration and international travel.
- ***T. asiatica*** infections have been reported from Korea, Taiwan, Indonesia, China, Malaysia, Philippines and Thailand, and is increasingly being recognised from other regions such as Nepal and India.

Risk Factors

Open defecation, lack of education, poor personal hygiene, the presence of infected pigs or cattle in the vicinity and proximity to tapeworm carriers contribute to the transmission of the infection.

MORPHOLOGY

Adult Worm

Tapeworms (Fig. 37.1a–d) are flat, elongated, white to greyish worms that measure up to several meters in length. They reside in the intestine of the definitive host. These worms lack a body cavity and a circulatory system. The adults of the three species can be differentiated based on several features (Table 37.2). The following are the morphological features of the adult worm:

- The **scolex** or the head has muscular suckers (**acetabula**) for attachment to the host's intestinal wall (Fig. 37.1d). There may be a round, retractable **rostellum** (Fig. 37.1b) on the head with two rows of 25–30 hooks, depending on the species.

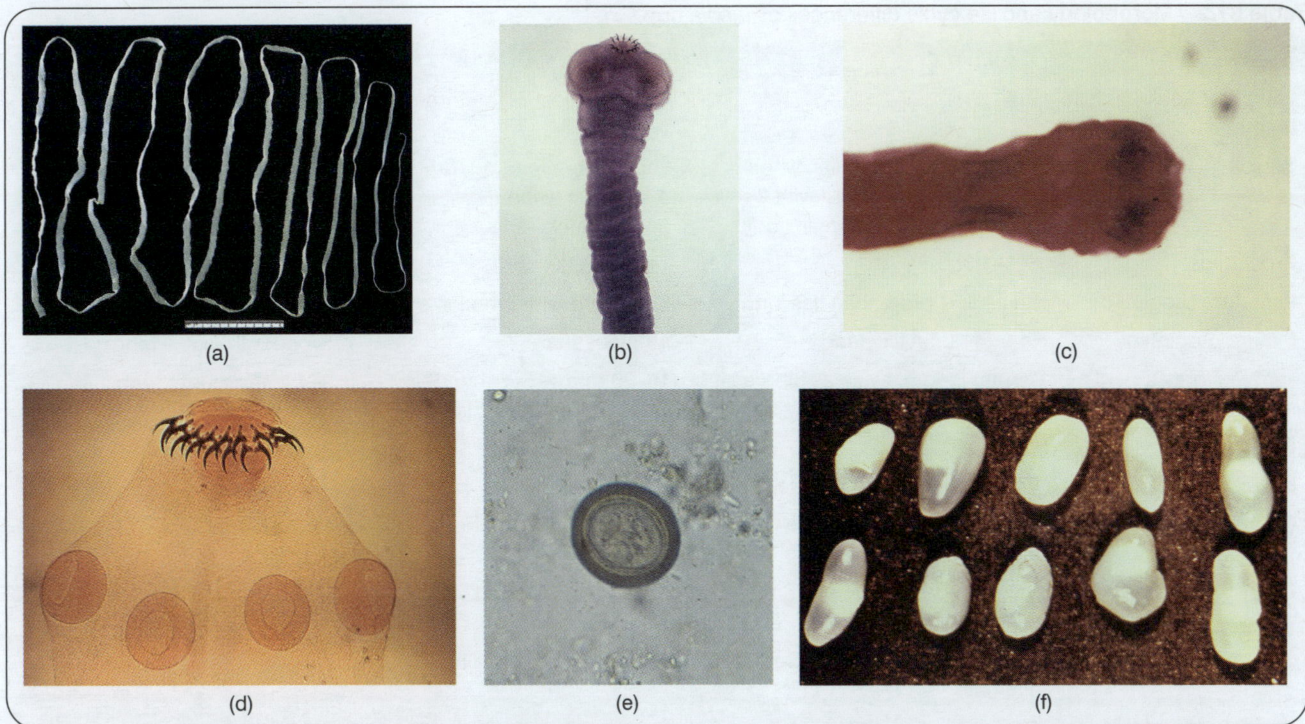

Fig. 37.1 Features of tapeworms: (a) *Taenia saginata* measuring about 4 metres in length, (b) *T. solium* scolex with a rostellum bearing the hooks, (c) *T. saginata* scolex without rostellum and hooklets, (d) *T. solium* scolex with 4 suckers and 2 rows of hooks (*Source [a-d]:* Centers for Disease Control and Prevention [CDC], Public Health Image Library [PHIL], Image IDs 5260, 14377, 10857, 5262), (e) egg of *Taenia* spp.—spherical with a thick, radially striated brown shell (*Source:* CDC, DPDx) and (f) cysticerci (larvae) of *Taenia solium* (*Source:* CDC, PHIL, Image ID 17539)

- The head is followed by a short neck which gives rise to proglottids or segments.
- The **proglottids** form the **strobila**. The initial segments are immature and become mature posteriorly as the sexual organs develop. Fertilisation may either be hermaphroditic or facilitated by another worm, following which the terminal segments become gravid or egg-laden. The eggs are released when the uterine wall ruptures during the shedding of the gravid proglottids. The proglottids are passed in stool either singly or in groups of three or four.
- The body wall (tegument) has microvilli-like structures that facilitate **absorptive nutrition** from the host's intestine.
- The movement of the worm is facilitated by two layers of muscles lying beneath the tegument, the outer circular and the inner longitudinal layer.
- The nervous system consists of a central nerve ring connected to the nerves traversing posteriorly.
- The excretory system comprising lateral canals is made up of **flame cells**. The excreta, which is carried through the canalicular network, is collected and released at the terminal segments.
- The reproductive system is **hermaphroditic (monoecious)**, with both male and female organs present in each segment (please refer to **Chapter 22**, *Helminths—Introduction and Classification*).

Eggs

The fertilised egg is **spherical** or slightly oval and light brown and measures **31–43 µm** in size. It has a radially striated, thick shell (Fig. 37.1e). Each egg contains a fully developed embryonic **oncosphere** or the **hexacanth** larval stage with six hooklets. Once shed, the eggs remain viable in soil for several weeks and contaminate water and vegetation.

Larvae

The larvae (Fig. 37.1f), which are **the infective forms**, **exist as milky white bladder-like cyst forms (cysticercus)** in the muscles or viscera of the intermediate host. These measure 8–10 × 5 mm in size and have a dense white body representing the head invaginated into the bladder.

LIFE CYCLE (Fig. 37.2a and b)

The various stages in the life cycle of *Taenia* species are as follows:

Table 37.2 Morphology and life cycle differences of *Taenia* spp.

Species	*T. solium*	*T. saginata*	*T. asiatica*
Length of adult parasite (in metres)	2–4	4–10; longest of the three	4–8
Scolex	Small – 1 mm, globular, with 4 suckers and rostellum with 2 rows of 25–30 large and small hooks	Large – 1–2 mm, quadrate, with 4 suckers, without rostellum and hooklets	Similar to *T. saginata*, but has rostellum and 2 rows of rudimentary hooklets
Proglottids	800–1,000	1,000–2,000	<1,000
Immature proglottids	Small and wider than it is long	Small and wider than it is long	Small and wider than it is long
Mature proglottids	Broader than it is long	Almost square	Broader than it is long
Terminal gravid proglottids	12 mm length, twice as long as it is broad	16–20 mm × 5–7 mm (3–4 times longer than it is broad)	3–4 times longer than it is broad
Eggs	Oval, light brown and 31–43 μm in size	Similar to *T. solium*	Similar to *T. solium*
Expulsion of proglottids	Expelled in chains of 5 or 6	Expelled singly	Expelled singly
Gravid uterus	7–13 thick lateral branches on each side	14–32 lateral branches	16–32 lateral branches
Ovary	Single and bi-lobed with an accessory lobe	Single and bi-lobed	Single and bi-lobed
Genital pore	Sub-median, unilateral, irregularly alternate	Lateral, irregularly alternate	Lateral, irregularly alternate
Vaginal sphincter	Absent	Small, well-developed	Similar to *T. saginata*
Larva	*Cysticercus cellulosae*, present in pig and also in humans	*Cysticercus bovis*, present in cattle but not in humans	*Cysticercus viscerotropica*, present in pigs
Tissue preference (larvae)	All tissues, especially the skeletal muscles, heart and brain	Skeletal muscles	Viscera, liver and lungs
Infective form	For intestinal taeniasis – larva (*Cysticercus cellulosae*) For cysticercosis – egg	Larva (*Cysticercus bovis*)	Larva (*Cysticercus viscerotropica*)
Mode of transmission	For intestinal taeniasis – ingestion of contaminated pork For cysticercosis – ingestion of contaminated food or water, autoinfection by fecal-oral route/ reverse peristalsis	Ingestion of contaminated beef	Ingestion of contaminated pork/beef

Definitive hosts: Human beings
Intermediate hosts: Mammals, depending on the tapeworm species (refer to Table 37.1)

Human cycle (intestinal): Humans are primarily infected by the **ingestion of cysticercus larvae** present in undercooked meat of infected intermediate hosts—cattle and pig. Once in the intestine, the scolex **evaginates**, **attaches** to the mucosa with the help of its suckers and hooklets, and **develops into an adult** worm in 5–12 weeks. There may be single or multiple worms in the intestine which start producing eggs on sexual maturation. These eggs and proglottids are shed in the host's feces.

Cattle/Pig cycle: The eggs, when ingested by the intermediate host while grazing, **hatch** in the first part of the small intestine to liberate oncospheres. These **oncospheres penetrate** the intestinal wall to **enter the mesenteric circulation** and are distributed throughout the body. They become **lodged in various organs** to develop into the cyst forms, preferentially in the muscles and nervous system of pigs (porcine cysticerci), as is the case with *T. solium* and the muscles of cattle (bovine cysticerci), as is the case with *T. saginata*. These cysts can persist in the flesh for many months until they are **ingested** by humans to continue the life cycle and become adult worms in the human intestine.

Human cycle (larval): Alternately, humans may also act as intermediate hosts and harbour *T. solium* cysticerci (**human cysticercosis**). In this case, humans may get exposed to the eggs via ingestion of **contaminated food or water**; or by **exogenous autoinfection**, wherein individuals harbouring the adult worm in their intestine release eggs in their feces and subsequently ingest them by the fecal-oral route; or by **endogenous autoinfection**,

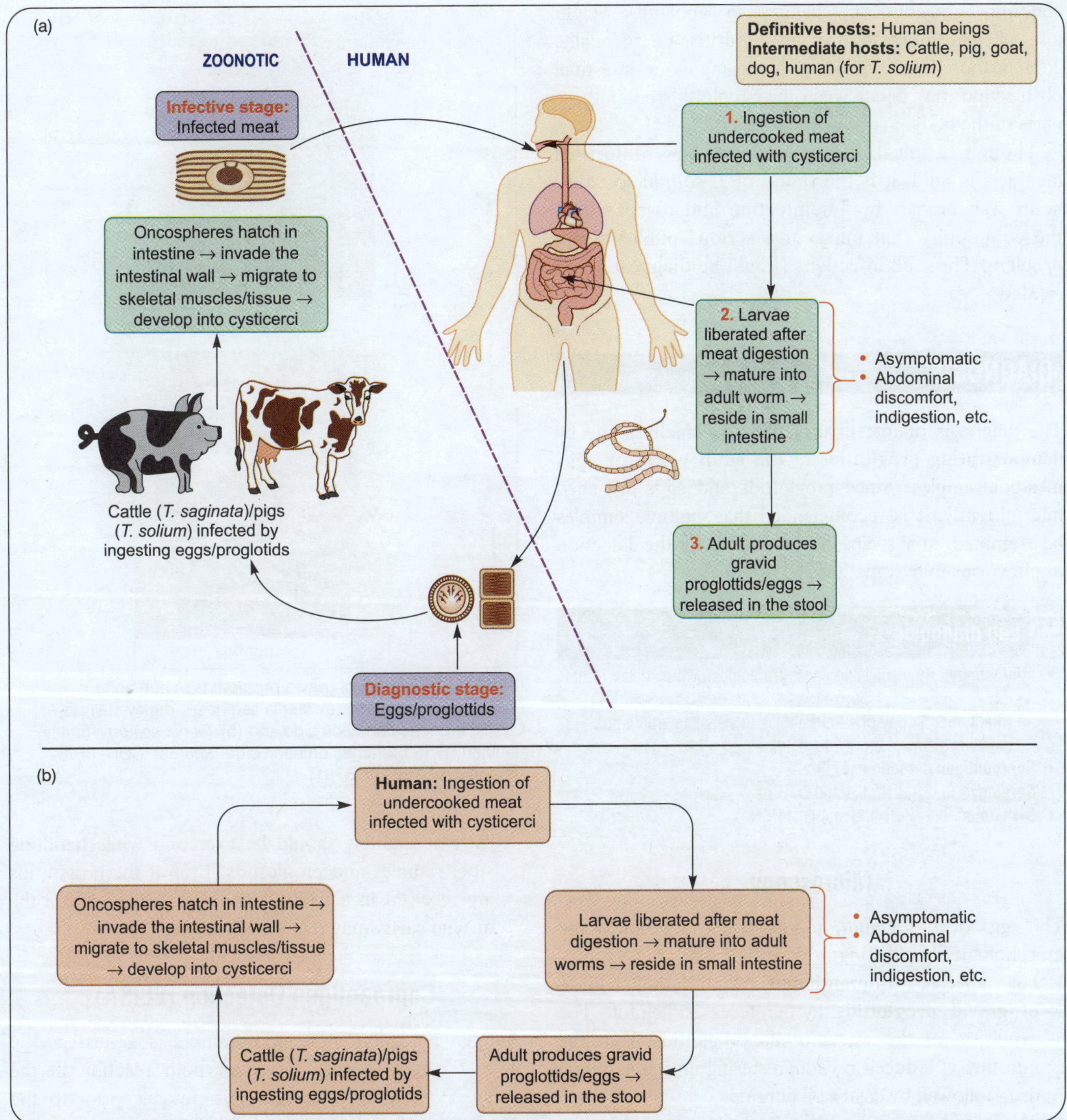

Fig. 37.2 Life cycle of *Taenia saginata/solium/asiatica* with humans as the definitive host: (a) detailed and (b) schematic

wherein the eggs are regurgitated into the stomach by reverse peristalsis. *T. solium* is the only *Taenia* species that is capable of causing cysticercosis in humans (refer to **Chapter 40**, *Cysticercosis*).

PATHOGENESIS

The adult worm attaching to the intestinal wall may cause irritation at the site of attachment. The worm does not affect the nutrition of the host unless the person is already malnourished. There may be mild eosinophilia and raised IgE levels.

CLINICAL FEATURES

Most people harbouring the adult *Taenia* are asymptomatic. When symptomatic, there may be nausea, abdominal discomfort, changes in appetite, weight loss, chronic indigestion or anal pruritis. Occasionally, complications like appendicitis, cholangitis or intestinal obstruction may occur when the proglottids enter these parts of the body.

Though clinical disease caused by intestinal taeniasis is mild, it is the ability of *T. solium* to cause neurocysticercosis by autoinfection and to spread to the community that makes it a serious public health problem. Thus, all infections should be diagnosed and treated.

DIAGNOSIS

The diagnosis of intestinal taeniasis is chiefly made by **demonstrating proglottids of the adult worm or eggs** in stool samples. Since proglottids and eggs are shed intermittently, it is recommended that multiple samples be examined. Anal swabs like those used for the detection of pinworms may sometimes be useful.

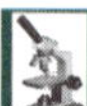

Lab diagnosis

- **Microscopy:** By visualising eggs, proglottids or the scolex of the worm
  - Direct microscopy of stool samples to visualise proglottids
  - India ink staining of gravid proglottids
- **Coproantigen detection:** ELISA
- **Serology:** ELISA, IHA, IFA and EITB
- **DNA detection:** PCR and real-time PCR

Microscopy

The **eggs** of *T. saginata*, *T. solium* and *T. asiatica* are morphologically indistinguishable (Fig. 37.1e).

- **For species differentiation, the demonstration of gravid proglottids** in the feces is helpful. The expulsion of the worm or its proglottids from the intestine is induced by administering an anthelmintic drug followed by castor oil purging.
- The lateral uterine branches in the proglottids can be stained by **injecting India ink through the genital pore**. Then, the number of branches can be counted. The number is generally >14 in *T. saginata* and <13 in *T. solium* (Table 37.2) (Fig. 37.3a and b).
- Rarely, the scolex is expelled in the patient's feces. This can help in species identification since *T. solium* has armed rostellum with hooks, whereas *T. saginata* has neither and *T. asiatica* has a rostellum but no hooks/only rudimentary hooks.
- The eggs and proglottids of *T. solium* are infectious and can potentially cause cysticercosis if ingested. Thus, extreme caution should be exercised while handling stool samples and proglottids. Even if the proglottids are received in a fixative, the eggs lodged inside the uterine cavity may remain infectious.

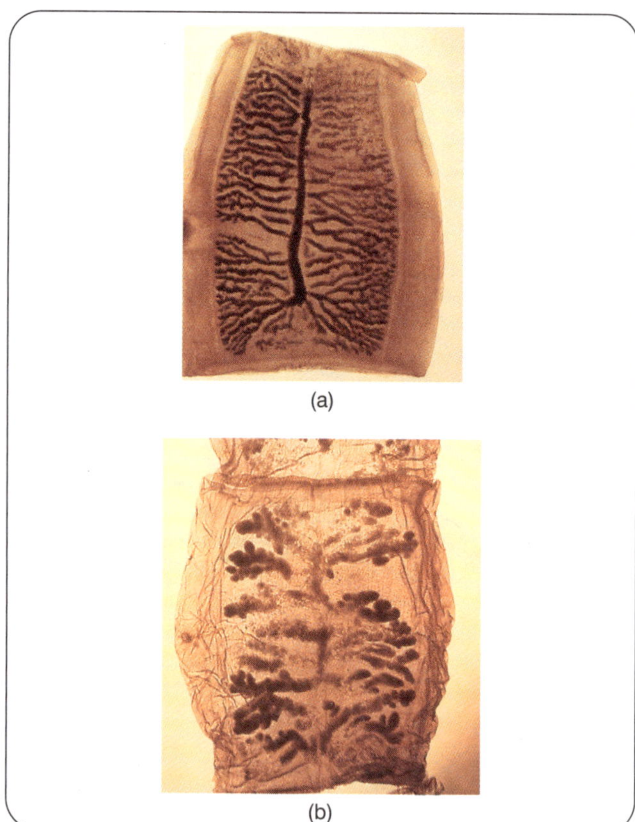

Fig. 37.3 Features of gravid proglottids of human tapeworms stained with India ink: (a) *Taenia saginata*—darkly stained, 15–20 branches on each side and (b) *Taenia solium*—darkly stained, 7–13 branches on each side (*Source:* CDC, PHIL, Image IDs 5259 and 5261)

Coproantigen Detection (ELISA)

Antigen detection in a stool sample is genus-specific with *T. saginata* and *T. solium* both reacting in the assay. Coproantigen detection is possible prior to the maturation of the worm's reproductive organs and thus, is independent of the presence of eggs. This makes it a very useful method of identifying carriers. High concentrations of coproantigens are present for about 1–2 weeks after treatment.

Antibody Detection

Serological tests for detecting antibodies are generally not used to diagnose intestinal taeniasis but play an important role in the diagnosis of cysticercosis. Indirect hemagglutination (IHA), indirect immunofluorescence

(IFA) and ELISA have been used for the demonstration of antibodies. Enzyme-linked immunoelectrotransfer blot (EITB) assay has been shown to have 95% sensitivity and 100% specificity.

Nucleic Acid-Based Detection

PCR and DNA probes may be used to detect as well as differentiate between various species and genotypes of *Taenia*. Different targets such as *ITS1*, *cox1* and *nad5* genes have been used.

TREATMENT

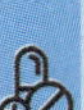

Drugs of choice

- *Niclosamide:* 2 g as a single dose for adults
- *Praziquantel:* 5–10 mg/kg as a single dose for both children and adults

With *T. solium* tapeworms, there is a potential for autoinfection leading to cysticercosis. Therefore, whenever any *Taenia* eggs are detected, treatment should be initiated without delay.

PREVENTION AND CONTROL

- Tapeworm carriers are a source of infection for themselves and the community. Thus, the identification and treatment of such carriers is very important.
- **Beef and pork should be inspected for cysticerci** before it is deemed ready for consumption.
- **Meat hygiene** should be practised. This consists of thoroughly cooking meat (at >65°C × 5 minutes or until it loses its pink colour) or freezing meat at –7°C for 6 days or –20°C for 24 hours. Pickling of meat is not effective in killing cysticerci.
- Proper **sanitary disposal of human feces** is important. Cattle and pigs should not be allowed to feed or graze on soil polluted with human feces or sewage.
- Hands should be thoroughly washed with soap and water after handling raw meat or defecating.

Questions

1. Describe the life cycle, pathogenesis and laboratory diagnosis of *Taenia solium/Taenia saginata*.
2. Discuss the laboratory diagnosis of intestinal taeniasis.
3. Discuss the management and preventive strategies for taeniasis and cysticercosis.
4. Differentiate between *Taenia solium*, *Taenia saginata* and *Taenia asiatica*.

Multiple Choice Questions

1. Humans are ________________ hosts in the natural life cycle of *Taenia solium*.
   a. Carrier b. Amplifier
   c. Definitive d. Reservoir
2. The reproductive system of *Taenia saginata* is ________ :
   a. Parthenogenetic b. Diecious
   c. Monoecious d. None of the above
3. The oncosphere of *Taenia solium* has ________ hooklets.
   a. Two b. Four
   c. Six d. Eight
4. *Taenia solium* eggs cannot be differentiated from ___________ eggs.
   a. *Diphyllobothrium latum*
   b. *Taenia saginata*
   c. *Hymenolepis nana*
   d. *Fasciola hepatica*
5. Gravid proglottids of *Taenia solium* and *Taenia saginata* can be stained with ________ :
   a. Iodine
   b. Calcofluor white
   c. India ink
   d. Trypan blue
6. The number of lateral uterine branches in gravid proglottids of *Taenia saginata* is ________ :
   a. 8–12
   b. 10–22
   c. 14–32
   d. 18–38

Chapter 38 Diphyllobothrium

([Form Greek] *di* = two + *phyllos* = leaf + *bothrium* = groove)

Case Study and Learning Goals

A 25-year-old male presents with megaloblastic anemia and pain abdomen. He has a history of eating pickled fish quite often. What are the parasitic causes of anemia? How would you approach the laboratory diagnosis in this case? How would you treat this patient?

INTRODUCTION

Diphyllobothrium latum (human **broad tapeworm** or **fish tapeworm**) is the largest parasite to inhabit the human intestine. It is a pseudophyllidean tapeworm characterised by the presence of a scolex with two atypical sucking organs called **bothria** instead of the four suckers typically seen in cyclophyllidean tapeworms (*Taenia*, *Echinococcus* and *Hymenolepis*). The most common species associated with human infections is *D. latum*.

D. latum has been described in classical ancient medical writings such as the Ebers papyrus, which dates back to 1500 BC, as well as the writings of Celsus and Avicenna. The disease caused by this entity was first described by the Swiss physician Felix Plater in the early 17th century, and the proglottids of the worm were first described in detail by the Swiss botanist Charles Bonnet in 1750. The role played by fish and copepods in the parasite's life cycle was elucidated by G. A. Braun, C. A. Janicki and E. Rosen in the late 19th and early 20th centuries.

EPIDEMIOLOGY

Although prevalent across the globe, human infections caused by *Diphyllobothrium* tapeworms are generally **associated with cold waters** and are more frequently reported from the Scandinavian region, western Europe, sub-Alpine areas, Swiss, Italian and French lakes, the Great Lakes of North America, Canada, Alaska, Japan and Russia. It is rarely reported from India.

Risk Factors

Diphyllobothriasis is associated with the cultural habit of eating raw, smoked, pickled or poorly cooked fish. The infection is common among fishermen. Diphyllobothriasis is also known as the **'Jewish housewives' disease'** because housewives would traditionally taste dishes while preparing them and acquire the infection in the process. In endemic areas, the **transmission of the disease is maintained by dogs, cats, foxes and other fish-eating animals.**

MORPHOLOGY

Adult Worm

D. latum is an ivory-coloured worm, ranging in length from **3–10 meters**. Its body consists of a head (scolex), a neck and several segments (proglottids). It is the **largest parasite found in humans**.

- The scolex is elongated and **spoon-shaped**, measuring 3 × 1 mm. The head has two shallow sucking grooves (**bothria**)—ventral and dorsal (Fig. 38.1a). Unlike cyclophyllidean worms, diphyllobothria do not have a rostellum or hooklets.
- The head is followed by a short neck.
- The adult worm's body has over 3,000 segments (proglottids). The mature gravid proglottids are wider than they are long, measuring 3 × 11 mm (which is why they are called **broad tapeworms**). Their reproductive structures are located in the central part of the proglottid in a conspicuous **rosette-like** structure which helps in the worm's identification (Fig. 38.1b). The uterine pore is situated mid-ventrally.

Eggs

The fertilised egg is **yellow-brown, broadly oval** and measures **60–70 × 40–50 µm** in size. It is **operculated and bile-stained,** with an inconspicuous **knob at the posterior end** (Fig. 38.1c). It is unembryonated when laid. Embryonation occurs in water, and the coracidium is released in about two weeks. The eggs can be confused with those of *Paragonimus westermani*.

Larvae

The first-stage larva, which is called the **coracidium,** contains the oncosphere with hooklets. It swims freely with the help of cilia. The second-stage larva, which is called

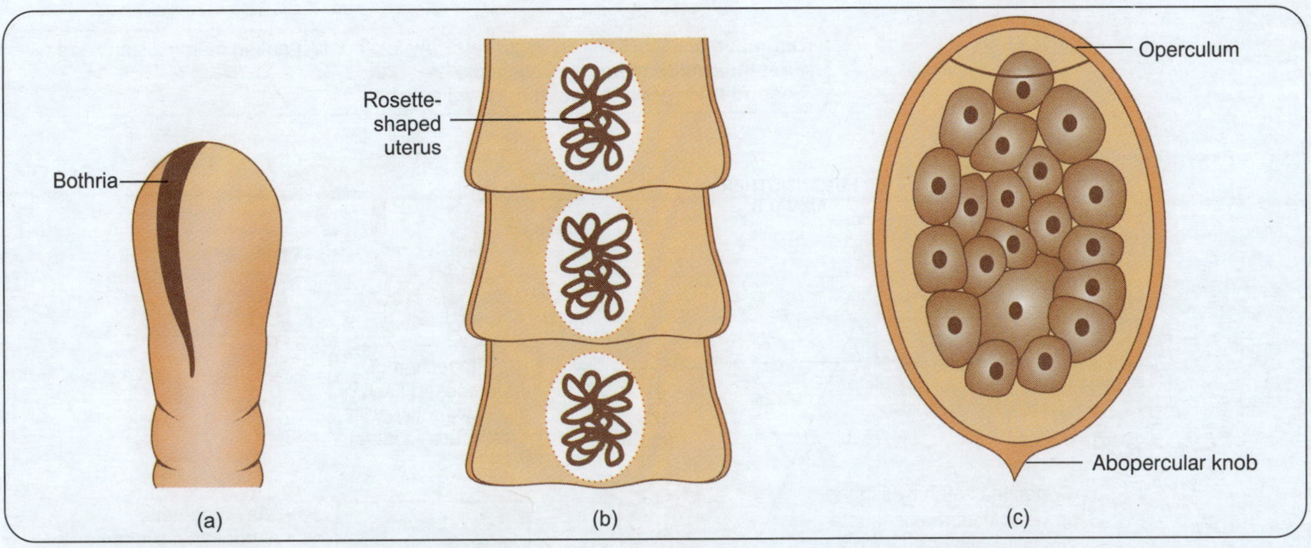

Fig. 38.1 Line diagrams of *Diphyllobothrium latum*: (a) scolex with two grooves, (b) broad proglottids with rosette-shaped uteri and (c) operculated egg with a small abopercular knob

the **procercoid**, measures 0.5 mm in size and is infective to fish. The third-stage larva—the **plerocercoid—**is infective to humans. It is 10–20 × 2–3 mm in size and has a partly invaginated scolex.

LIFE CYCLE (Fig. 38.2a and b)

> **Definitive hosts:** Humans, dogs, cats, foxes, other fish-eating mammals and birds
> **First intermediate hosts:** Copepods
> **Second intermediate hosts:** Freshwater fish

The various stages in the life cycle of *D. latum* are as follows:

Human cycle: Humans, **the definitive hosts**, acquire the infection by ingesting raw, poorly cooked or pickled freshwater fish containing the **plerocercoid larva**. The development after ingestion is as follows:

- The larva develops into an adult worm in the ileum or jejunum, where it attaches to the mucosa with the help of its bothria. It attains maturity and thereby, the egg-laying capacity, in about four weeks. The adult lays unembryonated fertilised eggs which are released in the host's feces. The adult worms can live in the human host for many years.
- The egg release leads to the degeneration and detachment of proglottids; this is known as **pseudoapolysis**.

Aquatic cycle: The eggs need water and a suitable temperature of 16–20°C for the development of the coracidium.

- On exposure to sunlight, the egg hatches to release the coracidium, which then swims freely with the help of cilia for about 12 hours, until it is ingested by suitable species of copepods (*Cyclops* and *Diaptomus*), the **first intermediate hosts**.
- The oncosphere is liberated in the intestine of the copepod. It penetrates the intestinal wall to reach the hemocoel, where it develops into a procercoid larva.
- When the copepod is are eaten by a **fish (like pike, perch, lawyer, salmon and trout)**, the **second intermediate host**, the procercoid larva penetrates its intestinal wall and grows into a plerocercoid larva which is infective to humans. It may stay in the gut wall, body cavity or the muscles of the fish.

If the infected fish is eaten by a larger fish, the plerocercoid larvae penetrate the intestine of the second host and survive there without developing further. Such a host, i.e., one in which the infective stage may accumulate but not develop, is called a **paratenic host**.

PATHOGENESIS

D. latum is associated with megaloblastic anemia which occurs due to competitive absorption, wherein the worm competes with the host for the absorption of vitamin B12. The reason for such anemia may also be the dissociation of vitamin B12 from the intrinsic factor in the host's intestine, resulting in decreased absorption by the host.

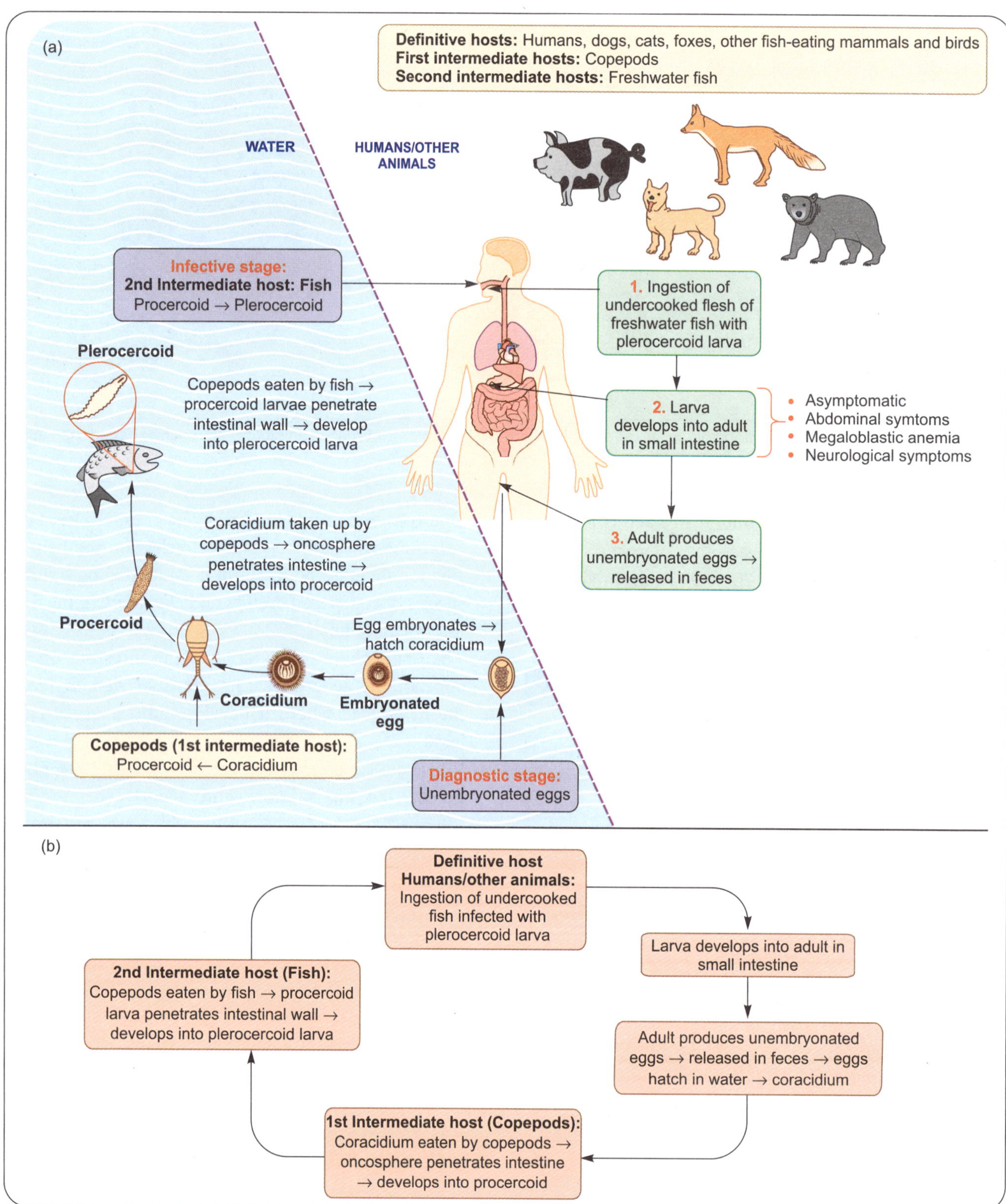

Fig. 38.2 Life cycle of *Diphyllobothrium latum*: (a) detailed and (b) schematic

CLINICAL FEATURES

Asymptomatic infections: The majority of infected individuals remain asymptomatic.

Symptomatic infections: About one-fifth of those infected may be symptomatic. These patients may report fatigue, diarrhea, dizziness, weakness, numbness in the limbs and a hunger sensation. There may be intestinal obstruction, abdominal pain and anemia. About 40% of infected people have reduced vitamin B12 but <2% develop anemia.

Heavy or long-term infections with *D. latum* may cause **megaloblastic anemia**. In persons who have a hereditary or racial predisposition, *D. latum* precipitates **Addisonian anemia (pernicious)**; this is especially seen in Finland. Pernicious anemia can cause permanent damage to the nerves and other organs if it is left untreated for a long period—neurological symptoms such as weakness, numbness, paresthesia, deficits in movement and co-ordination and impairment of deep sensation may occur.

DIAGNOSIS

The diagnosis of *Diphyllobothrium* infection and the detection of the sources of such human infection are important with respect to epidemiology. A stool sample is the specimen of choice.

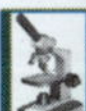

Lab diagnosis

- **Microscopy:** By visualising eggs or proglottids
- **Other diagnostic parameters:**
  - Mild to moderate eosinophilia
  - Evidence of megaloblastic anemia and B12 deficiency

Microscopy

The diagnosis of diphyllobothriasis is made by demonstrating the characteristic **eggs** or **proglottids** of the parasite in fecal samples (Fig. 38.3a and b). The proglottids are passed out in chains measuring a few inches to several feet and are identified by their broad shape and rosette-shaped central reproductive apparatus. *Diphyllobothrium* eggs may be confused with those of *P. westermani*. The difference between the two is that the latter have distinct opercular shoulders and marked thickening at the end opposite to the operculum (abopercular end), whereas *Diphyllobothrium* eggs have an indistinct operculum and a small knob-like structure at their abopercular end.

Nucleic Acid-Based Detection

PCR assays may be helpful for epidemiological studies to track the source of infection.

Other Diagnostic Parameters

- There may be mild to moderate eosinophilia.

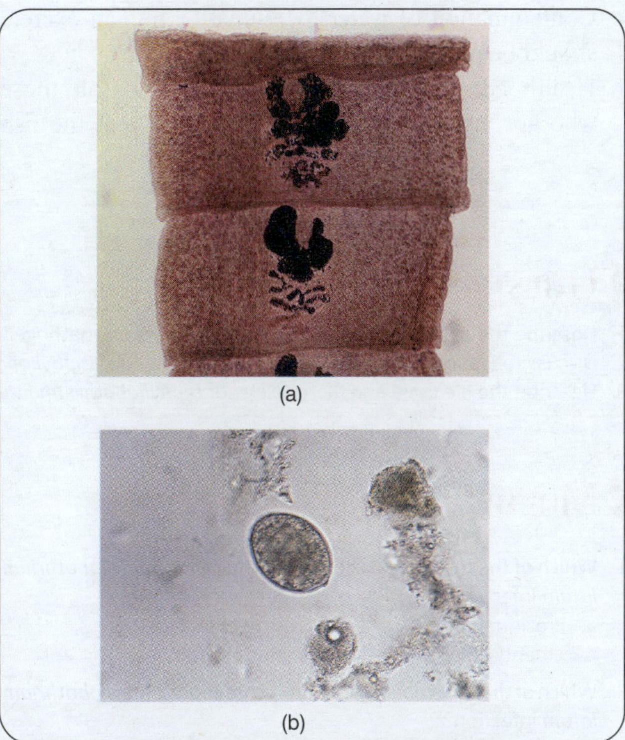

Fig. 38.3 *Diphyllobothrium latum*: (a) stained gravid proglottids and (b) oval operculated egg with a small knob (*Source:* Centers for Disease Control and Prevention [CDC], Public Health Image Library [PHIL], Image IDs 1516 and 1541)

- There is evidence of megaloblastic, macrocytic anemia, with increased MCV (mean corpuscular volume) and MCHC (mean corpuscular hemoglobin concentration).

TREATMENT

Drug of choice

- *Praziquantel:* 5–10 mg/kg body weight as a single oral dose for both adults and children

Alternate drug

- *Niclosamide:* For adults, as a single dose of 2 g (4 tablets chewed thoroughly); for children <6 years, 50 mg/kg as a single dose

Parenteral vitamin B12 should be given if B12 deficiency is documented.

PREVENTION AND CONTROL

- All freshwater **fish should be thoroughly cooked**.
- Fish intended for raw or semi-raw consumption should be blast frozen to –35°C for 15 hours or frozen to –20°C or below for seven days.

- Contamination of water by animal or human excreta should be prevented.
- Health education should be provided for all those who are involved in the various segments of the fish industry including consumers, fishermen and sellers. Rigorous sanitary inspections of fish products should be performed before they are transported across the globe.

Questions

1. Describe the parasitic etiology of anemia. Discuss the pathogenesis of anemia caused by *Diphyllobothrium latum.*
2. Discuss the laboratory diagnosis and management of *Diphyllobothrium latum* infection.
3. Describe the life cycle and morphology of *Diphyllobothrium latum.*

Multiple Choice Questions

1. Which of the following is the drug of choice for *Diphyllobothrium latum* infection?
   a. Praziquantel b. Ivermectin
   c. Albendazole d. Pyrantel pamoate
2. Which of the following statements is true about *Diphyllobothrium latum* infection?
   a. It requires one definitive and one intermediate host.
   b. It causes megaloblastic anemia.
   c. It is diagnosed by the demonstration of operculated eggs in feces.
   d. Fish is its definitive host.
3. Which parasite is known as fish tapeworm?
   a. *Taenia solium*
   b. *Taenia asiatica*
   c. *Diphyllobothrium latum*
   d. *Hymenolepis nana*
4. Which is the second intermediate host for *Diphyllobothrium latum*?
   a. Human being
   b. Fish
   c. Snail
   d. *Cyclops*
5. Humans acquire *Diphyllobothrium* infection by ____________ :
   a. Ingestion of raw or poorly cooked freshwater fish
   b. Ingestion of raw vegetables contaminated with eggs
   c. Ingestion of raw vegetables contaminated with larva
   d. Any of these

Chapter 39

Hymenolepis

([From Greek] *hymen* = thin membrane + *lepis* = cover)

Case Study and Learning Goals

A 10-year-old child presents with diffuse abdominal pain. His differential blood count shows eosinophilia and stool examination shows oval hexacanth eggs with polar filaments. What are the parasitic causes of eosinophilia? What are the modes of transmission of this infection?

INTRODUCTION

Hymenolepis (Rodentolepis) nana **(dwarf tapeworm)** is considered to be the most common tapeworm globally. It was first described in 1845 by Félix Dujardin in rats and mice. Though the reassignment of this parasite to the genus *Rodentolepis* is being considered, we are using the name *Hymenolepis nana* in this chapter.

H. diminuta (**rat tapeworm**) is larger than *H. nana* and rarely colonises humans.

HYMENOLEPIS NANA

EPIDEMIOLOGY

H. nana is cosmopolitan in distribution. It is the only human tapeworm that does not need an intermediate host and is transmitted from person to person. Children are more commonly infected than adults. The infection is highly prevalent in South Africa, southern Europe, Latin America, the Middle East and India. Severe infections are seen in malnourished and immunosuppressed individuals.

MORPHOLOGY

Adult Worm

It is the smallest tapeworm to be found in humans, ranging in size from **5–50 mm**. Other morphological features of the adult worm are as follows:

- The scolex is round, with four cup-shaped suckers and a prominent retractable rostellum with a single circle of small hooklets.
- The head is followed by a long and slender neck.
- The worm's body comprises around 200 segments (proglottids). These proglottids, which are arranged in an overlapping fashion, are known as **craspedote proglottids**. The mature gravid proglottids are four times wider than they are long. The genital pore of the adult worm opens up on the lateral border (Fig. 39.1a).

Egg

The egg is **round or oval, measures 30–45 μm** in size and has two membranes. The inner membrane has two polar thickenings, from which arise **4–8 polar filaments** (Fig. 39.1b). The egg is infectious when laid.

Larva

The larva is called a **cysticercoid.** It is a solid structure with a fully developed scolex.

LIFE CYCLE (Fig. 39.2)

> **Definitive hosts:** Human beings and rodents
> **Intermediate hosts:** Beetles and fleas

H. nana follows a different life cycle pattern than other tapeworms because it primarily **requires only one definitive host (direct life cycle)**, a human being or a rodent—either a mouse or a rat. However, beetles, fleas or other similar insects occasionally act as the **intermediate hosts (indirect life cycle)**.

Humans acquire the infection **feco-orally** by the **hand-to-mouth route**. In rare cases, they may **ingest the eggs directly** from the environment through contaminated

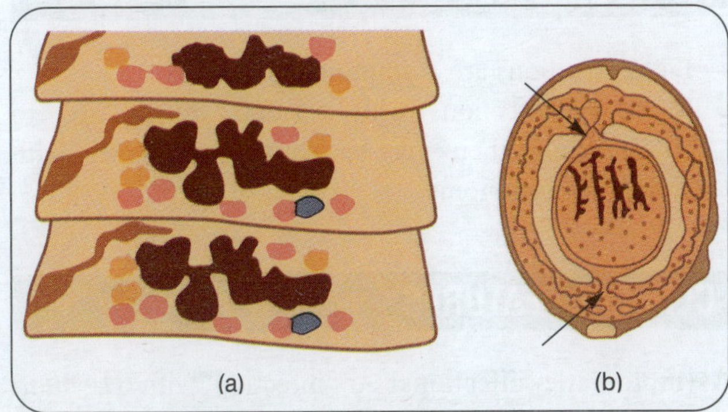

Fig. 39.1 Line diagrams of *Hymenolepis nana*: (a) overlapping proglottids and (b) egg with polar filaments (arrows)

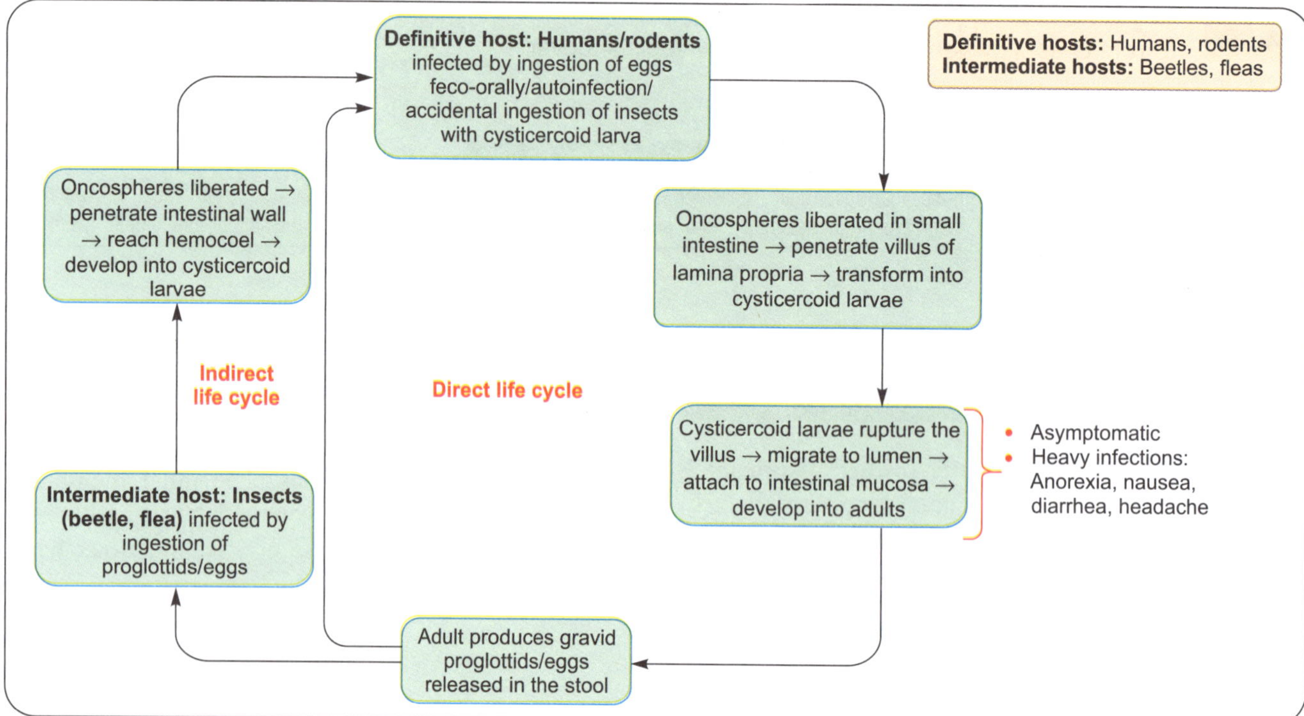

Fig. 39.2 Life cycle of *Hymenolepis nana* (schematic)

food and water or accidentally ingest infected insects. Once ingested, the oncosphere is liberated in the small intestine, where it penetrates a villus of the lamina propria, and subsequently transforms into a cysticercoid larva in four days. It then ruptures from the villus and attaches itself to the intestinal mucosa to develop into the adult worm in about 30 days. The sexually mature adults lay eggs which are shed in the environment along with the host's feces. The eggs are susceptible to environmental conditions and desiccate quickly.

Alternatively, the eggs may hatch in the same host and liberate the oncosphere to begin the life cycle afresh. In such **autoinfection**, a large number of worms accumulate in the intestine.

PATHOGENESIS

- Light infections are asymptomatic.
- In heavy infections with >1,000 worms due to autoinfection, there may be features of enteritis with abdominal symptoms.

CLINICAL FEATURES

Asymptomatic infections: An infection with *H. nana* may produce no symptoms, even when there is a heavy worm burden.

Symptomatic infections: The most common symptom is persistent abdominal pain. Other symptoms are headache, dizziness, anorexia and diarrhea. Severe and disseminated infections are seen in malnourished and immunosuppressed individuals.

Heavy human infections can be attributed to autoinfection, which can lead to complications in an immunocompromised host.

DIAGNOSIS

The approach to the diagnosis of *H. nana* infection is based on the detection of its characteristic eggs in stool specimens (Fig. 39.3a and b). The adult worm or its proglottids are rarely seen in fecal samples.

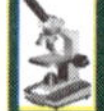

Lab diagnosis

- **Microscopy**: By visualising eggs with characteristic morphology in stool samples

Microscopy

In a **wet mount,** the characteristic *H. nana* eggs, which are non-bile-stained with polar filaments between the shell membranes, can be easily identified. The eggs of *H. diminuta* are larger and without polar filaments. (Note: The eggs are infectious and hence unpreserved stool samples should be handled carefully.)

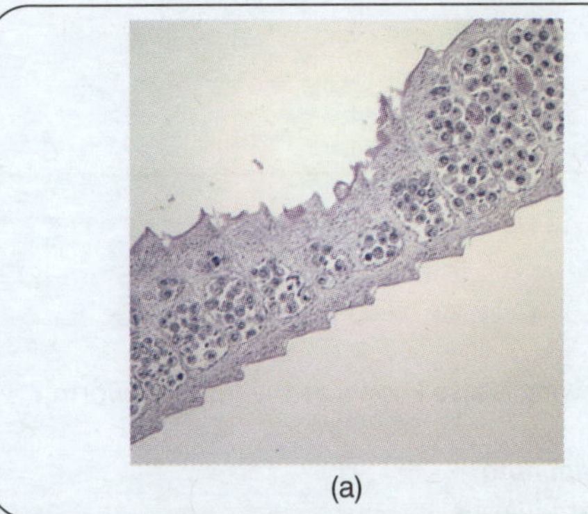
(a)

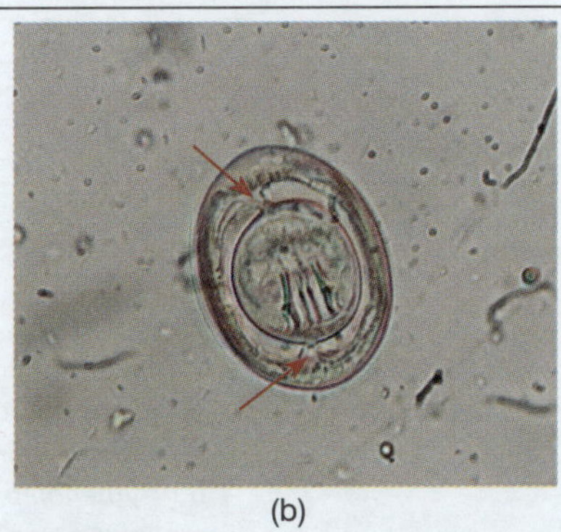
(b)

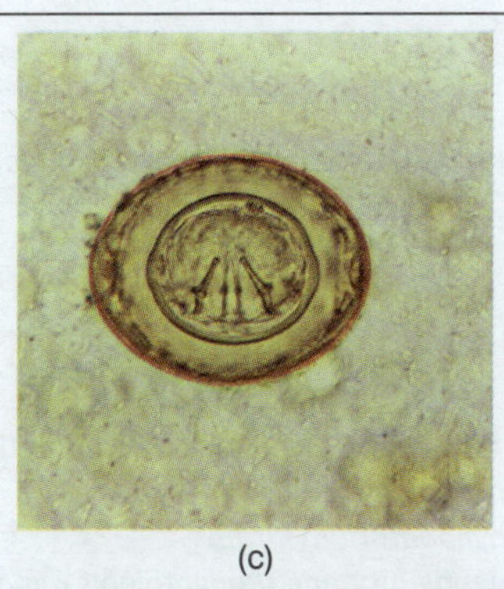
(c)

Fig. 39.3 Features of *Hymenolepis*: (a) overlapping proglottids of *H. nana* stained with hematoxylin and eosin, (*Source:* Centers for Disease Control and Prevention [CDC], DPDx), (b) the egg of *H. nana* in an unstained wet mount showing polar filaments (arrows) in the space between the oncosphere and outer shell, and (c) the egg of *H. diminuta* without polar filaments and with a clear space between the outer shell and the hexacanth oncosphere (*Source [c]:* CDC, Public Health Image Library [PHIL], Image ID 658)

Other Diagnostic Parameters

Low-grade **eosinophilia** of 5% or more is very common.

TREATMENT

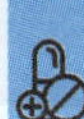

Drug of choice

Praziquantel: 25 mg/kg body weight as a single oral dose, both for adults and children; household contacts should also be treated

PREVENTION AND CONTROL

- Good **personal hygiene** is the most effective preventive measure.
- It is difficult to eradicate *H. nana* infections because of the zoonotic nature of the transmission; **rodent control** measures should be implemented.

HYMENOLEPIS DIMINUTA

H. diminuta is also called the '**rat tapeworm**'. It is a true **zoonosis**. It is similar to *H. nana*, but with the following differences:

- It rarely causes human infections.
- Its life cycle follows the pattern of the indirect life cycle of *H. nana*. The **arthropod intermediate host is necessary** for its transmission.
- The adult is larger (10–60 cm) than that of *H. nana* with more proglottids, and its scolex has no hooks on the rostellum.
- Its **eggs are larger** (60–85 μm) and **without polar filaments**.
- Infections are not transmitted from person to person.

LIFE CYCLE

The **definitive hosts, rodents,** acquire the eggs of this parasite by ingesting the **intermediate hosts—insects such as fleas and beetles** harbouring the 'cysticercoid stage'. Humans are accidental definitive hosts who are infected by the ingestion of cereals or other food items infested with insects. The development of the parasite in the intestine is similar to that of *H. nana*. However, unlike *H. nana* eggs, the eggs of *H. diminuta* are not infectious by the person-to-person route.

After the eggs are taken up by the insect host, the oncosphere is liberated. It then penetrates the intestinal wall to reach the hemocoel of the insect, where it develops into the cysticercoid larva.

CLINICAL FEATURES

The infection is usually asymptomatic. In symptomatic cases, anorexia, nausea, diarrhea and headache are usually reported, most often by children who have a heavy infection.

DIAGNOSIS

The diagnosis of *H. diminuta* infection is based on the demonstration of its characteristic eggs which are similar to those of *H. nana*, except that they are larger and without polar filaments (Fig. 39.3c).

TREATMENT

This is the same as that for *H. nana* infections.

Questions

1. Discuss the diagnosis and management of *Hymenolepis nana* infection.
2. Differentiate between *Hymenolepis nana* and *H. diminuta.*

Multiple Choice Questions

1. Which of the following is also known as the 'dwarf tapeworm'?
   a. *Taenia solium*
   b. *Diphyllobothrium latum*
   c. *Hymenolepis nana (Rodentolepis nana)*
   d. *Echinococcus oligarthus*
2. Which of the following is also known as the 'rat tapeworm'?
   a. *Taenia saginata*
   b. *Hymenolepis diminuta*
   c. *Echinococcus granulosus*
   d. *Taenia solium*

CHAPTER 40

Taenia solium – Cysticercosis

Case Study and Learning Goals

A 21-year-old male presents with multiple episodes of seizures, headaches and altered sensorium. The magnetic resonance imaging scans reveal a solitary cystic lesion in his left frontal lobe with perilesional edema and post-contrast ring enhancement. What will be your differential diagnosis for this case? What are the infectious causes of seizures? How would you approach the diagnosis in this case? What are the treatment options?

INTRODUCTION

Human cysticercosis is caused by the infection of the organs of the body by the **larval metacestodes of *Taenia solium*** when humans replace pigs as intermediate hosts in the natural life cycle of the parasite. These cysts may be present in any part of the body but have a predilection for the **central nervous system** (where they cause **neurocysticercosis [NCC]), subcutaneous tissue, skeletal muscles and eyes**.

Infestations of the human head and eyes with these parasites were described in ancient Vedic texts. The metacestode was named cysticercus (from the Greek words *kystic*, meaning bladder and *kercos*, meaning tail) by René-Théophile-Hyacinthe Laennec in 1818. In 1809, K. A. Rudolphi coined the term 'cellulosae' for the parasite's great affinity to connective tissue. Since then, the larvae of *T. solium* have been called *Cysticercus cellulosae*.

EPIDEMIOLOGY

Human cysticercosis is a major public health problem in many developing countries.

- NCC is considered the **most common parasitic infection** of the CNS in humans.
- It is the **most common cause of adult-onset epilepsy** globally, and the etiology of **seizures in about one-third of the cases of acquired epilepsy** in endemic regions.

Cysticercosis is typically more prevalent in countries where there is rampant poverty and poor sanitation and a lack of safe water supply. The endemic areas include Central and South America, sub-Saharan Africa, South-East Asia, India, China and Nepal. Differences are observed in the clinical and radiological presentation of NCC in different geographical areas.

- Intestinal infection (taeniasis) with *T. solium* occurs only in persons who eat undercooked pork. It largely affects those who live in poor sanitary conditions and is most prevalent in developing countries. Because of its association with the consumption of pork, taeniasis is uncommon among Jews and Muslims.
- Cysticercosis, on the other hand, may occur in any person residing in or visiting endemic areas (including vegetarians) because the infection is transmitted by the ingestion of food or water contaminated with *Taenia* eggs.
- Eggs of *T. solium* are infective to pigs and humans.

MORPHOLOGY

Adult Worm and Eggs

Please refer to **Chapter 37**, *Taenia*.

Larva

Cysticerci **commonly exist as milky white, bladder-like** cyst forms in the human muscles or viscera. The larval cyst measures 8–10 × 5 mm in size with a small, solid, eccentric scolex surrounded by a bladder wall (see Fig. 37.1e in **Chapter 37**, *Taenia*).

The other morphological form of the parasite is the **racemose cysticercus** (from the Latin word *racemus*, meaning bunch of grapes), which is composed of several bladders. It may be round, lobulated or in grape-like clusters, and is found in the more spacious areas of the body such as the subarachnoid space. It may be 10 to 20 cm in size and contains up to 60 ml of fluid. It does not have scolices.

LIFE CYCLE (Fig. 40.1a and b; also refer to Chapter 37, *Taenia*)

The **definitive hosts—humans—**who harbour the adult *T. solium*, release the extremely resistant eggs during defecation. These eggs are widely dispersed in the environment, from where pigs or other **humans may ingest** them through contaminated food and water. Alternately, human beings may be exposed to the eggs via autoinfection by the fecal–oral route or reverse peristalsis. These eggs hatch in the duodenum or jejunum and release oncospheres, which then penetrate the intestinal wall and are carried via the mesenteric veins to the systemic circulation and consequently, get distributed throughout the body. The oncospheres lodge themselves in various organs to form larval cysticerci. The commonly involved organs are the subcutaneous tissues and muscles, the eyes and the brain. Thus, in cysticercosis, **humans act as the intermediate host** and are a dead end in the life cycle of the parasite.

Definitive hosts: Humans
Intermediate hosts: Humans and pigs

PATHOGENESIS

The severity of the illness may depend on the number, size and location of the cysts, and the inflammatory response

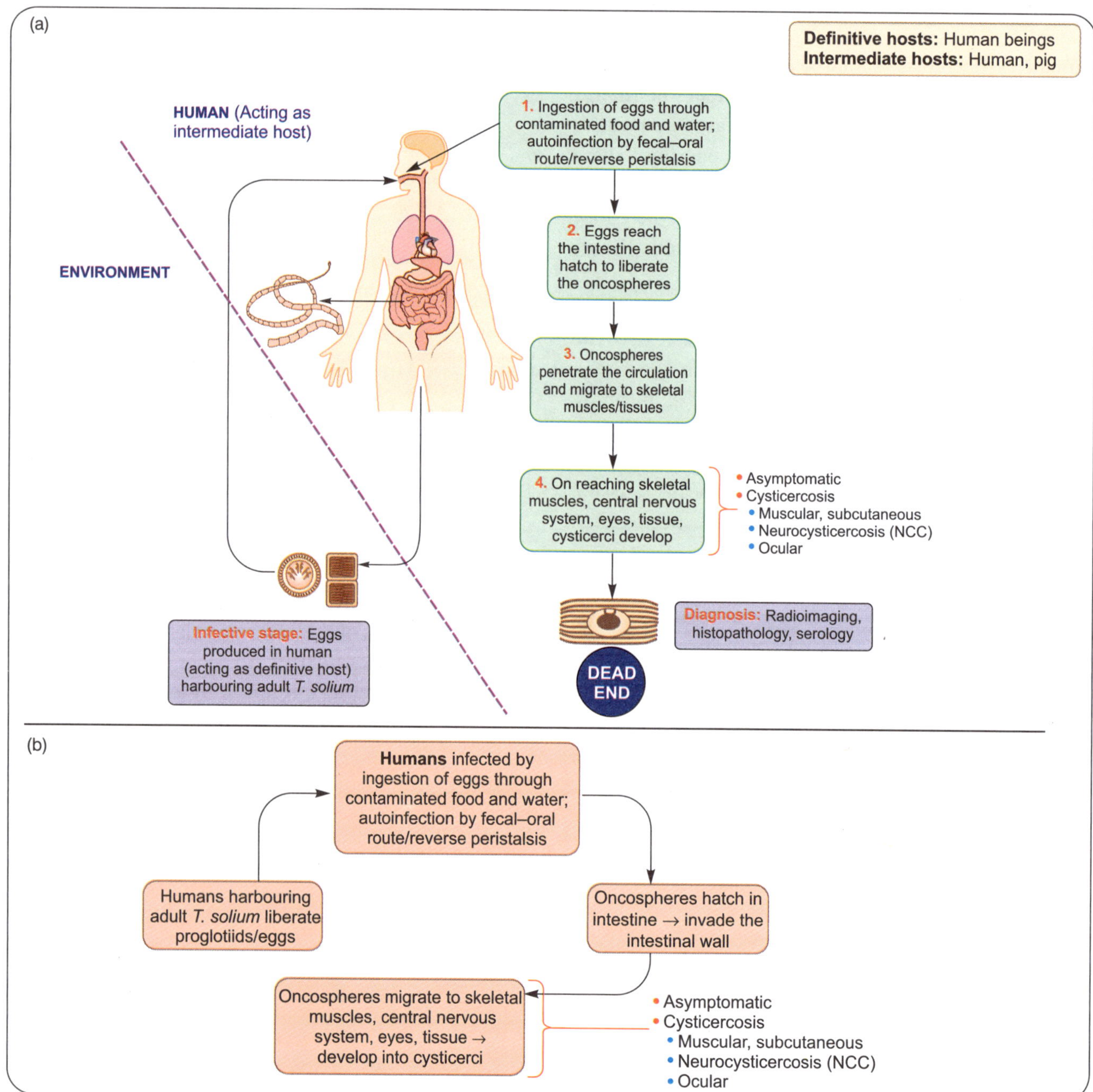

Fig. 40.1 Life cycle of *Taenia solium* with a human as the intermediate host instead of a pig: (a) detailed and (b) schematic

of the host. Though cysts may form in any organ of the body, the clinical manifestations are most commonly seen when the site of cyst formation is the central nervous system (which results in NCC), followed by the eyes and their adnexa. The cysts present in subcutaneous tissues and the muscles may often go unnoticed. **Based on the site of the brain involved**, one of the following two types of NCC may develop:

- **Parenchymal NCC:** Involves the brain parenchyma and causes seizures
- **Extra-parenchymal NCC:** Involves the meninges, ventricles and the spinal cord; mechanical obstruction to CSF circulation may ensue when the cyst is in contact with the meninges, which results in raised intracranial tension and hydrocephalus

The cysts in the brain exist in **four morphological stages.** The stage of the cyst is the key determinant of clinical features as inflammatory response against the dead or dying cysts is associated with symptoms which may sometimes be severe. The four stages are as follows:

- Initially, the cyst is a viable **vesicular** cyst with intact cyst walls. This stage is associated with minimal inflammation.
- Then, the lesion is surrounded by host inflammatory cells which start infiltrating the cyst, and it gradually enters the **colloidal** stage.
- This is followed by fibrosis, as a result of which, the cyst becomes **granular–nodular**.
- As the fibrosis progresses, the cyst finally becomes a **calcified** cyst.

Subarachnoid NCC

- This variety of extra-parenchymal NCC is characterised by the formation of a single giant cyst or a grape-like cluster of cysts (racemose).
- Such cysts are found in the more spacious areas of the body such as the subarachnoid space (basilar cisterns, Sylvian fissures and spinal cord).
- The incubation period before clinical presentation ranges from 10 to 25 years.
- In the early stage, there is proliferation of the cyst leading to invasion of the contiguous spaces. This causes mass effects with limited inflammation.
- In the later stages, an enormous amount of antigenic mass is generated and the cysts start degenerating. This leads to inflammatory arachnoiditis which can cause hydrocephalus, infarcts and other manifestations.
- Prolonged anthelmintic and anti-inflammatory treatment is required for the treatment of subarachnoid NCC. The mortality is very high.

CLINICAL FEATURES

The clinical features depend on the location, size, number and type of the cyst(s).

Neurocysticercosis (NCC)

Neural involvement is seen in about 60–80% of cases of cysticercosis. In some countries, NCC accounts for up to 50% of late-onset epilepsy cases. The clinical presentation is variable.

Asymptomatic NCC: Sometimes, a cyst may remain in the brain without causing any apparent symptoms.

Symptomatic NCC: Active NCC is usually associated with living cysts and is seen in about half of the NCC patients. Its features are as follows:

- **Seizure** is the most common manifestation (70–80% of cases), followed by headache
- Increased intracranial pressure, leading to vomiting, vertigo and papilledema
- Hydrocephalus may occur due to the cyst obstructing the CSF flow
- Meningitis symptoms
- Focal neurological deficits
- Cranial nerve palsy
- Gait abnormality
- Abnormal behaviour
- Visual disturbances

- A higher frequency of NCC caused by a single, parenchymal cysticercus is seen in patients in India as compared to patients in Latin America, who more frequently harbour multiple cysticerci in their ventricles or subarachnoid space.
- NCC is considered the second most common cause of intracranial space-occupying lesion (ICSOL) after tuberculosis in India.

Ocular Cysticercosis

The majority of ocular cysts are found in the posterior chamber, followed by the subretinal, subconjunctival, orbit or the anterior chamber. The symptoms may include proptosis, diplopia, loss of vision and slow-growing nodules with focal inflammation. The larvae are unencapsulated when found in the vitreous or anterior humor, and actively change shape. Permanent damage to the eye may occur, especially if the parasite dies and produces an intense inflammatory reaction in the process. Thus, it is imperative that the parasite be surgically removed.

Subcutaneous Cysticercosis

It is frequently asymptomatic and may present only as palpable nodules. Subcutaneous or muscular involvement has been detected in >75% of NCC patients across the world except in Latin America.

Muscular Cysticercosis

The majority of these infections are asymptomatic and generally involve the voluntary muscles. While the majority of muscular cysts die and become calcified, they may sometimes lead to myositis with accompanying fever and eosinophilia.

DIAGNOSIS

The diagnosis of cysticercosis is usually made by a combination of neuroimaging and clinico-epidemiological parameters along with laboratory tests.

A unified set of criteria for the diagnosis of NCC has been prepared to facilitate its diagnosis across different settings (Table 40.1).

Direct Demonstration

- **Stool microscopy** has little role in the diagnosis of cysticercosis since most patients do not harbour the adult worm at the time of larval infestation.

Table 40.1 Revised diagnostic criteria and degrees of diagnostic certainty for NCC (Adapted from Del Brutto's criteria, 2017*)

Absolute criteria		
1. **Histologic** demonstration (scolex with its suckers and hooks, or the presence of parasitic membranes) from a biopsy of a brain or spinal cord lesion 2. Conclusive demonstration of a cystic lesion with a scolex (bright nodule within the cyst) on **CT** or **MRI** 3. Direct visualisation of subretinal parasites (usually over the macula; yellowish with a central dark spot) by **fundoscopic** examination		
Neuroimaging criteria		
Major	**Confirmative**	**Minor**
1. Cystic lesions without scolex 2. Enhancing lesions 3. Multilobulated cystic lesions in the subarachnoid space 4. Typical parenchymal brain calcifications	1. Resolution of cystic lesions after cysticidal therapy (albendazole or praziquantel) 2. Spontaneous resolution of single, small (<20 mm) enhancing lesion 3. Migration of ventricular cysts on sequential neuroimaging studies	1. Obstructive hydrocephalus or abnormal enhancement of the basal leptomeninges

Clinical/Exposure criteria	
Major	**Minor**
1. Detection of specific anti-cysticercal antibodies or cysticercal antigens by immunodiagnostic assays 2. Cysticercosis outside CNS • Histologic demonstration from a biopsy of a subcutaneous nodule • X-ray showing multiple 'cigar-shaped' calcifications in the thigh and calf muscles • Direct visualisation of a cysticercus in the anterior chamber of the eye 3. Household contact with *T. solium* infection	1. Clinical manifestations suggestive of cysticercosis 2. Individuals travelling from or living in an endemic area (sub-Saharan Africa, Latin America, most parts of Asia)
Degree of diagnostic certainty	
Definitive diagnosis	**Probable diagnosis**
1. One absolute criterion 2. Two major neuroimaging criteria plus any clinical/exposure criteria 3. One major and one confirmative neuroimaging criteria plus any clinical/exposure criteria 4. One major neuroimaging criteria plus two clinical/exposure criteria (including at least one major clinical/exposure criterion) together with the exclusion of other pathologies producing similar neuroimaging findings	1. One major neuroimaging criteria plus any two clinical/exposure criteria 2. One minor neuroimaging criteria plus at least one major clinical/exposure criteria

*Del Brutto OH, Nash TE, White AC, et al. 2017. Revised diagnostic criteria for neurocysticercosis. *J Neurol Sci.* 372:202–210.

- **Histopathological examination** of surgically removed cysts from the muscles, eyes or subcutaneous tissues or brain biopsies may be done. In such cases, the suckers and hooks on the scolex may be visualised.
- On **FNAC** (fine-needle aspiration cytology), the characteristic morphology of parasitic tegument and parenchyma is helpful.
- On **fundoscopic examination**, the larval cyst in the eye may be identified by its morphology (translucent white cyst with a dense white spot) and characteristic undulating movement of the invaginated scolex when it is present in the posterior segment.

Neuroimaging

CT scan (Fig. 40.2a and b) and MRI are performed to demonstrate cystic lesions, the scolex and the surrounding inflammatory reaction. X-rays may show **'cigar-shaped' calcifications in the muscles**.

Antibody Detection

The detection of specific anti-cysticercal antibodies in serum or CSF by immunodiagnostic assays such as ELISA and western blot (enzyme-linked immunoelectrotransfer blot) is of value in the diagnosis of cysticercosis and NCC.

Enzyme-linked immunoelectrotransfer blot (EITB): The World Health Organization recommends the use of lentil lectin-purified glycoproteins (LLGP) in an EITB format for the serodiagnosis of cysticercosis and NCC. EITB assays for NCC available at reference laboratories use a semi-purified extract of *T. solium* cysticerci as the antigen with seven major glycoprotein bands (50 to 13 kDa) coated on a nitrocellulose membrane. A reaction of the patient's serum with any one of these bands is indicative of cysticercosis. The sensitivity and specificity of EITB are reported to be >98% for multiple cysts and somewhat lower for single cysts. EITB is more sensitive and specific than ELISA, but is cumbersome to perform.

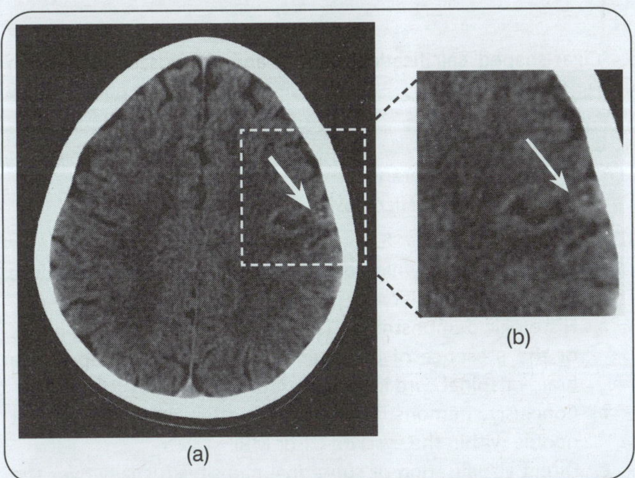

Fig. 40.2 Non-enhanced CT scan image of the brain showing (a) a single, rounded cystic lesion with a bright nodule (scolex within the cyst) in the left frontal lobe (white arrow) and (b) the area with cystic lesion shown as an inset (*Source:* Dr Ramesh Mangal, Consultant Radiologist, Zydus Hospital, Ahmedabad)

Antigen Detection

Antigens can be detected in serum or CSF by ELISA but these methods are not readily available commercially.

CSF Examination

The most characteristic features of NCC in the spinal fluid are atypical, reactive lymphoid cells with a mixed cell population.

TREATMENT

Anti-parasitic agents
- *Albendazole:* 15 mg/kg/day divided into 2 daily doses for 10–14 days for 1–2 viable parenchymal cysts
- *Praziquantel (in combination with albendazole):* 50 mg/kg/day for 10–14 days for more than 2 viable parenchymal cysts

Symptomatic treatment
- Anti-epileptic drugs for seizure control
- Adjunctive corticosteroid therapy
- Methotrexate may be considered as a steroid-sparing agent when prolonged anti-inflammatory therapy is required

The treatment should be individualised based on the number and location of cysts and their viability.

Medical treatment is more effective for parenchymal cysts and less effective for intraventricular, subarachnoid or racemose cysts, and has no effect on dead or calcified cysts. For 1–2 viable parenchymal cysts, albendazole monotherapy is recommended, whereas, for >2 viable parenchymal cysts, combination therapy of albendazole with praziquantel is recommended. High-dose glucocorticoids should be started prior to anti-parasitic drugs to reduce the acute inflammation that occurs following the degradation of viable cysts. Often, prolonged therapy for more than a year may be required, as in the case of subarachnoid cysts, especially the racemose type of cysts.

Surgical removal of cysts may be the best approach in the case of extensive infection or severe extra-parenchymal NCC and intraocular and spinal lesions where anti-cysticidal therapy is associated with a risk of extensive inflammatory damage, or in obstructive hydrocephalus where a shunt is required in addition to medical therapy.

PREVENTION AND CONTROL

- **Improved sanitation and hygiene** are among the most important prevention and control measures.
- Fruits and vegetables should be thoroughly washed before being consumed.
- Human feces should be disposed of in a sanitary manner. Cattle and pigs should not be allowed to feed on or graze on grounds polluted with human feces or sewage.
- Human carriers of *T. solium* must be identified and treated on public health grounds.
- Beef and pork should be subjected to inspection for cysticerci; infected meat in slaughterhouses should be discarded.
- The consumption of raw or undercooked beef and pork must be avoided.
- Meat should be thoroughly cooked (at >65 °C for 5 minutes) or frozen at –7°C for 6 days or –20°C for 24 hours. Pickling of meat is not an effective method of killing cysticerci.
- One option for the prevention and control of NCC is the development of vaccines for use in pigs. One such vaccine—the **TSOL18 vaccine**, which comprises a recombinant protein from a *T. solium* oncosphere—has shown promise.
- Treatment of pigs with oxfendazole has shown to eliminate cysticercosis in pigs.

Questions

1. Discuss the laboratory diagnosis of neurocysticercosis.
2. Discuss the clinical features and management of neurocysticercosis.
3. Discuss the prevention and treatment of cysticercosis.
4. Enumerate the space-occupying lesions of the brain. Discuss the lab diagnosis of NCC.

Multiple Choice Questions

1. Humans are ______________ hosts in neurocysticercosis.
   a. Definitive b. Intermediate
   c. Paratenic d. Reservoir
2. Neurocysticercosis is caused by the ingestion of ________.
   a. Beef containing *T. solium* cysts
   b. Pork containing *T. solium* cysts
   c. Food and water contaminated with *T. solium eggs*
   d. All these
3. Which is the most common parasitic cause of adult-onset epilepsy globally?
   a. Malaria
   b. Neurocysticercosis
   c. Amoebiasis
   d. Toxoplasmosis
4. The most common manifestation of neurocysticercosis is ___________:
   a. Stroke b. Coma
   c. Fever d. Epilepsy
5. 'Cigar-shaped' calcifications in thigh and calf muscles are seen in ____________.
   a. Trichinellosis
   b. Sarcocystosis
   c. Visceral larva migrans
   d. Subcutaneous cysticercosis
6. According to the 'Del Brutto' diagnostic criteria for neurocysticercosis, which of the following is NOT an absolute criterion for diagnosis?
   a. Histologic demonstration (scolex with its suckers and hooks or the presence of parasitic membranes) in a biopsy of a brain or spinal cord lesion
   b. Conclusive demonstration of cystic lesion with scolex (bright nodule within the cyst) on CT or MRI
   c. Direct visualisation of subretinal parasites (usually over the macula; yellowish with a central dark spot) by fundoscopic examination
   d. Detection of specific anti-cysticercal antibodies or cysticercal antigens by immuno-diagnostic assays

Chapter 41

Echinococcus

([From Greek] *echinos* = spine + *kokkos* = grain)

Case Study and Learning Goals

A 30-year-old male presents to the OPD with upper abdominal discomfort and poor appetite for the last six months. His sclera is yellowish on examination. The ultrasonography shows a round space-occupying lesion (SOL) in his liver measuring 6 cm in size with floating membranes. What are the parasitic causes of SOL in the liver? How would you approach the laboratory diagnosis in this case? How would you treat this patient?

ECHINOCOCCUS GRANULOSUS

INTRODUCTION

Humans are accidental hosts to the larval stage, i.e., hydatid cysts, of the **dog tapeworm *Echinococcus granulosus*** which causes a serious disease known as cystic echinococcosis or **'hydatid disease'** (from *hudatis* [Greek] = watery vesicle). The disease is present worldwide and has significant zoonotic importance. Chiefly, two *Echinococcus* species are of human importance. They are as follows:

- ***E. granulosus***, which causes **cystic echinococcosis (CE)**, is the most prevalent species.
- ***E. multilocularis***, which causes **alveolar echinococcosis (AE)**, is the most pathogenic species.

The other species, *E. vogeli* and *E. oligarthus*, are geographically limited to South America and are rarely reported to cause **polycystic echinococcosis**. They are also called 'neotropical echinococci'.

- ***E. vogeli*** has been reported in about 100 human cases.
- ***E. oligarthus*** is reported in less than 10 human cases.

The earliest reference to the large hydatid cysts formed inside the liver was made in the 4th century BC by Hippocrates, who observed these cysts in ritually slaughtered animals and animals slaughtered for meat in Babylon. Such cysts in humans were first described in the 2nd century AD by Galen. The parasitic nature of these cysts was first recognised by Francisco Redi in the 17th century. In 1766, Pierre Pallas showed that these cysts were the larvae of tapeworms, and in 1853, Carl von Siebold showed that the adult tapeworm grows in dogs that are fed infected sheep meat.

EPIDEMIOLOGY

E. granulosus is cosmopolitan in distribution. It is the more common species than *E. multilocularis*. The World Health Organization (WHO) has listed echinococcosis as one of the 17 neglected diseases targeted for control or elimination by 2050.

Based on the mitochondrial DNA sequences, ten genotypes of *E. granulosus* have been identified—genotypes G1 to G10. Each genotype has a particular host specificity and geographical distribution; these parasites generally infect sheep and other ungulates (Table 41.1). G1, the sheep strain, is the most common genotype in India. However, other genotypes may also cause human infections.

- **Worldwide:** Greater prevalence is reported from western China, Central and South-East Asia including India and Nepal, South America, Mediterranean countries and eastern Africa. Cystic echinococcosis (CE) has been declared eliminated from New Zealand and Tasmania in Australia.
- **India:** CE is endemic in many regions in India and is frequently reported from various states like Jammu and Kashmir, Uttar Pradesh, Tamil Nadu, Andhra Pradesh, Punjab and Himachal Pradesh.

Risk Factors

E. granulosus infections are most common in pastoral communities that rear sheep and cattle, and live in close

Table 41.1 Host preferences of *Echinococcus* species

Species	Definitive hosts	Intermediate hosts
E. granulosus	Dog, wolf and jackal	Sheep, buffalo, horse, cattle, camel, pig, cervid and human being
E. multilocularis	Red fox and arctic fox	Rodents, small mammals and human being
E. vogeli	Bush dog	Paca (forest rodent) and human being
E. oligarthus	Jaguar and bobcat	Rodent and human being

proximity to dogs. There is a greater risk of infection when dogs have unrestricted access to homes and regularly feed on sheep offal.

MORPHOLOGY

Echinococci exist in three developmental stages—the adult, egg and larva (Fig. 41.1a–e).

Adult Worm

It is **3–6 mm long** (Fig. 41.1a), consisting of a head (scolex), neck and segments (proglottids).

- The **scolex** has four muscular suckers (**acetabula**) for attachment to the intestinal wall and a rostellum with a double row of hooklets. The shape and size of the hooks help in differentiating *Echinococcus* species.
- The head is followed by a short neck.
- The adult worm's body comprises **2–5 segments (proglottids)** depending on the species. *E. granulosus* has three proglottids—the proximal segment is immature; the second segment is mature and bears the sexual organs and the terminal segment is gravid or egg-laden.

Egg

The fertilised egg (Fig. 41.1b) is **spherical** and light brown with a radially striated thick shell. It cannot be morphologically differentiated from the egg of *Taenia*. It contains the embryonic **oncosphere** or the **hexacanth** larval stage with six hooklets (Fig. 41.1c). The eggs are highly resistant and disperse widely in the environment. The oncospheres grow and develop into larvae or hydatid cysts in the intermediate host.

Larva

The metacestode larva or the hydatid cyst (Fig. 41.1d and e) ranges in size from a few millimetres to several centimetres, is typically unilocular and is filled with **hydatid fluid** (see box). The cyst wall can be differentiated into three layers, which are as follows:

- **Endocyst:** Inner **nucleated, germinal** layer
- **Ectocyst:** Middle **acellular, laminated** layer
- **Pericyst:** Outer **host-derived, fibrous, adventitial** layer

The cyst derives its nutrition by diffusion through the cyst wall. The inner germinal layer undergoes asexual proliferation endogenously to produce many **daughter cysts (brood capsules)** by budding. These daughter cysts (Fig. 41.1e) may stay attached to the inner layer or detach in the cyst cavity, eventually giving rise to protoscolices, each of which is capable of giving rise to an adult worm. The several protoscolices generated inside the brood capsule are found to be in different stages of development. Large cysts may contain thousands of protoscolices. As the cyst grows, internal septations develop. Such a cyst may be erroneously thought to be multiloculated. Cysts without any brood capsules and scolices (sterile) are known as acephalocysts.

Hydatid fluid

- Hydatid fluid is clear to pale yellow and has a neutral pH ranging from 6.7–7.2 and a specific gravity of 1.012.
- It contains NaCl, phosphates, proteins, creatinine, urea, glucose, polysaccharides, lipids, etc.
- The fluid also contains scolices and hooklets which are released upon the rupture of brood capsules and protoscolices. These settle down at the bottom of the cyst and are collectively known as **'hydatid sand'**.
- The fluid is antigenic and anaphylactic. *Echinococcus* allergens include AgB (protease inhibitor), Ag5, a serine protease, EA 21 and Eg EF-1 beta/delta, an elongation factor.

LIFE CYCLE (Fig. 41.2a and b)

Definitive host: Dog
Intermediate hosts: Cattle, goat, sheep, camel, horse, pig and human beings (accidental)

Two mammalian hosts are involved in the life cycle of *E. granulosus*—dogs (the **definitive hosts**) harbour the adult worm and sheep and cattle (the **intermediate hosts**) harbour the larval form.

Dog cycle: Typically, dogs acquire the infection by ingesting the meat of sheep or cattle infested with hydatid cysts. Subsequently, the protoscolices are released; these develop into adult worms in the dog's intestine. The worm may survive for about 20 months. Canines may harbour hundreds of worms in their intestines. After fertilisation, the gravid proglottid produces 100 to 1,500 eggs which are passed out along with the dog's feces.

Sheep/cattle cycle (larval stage): Sheep, cattle or other intermediate hosts ingest the eggs of the parasite, which then hatch in their duodenum and release oncospheres. These oncospheres penetrate the intestinal wall to enter the mesenteric circulation and may lodge themselves in various body organs. Though they principally settle in the liver, and less commonly, the lungs, any body organ may be infected. The hydatid cyst develops in the intermediate

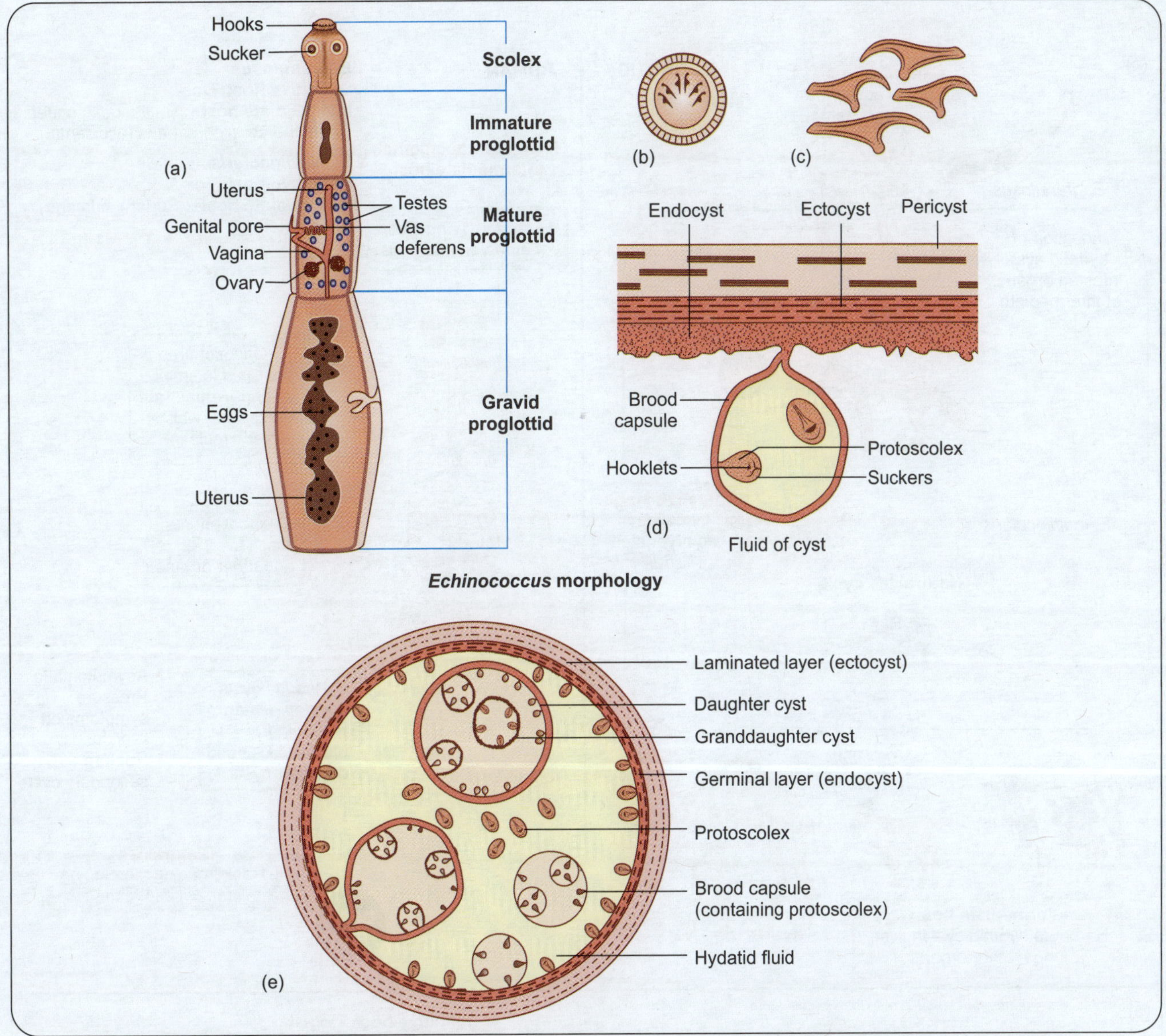

Fig. 41.1 Line diagrams of *Echinococcus granulosus*: (a) the adult worm, (b) egg containing the oncosphere, (c) hooks, (d) a section of the hydatid cyst showing layers of the cyst and brood capsule and (e) a complete hydatid cyst showing the development of endogenous daughter and granddaughter cysts

host and is well-differentiated into the three-layered cyst in about six months. It increases in diameter by about 1 cm per month and can survive for several years until it is consumed by the definitive host to continue its life cycle.

Humans act as **accidental hosts** when they replace the natural intermediate host in the life cycle. Human infections are the **dead end** in the life cycle of the parasite.

PATHOGENESIS

Human beings acquire *Echinococcus* infection by ingesting food or water contaminated with the eggs of *E. granulosus*. The cyst remains asymptomatic for years and keeps growing. Spontaneous regression, involution and calcification of the cyst may occur. The clinical symptoms usually appear due to the following:

- **Pressure effect:** When a cyst reaches a size of >10 cm in diameter in the liver or when more than two-thirds of the organ is occupied by a cyst, it results in physical compression. Damage to bile ducts, hepatic veins, portal vein, or the hepatic artery or damage to bronchia in the lungs or various structures of other involved organs is seen.
- **Anaphylactic reaction:** There may be minor fluid leaks from the cyst into the systemic circulation; this sensitises the patient. If such sensitisation is followed by a cyst rupture or a large leak, life-threatening

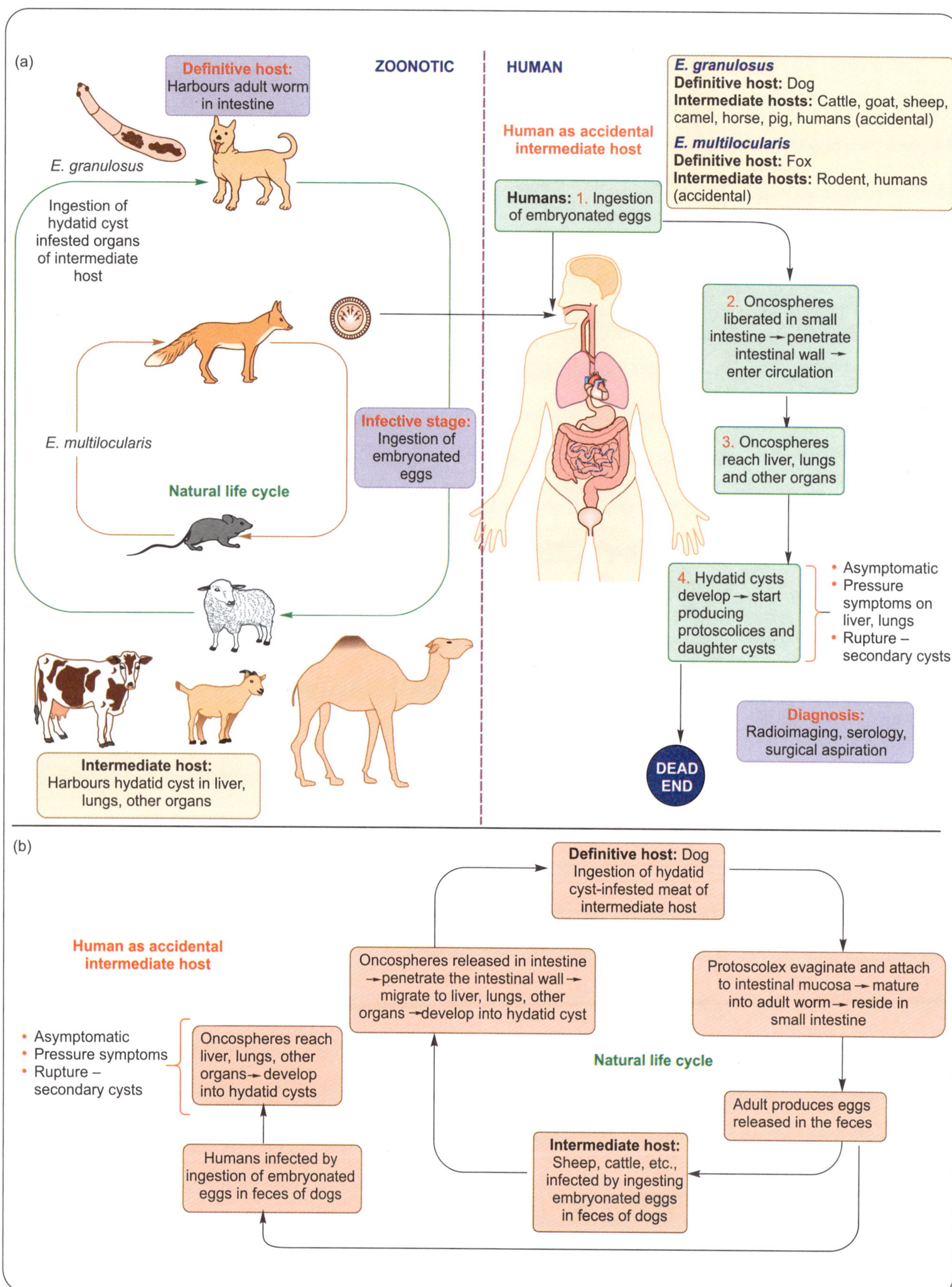

Fig. 41.2 Life cycle of *Echinococcus granulosus* and *Echinococcus multilocularis*: (a) detailed and (b) schematic

immune reactions including anaphylaxis may occur. This may also lead to the secondary spread of cysts to other organs.

- **Bacterial superinfections:** Sometimes, cysts may be complicated by bacterial superinfections.

CE is predominantly associated with the T_{h2} type of immune response, with high levels of interleukin-5 in both AE and CE. *Echinococcus*-specific IgE is present in most of the patients and is linked with the severity of the disease.

CLINICAL FEATURES

The incubation period ranges from months to several years. CE in humans is potentially dangerous. The clinical features are associated with damage or malfunction of the affected organs. The most commonly affected organs are the liver (70%) and lungs (20%); however, the brain, spleen, kidney, heart or any other organ may also be affected. While most patients have single cysts, the presence of multiple cysts or the involvement of multiple organs has been reported in 20–40% of cases. The mortality rate is low, ranging from 2–4%. The various stages of CE are as follows:

- **Early stages:** No significant symptoms are noted in the early stages of CE. The cysts can remain asymptomatic for 10 to 15 years.
- **Late stages:** CE liver cysts in humans grow very slowly, with more than half of the cysts showing no change in size after 10 years and one-third growing less than 3 cm. Thus, most patients present late.
- **Liver cysts:** These most often present with upper abdominal discomfort and poor appetite. The compression of bile ducts may lead to jaundice. On palpation, a tumour-like mass, hepatomegaly or abdominal distension may be found. Hydatid cysts in the liver may be confused with congenital liver cysts, amoebic abscesses or hepatic tumours. A liver cyst can cause complications such as communication with the biliary tree, intra-biliary rupture producing clinical features such as abdominal pain, cholestasis, obstructive jaundice, cholecystitis, cholangitis and fistula formation.
- **Lung cysts:** Chest pain, cough or hemoptysis may occur due to the rupture of a cyst into the bronchi. Pulmonary symptoms may be confused with tuberculosis.
- **Other organs:** Other neurological features such as signs of raised intracranial pressure, epilepsy, paralysis, etc., may be observed in patients with brain cysts.
- **Hypersensitivity reactions:** In any organ, a cyst rupture can induce fever, urticaria, eosinophilia and anaphylactic shock, which can be lethal.

DIAGNOSIS

The approach to the diagnosis of CE is based on radiological examination supported by serological evidence of hydatid disease.

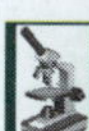

Lab diagnosis

- **Imaging:** USG, CT or MRI to visualise cysts
- **Serology:** Specific antibody recognition of AgB, Ag5, 8- and 116-kDa hydatid antigens and EITB
- **Casoni skin test**
- **Antigen detection:** ELISA
- **Microscopy:** By visualising hydatid sand or cyst
  - Direct microscopy of cyst fluid
  - Histopathology: Of cyst membranes
- **DNA detection:** PCR

Radioimaging

Imaging techniques are essential for the diagnosis of CE.

- Ultrasonography (USG) is widely used to diagnose liver cysts, whereas X-ray is preferred for lung cysts. The **water-lily sign** is seen when there is detachment of the endocyst membrane resulting in floating membranes within the pericyst, giving it the appearance of a water lily. This sign is classically described on plain radiographs (mainly chest X-ray) when the collapsed membranes are calcified but may also be seen on USG, CT and MRI. Daughter cysts appear as cysts within a cyst, giving cysts a characteristic **cartwheel or honeycomb appearance**.
- Based on cyst characteristics on USG imaging, the **WHO Informal Working Group on Echinococcosis (WHO-IWGE)** has classified hepatic CE cysts into five types—CE1 to CE5. This classification provides basic information for physicians to make treatment decisions.
- CT or MRI may be used for diagnosis, population screening and follow-up.

Serodiagnosis

Antibody detection: The detection of specific antibodies against *Echinococcus* antigens is a confirmatory step with various levels of sensitivity and specificity depending on the cyst location and number and the antigen used. Hydatid cyst fluid is the major antigenic source for echinococcosis immunodiagnosis, with the lipoprotein **antigen B (AgB)** and **antigen 5 (Ag5)** widely used in serological assays for CE. Recombinant antigens are increasingly being used now. Enzyme-linked immunoelectrotransfer blot (EITB) assays are better than ELISA. However, these are more cumbersome to perform. Specific antibody recognition of **8- and 116-kDa** hydatid antigens by EITB western blot in serum samples from patients with hydatid disease is considered confirmatory.

- The sensitivity and specificity of serological methods ranges from 60–90%.
- A good correlation is seen between radiologic and serologic detection; however, serology is more specific but less sensitive than imaging.
- Patients with liver cysts show better serological response than extrahepatic cysts.
- Antibody detection tests cannot differentiate between recent and past infection.

Casoni intradermal test: It is an immediate hypersensitivity reaction to hydatid fluid antigens administered intradermally. Patients exposed to the parasite develop large wheals (>5 cm) on their skin with pseudopodia formation within 30 minutes. This test exhibits low specificity and sensitivity and thus is no longer used by most laboratories.

Antigen Detection

Specific echinococcal antigens in serum, urine and CSF can be detected and may be used in addition to antibody detection for improved sensitivity and specificity. Antigen detection can be used to differentiate recent from past infection and can be used as a prognostic marker.

Microscopy

Aspirated hydatid cyst fluid can be examined microscopically for brood capsules, protoscolices or **'hydatid sand'** by direct microscopy or after staining with acid-fast stain (Fig. 41.3a–d). Hydatid sand comprises broken brood capsules and protoscolices, which get deposited at the bottom of the cyst as a granular deposit. However, if the cyst is old, the daughter cysts or scolices may have disintegrated, and only hooklets may be present.

Method: A drop of centrifuged fluid is placed between two slides. The slides are then rubbed together. A perception akin to the grating of sand grains between the slides indicates the presence of hydatid sand.

Purulent material can be examined after treating it with concentrated hydrochloric acid and subsequently boiling it for 10 minutes or leaving it at room temperature for one hour.

***Caution*:** Surgical aspiration of hydatid cyst is associated with a risk of hydatid fluid leakage which can cause a hypersensitivity reaction or dissemination.

Nucleic Acid-Based Detection

Recently developed DNA-based methods such as PCR and loop-mediated isothermal amplification (LAMP) assays may be performed on surgically obtained hydatid cysts or fluid, but are yet to find use in preoperative diagnosis. These tests are sensitive, specific and can discriminate between various genotypes of *E. granulosus*.

Histopathology

Surgically removed cysts can be stained with Giemsa, hematoxylin and eosin (H&E) or periodic acid–Schiff (PAS) stain to demonstrate the layers of the cyst wall and attached brood capsules.

Other Diagnostic Parameters

- **Eosinophilia** is present in 20–25% of patients. It is especially seen in cases where the cyst ruptures.

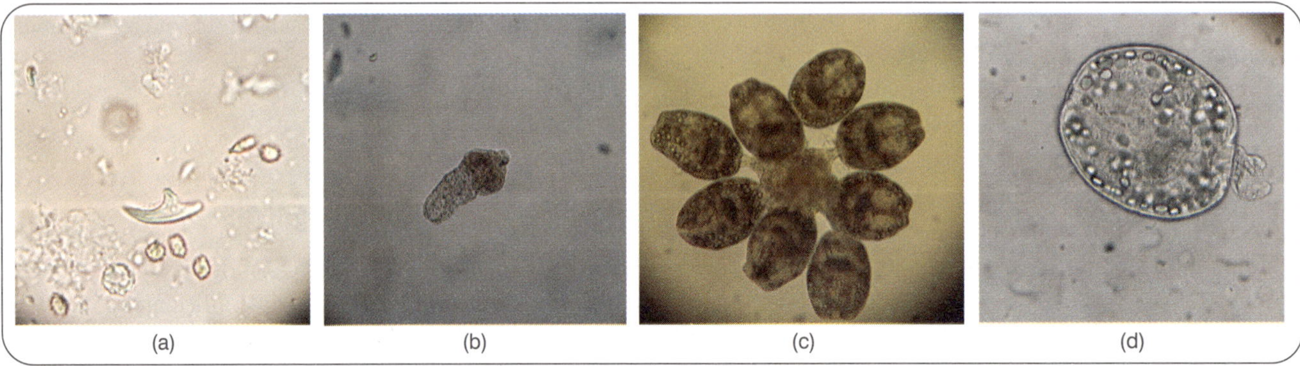

Fig. 41.3 Features of *Echinococcus granulosus* elements in surgically aspirated cyst fluid: (a) free hooklet, (b) evaginated protoscolex, (c) a bunch of protoscolices and (d) protoscolex showing conspicuous calcareous corpuscles and hooklets

- *Echinococcus*-specific IgE is present in most patients.

TREATMENT

For cystic echinococcosis, there are broadly **four treatment and management modalities** which may be used in combination; there is no optimum treatment. The WHO-IWGE classification of the type of cyst based on USG findings of cyst size, location and presence/absence of complications determines the choice of management option.

These broad modalities are drug treatment, surgery, percutaneous sterilisation (puncture, aspiration, injection and re-aspiration [PAIR]) and observation (wait and watch).

Drug Treatment

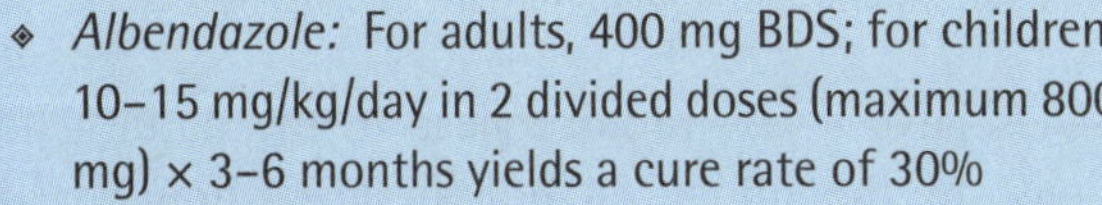

Drug of choice
- *Albendazole:* For adults, 400 mg BDS; for children, 10–15 mg/kg/day in 2 divided doses (maximum 800 mg) × 3–6 months yields a cure rate of 30%

Alternate drug
- *Mebendazole*: 40–50 mg/kg/day in 3 divided doses (if albendazole is not well-tolerated)

Drug treatment is recommended for **small or medium-sized, isolated cysts** or **multiple and inoperable cysts** in the liver and/or in multiple organs.

- Administration of albendazole or mebendazole for 3–6 months or more is the mainstay of drug therapy. However, optimum dosage and treatment have not been formally assessed. In general, a longer duration yields better improvement.
- Patients must be monitored for side effects which may arise from the prolonged administration of albendazole.
- A combination of interventional techniques with albendazole is recommended to be used routinely with PAIR and less commonly, with surgery.

Surgery

Total or partial cystectomy or hepatectomy is recommended as definitive treatment of **large or operable cysts**. For pulmonary cysts, treatment consists of wedge resection or lobectomy.

Indications

- Liver cyst >10 cm with multiple daughter cysts
- Superficial, single liver cyst (rupture or trauma)
- Secondarily infected cyst
- Cyst located in certain organs like the brain, lung or kidney
- Cyst communicating with the biliary tree/exerting pressure on an adjacent organ

Contraindications

- Multiple cysts in various locations
- Concomitant severe disease (cardiac, renal, etc.)
- Cysts that are difficult to access
- Dead cysts or very small cysts

PAIR (Puncture, Aspiration, Injection and Re-aspiration)

In this method, the cyst is percutaneously punctured under USG guidance, and fluid is aspirated (10–15 ml). Then, a **protoscolicidal agent** (95% ethanol or 20% hypertonic NaCl) is injected to destroy the germinal layer. After another 15–20 minutes, fluid is re-aspirated from the cyst.

Advantages

- Higher cure rates and lower rates of recurrence
- Lower complications rates and mortality
- Lesser duration of hospitalisation as compared to surgery

Contraindications

- Superficially located cysts
- Cysts with multiple, thick internal septal divisions (honeycomb pattern)
- Cysts communicating with the biliary tree

Note: Great care should be taken to avoid spillage of fluid during PAIR. Albendazole is initiated one week before the procedure and continued for two months post-intervention.

Percutaneous Thermal Ablation

The germinal layer of the hydatid cyst may be destroyed using a radiofrequency ablation device. This method is being explored as a promising new modality.

Wait and Watch

This approach is used for biologically inactive or degenerative cysts on imaging. Follow-up of patients by imaging is recommended at 3–6 monthly intervals.

PREVENTION AND CONTROL

- **Fruits and vegetables eaten raw should be washed** thoroughly to get rid of eggs. The eggs are resistant to commonly used disinfectants.

- Good personal hygiene is important.
- Livestock slaughtering conditions in abattoirs should be regulated (by the destruction of offals and preventing dogs from feeding on infected organs of ungulates).
- There should be strict dietary regulation of pet dogs. Intimate contact with dogs should be restricted.
- Dogs should be periodically treated with a single dose of praziquantel.
- A vaccine called **EG95 recombinant vaccine** is commercially available for **use in sheep**.

ECHINOCOCCUS MULTILOCULARIS

INTRODUCTION

Alveolar echinococcosis is one of the most fatal parasitic diseases. It chiefly exists in a sylvatic cycle involving foxes and rodents, and humans are accidental hosts. For a long time, AE was considered a multi-cystic variant of *E. granulosus* disease. It only in the 1950s that *E. multilocularis* was identified as a separate species by H. Vogel.

EPIDEMIOLOGY

It is reported from Eurasia, north and central United States, northwestern Alaska, northwestern Canada, China and Japan. It is not known to be prevalent in India.

Risk Factors

Hunters and persons who work with fox fur, those involved in farming and agricultural occupations and those who live in the vicinity of dogs that regularly feed on rodents are especially at risk.

MORPHOLOGY

Adult Worm

It is smaller than *E. granulosus*, measuring **1.2–3.7 mm** in length.

Larva

The metacestode larva ranges in size from 1 mm to several centimetres. It is multi-vesicular with a semi-solid connective tissue and little or no fluid (Fig. 41.4). The

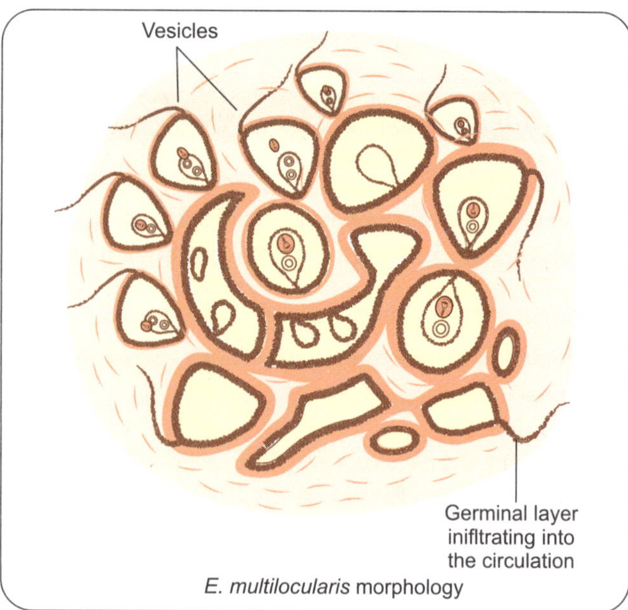

Fig. 41.4 Line diagram of *Echinococcus* multilocularis: multi-cystic vesicles showing the germinal layer infiltrating the circulation

vesicles have a few protoscolices in the natural host—rodent. In the unnatural human host, however, these vesicles are typically sterile with no scolices.

- The **germinal layer grows both endogenously and exogenously**, creating a network of tube-like and cystic structures with no adventitial layer to limit its growth and spread.
- The cystic vesicles and germinal cells may detach and metastasise to different body sites hematogenously or through lymph.

Egg

The eggs of *Echinococcus* are similar to those of *Taenia*.

LIFE CYCLE (Fig. 41.2)

E. multilocularis follows a life cycle similar to that of *E. granulosus* with a few differences, which are as follows:

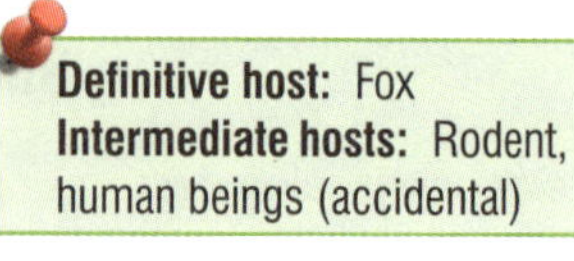

- The transmission of *E. multilocularis* is mainly sylvatic.
- The definitive hosts of *E. multilocularis* are the red fox (*Vulpus vulpes*) and the arctic fox, and rarely, wolves, coyotes, dogs and cats. The natural intermediate hosts are rodents, voles, hamsters, gerbils, squirrels and similar small mammals.

Humans are the **accidental dead-end** hosts and are affected when there is an **overlap in the sylvatic cycle of the parasite and the domestic environment of the human** by the involvement of dogs and cats as definitive hosts when they regularly feed on rodents. In humans, no protoscolices are found in the cysts. This indicates that humans are not very good hosts for this parasite.

PATHOGENESIS

Human beings acquire the infection by ingesting the eggs of *E. multilocularis*. The alveolar cyst behaves like a slow-growing malignancy and remains asymptomatic for several years. The larval mass spreads by proliferating at the margins and invading the surrounding tissue. It also metastasises to distant organs like the lungs and brain. The protein 14-3-3 found in the germinal layer is associated with the progressive and unlimited growth of the AE cyst.

CLINICAL FEATURES

Almost all primary AE lesions are found in the **liver (98%)**. However, extensive proliferation and metastases could involve other organs. No significant symptoms are seen in the early stages of the disease, and patients may remain asymptomatic for 10–15 years. For this reason, patients usually present late. However, in immunosuppressed individuals, the rate of growth of the metacestode is faster.

- The clinical features mimic those of hepatic malignancy. The multilocular infiltrating lesion appears like a grossly invasive growth without any fluid, free brood capsule or scolices, which can result in it being mistaken for a malignant tumour.
- Patients present with upper quadrant and epigastric pain. Hepatomegaly and obstructive jaundice may also be present. The lesion may also metastasise to the spleen, lungs and brain in a few cases.
- If left untreated, AE has a **mortality of more than 90%** within 10–15 years of diagnosis.

DIAGNOSIS

The approach to the diagnosis of AE is based on radiological examination and supported by serological evidence of echinococcal disease.

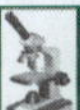

Lab diagnosis

- **Imaging:** USG, CT or MRI to visualise cysts
- **Serology:** Detection of specific antibodies against Em2 and Em18 antigens
- **Microscopy:** By visualising cysts
  - Histopathology: Cyst morphology
- **DNA detection:** PCR

Radioimaging

Imaging is most sensitive and specific for the diagnosis of AE. Based on USG imaging, WHO-IWGE has classified hepatic AE lesions into different PNM (**p**arasitic lesion, involvement of **n**eighbouring organs and distant **m**etastases) types which provide the basis for treatment decisions. Complementary imaging techniques include CT, PET scan and MRI, which help to determine whether the cyst is metabolically active or inactive.

Contrast-enhanced ultrasonography (CEUS) may be used for detecting small AE lesions and differentiating them from abscesses and tumours.

Serodiagnosis

Antibody detection: AE serology is quite reliable. ELISA tests based on antibody detection against **Em2** and **Em18** are available; they are specific for *E. multilocularis* infection and can differentiate it from *E. granulosus*. However, imaging remains the mainstay of diagnosis. Serology is used only to confirm the imaging results for both CE and AE; it cannot be used as a first-choice diagnostic tool for mass screening in endemic areas where a certain proportion of the population is expected to yield positive serology without AE lesions.

Nucleic Acid-Based Detection

DNA-based methods are highly sensitive, specific and can distinguish between *Echinococcus* species.

Histopathology

Surgically removed cysts can be stained with Giemsa, H&E or PAS stain.

TREATMENT

The treatment of AE depends on the size of the lesion, the extent of involvement of the neighbouring organs and the surgical expertise available.

Surgery

Surgical resection of early lesions may be curative. Due to the absence of a limiting capsule, the complete removal of an AE cyst is not possible. Hence there are high rates of relapses. Since AE lesions are most often located in the right lobe of the liver and invade the major bile ducts and vessels in advanced cases, surgery is associated with significant morbidity and mortality due to uncontrolled bleeding or liver failure. Liver transplantation may also be desirable in few cases.

Note: Unlike CE, injection of protoscolicidal agents should never be used in AE.

Drug Treatment

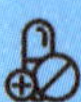

Drug of choice

- *Albendazole:* For adults, 400 mg BDS; for children, 10–15 mg/kg/day in 2 divided doses (maximum 800 mg) for at least 2 years or longer

Alternate drug

- Patients must be monitored for side effects of prolonged administration of albendazole; if such side effects are noted, they should be switched to mebendazole, 40–50 mg/kg/day in 3 divided doses

Wait and Watch

This approach may be used for calcified or metabolically inactive cysts.

Follow-up: All AE patients should receive follow-ups after the initiation of treatment for at least ten years by imaging and/or serological methods.

PREVENTION AND CONTROL

- Standards of sanitation and hygiene should be improved.
- Food like fruits and vegetables which are eaten raw should be thoroughly washed before consumption.
- Contact with dogs and foxes should be avoided in endemic areas.
- Dogs should be periodically treated with a single dose of praziquantel.
- Fox baits should be laced with praziquantel.

Questions

1. Enumerate the types of space-occupying lesions of the liver. Discuss the lab diagnosis and management of cystic echinococcosis.
2. Discuss the life cycle of *E. granulosus* and the morphology of hydatid cysts (cystic echinococcosis).
3. Discuss the laboratory diagnosis and management of alveolar echinococcosis.

Multiple Choice Questions

1. Cystic echinococcosis is caused by ____________:
   a. *Echinococcus granulosus*
   b. *Echinococcus multilocularis*
   c. *Echinococcus vogeli*
   d. *Echinococcus oligarthus*
2. Alveolar echinococcosis is caused by ____________:
   a. *Echinococcus granulosus*
   b. *Echinococcus multilocularis*
   c. *Echinococcus vogeli*
   d. *Echinococcus oligarthus*
3. Humans serve as the ____________ host in hydatid disease.
   a. Definitive
   b. Intermediate
   c. Carrier
   d. Paratenic
4. Humans acquire hydatid disease by the ingestion of _________:
   a. Contaminated fruits and vegetables
   b. Infected pork containing cysts
   c. Infected beef containing cysts
   d. All these
5. PAIR (puncture, aspiration, injection and re-aspiration) technique is recommended for the management of cystic echinococcosis having ____________:
   a. Degenerative cysts
   b. Cysts with multiple thick internal septal divisions
   c. Cysts communicating with the biliary tree
   d. Single, uncomplicated cysts in the liver
6. Which protoscolicidal is used for the PAIR technique?
   a. 95% ethanol
   b. 40% formalin
   c. 10% phenol
   d. Xylene

7. Surgery is recommended for the management of all the following cystic echinococcus cysts EXCEPT ____________ :
   a. Liver cyst <5 cm
   b. Secondarily infected cyst
   c. Cyst located in certain organs like the brain, lung or kidney
   d. Cyst communicating with the biliary tree/exerting pressure on an adjacent organ
8. All the following statements about cystic echinococcosis are true EXCEPT ____________ :
   a. Cysts are most commonly located in the liver.
   b. Most patients have a single cyst.
   c. Microscopic examination of aspirated fluid is the test of choice.
   d. It is caused by *Echinococcus granulosus.*
9. Alveolar echinococcosis is ____________ :
   a. Most commonly reported from India
   b. Most commonly located in the lungs
   c. Associated with a very high mortality
   d. Acquired by the ingestion of meat contaminated with cysts
10. The treatment of alveolar echinococcosis includes all the following modalities EXCEPT:
   a. Albendazole
   b. Surgical resection
   c. PAIR (puncture, aspiration, injection of protoscolicidal agent and re-aspiration)
   d. All these

Chapter 42 Fasiolopsis and Other Intestinal Trematodes

([From Greek] *fasciola* = small band + *opsis* = resembling)

Case Study and Learning Goals

A 25-year-old male presents with chronic diarrhea and eosinophilia. What are the parasitic causes of chronic diarrhea with eosinophilia? How would you approach the laboratory diagnosis in this case? How would you treat this patient?

INTESTINAL TREMATODES

INTRODUCTION

These parasites of vertebrates are hermaphrodites, dorsoventrally flattened (**leaf-like**) and require one or more intermediate hosts to complete their life cycles. More than 60 species of trematodes have been described in the intestinal tracts of humans. The majority of these infections are **zoonotic and foodborne** and have a **restricted geographic distribution**, largely because of specific food preferences. Often, the clinical reports consist of single cases or a small cluster of cases.

EPIDEMIOLOGY

Approximately 100 million people are estimated to be infected with intestinal trematodes worldwide. These infections are foodborne and are emerging as a major public health problem. Most of those infected are from the Far East and parts of South-East Asia including Korea, China, Thailand, Vietnam, Lao PDR, the Philippines, Indonesia and India.

Of the several fluke species which can infect humans, the most important genera are *Fasciolopsis, Heterophyes, Gastrodiscoides, Metagonimus, Echinostoma* and *Watsonius* (Table 42.1).

Human infections: Various types of foods are sources of human infections. They include freshwater or brackish-water fish, freshwater snails, oysters, amphibians, snakes, aquatic insects and aquatic plants. The reservoir hosts include various species of mammals and birds. All intestinal flukes require a freshwater snail as an intermediate host.

FASCIOLOPSIS BUSKI

INTRODUCTION

It is the **largest trematode found in humans** and is also known as the **giant intestinal fluke.** It was first discovered by George Busk in 1843 in the duodenum of an East Indian sailor who died in London.

EPIDEMIOLOGY

It is a common parasite of **humans and pigs** in South and South-East Asia, viz. India, China, Pakistan, Bangladesh, Thailand, Malaysia and Indonesia. The risk factors that predispose to acquiring the infection are poverty, poor hygiene and the habit of eating **raw or pickled water plants.** The infections are most common in school-age children.

India: *F. buski* infections have been reported from many parts of the country, viz. the north and north-eastern states, especially Assam, Bengal, Uttar Pradesh, Bihar, Odisha and Madhya Pradesh. Recent epidemiological investigations of human infections point towards a focus in the East Champaran district of Bihar. A high prevalence of the infection in livestock is reported in many studies indicating a wide reservoir in the country.

MORPHOLOGY

For general morphological features of trematodes, refer to **Chapter 22**, *Helminths – Introduction and Classification*.

Adult Worm

It is the largest trematode to infect humans (Fig. 42.1a, b and c).

- It is dark red, fleshy, ovoid and measures 20–75 mm in length and 8–20 mm in width.
- It is similar in external morphology to *Fasciola hepatica*, except that the **ventral sucker is much larger than the oral sucker and there is no cephalic cone.**
- The adults are monoecious.

Eggs

The eggs are large, ellipsoidal, yellow-brown and measure 130–140 × 80–85 μm in size (Fig. 42.3a).

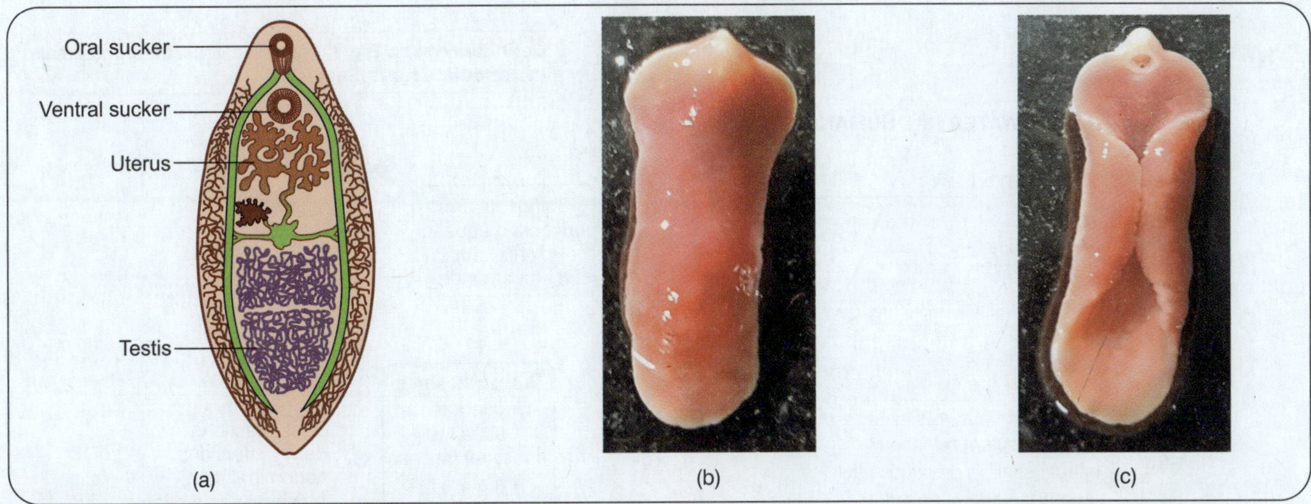

Fig 42.1 Adult of *Fasciolopsis buski*: (a) line diagram, (b) dorsal view of a red, fleshy adult fluke and (c) ventral aspect with sides folded, showing a large ventral sucker

They have a clear, thin shell and are operculated at the top and unembryonated. The operculum is difficult to see and does not have any distinct opercular shoulders. The egg releases the miracidium, which develops into the subsequent larval stages of sporocyst, redia, cercaria and finally, the metacercaria.

LIFE CYCLE (Fig. 42.2a and b)

> **Definitive hosts:** Pigs, humans, livestock and other mammals
> **Intermediate hosts:** Snails

Humans are infected when they **consume uncooked aquatic plants (water caltrops, water chestnuts, water bamboo, lotus)** infected with encysted metacercariae. The various life cycle stages of *F. buski* are as follows:

Excystation: Once ingested, the metacercariae excyst in the duodenum of the host and become attached to the intestinal mucosa. There, they develop into adult worms in three months.

Sexual phase: The adult lives in the small intestine and produces eggs which are excreted along with the host's feces and eventually reach freshwater bodies.

Asexual phase: The miracidium develops in the egg for 3–7 weeks. It then escapes the egg to find the **intermediate host, a species-specific snail (*Segmentina*),** in which it passes through the sporocyst stages, 2–3 generations of redia, and finally develops into cercariae.

Free-living stage: The cercariae are released out of the snail after 4–7 weeks. They encyst on aquatic plants, where they develop into metacercariae in about four weeks to once again infect a definitive host.

PATHOGENESIS

The attachment of the adult worm to the intestinal mucosa causes inflammation, hemorrhage, ulceration and abscesses. Heavy infections tend to cause intestinal obstruction. The absorption of the worm's toxic metabolites may cause allergic reactions, generalised edema and ascites.

CLINICAL FEATURES

Flukes predominantly reside in the duodenum and jejunum but may be found in other parts of the intestine, especially in heavy infections.

Light infections: Light infections are usually asymptomatic. Anemia, eosinophilia, headache, dizziness, gastric pain and loose stools are the commonest features of such infections.

Heavy infections: Heavy infections may manifest as abdominal pain, diarrhea, intestinal obstruction, acute ileus, etc. Ascites, general edema, anemia and asthenia may occur. Chronic heavy infections may result in chronic diarrhea leading to malabsorption, protein-losing enteropathy or vitamin B12 deficiency.

DIAGNOSIS

The diagnosis is made by demonstrating eggs in stool (Fig. 42.3a).

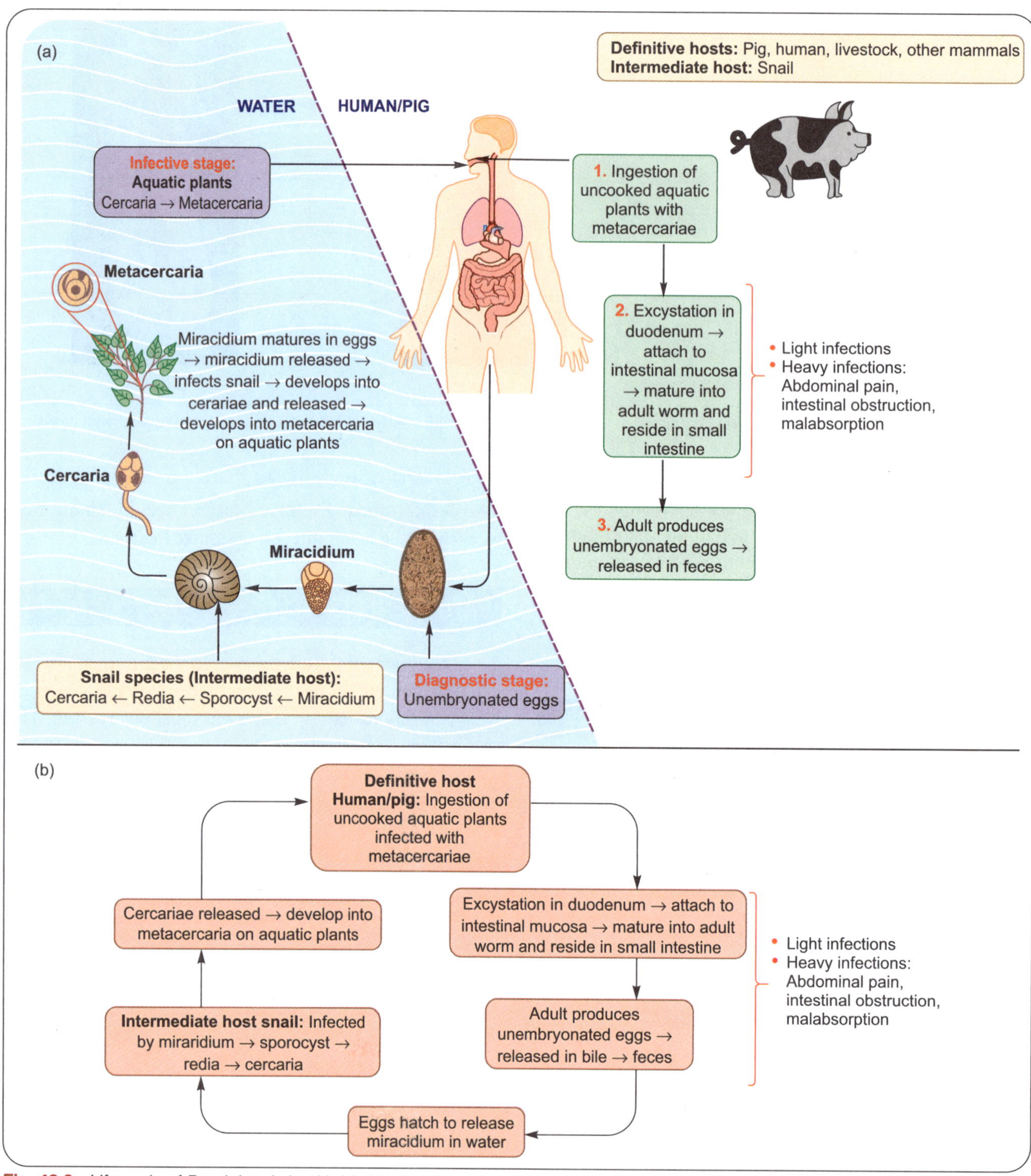

Fig. 42.2 Life cycle of *Fasciolopsis buski*: (a) detailed (b) schematic

Lab diagnosis

- **Microscopy:** By visualising eggs in stool samples and rarely, the adult worm
- **Other diagnostic parameters:**
  - Persistent eosinophilia
  - Anemia

Microscopy

Eggs are operculated and thus, should be concentrated by the sedimentation technique; floatation is not effective since the eggs do not float.

The problem with this modality is that the eggs of *Fasciolopsis buski* cannot be differentiated from

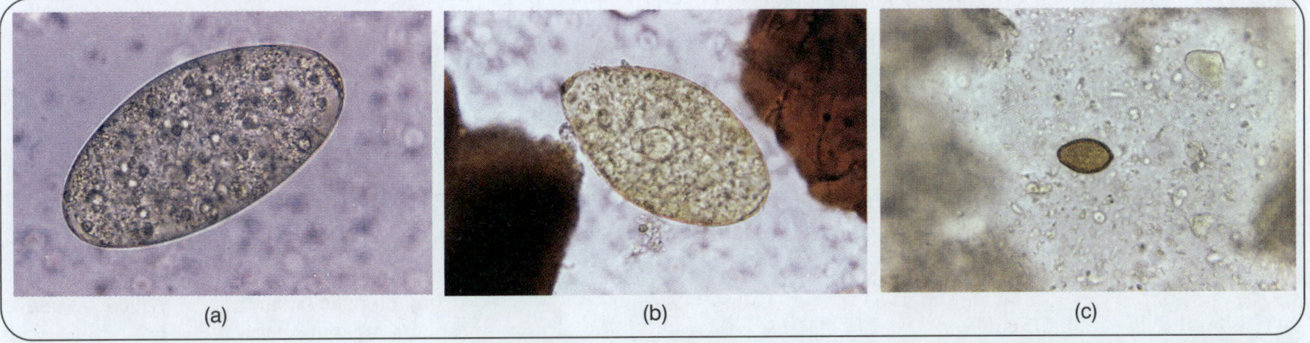

Fig. 42.3 Eggs of intestinal flukes: (a) broadly ellipsoidal, operculated and unembryonated *Fasciolopsis buski* egg, (b) *Echinostoma* spp. egg and (c) *Heterophyes* spp. egg (*Source:* Centers for Disease Control and Prevention [CDC], Public Health Image Library [PHIL], Image IDs 15219, 655 and 657)

the morphologically similar eggs of *Echinostoma ilocanum*, *Gastrodiscoides hominis* and *Fasciola hepatica* (Table 42.1).

Adult worms, when recovered, can rarely confirm the diagnosis.

Other Diagnostic Parameters

Marked eosinophilia and leukocytosis are usually seen.

TREATMENT

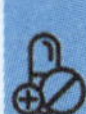

Drug of choice
- *Praziquantel:* 25 mg/kg/day TDS × 1 day for both children and adults

PREVENTION AND CONTROL

- **Water plants should be cooked** or immersed in boiling water for a few seconds before they are eaten or peeled.
- The use of unsterilised night soil as fertiliser should be prohibited.
- The chain of infection should be broken by prompt diagnosis and treatment of infected humans and livestock.

LESS COMMON INTESTINAL FLUKES

Other trematodes which infect the human intestine less commonly are *Heterophyes, Gastrodiscoides, Metagonimus, Echinostoma* and *Watsonius* (Table 42.1). The habitat of all intestinal flukes in humans is the small intestine. The exception is *Gastrodiscoides*, which inhabits the large intestine. *Heterophyes* is the **smallest** trematode to infect humans.

CLINICAL FEATURES

Most light infections are asymptomatic or present with only minor symptoms. Heavy infections may lead to intestinal inflammation and mild ulceration, and the patient may have abdominal pain or diarrhea.

DIAGNOSIS

The diagnosis of intestinal fluke infection is made by demonstrating eggs in stool (Fig. 42.3a, b and c). These eggs are similar in appearance for different species and difficult to differentiate except on the basis of their size (Table 42.1). The eggs are operculated and thus should be concentrated by the sedimentation technique; floatation is ineffective since they do not float. The eggs of *Heterophyes* and *Metagonimus* are minute and may be missed if the specimen is not examined carefully.

TREATMENT

It is the same as that for *Fasciolopsis buski* infections.

PREVENTION AND CONTROL

- Vegetables that grow in water should be thoroughly washed, preferably in hot water.
- The contamination of ponds and other water bodies with pig or human excreta should be prevented.
- Night soil should be sterilised before using it as a fertiliser.
- The population of molluscs and snails should be controlled.

Table 42.1 Characteristics of important trematodes

Parasite	Distribution	Agent of infection	Reservoir hosts	Adult worm and habitat in humans	Egg
Fasciolopsis buski	Far East, South-East Asia, India	Freshwater plants, water caltrop, waterlily, watercress	Dogs, pigs	Largest trematode 20–75 mm × 8–20 mm Small intestine (duodenum and jejunum)	130–140 × 80–85 μm Operculum difficult to see
Echinostoma ilocanum	Far East, South-East Asia	Molluscs, fish, tadpoles	Dogs, rats	10 × 2 mm Small intestine Characteristic collar of spines present on the lateral and dorsal sides of the oral sucker	100 × 60 μm Operculum difficult to see
Heterophyes heterophyes, Metagonimus yokogawai	Far East, Middle East	Freshwater fish	Fish-eating mammals	Minute 5 × 1 mm Small intestine (jejunum and upper ileum)	30 × 15 μm Operculum difficult to see
Gastrodiscoides hominis	Far East, Middle East, former USSR	Freshwater fish	Pigs, deer, mice, rats	5 × 10 mm Pyriform Large intestine (caecum and ascending colon)	60 × 150 μm Operculum difficult to see

Questions

1. Describe the morphology and life cycle of *Fasciolopsis buski*.
2. Discuss the diagnosis, management and prevention of intestinal trematode infections.
3. Describe the general characteristics of intestinal trematodes.

Multiple Choice Questions

1. The smallest intestinal trematode is ____________:
   a. *Fasciolopsis buski*
   b. *Metagonimus metagoni*
   c. *Heterophyes heterophyes*
   d. *Clonorchis sinensis*
2. Which of the following is NOT a characteristic of intestinal trematodes eggs?
   a. Operculated
   b. Measure 130–140 × 80–85 μm in size
   c. Thick outer shell with striate radiations
   d. Unembryonated
3. The drug of choice for intestinal fluke infections is ____________:
   a. Ivermectin
   b. Albendazole
   c. Praziquantel
   d. Metronidazole
4. The largest and the most common intestinal fluke to infect humans is ____________:
   a. *Fasciola hepatica*
   b. *Fasciolopsis buski*
   c. *Metagonimus yokogawai*
   d. *Heterophyes heterophyes*
5. Humans are infected with *Fasciolopsis buski* when they consume ____________:
   a. Uncooked aquatic plants (like water caltrops, water chestnuts and lotus) infected with encysted metacercariae
   b. Snails containing metacercariae
   c. Snails harbouring miracidia
   d. Uncooked aquatic plants (water caltrops, water chestnuts, lotus) infected with encysted miracidia
6. Which of the following statements about intestinal trematodes is NOT TRUE?
   a. These infections are most common in Far Eastern and South-East Asian countries.
   b. All these parasites produce operculated eggs but the operculum may not be conspicuous.
   c. The only sources of infection are infected snails, molluscs and fish.
   d. The infections do not disseminate to extraintestinal sites.

CHAPTER 43

Fasciola

(*fasciola* [From Greek] = small band; *hepatica* from *hepai* [Greek] = liver)

Case Study and Learning Goals

An 18-year-old female presents with recurrent anorexia, nausea and flatulence with features of jaundice. On endoscopic exploration, a leaf-like worm is recovered from her biliary aspirate. Which parasites can be found in the biliary tract? How would you approach the laboratory diagnosis in this case? How would you treat this patient?

INTRODUCTION

Chiefly, two species of the genus *Fasciola* are of medical importance to humans—***Fasciola hepatica***, also known as the **common liver fluke or sheep liver fluke,** and ***F. gigantica***, the **giant liver fluke.** Apart from being foodborne trematodes of human importance, the liver flukes also have immense veterinary importance as they infect domestic livestock such as sheep, goats, camels and cattle.

Liver fluke infections were first described in sheep as '**liver rot**' by Jehan de Brie in 1379, but the organism was named by Carl Linnaeus only in 1758. The human infections caused by these parasites were documented in 1760 by P. S. Pallas. *Fasciola* was the first trematode whose life cycle was described; this was done independently by Rudolf Leuckart and Algernon Thomas in 1880.

EPIDEMIOLOGY

Across the world, approximately 5–17 million people are infected with liver flukes, i.e., *Fasciola, Opisthorchis* and *Clonorchis* (Table 43.1).

- *F. hepatica* has a worldwide distribution and is a common zoonosis throughout Eurasia and parts of South America and Africa. Infections are most common in areas where there is close association between livestock, humans and snails.
- *F. gigantica* is known to be endemic in Africa and Asia along with *F. hepatica*.

India: Liver flukes are relatively rare in India; there are only some reports of *F. hepatica* and *F. gigantica*. *Clonorchis* and *Opisthorchis* infections are not reported from India.

MORPHOLOGY

For the general morphological features of trematodes, please refer to **Chapter 22**, *Helminths – Introduction and Classification*.

Adult Worm

It is one of the largest trematodes to infect humans. The two species, *F. hepatica* and *F. gigantica,* are difficult to differentiate morphologically, except on the basis of their size.

- Liver flukes are **leaf-shaped**, have highly branched testes and intestinal caeca. *F. hepatica* measures 30 × 12 mm, while *F. gigantica* measures 25–75 × 12 mm in size.
- A distinct identifying feature of *Fascicola* is the presence of a '**shoulder**' and an anterior prominence called the **cephalic cone** (Fig. 43.1a and b).
- The oral sucker is situated on the cephalic cone. The **equally-sized ventral sucker** is also situated in the anterior portion of the fluke's body, close to the genital pore.
- The adults are monoecious.

Eggs

The eggs of *F. hepatica* are large, yellowish-brown, bile-stained, ovoid and measure 130–150 × 60–90 μm in size.

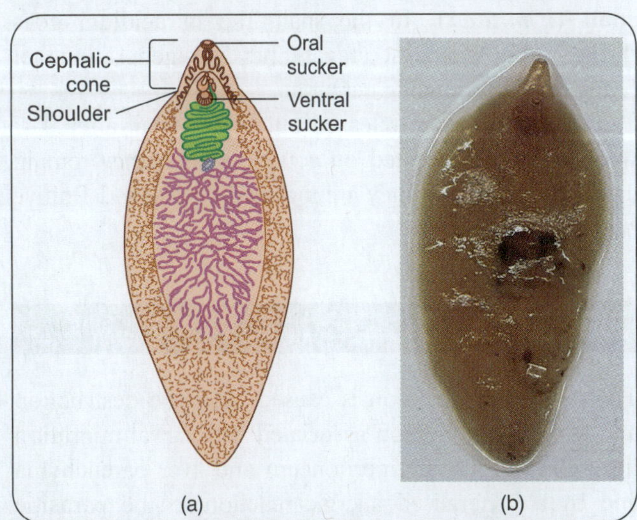

Fig. 43.1 Adult of *Fasciola hepatica*: (a) line diagram and (b) unstained adult fluke showing a prominent cephalic cone and equally-sized oral and ventral suckers

They are operculated and unembryonated. The eggs of *F. hepatica* are very similar to those of *Fasciolopsis buski*. The eggs of *F. gigantica* measure 160–190 × 70–90 µm. The eggs release miracidium-stage larvae, which develop into the subsequent larval stages of sporocyst, redia, cercaria and finally, the metacercaria.

LIFE CYCLE (Fig. 43.2a and b)

> **Definitive hosts:** Sheep, goat, camel, cattle and humans
> **Intermediate host:** Snail

Humans are infected when they consume **uncooked aquatic plants (watercress) infected with metacercariae** of the liver fluke. The various life cycle stages of *F. hepatica* are as follows:

Migratory phase: Once ingested, the metacercariae excyst in the host's duodenum and penetrate the intestinal wall to reach the peritoneum. Then, they further burrow into the Glisson's capsule and enter the liver tissue and finally, infiltrate the bile ducts in about 6–7 weeks.

Sexual phase: The metacercariae settle and mature into adult flukes in the bile ducts, gallbladder and liver tissue of mammalian hosts including humans. After maturation, they start producing eggs. They have a long life span of more than ten years. The unembryonated eggs are carried by bile to the intestinal tract, from where they are released into the environment along with the host's feces in about 3–4 months after infection.

Asexual phase: In freshwater bodies, the miracidium develops in the egg in about two weeks and then escapes the egg to find the **intermediate host, a species-specific snail (*Lymnaea*).** In the snail, the miracidium goes through the sporocyst stages and 2–3 generations of redia, finally producing cercariae.

The cercariae are released out of the snail after 4–7 weeks and get encysted on aquatic plants; they remain in such a state until they are ingested by a new definitive host.

PATHOGENESIS

The disease progression is caused by tissue destruction and acute inflammation associated with larval migration through the intestine, peritoneum and liver parenchyma and by a generalised allergic reaction to the parasitic antigens. The following features are seen:

- The worms reside in the bile duct and stimulate chronic inflammation and fibrosis.
- There is granuloma formation around the eggs and worms which develops into abscesses. This is followed by fibrosis, bile duct hyperplasia and deposition of collagen.

CLINICAL FEATURES

The incubation period of fascioliasis varies from days to a few months. Infections with *F. hepatica* and *F. gigantica* are clinically indistinguishable and can be divided into acute, latent (the stage at which the parasites mature into adults) and chronic phases.

Acute Infection

Acute clinical features usually represent metacercarial migration through the host's tissues. Fever and abdominal pain, which may be severe, are the most frequently reported symptoms. Anorexia, nausea, diarrhea, flatulence, urticaria and cough are also common. Sometimes, hepatomegaly, splenomegaly, jaundice and ascites occur. Leukocytosis, eosinophilia, mild to moderate anemia and hypergammaglobulinemia are frequently observed.

Acute symptoms may last 2–4 months, but in endemic areas, re-infection is known to cause episodic symptoms and overlap of acute and chronic symptoms.

> **Halzoun syndrome**
> In some endemic areas where uncooked goat liver or sheep liver is eaten, the adult worms may, in rare cases, get attached to the pharyngeal mucosa and cause the swelling of the soft palate, laryngopharynx, nasal fossae and the eustachian tube. This may lead to dyspnea, dysphagia, deafness or suffocation.

Chronic Infection

The adult flukes can live in humans for up to 15 years. They cause inflammation and obstruction of the large biliary ducts. Cholangitis, cholecystitis, cholelithiasis, subcapsular hemorrhages and abscesses (called **liver rot**), cirrhosis and pancreatitis are known complications. There is no known association between *Fasciola* infection and cholangiocarcinoma.

DIAGNOSIS

Direct microscopic demonstration of eggs in stool samples, duodenal aspirates, bile specimens or surgical samples may be useful in the late phase of

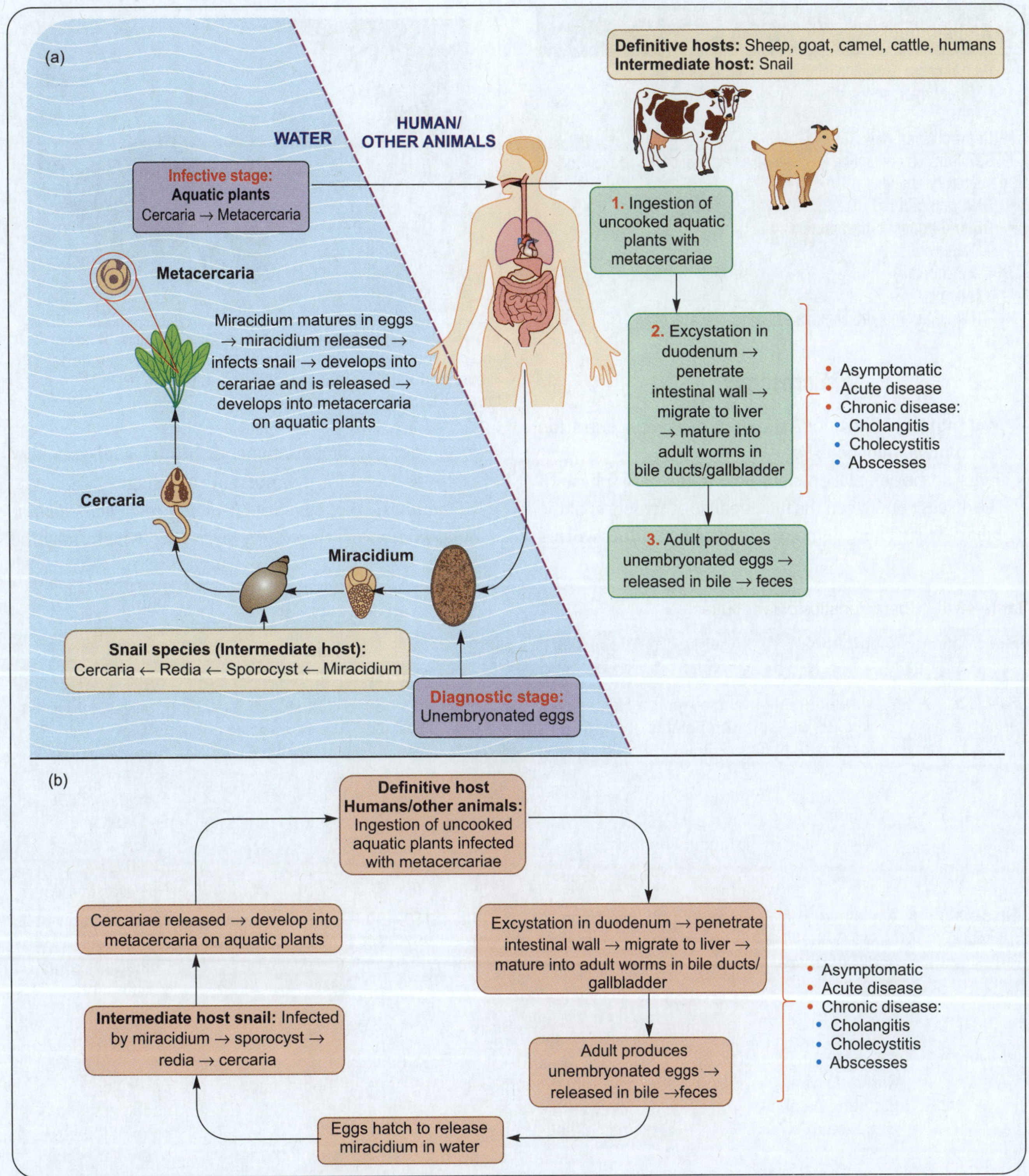

Fig. 43.2 Life cycle of *Fasciola*: (a) detailed and (b) schematic

the infection (Fig. 43.3). Multiple stool samples may be required to find the eggs. Since *Fasciola* eggs do not float, the zinc sulphate floatation method is not an effective concentration technique. Instead, stool samples should be concentrated by the sedimentation technique. Egg morphology alone is not enough to differentiate between various flukes as the **eggs of *F. hepatica* resemble those of *F. gigantica* and some intestinal flukes like *F. buski*, *Gastrodiscoides*,** etc. (Table 43.1).

Lab diagnosis

- **Microscopy:** By visualising eggs or adult worms
  - Direct microscopy of stool, duodenal aspirate or bile
  - ERCP
- **Coproantigen detection:** ELISA
- **Serology:** By detecting IgG antibodies against crude or excretory–secretory antigens
- **DNA detection:** PCR
- **Other diagnostic parameters:**
  - Radioimaging
  - Eosinophilia
  - Anemia
  - Hypergammaglobulinemia

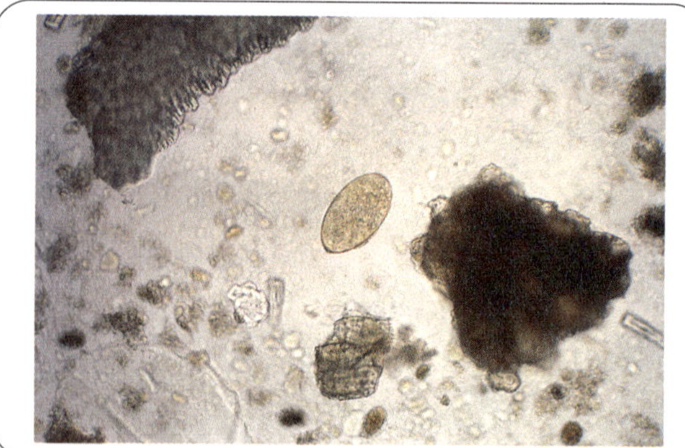

Fig. 43.3 Egg of *Fasciola hepatica*: broadly ellipsoidal and operculated (*Source:* Centers for Disease Control and Prevention [CDC], Public Health Image Library [PHIL], Image ID 1540)

Microscopy

- **Wet mount** preparations and preferably, concentration techniques, may be used.
- Eggs do not appear in stool during the early phase of the disease and when the flukes cause obstruction of the biliary tree. Thus, demonstrating **ova or adult worms** in endoscopic or percutaneous **biliary aspirates** may be more useful for diagnosis at such stages.
- Sometimes, the eggs of *F. hepatica*, *Dicrocoelium dendriticum* or *Capillaria hepatica*, which may be

Table 43.1 Characteristics of liver flukes

Species	Distribution	Agent of infection	Reservoir host	Adult worm	Egg		Comments
					Size (μm)	Morphology	
Fasciola hepatica	Worldwide	Uncooked water plants	Herbivores	3 cm long × 1.2 cm wide Prominent shoulders	130–150 × 60–90	Unembryonated and operculated	Operculum difficult to see Eggs resemble those of *Fasciolopsis buski, Echinostoma, Fasciola gigantica* and *Gastrodiscoides*
Fasciola gigantica	Africa and Asia Mixed *F. hepatica* and *F. gigantica* infections frequently reported	Uncooked water plants	Herbivores	2.5–7.5 cm long × 1.2 cm wide	160–190 × 70–90	Unembryonated and operculated	Operculum difficult to see The egg is larger than that of *F. hepatica*
Clonorchis sinensis	China, South Korea, Taiwan, northern Vietnam and eastern Russia	Uncooked fish	Dogs, cats, other fish-eating mammals	10–20 mm long × 3–5 mm wide	20–30 × 15	Embryonated and operculated	Very prominent opercular shoulders, and a knob at the ab-opercular end
Opisthorchis viverrini	Northern Thailand, Laos, Cambodia and central and south Vietnam	Uncooked fish	Dogs, cats, other fish-eating mammals	8–12 mm long × 3–5 mm wide	20–30 × 15	Embryonated and operculated	Prominent opercular shoulders
Opisthorchis felineus	Soviet Union, including Belarus, Kazakhstan and Ukraine	Uncooked fish	Dogs, cats, other fish-eating mammals	Same as *O. viverrini*	20–30 × 11	Unembryonated and operculated	Prominent opercular shoulders

present in the liver of cattle, sheep and rodents respectively, may be observed in human stool samples due to the ingestion of the uncooked infected liver of these animals, which results in the passage of the eggs in the feces. Such spurious infections (**pseudofascioliasis**) can be ruled out by repeated ova and parasite examinations for a few days.

Adult flukes can be visualised on examining stool after their expulsion from the biliary tree post-treatment.

Histopathology

Parasite fragments and eggs can sometimes be seen in surgical tissue or biopsies.

Serology

Commercially available serological tests for the detection of serum antibodies against crude or excretory–secretory antigens help in early diagnosis, before the eggs are detected in stool. These are also useful for epidemiological purposes.

Coproantigen Detection

ELISA-based tests have been used with higher sensitivity than stool microscopy. These could be of use to detect light infections and to assess treatment success.

Nucleic Acid-Based Detection

PCR assays performed on fecal samples are chiefly employed at research centres to speciate the parasite.

Other Diagnostic Parameters

- **Radioimaging:** Ultrasound, CT or MRI may be useful in diagnosis.
- **Hematological and biochemical abnormalities:** Eosinophilia, anemia and hypergammaglobulinemia related to chronic blood loss from damaged biliary epithelia, and deranged liver function tests are common.

TREATMENT

Fasciola is the only trematode that does not respond to praziquantel.

Drug of choice

- *Triclabendazole:* 10 mg/kg as a single dose

Alternate drugs

- *Nitazoxanide:* 500 mg/day BDS × 7 days
- *Bithionol:* 30–50 mg/kg on alternate days × 10–15 doses

Surgical management: Endoscopic retrograde cholangiopancreatography (ERCP) is particularly useful for the treatment of biliary obstruction and could be of use in any liver fluke infection causing biliary obstructive cholangitis or in cholecystitis due to flukes.

PREVENTION AND CONTROL

- The consumption of **raw or undercooked fish should be avoided.**
- Stool and sewage should be disposed of in a sanitary manner.
- The WHO recommends mass treatment with 10 mg/kg triclabendazole as a single dose for school-age children or the entire community in areas where cases of fascioliasis appear to be clustered.
- Drug resistance to *F. hepatica* from farm animals has been reported. Good practices for the management of livestock need to be put in place for the control of fascioliasis.

Questions

1. Discuss the epidemiology of liver flukes.
2. Discuss the laboratory diagnosis and management of liver fluke infections.
3. Describe the morphology and life cycle of *Fasciola hepatica*.

Multiple Choice Questions

1. The first-line treatment for fascioliasis is ________________ :
   a. Praziquantel
   b. Albendazole
   c. Triclabendazole
   d. Ivermectin

2. All liver flukes produce eggs which are ________________ :
   a. Operculated
   b. Non-operculated
   c. Float in saline solution
   d. Covered by a thick outer albuminous coat

3. Carcinoma is associated with all the following parasites EXCEPT ____________ :
   a. *Fasciola hepatica*
   b. *Opisthorchis viverrini*
   c. *Clonorchis sinensis*
   d. *Schistosoma haematobium*

CHAPTER 44

Clonorchis and Opisthorchis

(*Clonorchis* from *chlon* [Greek] = branching; *Opisthorchis* from *opisthos* [Greek] = behind + *orchis* [Greek] = testis)

Case Study and Learning Goals

A 55-year-old male from Thailand has obstructive jaundice and periportal fibrosis. His stool examination shows ovoid operculated eggs measuring 25 μm in size with knobs at the posterior ends. Which of the parasites affecting the hepatobiliary system are endemic in South-East Asia? How would you approach the laboratory diagnosis in this case? How would you treat this patient?

INTRODUCTION

Clonorchis sinensis is also called the **Chinese liver fluke**. It is the only species in this genus of medical importance in humans. It was first discovered in 1874 by James McConnell while he was performing an autopsy on a Chinese worker who had died in a medical college in Kolkata. The parasite was named by Thomas Spencer Cobbold in 1875.

There are mainly two ***Opisthorchis*** species of medical importance in humans—***O. viverrini*** and ***O. felineus***. Both species were first described in cats; human infections were reported later.

The three flukes—*C. sinensis, O. viverrini* and *O. felineus*—are maintained in the environment in pigs, dogs, cats, rats and other mammals, all of which they infect.

EPIDEMIOLOGY

People who live in geographical areas endemic for infections caused by these flukes often consume uncooked, pickled, smoked, salted or dried freshwater fish which are infested with the metacercaria. These infections are not reported in India.

C. sinensis and ***O. viverrini*** are listed as **'Class 1' biological carcinogens** (carcinogenic to human beings) by the International Agency for Research on Cancer (IARC) and cause **cholangiocarcinoma (bile duct cancer)**. *O. felineus* is usually not associated with this cancer.

- *C. sinensis* is endemic in China, South Korea, Taiwan, northern Vietnam and eastern Russia.
- *O. viverrini* is endemic in Thailand, Laos, Cambodia and central and south Vietnam. In certain areas, its prevalence may be as high as 90%.
- *O. felineus* is found in the former Soviet Union, including Belarus, Kazakhstan and Ukraine.

MORPHOLOGY

For the general morphological features of trematodes, please refer to **Chapter 22**, *Helminths – Introduction and Classification.*

Adult Worm

These are very small, elongated and **lance-shaped**, i.e., tapered anteriorly.

- *C. sinensis* measures 10–20 × 3–5 mm, while *Opisthorchis* is smaller, measuring 8–12 × 3–5 mm.
- The oral sucker is situated on the anterior end. The ventral sucker is smaller and located in the anterior portion, close to the genital pore.
- The adults are monoecious.

Eggs

The eggs are small, yellowish-brown, ovoid and measure 20–30 × 15 μm. They have a distinct operculum with shoulders (**flask-shaped**) and a comma-shaped knob at their posterior end. The eggs of *O. viverrini* have less prominent shoulders than *C. sinensis* and may or may not have the abopercular knob. These are embryonated when laid and contain a fully developed miracidium. The eggs release the miracidia, which develop into the subsequent larval stages of sporocyst, redia, cercaria and finally, the metacercaria.

LIFE CYCLE (Fig. 44.1a and b)

Humans are infected when they **consume raw or undercooked freshwater fish** infected with the flukes' metacercariae. The following are the various life cycle stages of these flukes:

Definitive hosts: Pig, dog, cat, rat and other mammals
1st intermediate host: Snail
2nd intermediate host: Freshwater fish

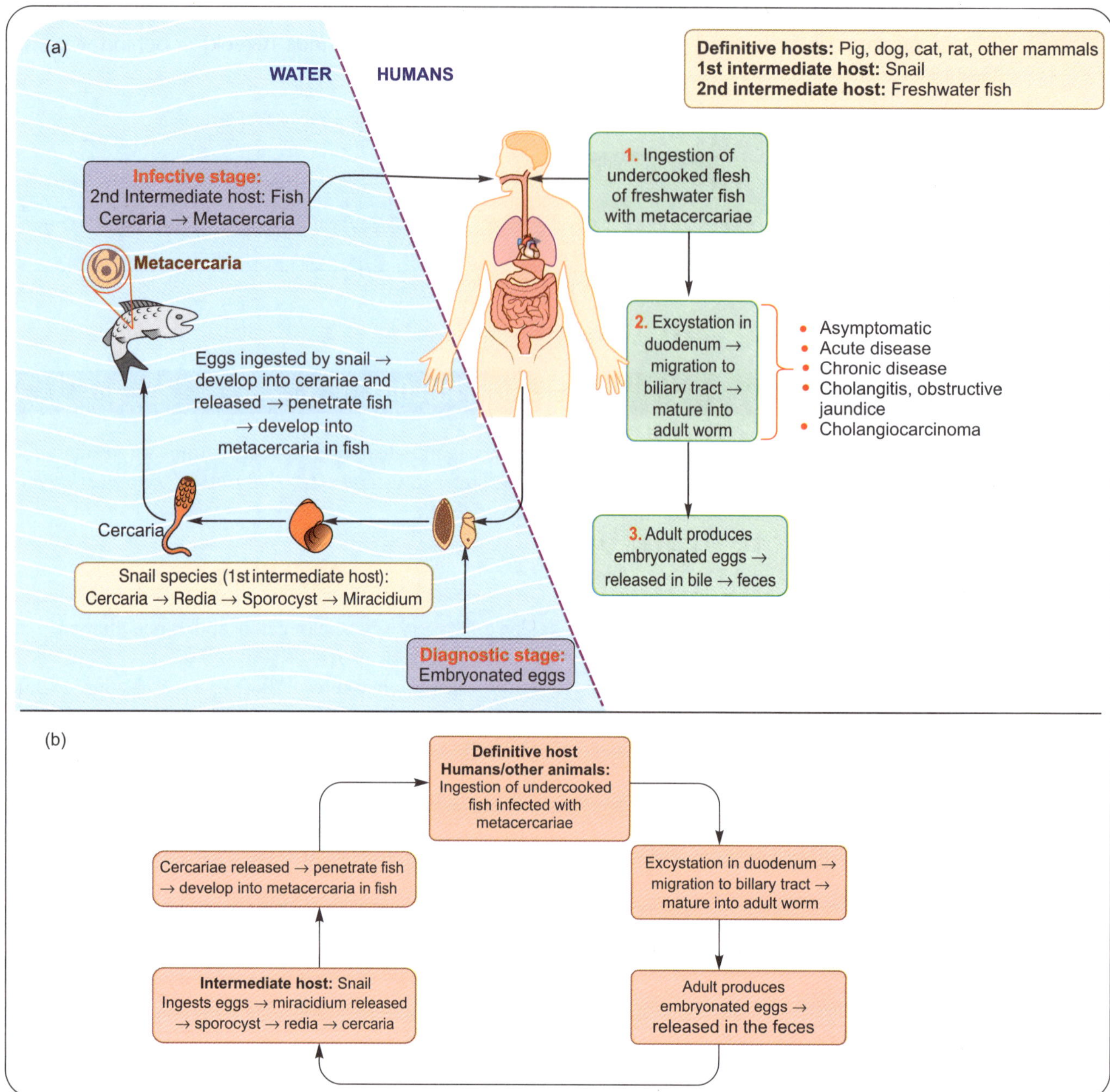

Fig. 44.1 Life cycle of *Clonorchis* and *Opisthorchis*: (a) detailed and (b) schematic

Migratory phase: After ingestion, the metacercariae excyst in the duodenum and enter the ampulla of Vater to reach the biliary duct system. They finally reach the intrahepatic ducts and mature there in about a month.

Sexual phase: The adult fluke starts producing 1,000 to 4,000 eggs per day which escape the bile ducts to be released into the environment along with the host's feces. The flukes usually live for about 10 years; the longest life span recorded in *Clonorchis* is 26 years.

Asexual phase: The eggs, which contain the mature miracidium, are ingested by the **first intermediate host, a species-specific snail (*Bithynia*).** In the snail, they pass through the sporocyst stages, 2–3 generations of redia, and finally produce cercariae.

The cercariae are released by the snail and are taken up by the **second intermediate host, a freshwater fish.** In the fish, they encyst into metacercariae and are ready to infect another definitive host.

PATHOGENESIS

Acute infections: The parasitic antigens elicit an inflammatory response which leads to local dilation and thickening of the bile ducts. There is proliferation of the epithelium, goblet cell metaplasia and infiltration of lymphocytes, monocytes and eosinophils, causing periductal fibrosis. Eventually, there may be strictures and enlargement of the gallbladder, leading to bile stasis.

Chronic infections: There is an increased risk of cholangiocarcinoma in chronic infections. Various mechanisms of carcinogenesis are postulated and are as follows:

- The migratory and feeding activities of the flukes lead to **mechanical damage of the tissues**. The fluke may partially obstruct the bile duct, leading to increased biliary pressure. The eggs are engulfed by granulomatous inflammation.
- The **release of excretory–secretory products** of the fluke induces chronic irritation and inflammation in the biliary system. **Remodelling of the extracellular matrix and enhanced fibrosis** are seen. The parasitic proteins also promote cell proliferation and carcinogenesis.
- Epithelial cell proliferation **increases the host's susceptibility to carcinogens** such as N-nitrosodimethylamine, which is also boosted by exposure to high levels of nitrosamines in diet or tobacco. The amines combine with nitric oxide generated by the chronic inflammation to **produce carcinogenic nitrosamines**.
- In fluke infections, there are increased levels of hepatic cytochrome P450 isoenzymes which enhance the production of toxic substances and promote the proliferation of the epithelium.
- Interleukin-6, transforming growth factor-beta (TGF-β), tumour necrosis factor-alpha (TNF-α) and platelet-derived growth factor (PDGF) are thought to play a key role in the proliferation of biliary epithelial cells or cholangiocytes, ultimately leading to cholangiocarcinoma.

CLINICAL FEATURES

Acute as well as chronic infections with *C. sinensis, O. viverrini* or *O. felineus* are usually asymptomatic; symptoms are reported in only 5–10% of infections.

Acute Infections

Malaise, anorexia, nausea, vomiting, abdominal pain, flatulence and diarrhea are the usual features of acute infections. Acute symptoms usually resolve within a few weeks.

Obstructive jaundice can occur in heavy infections. Hepatomegaly is common.

Chronic Infections

These parasites cause long-lasting infections and can persist for decades in human beings. Although chronic infections are usually asymptomatic, the chronicity may lead to complications such as cholangitis, cholecystitis, fluctuating obstructive jaundice, periportal fibrosis, cholelithiasis, pancreatitis and cholangiocarcinoma. Recurrent pyogenic cholangitis is also a common complication.

Cholangiocarcinoma

The most serious complication of chronic liver fluke infection is cholangiocarcinoma, which is associated with a high mortality rate. It seems to have a direct association with *C. sinensis* and *O. viverrini*. It is the second most prevalent liver cancer after hepatocellular carcinoma which arises from the bile duct epithelium. It is commonly seen in 60–80-year-old patients and rarely, in younger patients.

DIAGNOSIS

The approach to the diagnosis of infections caused by *Clonorchis* and *Opisthorchis* is similar to the diagnostic approach to infections caused by *Fasciola hepatica*, i.e., it is based on the direct microscopic demonstration of the eggs (Fig. 44.2a and b). However, egg morphology may not reliably differentiate the various liver flukes.

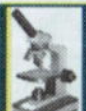
Lab diagnosis

- **Microscopy:** By visualising eggs or adult worms
  - Direct microscopy of stool, duodenal aspirate or bile
  - ERCP
- **Serology:** By detecting antibodies against crude or excretory–secretory antigens
- **Histopathology:** To visualise parasite fragments or eggs
- **DNA detection:** PCR
- **Other diagnostic parameters:**
  - Radioimaging
  - Eosinophilia

Microscopy

- **Wet mount** preparations and, preferably, concentration techniques like the Kato–Katz method or formalin-ethyl acetate may be used. Sedimentation techniques

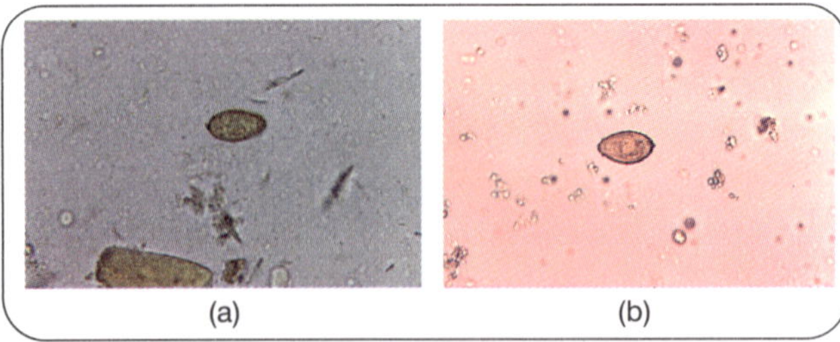

Fig. 44.2 Unstained eggs of liver flukes: (a) *Clonorchis sinensis* egg and (b) *Opisthorchis* spp. egg (*Source:* Centers for Disease Control and Prevention [CDC], Public Health Image Library [PHIL], Image IDs 650 and 15715)

are preferred over floatation since eggs are operculated and do not float in the zinc sulphate solution. Multiple stool samples may be required for the diagnosis, especially in early or light infections.

- Eggs do not appear in stool during the early phase of the disease; the detection of ova or worms in endoscopic or percutaneous biliary aspirates may be more useful in such cases.

  Adult flukes can be seen on stool examination.

Antigen Detection

ELISA assays to detect circulating antigens in the blood or coproantigen in stool have been developed with higher sensitivity than stool microscopy.

Serology

Serological tests for the detection of antibodies against excretory–secretory antigens are mainly used for seroepidemiological purposes. Specific IgE and IgG4 antibodies may act as infection markers.

Histopathology

The common histological findings include biliary epithelial adenomatous proliferation and goblet cell metaplasia. Granulomatous inflammation is frequently seen. Necrotising arterial vasculitis and portal venous thrombosis have also been described.

Nucleic Acid-Based Detection

PCR assays for the detection of the parasite's DNA in fecal samples are mainly employed by research centres to speciate the parasite. The PCR assay is also able to detect cercaria and metacercaria in artificially inoculated snails and fish. These tests are useful in large-scale field studies and control programmes.

Other Diagnostic Parameters

- **Radioimaging modalities** like ultrasound, CT or MRI may be useful in diagnosis.
- **Endoscopic retrograde cholangiopancreatography (ERCP)** may show elliptic filling defects and is particularly useful.
- Peripheral eosinophilia is frequently seen.

TREATMENT

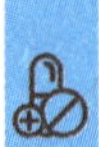

Drug of choice
- *Praziquantel:* 25–75 mg/kg TDS × 2–3 days

Alternate drug
- *Albendazole:* 10 mg/kg/day × 7 days

Surgical management: Once cholangiocarcinoma is diagnosed, complete resection is the best line of treatment. Chemotherapy does not prove to be useful.

PREVENTION AND CONTROL

- The consumption of raw or undercooked fish, crabs and crustaceans should be avoided.
- Stool and sewage should be disposed of in a sanitary manner.
- Mollusc control is an important aspect of controlling fluke infections.
- The WHO recommends mass treatment with 40 mg/kg praziquantel at 12- or 24-month intervals in populations endemic for clonorchiasis or opisthorchiasis.

Questions

1. Discuss the laboratory diagnosis and management of liver fluke infections.
2. Describe the morphology and life cycle of *Clonorchis sinensis.*
3. Discuss parasites and carcinogenesis.

MULTIPLE CHOICE QUESTIONS

1. **Cholangiocarcinoma is associated with which of the following parasites?**
   a. *Fasciola hepatica*
   b. *Opisthorchis viverrini* and *Clonorchis sinensis*
   c. *Fasciolopsis buski*
   d. *Schistosoma haematobium*

2. **The first-line treatment for opisthorchiasis is ____________:**
   a. Praziquantel
   b. Albendazole
   c. Triclabendazole
   d. Ivermectin

3. **Mass treatment with praziquantel at 12- or 24-month intervals is recommended in populations endemic for ____________ :**
   a. Hookworm infections
   b. Clonorchiasis or opisthorchiasis
   c. Onchocerciasis
   d. Lymphatic filariasis

4. **Humans acquire *Clonorchis* infection by the ____________ :**
   a. Ingestion of raw or undercooked freshwater fish
   b. Ingestion of raw or undercooked snails
   c. Ingestion of raw or undercooked beef
   d. Ingestion of raw or undercooked aquatic plants

CHAPTER 45

Paragonimus

([From Greek] *para* = besides + *gonimos* = reproducing)

Case Study and Learning Goals

A 45-year-old male from Manipur visits the OPD with a fever and coughing along with blood-tinged sputum and chest pain. He has a history of eating raw crabs a few months back. What are the parasitic causes of hemoptysis? How would you approach the laboratory diagnosis in this case? How would you treat this patient?

INTRODUCTION

Paragonimus westermani, which causes paragonimiasis, along with other species, forms an important group of foodborne trematodes that cause human infections. These are commonly known as **'lung flukes'** because they reside in the lungs of the reservoir hosts—tigers, cats, dogs, rats, wolves and foxes; **humans are accidental hosts**.

Paragonimus was first discovered in the lungs of a Bengal tiger by Coenraad Kerbert in 1878. Later, it was also found in human autopsies.

There are about 50 species in the genus *Paragonimus*, of which about 11 cause infection in humans. *P. westermani* is the most common and widely distributed human pathogen, followed by *P. heterotremus*. North American paragonimiasis, caused by *P. kellicotti*, is a rare human infection which appears to be emerging in the United States.

EPIDEMIOLOGY

Paragonimiasis is also known as **endemic hemoptysis**, **oriental lung fluke infection** or **pulmonary distomiasis**. It is endemic in many parts of the Far East, Asia, Africa and North America but not in Europe and South America.

Infections are acquired by the consumption of infected crabs and crayfish. The cultural practices of eating certain dishes containing raw, uncooked, pickled or wine-soaked crabs and crayfish are associated with the transmission of the infection. The raw juice of crushed crabs or crayfish has also been used in traditional medicine for the treatment of measles, diarrhea and urticaria in some countries, and is linked to the transmission of the disease.

Food preparations associated with *Paragonimus*
- Ke jang: Crab immersed in soy sauce
- Drunken crab: Live crabs immersed in wine
- Nam prik poo: Crab sauce

India: Paragonimiasis is endemic in the northeastern states of India, especially Manipur.

MORPHOLOGY

For the general morphological features of trematodes, please refer to **Chapter 22**, *Helminths – Introduction and Classification.*

Adult Worm

- The lung fluke is oval, measures 16 × 8 mm and is reddish-brown (Fig. 45.1).
- It has an oral sucker on the anterior end of its body and a **ventral sucker located in the middle** of its body.
- The adults are monoecious.

Eggs

These are dark golden-brown, oval, measure 90 × 55 μm and have a **flat operculum** and **raised opercular shoulders.** They

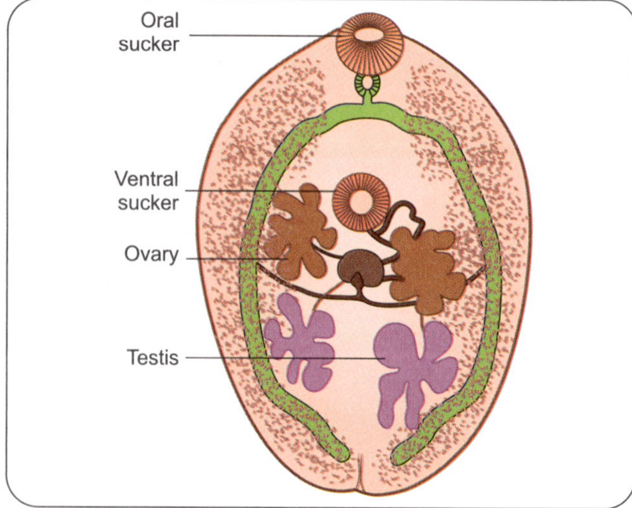

Fig. 45.1 Line diagram of the adult stage of *Paragonimus westermani*

are unembryonated when laid. The eggs release miracidium larvae which develop into the subsequent larval stages of sporocyst, redia, cercaria and finally, the metacercaria.

LIFE CYCLE (Fig. 45.2a and b)

Definitive hosts: Tiger, cat, dog, rat and other mammals; humans (accidental)
1st intermediate host: Snail
2nd intermediate host: Crab, crayfish
Paratenic host: Wild boar

Humans acquire the **infection when they consume raw/undercooked/pickled crabs or crayfish** infected with the encysted metacercariae. In oriental countries, live crabs are immersed in wine. These 'drunken crabs' are consumed as part of treatment in traditional medicine. Humans acquire the infection by ingesting infected crabs in this manner. The infection may also be acquired by the ingestion of developing metacercariae in the raw meat of **paratenic hosts such as wild boars.**

Migratory phase: The metacercariae excyst in the duodenum and penetrate the intestinal wall to reach the abdominal cavity, where they stay for some time. They then further penetrate the diaphragm and the pleural cavity, the lung tissue and finally enter the terminal alveoli or reach underneath the pleura. Occasionally, the worm may aberrantly migrate to extrapulmonary sites like the heart, brain or abdominal cavity.

Sexual phase: In the lungs, the metacercariae mature into adult flukes which are encapsulated by the inflammatory response of the host. The adults mature and start producing eggs which are liberated in the sputum. The lung fluke lives for about six years, the longest documented life span being 20 years.

Asexual phase: In freshwater, the miracidium develops in the egg for about three weeks and then escapes the egg to find the **first intermediate host, a species-specific snail (*Oncomelania, Semisulcospira*).** In the snail, the miracidia develop into sporocysts and 2–3 generations of redia and finally, cercariae.

The cercariae are released from the snail after 4–7 weeks and subsequently enter the gills and muscles of the **second intermediate host, the crab or crayfish.** In the muscles and viscera of the second intermediate host, they encyst into metacercariae and go on to infect the definitive host when they are consumed.

PATHOGENESIS

The disease process relates to adult worms and eggs trapped in the lung tissue. The various mechanisms of pathogenesis are as follows:

- The worms and eggs stimulate an inflammatory response and the formation of a **granuloma**, which consists of eosinophils and neutrophils. A cyst-like capsule forms around the developing parasite. The various chemokines released play a role in the worm's pathogenesis.
- The leakage of pleural fluid in the bronchioles causes **cough and hemorrhage**.
- Later in the course of the disease, **nodular and cavitating lesions** develop in the lung.

CLINICAL FEATURES

The incubation period of paragonimiasis ranges from 1–2 months or longer.

Acute Infections

Larval migration through the intestine and abdomen may produce some clinical features. These are characterised by diarrhea, abdominal pain, fever, cough, urticaria, hepatosplenomegaly, pulmonary features and eosinophilia.

Chronic Infections

Clinically, the disease may be broadly classified into pulmonary and extrapulmonary forms.

Pulmonary paragonimiasis: This is the **commonest** clinical form of paragonimiasis, occurring in 75–90% of cases. Initially, patients may present with mild pleural effusion, pneumonitis, bronchiectasis or bronchopneumonia, the major presenting symptoms being chest pain, difficulty in breathing and **cough with rusty brown or bloodstained sputum that has a foul, fishy odour. Hemoptysis** may be exacerbated on physical exertion and may be massive, requiring immediate medical attention and hospitalisation. The chronic infection may be associated with fever, anemia, weakness and weight loss.

Extrapulmonary paragonimiasis: Sometimes, juvenile worms migrate aberrantly to extrapulmonary organs such as the intestine, abdominal cavity, diaphragm, pleural cavity, heart and brain. This is most likely to occur in children and in heavy infections.

The following may be the manifestations of extrapulmonary paragonimiasis:

- **Pleural effusion:** The migrating worms in the pleural cavity produce pleuritis and effusion which may be minimal to massive depending on the number of worms, frequency of migration and duration of infection.

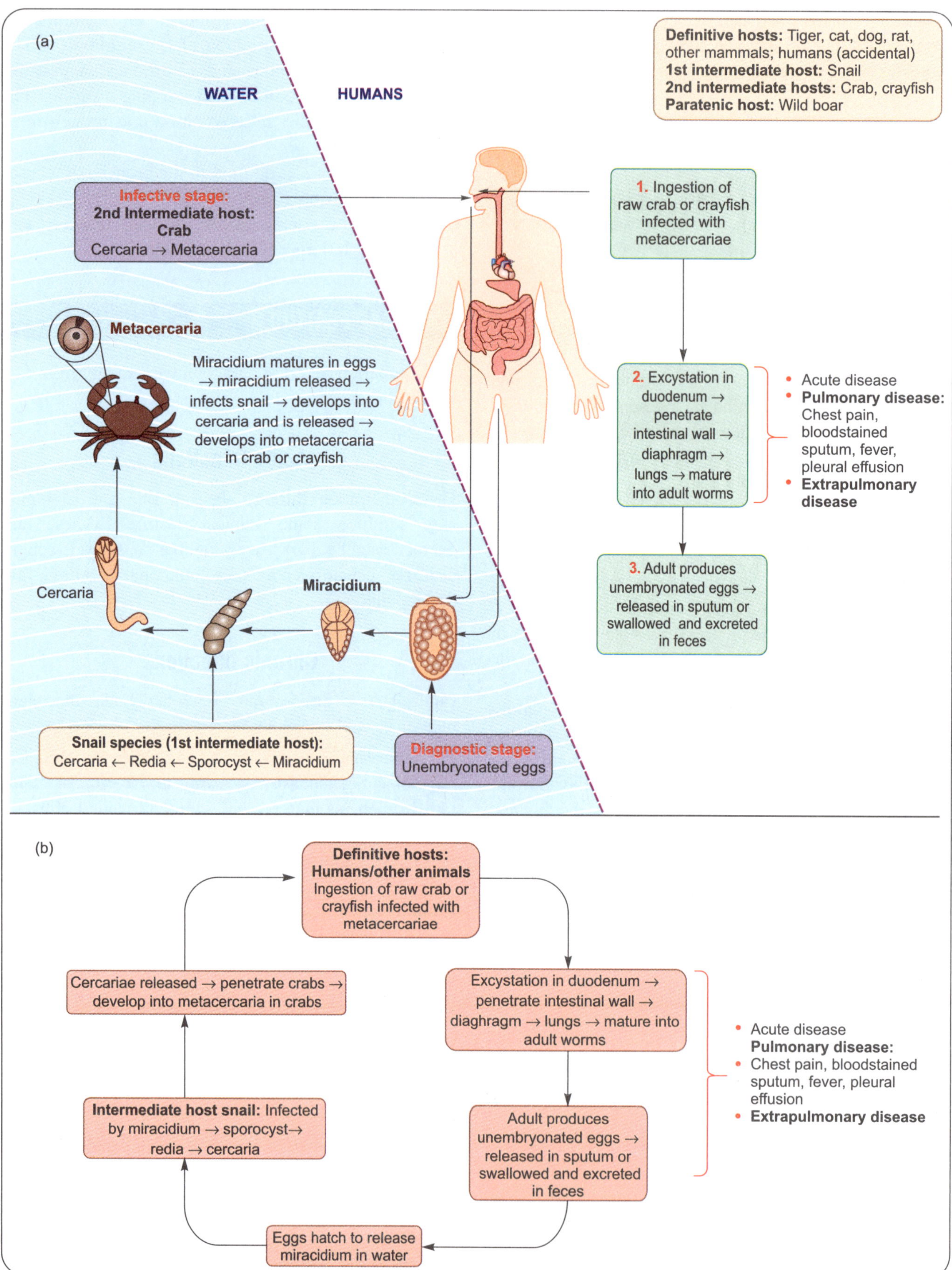

Fig. 45.2 Life cycle of *Paragonimus westermani*: (a) detailed and (b) schematic

- **Cutaneous paragonimiasis:** Skin is a common site of ectopic paragonimiasis. The typical lesion is a migratory subcutaneous nodule which usually appears on the anterior chest wall and then migrates through the abdominal wall to the pelvic region or lower limbs. It does not cause much discomfort to the patient except for mild pain and itching.
- **Cardiovascular paragonimiasis:** This is a rare but serious condition which may be associated with pleuropulmonary paragonimiasis.
- **Cerebral paragonimiasis:** This entity has been described as the most common and serious form of extrapulmonary paragonimiasis. The condition may be confused with tubercular meningitis or tuberculoma or other space-occupying lesions in the brain. It is seen in endemic regions in young adults, commonly presenting with seizures, fever, headache, nausea, vomiting, visual disturbance and motor weakness.

DIAGNOSIS

The diagnosis of paragonimiasis chiefly depends on the demonstration of eggs in sputum and radiological evidence of the disease. Deeply coughed out morning sputum samples are ideal for a direct wet smear examination. Other samples include pleural fluid and other aspirated fluids, stool or excision biopsy.

The **rusty brown or bloodstained sputum** usually contains numerous *Paragonimus* ova and Charcot–Leyden crystals. Blood-tinged flecks of sputum should be carefully examined as clusters of eggs typically look like **'iron filings'**.

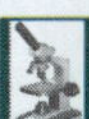

Lab diagnosis

- **Microscopy:** Visualising eggs and Charcot–Leyden crystals
  - Direct microscopy of sputum
- **Serology:**
  - IgG antibody against excretory–secretory antigen
- **Intradermal test**
- **DNA detection:** PCR
- **Other diagnostic parameters:**
  - Radioimaging: Pulmonary lesions
  - Leukocytosis with relative lymphocytosis and eosinophilia
  - Increased ESR

Microscopy

- A definitive diagnosis can be made by the demonstration of characteristic eggs on wet mounts of the clinical specimens (Fig. 45.3). The adult worms may occasionally be detected in excised tissue or pleural aspirate or may be expectorated in the sputum.

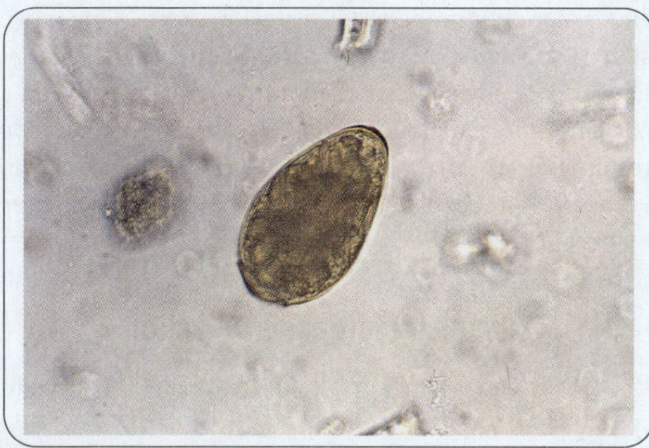

Fig. 45.3 Egg of *Paragonimus westermani* (*Source:* Centers for Disease Control and Prevention [CDC], Public Health Image Library [PHIL], Image ID 1534)

However, in lighter infections, multiple (up to seven) sputum samples should be examined.
- Paragonimiasis is frequently confused with pulmonary tuberculosis. The Ziehl-Neelsen staining method for detecting mycobacteria destroys *Paragonimus* eggs.

Serology

When neither the ova nor the worms are detectable, serological tests play an important but adjunctive role in the diagnosis of extrapulmonary paragonimiasis.

- Serology also helps in differentiating paragonimiasis from tumours, cysts, other infections like tuberculosis and non-infectious causes.
- Various tests like the complement fixation test (CFT), immunodiffusion, indirect hemagglutination test (IHA), enzyme-linked immunosorbent assay (ELISA), dot-ELISA, and Western blot can be used. A rapid point-of-care test (dot-immunogold filtration assay [DIGFA]) has been developed for anti-*P. westermani* antibody detection. This test has good sensitivity and specificity and yields results within ten minutes.
- Serology is useful especially for the **mass screening** of a population.

Intradermal Test

This is a simple, easy, cheap, rapid and highly sensitive **immediate hypersensitivity reaction-**based test used for mass screening and laboratory diagnosis.

The test is performed by intradermally inoculating 0.01 to 0.1 ml of the saline extract or purified antigen of adult *P. westermani* on the volar aspect of the forearm. The diameter of the wheal formed on the skin is measured immediately and 15 minutes after the inoculation. A differential wheal diameter of ≥5 mm with erythema and pseudopodia indicates a positive test. A negative skin test almost certainly rules out paragonimiasis. However, a positive test cannot differentiate between a past and a present infection as the test may yield positive results for as long as 10–20 years of the infection even after successful chemotherapy or spontaneous recovery.

Nucleic Acid-Based Detection

PCR assays are mainly employed by research centres to speciate the parasite.

Other Diagnostic Parameters

- **Radioimaging:** MRI, CT scan or chest X-ray may demonstrate the characteristic pulmonary lesions, including patchy consolidation or opacity with associated pleural reaction or thickening, cystic or cavitary lesions, pleural effusion and nodular opacities. However, it may be difficult to differentiate these lesions from similar tubercular lesions radiologically.
- **Hematological and biochemical abnormalities:** Leukocytosis with relative lymphocytosis, eosinophilia and increased ESR may be noted.

TREATMENT

Drug of choice
- *Praziquantel:* 25 mg/kg body weight orally TDS × 3 days

Alternate drug
- *Bithionol:* 30–50 mg/kg on alternate days × 10–15 doses

PREVENTION AND CONTROL

- The consumption of raw or undercooked fish, pickled crabs, crayfish, shrimp and raw boar meat should be avoided.
- Utensils, cutting boards, cutlery, etc., should be maintained in sanitary conditions.
- Controlling the population of snails also helps in the prevention and control of the infection.

Questions

1. Discuss the laboratory diagnosis and management of lung fluke infections.
2. Describe the morphology and life cycle of *Paragonimus*.

Multiple Choice Questions

1. The oriental lung disease is caused by __________ :
   a. *Mycobacterium tuberculosis*
   b. *Paragonimus* spp.
   c. *Clonorchis* spp.
   d. All these
2. The clinical manifestations of paragonimiasis are most frequently confused with __________ :
   a. Coccidioidomycosis
   b. Cryptococcosis
   c. Tuberculosis
   d. Cryptosporidiosis
3. *Paragonimus* typically produces eggs which are __________ :
   a. Non-operculated
   b. Embryonated when laid
   c. 20–30 microns in size
   d. Dark golden-brown and oval
4. The diagnosis of paragonimiasis is usually made by __________ :
   a. The demonstration of eggs in sputum on the basis of their characteristic morphology and the colour of the wet mount
   b. The demonstration of eggs in sputum by Ziehl-Neelsen staining
   c. The demonstration of larvae in sputum on the basis of their characteristic morphology and the colour of the wet mount
   d. All these
5. Humans are infected by the consumption of __________ :
   a. Raw/undercooked/pickled crabs or crayfish
   b. Raw or undercooked beef
   c. Raw or undercooked aquatic plants
   d. Water contaminated with infected cyclops

Chapter 46

Schistosoma

([From Greek] *schisis* = division + *soma* = body)

Case Study and Learning Goals

A 40-year-old male presents to the hospital with fever and hematuria. He has a history of a 6-month-stay in Egypt about three months back. What are the parasitic causes of hematuria? How would you approach the laboratory diagnosis in this case? How would you treat this patient?

INTRODUCTION

Schistosomes are trematodes that reside in the blood vessels (**'blood flukes'**) of the intestinal tract or the urinary bladder of mammals and cause **schistosomiasis** or **'bilharziasis'**. A few species are of human importance, viz. *Schistosoma haematobium, S. mansoni, S. japonicum, S. intercalatum* and *S. mekongi*. These species have a specific geographical distribution (Table 46.1).

The earliest evidence of the characteristic terminal-spined egg of *S. haematobium* was found in human skeletal remains recovered from Syria which date back to 5800–4000 BC. The eggs have also been recovered from Egyptian mummies at different times in history. However, attempts to demonstrate descriptions of schistosomiasis in ancient medical literature have been controversial. In 1798, the soldiers of Napoleon's army were documented to be afflicted by the disease. The adult *S. haematobium* worm was first described by Theodor Maximilian Bilharz and Carl Th. von Siebold in 1851; the complete life cycle of the parasite involving aquatic snails was first demonstrated by Robert Thomson Leiper in 1915.

EPIDEMIOLOGY

About 85% of schistosome infections are reported from the African continent; countries of South-East Asia, the Far East and South America contribute to 15% of the infections (Table 46.1). Aquatic snails play an important role in the life cycle of schistosomes. **Each species has a specific snail as an intermediate host**. The distribution of that particular snail species determines the geographical spread of the schistosome species. Areas

Table 46.1 Characteristics of blood flukes

Species	Distribution	Definitive host	Intermediate host (snail)	Diagnostic specimen	Egg morphology	Habitat
Schistosoma haematobium	Africa and the Middle East	Humans, monkeys and chimpanzees	*Bulinus*	**Urine**, bladder biopsy and serology	Oval with a sharp terminal spine at the posterior end, 110–170 × 40–70 μm	Veins of vesical and pelvic plexus
S. mansoni	Africa, Brazil, Venezuela and the Caribbean	Humans, non-human primates	*Biomphalaria*	Stool, rectal biopsy and serology	Elliptical with sharp lateral spine, 110–180 × 45–70 μm	Inferior mesenteric veins draining sigmoido-rectal region
S. intercalatum	Western and Central Africa	Humans	*Bulinus*	Stool, rectal biopsy and serology	Elongated, terminal spine, 140–240 × 50–85 μm	Inferior mesenteric veins draining sigmoido-rectal region
S. japonicum	China, Indonesia, Japan and the Philippines	Humans, dogs, cats, cattle, rodents, etc.	*Oncomelania*	Stool, rectal biopsy, serology	Oval to almost spherical with a rudimentary lateral knob, 70–100 × 50–70 μm	Superior mesenteric veins draining the ileocaecal region
S. mekongi	Mekong river basin of Cambodia, Laos and Thailand	Humans and dogs	*Neotricula*	Stool, rectal biopsy, serology	Sub-spherical, minute lateral spine, 50–65 × 30–55 μm	Superior mesenteric veins draining the ileocaecal region

where artificial water bodies such as dams and water canals are constructed have a greater population of snails and consequently, greater incidence of schistosomiasis.

The parasite transmission in the environment is maintained by open defecation or urination by the definitive host in close proximity to the snail's aquatic habitat. A single infected snail sheds enough cercariae to infect people exposed to such water bodies. Humans are important in the sustained transmission of the parasite in a particular area. However, some schistosome species also have animal reservoirs such as cattle, dogs, cats, horses, rats, etc.

India: Schistosomiasis is reported in animals in India but very rarely in humans. A confirmed endemic focus of urinary schistosomiasis was demonstrated in the Gimvi village of Ratnagiri district, Maharashtra, in 1953. However, no cases have been reported since then. Only cercarial dermatitis, which is an immunological reaction to skin penetration by cercariae of non-human *Schistosoma* species, is reported from Assam and parts of central India. The species documented in human cases in India is *Schistosoma spindale*, the definitive hosts for which are cattle, sheep and goat.

Very recently, urinary schistosomiasis caused by *S. haematobium* was reported in the Terai region of Nepal in a fisherman who had no history of travelling outside the Indian subcontinent.

MORPHOLOGY

The morphologies of the schistosomes of human importance are quite similar, with a few species-specific differences.

Adult Worm

The males and females are separate (**diecious**) in contrast to all other trematodes of human importance, which are monoecious.

- The male is short, about 1–1.5 cm long and 0.8–1.0 mm wide (*S. japonicum* is longer and thinner, measuring about 1.2–2.0 cm × 0.5 mm).
- The male has a **gynecophoric canal** to hold the slenderer female worm (Fig. 46.1a), which is about 2 cm long and 0.25 mm wide (*S. japonicum* measures about 2.5 cm × 0.3 mm).
- The tegument of the male worm is tuberculated in *S. mansoni* and *S. haematobium* and smoother in *S. japonicum*. The suckers are armed with delicate spines.

Eggs

The eggs are yellowish-brown, generally elongated (oval to round in *S. japonicum*) and non-operculated (Fig. 46.1b, c and d). Each egg **possesses a spine**, the position and size of which vary in different species (Table 46.1).

Miracidium

It is a non-feeding larva which swims freely with the help of cilia (Fig. 46.1e).

Cercaria

It is a 400 μm long larva with a **bifurcated tail** (Fig. 46.1f). It is equipped with glands containing proteolytic enzymes which help in penetrating the host skin.

LIFE CYCLE (Fig. 46.2a and b)

The definitive hosts, humans or other animal hosts, get **infected by the cercarial stages** of schistosomes in water. The various life cycle stages of schistosomes are as follows:

> **Definitive hosts:** Humans and other animals, depending on the species (see Table 46.1)
> **Intermediate hosts:** Snail species, depending on the *Schistosoma* species (see Table 46.1)

Skin penetration: The free-swimming cercariae penetrate the host's skin in about 30 minutes with the help of their proteolytic enzymes, and subsequently drop off their tails to become **schistosomulae.**

Migratory phase: The schistosomulae enter the venules in the skin and migrate through the circulation or lymphatics to the right side of the heart and then to the lung vasculature in about 3–4 days. Here, they stay for another 3–4 days before continuing their journey to the left side of the heart. Then, they are pumped to the systemic circulation of the body to reach the mesenteric arteries and the hepatoportal system.

Sexual phase: In the intrahepatic portion of the portal bloodstream, the schistosomulae develop into **young adults** in about three weeks. The male and female then pair and migrate against the blood flow to their final abode in the venous plexuses in 1–3 months. Here, they fertilise and lay hundreds of **eggs** per day. The final destination of the worm depends on the species—***S. mansoni* migrates to the inferior mesenteric plexus, *S. japonicum* to the superior**

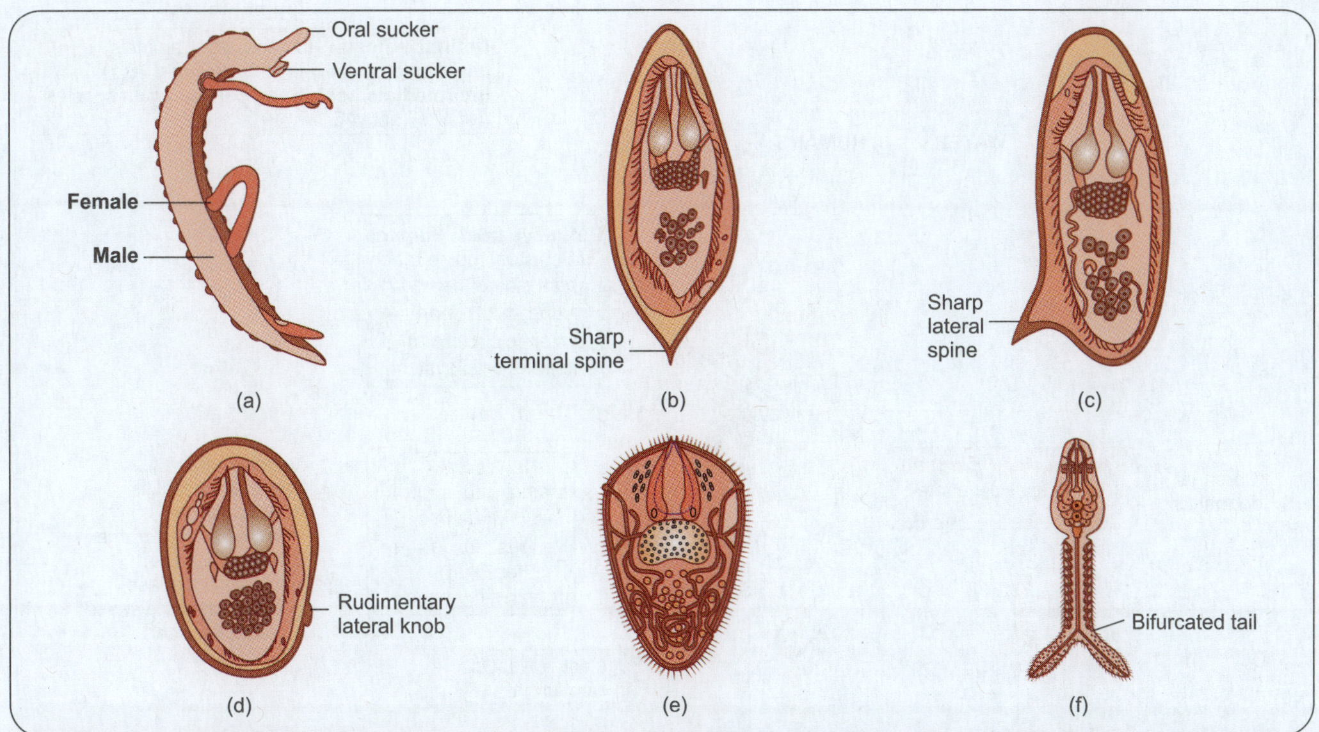

Fig. 46.1 Line diagrams of the different developmental stages of *Schistosoma*: (a) adults in a pair; male holding the female in its gynecophoric canal, (b) *S. haematobium* egg, (c) *S. mansoni* egg, (d) *S. japonicum* eggs, (e) miracidium and (f) cercaria

mesenteric plexus and *S. haematobium* to the vesicular plexus. Adult worms can live for up to 20–30 years.

Escape from the definitive host: The eggs, once laid, elicit a granulomatous immune response in the host. Aided by the host's immunity and some enzymes released by the miracidium which help to digest the surrounding tissue, about half to one-third of the eggs are able to gradually traverse the vessel walls, tissue and the mucosa and reach the lumen of the intestine or the urinary bladder to be finally released into the environment along with feces or urine (depending on the species) in a completely embryonated state containing the ciliated embryo.

Asexual phase: In response to the lower osmolarity and salinity of freshwater, the **eggs hatch to liberate the free-swimming miracidia** which swim rapidly to find the **snail host** within a few hours. After penetrating the exposed surface of the snail, the miracidium sheds its epithelium and transforms through two generations of mother and daughter sporocysts to generate the cercariae in about four weeks. Thousands of cercariae are generated from one miracidium.

Infective stage: The cercariae exit the snail musculature and swim in water with the help of their **forked tails**. They can live in water for about 1–3 days until they either find a host or degenerate. Upon finding a suitable host, the life cycle of the worm continues.

PATHOGENESIS

The pathogenesis of schistosomiasis is related to the migration of the parasite and the immune response of the host to the antigens of the worm and the deposited eggs.

Skin penetration: In endemic regions, the host is sensitised by **repeated exposure to cercariae**. Both humoral and cellular responses are elicited, leading to more intense inflammation and related clinical features on subsequent exposures. Once the host is sensitised, most newly penetrating cercariae die in the skin due to the intense immune response.

Acute infection: A heavy infection in previously unexposed persons leads to a febrile illness mediated by immune-complex formation and the release of pro-inflammatory cytokines in response to the antigens of schistosomulae. The more mature worms are better adjusted to the host machinery and coat themselves with host antigens (antigen mimicry), thus evading the immune response.

Chronic infection: The immune reaction is dependent on past exposure of the host to the parasite.

- In people who live in endemic areas and develop chronic infections, there is T cell-mediated immune response to the soluble antigens of the eggs. This leads to the formation of **granulomas** composed of phagocytes, neutrophils, lymphocytes, eosinophils,

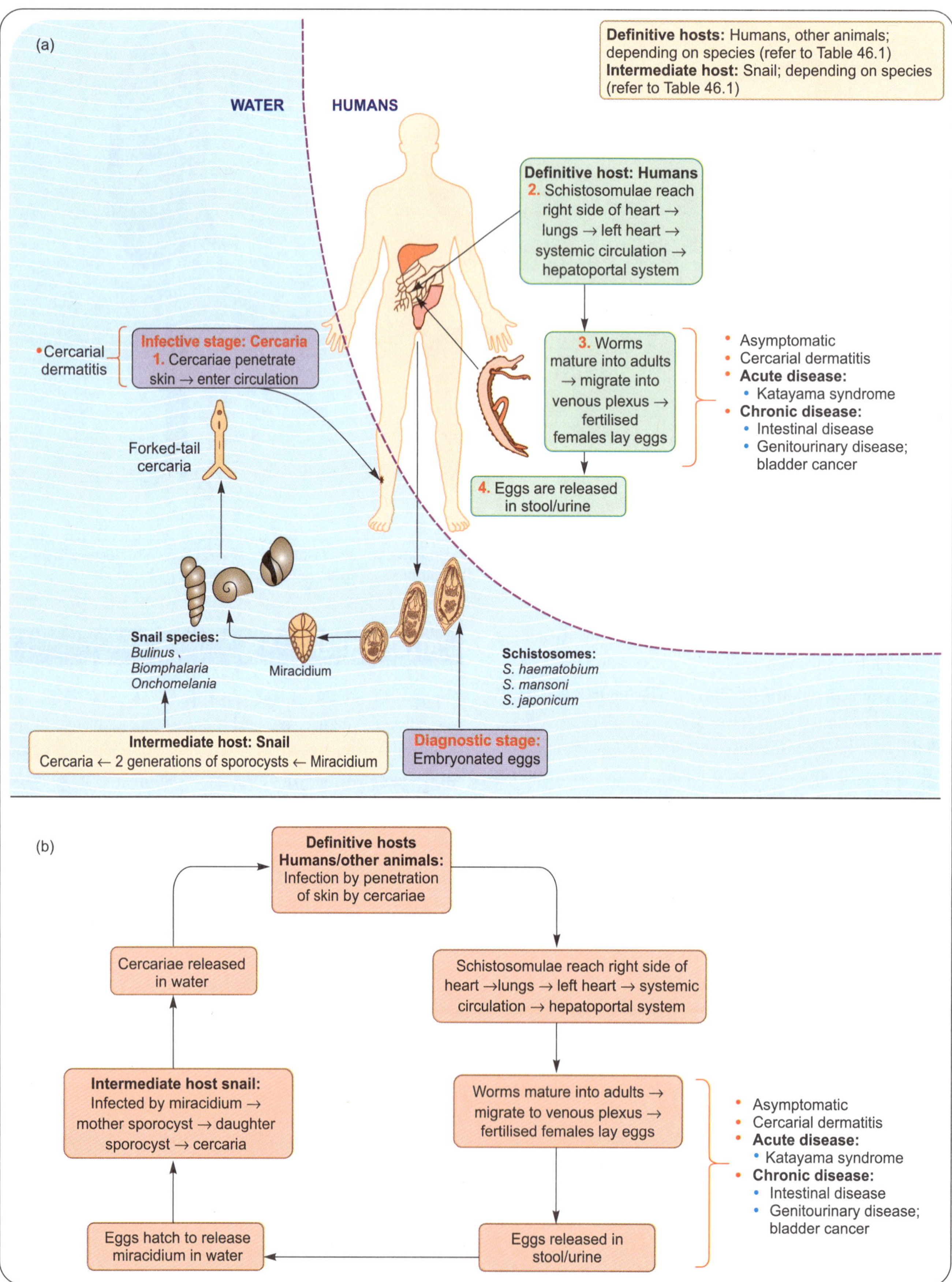

Fig. 46.2 Life cycle of *Schistosoma* spp.: (a) detailed and (b) schematic

fibroblasts and multinucleated giant cells (also known as **pseudotubercles**). The eggs, which are not able to escape the host, eventually die, calcify or get absorbed.

- The eggs retained in the gut wall induce inflammation, hyperplasia, ulcerations, micro-abscess formation, polyposis, fibrosis and thickening in the intestinal wall along the entire length of the colon and rectum. This may lead to intestinal obstruction.
- The eggs of *S. mansoni* and *S. japonicum* embolise to the liver where the granulomatous inflammatory response induces pre-sinusoidal inflammation and the replacement of normal tissue with fibrosis, collagen deposition and scarring. This leads to **periportal or clay pipestem fibrosis**. Embolisation may also involve the lungs, brain, spinal cord and other organs.
- Infection with *S. haematobium* leads to granulomatous inflammation in the urinary tract tissues. The terminal spine may cause hemorrhage by directly damaging the blood vessels and cause hematuria.
- *S. haematobium* is implicated in **bladder carcinoma**. The production of nitrosamines and β-glucuronidases in the tissue and inflammatory gene damage have been proposed as possible carcinogenic factors. The lesions also intensify the exposure of the bladder epithelium to mutagenic substrates from tobacco or chemicals.

CLINICAL FEATURES

Schistosomiasis progresses in three distinct phases—acute, chronic and advanced disease.

Early Manifestations

Maculopapular **rashes** with discrete, erythematous, raised lesions that vary in size from 1–3 cm may arise at the site of skin penetration by schistosomal cercariae. People infected for the first time may develop a skin reaction within a few hours, although a rash may appear up to a week later.

A more severe form of the rash, generally described as **'cercarial'** or **'swimmer's'** or **'paddy field' dermatitis,** occurs on exposure to the cercariae of animal schistosomes which are not infective to humans. This is considered a re-emerging disease. Human cases have been described from all continents, and tourism-threatening outbreaks are reported. These parasites of animals usually do not progress beyond the skin; cercarial death occurring in subcutaneous tissues leads to immediate hypersensitivity reactions at the invasion sites.

Acute Schistosomiasis (Katayama Syndrome)

This is seen in people who are infected for the first time while travelling to endemic areas. The symptoms resemble serum sickness and include fever, malaise, myalgia, fatigue, non-productive cough, diarrhea or dysentery, hematuria (*S. haematobium*), enlarged, tender liver, palpable spleen and right upper quadrant pain. Eosinophilia is common. These manifestations are a result of the toxic metabolic products of schistosomulae growing in the portal circulation and are more commonly seen with *S. japonicum* and rarely with *S. haematobium*.

Chronic and Advanced Disease

The features of chronic disease depend upon the infecting species and usually coincide with the release of eggs.

- *S. mansoni*, *S. japonicum*, *S. intercalatum*, and *S. mekongi* lead to gastrointestinal and hepatosplenic manifestations.
- *S. haematobium* involves the genitourinary tract system.

Gastrointestinal disease

- Symptoms include colicky hypogastric pain or pain in the left iliac fossa, diarrhea that may alternate with constipation and hematochezia (blood in the feces). Severe chronic intestinal disease may result in colonic or rectal stenosis. The disease may present as protein-losing enteropathy. An inflammatory mass in the colon may even mimic cancer.
- A considerable body of evidence points towards an **etiological link between *S. japonicum* and colorectal cancer** but the evidence is not conclusive.

Hepatosplenic disease

- A number of eggs escape through the circulation and get trapped in the liver, evoking an immune reaction.
- Hepatomegaly, portal hypertension, splenomegaly and hypersplenism may be seen.

Genitourinary disease

- Painless terminal hematuria, appearing 10–12 weeks after infection, is the first sign of established disease.
- Late manifestations include proteinuria, bladder calcification, ureteric obstruction, secondary bacterial infection in the urinary tract, renal colic, hydronephrosis and renal failure.
- Epidemiological studies have associated chronic urinary schistosomiasis (*S. haematobium*) with **squamous cell carcinoma of the bladder**.

- *S. haematobium* causes genital disease in about a third of infected women. Vulval schistosomiasis may also facilitate the transmission of HIV.

Involvement of other organs

- **Neuroschistosomiasis** leads to signs and symptoms of increased intracranial pressure, myelopathy and radiculopathy. These manifestations result from egg deposition in the brain or spinal cord following the aberrant migration of worms.
- In **renal disease**, the circulating immune complexes get deposited on the basement membrane and in the glomerular capillaries and may lead to renal failure.
- Schistosome infection can cause growth retardation and anemia as well as possible cognitive and memory impairment.

Chronic bacteremic infections with *Salmonella* species have been associated with *S. haematobium*, *S. japonicum* and *S. mansoni* infections. If schistosome infections are not treated, *Salmonella* infections continue to recur.

DIAGNOSIS

The diagnosis of *Schistosoma* infections is made by demonstrating eggs in urine (for *S. haematobium*), or rarely, in stool samples (for schistosomes other than *S. haematobium*) (Fig. 46.3a, b and c). The examination of multiple samples increases the sensitivity of detection. The sensitivity of microscopy depends on the worm load and the duration of infection. The eggs cannot be detected in stool for at least 4–7 weeks after infection. Old or chronic infections may be associated with the production of very few eggs.

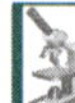

Lab diagnosis

- **Microscopy:** By visualising eggs
  - Direct microscopy of stool and urine
  - Hatching test
  - Histopathology: Biopsy of the bladder/GIT
- **Serology:** IgG antibody
- **Antigen detection:** ELISAs of circulating cathodic antigen (CCA) and circulating anodic antigen (CAA) in blood/urine
- **DNA/RNA detection:** PCR and real-time PCR
- **Other diagnostic parameters:**
  - Urinalysis for hematuria
  - Eosinophilia and ↑ IgE
  - Radiology: USG chest/pelvis

Microscopy

Urine: The **terminal hematuric portion** of urine contains the maximum number of eggs. The peak egg excretion occurs between noon and 3 p.m. Concentration by centrifugation or filtration (not floatation) is advisable, especially for urine samples.

Stool: Stool samples may be examined for the presence of eggs. In active infections, the eggs contain mature miracidia which can be detected in unpreserved, fresh samples by examining flame cell activity or by performing the hatching test. The presence of flame cell activity is proof of viability.

Hatching test: When feces containing mature living schistosome eggs is diluted with water, the eggs hatch within a few hours at room temperature. The released miracidia tend to collect in the upper layers of water where they may be located with a hand lens as minute, white organisms swimming rapidly in a straight course. This test can be performed on unpreserved samples only.

Biopsy

A biopsy of the bladder or intestinal tract may be performed for the identification of eggs if schistosomiasis is strongly suspected.

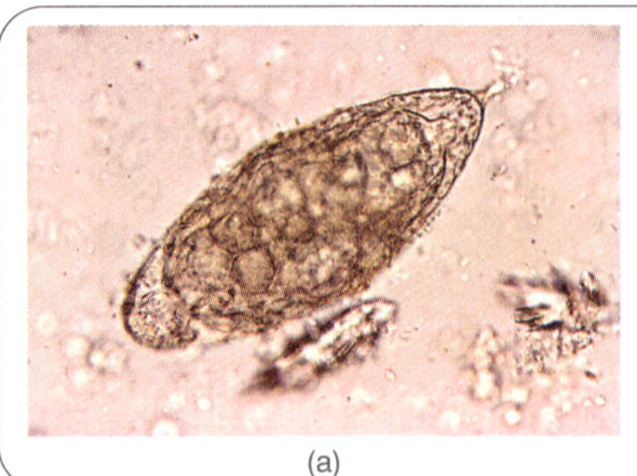

(a)

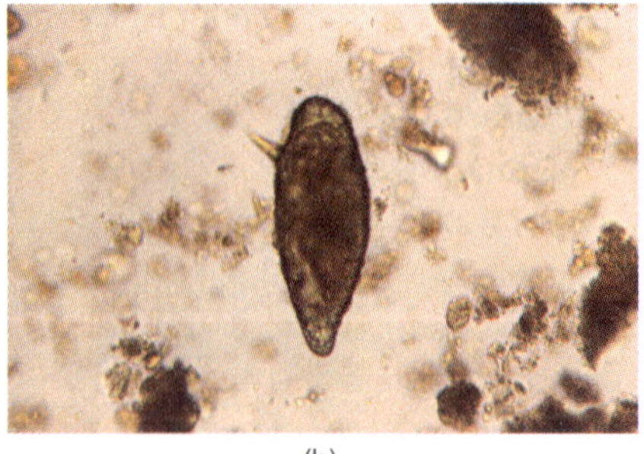

(b)

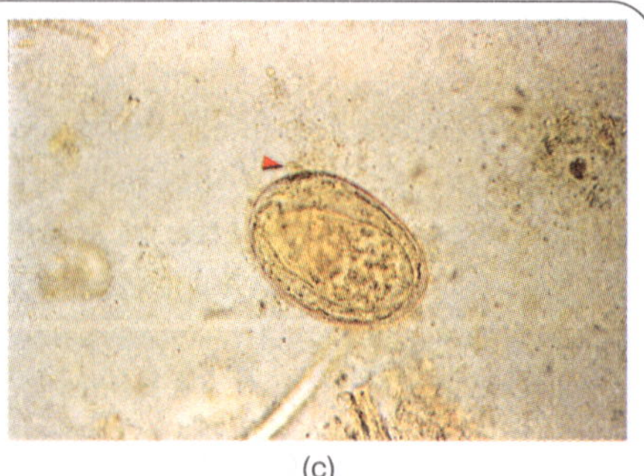

(c)

Fig. 46.3 Eggs of *Schistosoma*: (a) *S. haematobium* egg, elongated with a terminal spine, (b) *S. mansoni* egg, elongated with a lateral spine and (c) *S. japonicum* egg, spherical with a lateral rudimentary knob indicated by the red arrowhead (*Source:* Centers for Disease Control and Prevention [CDC], Public Health Image Library [PHIL], Image IDs 622, 17940 and 649)

Serology

Antibody detection: Immunological methods are particularly useful in cases where no eggs are present, such as patients who have Katayama syndrome. The serum IgG levels are significantly higher in chronic *S. japonicum* infection than they are in acute ones. On the other hand, IgM, IgA and IgE levels are higher in acute infections than they are in chronic infections. Enzyme-linked immunoelectrotransfer blot (EITB) can be used to confirm the diagnosis. Antibody detection, however, has the following drawbacks:

- Difficulty in differentiating active from past infection and re-infection
- Antibody cross-reactivity with different species of schistosomes including animal schistosomes and other helminth parasites

Antigen detection: The detection of schistosomal antigens (from schistosomula, adult worms or eggs) in blood, urine or sputum is considered a sensitive and specific test for diagnosis. Two major components that have been targeted are circulating cathodic antigen (CCA) and the circulating anodic antigen (CAA). Both antigens can be demonstrated in blood at around three weeks post-infection and are also excreted in the host's urine. They can be detected by different types of ELISA and lateral flow assay formats. In addition to diagnosis, antigen levels are also used to assess the severity of the disease and monitor the patient's response to treatment.

Nucleic Acid-Based Detection

The detection of schistosome DNA by conventional or advanced PCR-based techniques is promising. Recent advances include the detection of egg DNA and circulating cell-free parasitic DNA.

Other Diagnostic Parameters

- **Rapid tests:** Urinalysis to detect hematuria and proteinuria provides important clues for the diagnosis of urinary schistosomiasis.
- **Eosinophilia:** It is seen in >80% of patients with acute infections.
- **Anemia and thrombocytopenia:** These may be present in chronic and advanced schistosomiasis.
- **Coagulation profile:** Prolonged prothrombin time may be evident in chronic and advanced schistosomiasis.
- **Urea, electrolytes and liver function:** Raised urea, hyperglobulinemia and hypoalbuminemia may be present in chronic and advanced schistosomiasis.
- **Radioimaging:**
  - ***Chest radiograph:*** Pulmonary infiltrates are common in acute cases (Katayama syndrome).
  - ***Pelvic ultrasound:*** It helps to establish the extent of bladder, ureteral and renal pathology in urinary schistosomiasis.
  - ***Abdominal ultrasound:*** It is useful for detecting liver and gastrointestinal lesions.

TREATMENT

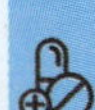

Drug of choice

- *Praziquantel:* 40–60 mg/kg in a single dose or 1–3 divided doses in one day
- Corticosteroids may be required in life-threatening cases of Katayama fever and in the case of CNS involvement

A single dose of praziquantel has cure rates of 65–90% and reduces the egg excretion by >90%. However, the early schistosomulae are unaffected by praziquantel and hence follow-up ova and parasite examinations should be done for a year. Repeated treatment may be required.

PREVENTION AND CONTROL

- **Mass drug administration (MDA) programmes** are designed to target both soil-transmitted helminths infections and schistosomiasis since these coexist. MDA with praziquantel is most appropriate in populations with prevalence rates of >30%.
- Water supplies, sanitation and hygiene (WASH) programmes are effective.
- **Molluscicidal agents** are used to reduce the numbers of intermediate host snails. These include chemical control (niclosamide), biological control (ducks, fish, turtles, fungi and other snail species) or environmental and engineering modifications of dams and water canals to reduce breeding sites of snails.
- No effective vaccine is available yet.

Questions

1. Describe Katayama syndrome.
2. Discuss the life cycle of *Schistosoma mansoni*.
3. Discuss the laboratory diagnosis and management of urinary schistosomiasis.

Multiple Choice Questions

1. Bilharziasis is caused by __________ :
   a. *Leishmania infantum*
   b. *Schistosoma* spp.
   c. *Toxocara canis*
   d. *Fasciolopsis buskii*
2. Elongated eggs with terminal spines are a feature of ________ .
   a. *Schistosoma haematobium*
   b. *Schistosoma japonicum*
   c. *Toxocara canis*
   d. *Fasciolopsis buskii*
3. Cercariae are the infective form of __________ .
   a. *Paragonimus*
   b. *Strongyloides*
   c. *Schistosoma*
   d. *Fasciola*
4. Elongated eggs with lateral spines are a feature of __________:
   a. *Schistosoma haematobium*
   b. *Schistosoma japonicum*
   c. *Toxocara canis*
   d. *Fasciolopsis buskii*
5. Which of the following are the intermediate hosts for *Schistosoma* spp.?
   a. Fish
   b. Crabs
   c. Snails
   d. Mammals
6. Adult worms of *Schistosoma haematobium* reside in the ________ plexus.
   a. Superior mesenteric
   b. Inferior mesenteric
   c. Vesicular
   d. All these
7. Adult worms of *Schistosoma mansoni* reside in the __________ plexus.
   a. Superior mesenteric
   b. Inferior mesenteric
   c. Vesicular
   d. All these
8. The route of transmission of schistosome infections to humans is by __________ :
   a. The ingestion of uncooked aquatic plants (water caltrops, water chestnuts or lotus) infected with encysted metacercariae
   b. The ingestion of snails containing metacercariae
   c. The ingestion of snails harbouring miracidia
   d. The penetration of the skin by cercariae
9. Which species of *Schistosoma* is implicated in causing bladder cancer?
   a. *Schistosoma haematobium*
   b. *Schistosoma japonicum*
   c. *Schistosoma mansoni*
   d. *Schistosoma japonicum*
10. Swimmer's itch is caused by __________ :
    a. Hookworms
    b. Schistosomes
    c. Roundworms
    d. Pinworms
11. The drug of choice for the treatment of *Schistosoma* infections is __________ :
    a. Albendazole
    b. Praziquantel
    c. Ivermectin
    d. Thiabendazole
12. The diagnosis of *Schistosoma haematobium* infection is made by __________ :
    a. Demonstrating adult worms in the urinary bladder
    b. Demonstrating eggs in urine samples
    c. Demonstrating adult worms in stool samples
    d. Demonstrating eggs in stool samples

Chapter 47

Gastrointestinal and Hepatobiliary System Infections

Learning Goals

- What are the organ systems affected by infectious diseases?
- What are the clinical manifestations of infectious diseases?
- What are the parasitic and other microbiological causes of various disease manifestations?
- What are the underlying disease processes of infectious disease manifestations?

INTRODUCTION TO SECTION IV (Chapters 47–54)

Infectious diseases are a major cause of morbidity and mortality globally, more so in the tropical and subtropical regions of the world and poor communities. Typically, individuals with intact immunities remain asymptomatic for most infections. When symptomatic, the disease presentation ranges from a mild to severe illness, uncomplicated to complicated course of disease, local to systemic infliction, and acute to chronic disease. Some infections confer lifelong immunity on the host while some others persist as latent infections, with the infectious organism persisting in the body for months to years.

The clinical presentation of an infection may be non-specific with features such as fever and malaise, but quite often there are symptoms and signs specific enough to point towards a few etiological agents. This section provides a bird's eye view of the major infectious syndromes and their infectious agents with respect to the various organ systems of the human body. The aim of this section is to impart a clinical orientation of infectious diseases to students of medicine. In addition to parasitic etiology, the other important microbiological causes of diseases, i.e., bacteria, viruses and fungi are also listed in this section for a wholesome grasp of the wide etiological range of various infectious disease syndromes. It should be noted, however, that these lists are not comprehensive and that the main focus of the text remains on parasitic diseases. A brief background of the disease process is also included in this section, the detailed versions of which are discussed in the organism-specific chapters that preceded this section.

GASTROINTESTINAL SYSTEM INFECTIONS

Parasitic infections of the **gastrointestinal tract** may clinically present as alterations of bowel movements in the form of diarrhea and dysentery or sometimes, as constipation along with a variety of other disease manifestations (see box).

Disease manifestations of gastrointestinal system infections

- Diarrhea
- Constipation
- Fever
- Vomiting
- Steatorrhea
- Malnutrition
- Stunting
- Dysentery
- Abdominal pain
- Nausea
- Bloating
- Lactose intolerance
- Failure to thrive
- Growth retardation

Diarrhea is defined as the passage of **unformed or abnormally liquid stools at an increased frequency**. When diarrhea is accompanied by **blood and mucus**, it is called **dysentery**.

Diarrheal illnesses may be categorised on the basis of the duration of the illnesses as follows:

- **Acute:** Less than two weeks
- **Persistent:** Two to four weeks
- **Chronic:** More than four weeks

Acute Diarrhea

More than 90% of cases of acute diarrhea are caused by infections. Microorganisms may cause diarrhea/dysentery by various mechanisms; the pathophysiology differs depending on the infectious agent (Table 47.1) and ranges from profuse **watery diarrhea** to frank **bloody diarrhea.**

- **Watery diarrhea:** Profuse watery diarrhea with marked vomiting with or without fever may be the result of the ingestion of **preformed bacterial toxins** in food (e.g., *Staphylococcus aureus*) or infection with **enterotoxin-producing** bacteria (e.g., *Vibrio cholerae*) and entero-adherent pathogens causing **mechanical damage** to the epithelium (e.g., *Giardia duodenalis*). These toxins cause alterations in ion transport and epithelial barrier

Table 47.1 Infectious causes and pathobiologies of acute diarrhea

Pathobiology/agents	Vomiting	Fever	Blood in stool	Stool examination
Preformed toxin: *Bacillus cereus* *Staphylococcus aureus* *Clostridium perfringens* *Clostridium botulinum*	+++	Less likely	–	No fecal leukocytes Mild or no ↑ in lactoferrin
Enterotoxin production: *Vibrio cholerae* Enterotoxigenic *Escherichia coli* Rotavirus	++	Less likely	–	No fecal leukocytes Mild or no ↑ in lactoferrin
Enteroadherence: *Giardia duodenalis* *Cryptosporidium* Enteropathogenic *Escherichia coli* Enteroadherent *Escherichia coli* Helminths	–/++	Common	–	No fecal leukocytes Mild or no ↑ in lactoferrin Parasitic cysts demonstrated
Cytotoxin/lytic enzyme production: *Entamoeba histolytica* *Balantidium coli* *Clostridium difficile* Enterohemorrhagic *Escherichia coli*	–/+	Common	Usual	↑ Fecal leukocytes ↑ Lactoferrin Parasitic trophozoites and cysts demonstrated
Invasion: **a. Minimal/variable inflammation:** *Salmonella* *Campylobacter* Rotavirus Norwalk-like virus **b. Intense inflammation:** *Entamoeba histolytica* *Shigella* Enteroinvasive *Escherichia coli* **c. Inflammation (with eosinophilia):** *Schistosoma mansoni* *Schistosoma japonicum* *Trichuris trichiura*	–/+	Common	Usual	↑ Fecal leukocytes ↑ Lactoferrin Parasitic trophozoites, cysts or ova/eggs demonstrated Predominant eosinophilia (helminths)

functions, leading to the hypersecretion of fluids in the small bowel.

- **Dysentery:** Bloody diarrhea along with fever and abdominal pain may be manifestations of damage to the gut epithelial lining. This may be caused by **lytic enzymes** of the invading pathogen and the host inflammatory response (e.g., *Entamoeba histolytica, Shigella*) or the production of **cytotoxins** causing cell damage (e.g., *Clostridium difficile*).

Chronic Diarrhea

Most of the causes of chronic diarrhea are non-infectious. However, amongst the infectious causes, parasitic agents are the most important (Table 47.2). In helminthic infections, diarrhea is often associated with intermittent periods of constipation.

Traveller's Diarrhea

Over one-third to half of those who travel from temperate industrialised countries to tropical and underdeveloped countries experience diarrhea/ dysentery (Table 47.3).

Diarrhea in the Immunocompromised Host

Any infection has the potential to cause more severe disease in an immunocompromised host. However, the etiology depends on the type of immunosuppression and individual lifestyle and risk factors such as travel-associated exposures, sexual practices, etc. (Table 47.4). Diarrhea tends to be more severe and prolonged in immunocompromised patients.

Table 47.2 Infectious causes of chronic diarrhea

Protozoa	Helminths	Bacteria
• *Entamoeba histolytica* • *Giardia duodenalis* • *Cryptosporidium, Cyclospora* and *Cystoisospora* (opportunistic agents)	• *Strongyloides stercoralis* • Hookworms • *Ascaris lumbricoides*	• Enteroaggregative *Escherichia coli* (EAEC) • *Yersinia* • *Aeromonas* • Recurrent *Clostridium difficile* infection • *Tropheryma* (Whipple's disease) • Tuberculosis • SIBO (small intestinal bacterial overgrowth): presence of $>10^5$ CFU/ml bacteria in the proximal small intestine

Table 47.3 Infectious causes of traveller's diarrhea

Parasites	Bacteria	Viruses
• *Giardia duodenalis* • *Cryptosporidium* • *Entamoeba histolytica* • *Cyclospora*	• Enterotoxigenic *Escherichia coli* • Enteroaggregative *Escherichia coli* • *Campylobacter* • *Shigella* • *Salmonella*	• Norovirus • Rotavirus

Table 47.4 Infectious diarrhea in immunocompromised patients

Protozoa	Helminths	Bacteria	Viruses	Fungi
• *Cryptosporidium* • *Cystoisospora* • *Cyclospora* • *Giardia duodenalis* • *Entamoeba histolytica* • *Blastocystis hominis* • Microsporidia	• *Strongyloides stercoralis*	• *Salmonella* • *Shigella* • *Campylobacter* • *Clostridium difficile* • *Chlamydia trachomatis* • *Escherichia coli* • *Mycobacterium avium* complex • Tuberculosis	• Cytomegalovirus • Adenovirus • Norovirus • Herpes simplex • Human immunodeficiency virus	• *Histoplasma* • *Candida*

HEPATOBILIARY SYSTEM INFECTIONS

The **hepatobiliary system** may be affected by several parasites; these infections may have myriad clinical manifestations (see box).

Disease manifestations of hepatobiliary system infections

- Abdominal pain
- Vomiting
- Hepatomegaly
- Space-occupying lesions
- Weight loss
- Fever
- Jaundice
- Altered liver enzymes
- Obstruction

- **Abscesses** may form due to a composite effect of the lytic enzymes released by the parasite and the inflammatory response of the host (e.g., amoebic liver abscess) or when the liver is secondarily infected with bacteria.
- **Space-occupying lesions** caused by parasites (e.g., *Echinococcus*) usually go unnoticed when small but they may cause pressure symptoms when they become large.
- **Obstruction** due to the blockage of the biliary passage is seen when a parasite resides in the ducts (e.g., liver flukes) or enters the hepatobiliary–pancreatic system aberrantly (e.g., *Ascaris lumbricoides*).
- Vascular congestion and proliferation of reticuloendothelial cells leads to **hepatomegaly** (e.g., malaria and kala-azar) (Table 47.5).
- **Granuloma** formation may occur in response to the eggs laid by the parasite (e.g., *Fasciola hepatica*).
- **Carcinomatous** changes may occur due to chronic irritation of the liver parenchyma and the formation of N-nitroso compounds locally (e.g., *Clonorchis sinensis*).
- **Allergic** features may be seen in the case of the rupture of a hepatic cyst (e.g., *Echinococcus*) or in reaction to a passing aberrant larva (e.g., visceral larva migrans).

Parasitic Causes of Cholangiocarcinoma

Cancer of the gallbladder can be attributed to some infections. Liver flukes, specifically *Opisthorchis viverrini* and *Clonorchis sinensis,* are strongly associated with the induction of cholangiocarcinoma (bile duct cancer).

Table 47.5 Infectious causes of hepatomegaly

Parasites	Bacteria	Viruses
• *Entamoeba histolytica* (amoebic liver abscess) • *Leishmania donovani* (kala-azar, usually associated with massive splenomegaly) • Malaria (usually associated with massive splenomegaly) • *Echinococcus* • *Toxocara* (visceral larva migrans) • *Trypanosoma cruzi* (not prevalent in India) • *Fasciola hepatica, Clonorchis sinensis, Opisthorchis* (liver flukes) • *Schistosoma* spp.	• *Leptospira* • *Brucella* • *Yersinia* • *Bartonella*	• Viral hepatitis (hepatitis A–E) • Cirrhosis subsequent to any cause including hepatitis B infection • Epstein-Barr virus (EBV) • Human immunodeficiency virus (HIV)

CHAPTER 48

Cardiovascular and Hemolymphatic System Infections

CARDIOVASCULAR SYSTEM INFECTIONS

Parasitic infections of the heart involve both the **myocardium (myocarditis) and the pericardium (pericarditis) in the inflammatory processes of the disease** to a variable degree and extent with myriad clinical manifestations (see box). Myocarditis and pericarditis may be caused by a variety of infectious and non-infectious etiologies.

Disease manifestations of cardiovascular infections

- Cardiomyopathy
- Conduction abnormalities
- Aneurysms
- Fever
- Dyspnea
- Heart failure
- Sudden death
- Thromboembolism
- Chest pain

Myocarditis

Inflammation of the myocardium is known as myocarditis (Table 48.1). It may be asymptomatic initially and present later with unexplained heart failure, arrhythmias, fever, chest pain and sudden death. The various mechanisms involved in the pathogenesis of myocarditis are as follows:

- **Direct myocyte damage** by the pathogen (e.g., Coxsackievirus B, *Trypanosoma cruzi* and *Toxoplasma gondii*)
- **Cytotoxicity** due to a circulating toxin (e.g., *Corynebacterium diphtheriae*)
- **Immune response-mediated damage** or antigenic mimicry (e.g., *Streptococcus pyogenes* and *T. cruzi*) or intense inflammatory damage due to migrating larvae (e.g., *Trichinella spiralis* and *Toxocara* spp.)
- **Helminth-induced hypereosinophilia** has been associated with **'tropical endomyocardial fibrosis'**; some helminths frequently induce chronic eosinophilia with consequent endomyocardial fibrosis which manifests clinically as restrictive cardiomyopathy (e.g., filarial worms and *Schistosoma*)
- **Damage to the vascular endothelium** (e.g., cytomegalovirus, hepatitis virus, fungi and rickettsiae)

Pericarditis

Pericardial inflammation is known as pericarditis (Table 48.1). The clinical features of pericarditis are chest pain, fever, dyspnea, tachycardia and flu-like symptoms; its onset may be either acute or insidious. While viral pericarditis generally has a benign course, pericarditis caused by other agents may lead to significant morbidity and mortality. The following are the mechanisms involved in pericarditis:

Table 48.1 Infectious causes of myocarditis and pericarditis

Protozoa	Helminths	Bacteria	Viruses	Fungi
• *Trypanosoma cruzi* (Chagas' disease) • *Trypanosoma brucei* (African trypanosomiasis) • *Toxoplasma gondii* • *Entamoeba histolytica* • *Sarcocystis*	• *Trichinella spiralis* • *Toxocara* • *Schistosoma* • *Echinococcus*	• *Corynebacterium diphtheriae* • *Mycobacterium tuberculosis* • *Clostridium perfringens* • *Neisseria meningitidis* • *Salmonella* • *Shigella* • *Campylobacter* • *Streptococcus pyogenes* • *Staphylococcus aureus* • Non-tubercular mycobacteria • *Mycoplasma pneumoniae* • *Rickettsiae* • *Borrelia burgdorferi* • Anerobic bacteria	• Coxsackievirus B • Echoviruses • Poliovirus • Non-polio enteroviruses • Adenovirus • Mumps • Influenza A and B • Dengue • Chikungunya • Varicella-zoster virus (VZV) • Cytomegalovirus (CMV) • Epstein-Barr virus (EBV) • Hepatitis viruses • Parvovirus B19 • Human immunodeficiency virus (HIV)	• *Aspergillus* • *Candida* • *Blastomyces* • *Coccidioides* • *Cryptococcus* • *Histoplasma*

- **Direct damage** of the pericardium by the pathogen by the hematogenous route as part of systemic involvement (this is the case with most viral agents)
- **Spread from a contiguous focus** of infection in the chest (e.g., *Entamoeba histolytica* and *Staphylococcus aureus*)
- **Spread from a focus of infection within the heart** (as is the case with most viruses)
- **Penetrating injury to the pericardium** (as is the case with anerobic bacteria)

Diseases of the Ventricles and Blood Vessels

The disease processes involving the heart may cause the **thinning of the ventricular walls** (e.g., *T. cruzi*), **aneurysms** (e.g., syphilis, tuberculosis and *T. cruzi*) and the formation of **thrombi** (as with any bacterial or fungal endocarditis and *T. cruzi*), which may embolise to the pulmonary or systemic circulation and cause complications. A number of parasitic agents **reside in the blood vessels** (like schistosomes).

HEMOLYMPHATIC SYSTEM INFECTIONS

Hemolymphatic system infections comprise diseases of the blood and bone marrow components, lymph nodes and lymphatics. A number of microbial agents infect the blood either **transiently** (as in bacteremia, viremia and fungemia) or **reside in plasma** (e.g., microfilariae of filarial nematodes, trypanosomes) or **inside blood components** (e.g., *Plasmodium* in RBC, *Leishmania* in macrophages).

The clinical features are non-specific, ranging from non-specific fever of unknown origin (FUO) to anemia, thrombocytopenia, alterations in leukocyte counts, hepatomegaly, splenomegaly, etc. (see box).

Disease manifestations of hemolymphatic infections

- Fever
- Anemia
- Pallor
- Malaise
- Hepatomegaly
- Splenomegaly
- Lymphadenopathy
- Lymphangitis
- Lymphedema
- Elephantiasis
- Hydrocele

Fever of Unknown Origin (FUO)

Multiple episodes of **fever >38.3°C over a span of more than three weeks for which no diagnosis is arrived at despite one week of investigations after hospitalisation** is classically defined as FUO. It is also known as pyrexia of unknown origin (PUO). FUO has been further classified as classic FUO, nosocomial FUO (infection not apparent at admission), neutropenic FUO (neutrophil count <500/μl) and FUO associated with HIV infection. The majority of FUOs have non-infectious etiologies (inflammation, neoplasms and undiagnosed causes); however, several pathogens are also implicated as the cause, especially in tropical and subtropical countries (Table 48.2).

Infections Causing Anemia

Anemia is a very common manifestation observed in the tropics; the higher incidence is attributed to widespread **malnutrition compounded by infections** leading to malabsorption (e.g., *Giardia duodenalis*, acute enteric infections and tuberculosis) (Table 48.3). Anemia may occur due to a number of non-infectious and infectious causes which are as follows:

- **Marrow production defects or hypoproliferation** (e.g., kala-azar, tuberculosis and HIV)
- **Decreased red cell survival (hemolysis) or disorders of hemostasis** (e.g., malaria, *Babesia*, typhus,

Table 48.2 Important infectious causes of fever of unknown origin

Protozoa	Helminths	Bacteria	Viruses	Fungi
• *Plasmodium* (malaria) • *Entamoeba histolytica* • *Leishmania* (kala-azar) • *Toxoplasma gondii* • *Trypanosoma cruzi* • *Trypanosoma brucei*	• *Strongyloides stercoralis* hyperinfection syndrome • *Toxocara* (visceral larva migrans) • *Trichinella spiralis* • *Schistosoma* (Katayama fever)	• *Salmonella typhi* (typhoid/enteric fever) • Scrub typhus • Extrapulmonary tuberculosis • Non-tubercular mycobacteria • *Brucella* • *Leptospira* • *Streptococcus pneumoniae* • *Legionella* • *Rickettsiae* • *Francisella* • Septicemia (gram-positive or -negative bacteria) • Urinary tract infection	• Respiratory viruses • Dengue • Chikungunya • Viral hepatitis • Epstein-Barr virus (EBV) • Human immunodeficiency virus (HIV) • Cytomegalovirus (CMV) • Viral hemorrhagic fevers (Lassa, Ebola, Marburg, etc.)	• *Candida* • *Cryptococcus* • *Histoplasma* • *Coccidioides* • *Mucor* • *Rhizopus* • *Pneumocystis*

meningococcemia, viral hemorrhagic fevers and septicemia)

- **Blood loss** (as seen with hookworms and *Trichuris trichiura*); hookworms damage the intestinal mucosa and ingest blood
- **Competition for components** essential for RBC production (e.g., *Diphyllobothrium latum* competes with the host and usurps intestinal vitamin B12, leading to megaloblastic anemia)

Infections of the Spleen

An increased activity of the cells of macrophages and lymphocytes may lead to the enlargement of the spleen and liver. A palpable spleen is a common clinical finding in the tropics, especially in regions where diseases such as malaria and kala-azar are endemic. In many instances, splenomegaly is accompanied by pancytopenia, anemia, granulocytopenia and thrombocytopenia (features of hypersplenism) (Table 48.4).

Infections of the Lymph Nodes and Lymphatics

Lymph nodes are a major component of the body's defence against bacteria, parasites, viruses and fungi and are frequently found enlarged **(lymphadenitis)** in various infections (Table 48.5). Some parasites have a special predilection for the lymphatic system and lymph nodes.

- **Filarial worms are notable in choosing the lymphatics and lymph nodes** as their primary abode, inciting host inflammatory response and leading to various manifestations. The early disease may present as fever, lymphangitis and lymphadenitis, whereas chronic infections may cause serious debilitating illness and present as lymphedema, lymphatic obstruction, elephantiasis and hydrocele.
- The intracellular protozoan *Leishmania* resides inside the macrophages and **causes localised or generalised lymphadenopathy** in cutaneous leishmaniasis and kala-azar respectively.

Table 48.3 Infectious causes of anemia

Acute	Chronic
• Malaria • Shiga toxin-producing *Escherichia coli* O157:H7 (hemolytic uremic syndrome) • *Clostridium perfringens* sepsis • Dengue • Bleeding diathesis	• Hookworm • *Trichuris trichiura* • *Schistosoma* • *Plasmodium* (malaria) • *Leishmania donovani* (kala-azar) • *Diphyllobothrium latum* (megaloblastic anemia) • Tuberculosis • *Brucella* • Human immunodeficiency virus (HIV) • Parvovirus B19

Table 48.4 Infectious causes of splenomegaly

Protozoa	Helminths	Bacteria	Viruses
• *Plasmodium* (malaria) • *Leishmania donovani* (kala-azar) • *Toxoplasma gondii* • *Trypanosoma*	• *Echinococcus* • *Schistosoma*	• *Salmonella typhi* (enteric fever/typhoid) • Scrub typhus • Septicemia • *Mycobacterium tuberculosis* • *Brucella*	• Viremia

Table 48.5 Infectious causes of lymphadenitis

Protozoa	Helminths	Bacteria	Viruses	Fungi
• *Toxoplasma gondii* • *Leishmania donovani* (kala-azar)	• *Wuchereria bancrofti* • *Brugia malayi* • *Loa loa* • *Trypanosoma brucei* (Winterbottom sign)	• Pyogenic bacteria (*Streptococcus pyogenes, Staphylococcus aureus*) • Tuberculosis • *Brucella* • *Treponema* • *Bartonella* (cat-scratch disease) • Other bacterial infections	• Cytomegalovirus • Epstein-Barr virus • Herpes simplex virus (HSV) • Human immunodeficiency virus • Human herpesvirus - 6 • Measles	• *Cryptococcus* • *Histoplasma*

Chapter 49 Central Nervous System Infections

The **central nervous system** (CNS) may be affected by a number of microorganisms. The clinical manifestations of these infections are non-specific and depend on the area of the CNS involved (leptomeninges, cerebral parenchyma, cerebellum, brainstem, cerebrovascular drainage or the spinal cord), and whether there is focal infection or generalised brain tissue involvement (see box). The clinical features often point specifically towards the underlying disease process (e.g., meningitis or encephalitis); however, a mixed picture is not uncommon (e.g., meningitis with seizures or signs of focal deficit).

Disease manifestations of the central nervous system

- Fever
- Nuchal rigidity
- Vomiting
- Seizures
- Coma
- Headache
- Altered mental state
- Personality changes
- Focal neurologic deficits

The pathology in CNS infections is caused by the invasion of the microorganism, the release of toxins or microbial components, the production of host inflammatory cytokines and pressure effects of the infective mass. These result in increased blood–brain barrier permeability, altered cerebral blood flow, congestion, ischemia and cell death, which, in turn, produce varied disease manifestations depending on the site involved.

- **Parenchymal involvement** may cause focal neurological deficits or generalised encephalopathic features depending on the underlying disease process. The disease manifestations in such cases are as follows:
  - **Hypoxia and ischemia** of the brain tissue due to the sequestration of RBCs in capillaries and pro-inflammatory cytokine storm in response to the pathogen (e.g., cerebral malaria)
  - **Granulomatous tissue reaction** elicited by the parasite (e.g., *Mycobacterium tuberculosis, Balamuthia mandrillaris*)
  - **Multiple necro-hemorrhagic lesions** with perilesional edema and congestion (e.g., *Toxoplasma gondii, Acanthamoeba*)
  - **Brain abscess** formation due to lytic enzymes released by the pathogen (e.g., bacterial abscess, tuberculoma, *Toxoplasma gondii*)
  - **Space-occupying lesions** may cause pressure symptoms or remain asymptomatic (e.g., the larval cyst of *Taenia solium*)
- **Extra-parenchymal involvement** may affect the ventricles, leptomeninges and the spinal cord.
  - **The leptomeninges and cerebrospinal fluid** (CSF) may be invaded by microorganisms which release their cell wall components to incite the inflammatory process (e.g., the lipopolysaccharides of gram-negative bacteria).
  - Any **obstruction in the CSF flow** can raise the intracranial pressure and cause hydrocephalus (e.g., the ventricular cysts of *T. solium* larva).

The diagnosis of CNS infections is made based on clinical presentation, radioimaging and CSF examination (Table 49.1). In rare cases, when all these are inconclusive, a biopsy may have to be performed.

The disease presentation may be **acute, subacute or chronic**. Occasionally, there may be **residual** neurological sequelae of the disease.

Acute Meningitis

Meningitis refers to the **inflammation of the leptomeninges and CSF** caused by infectious agents. Acute meningitis **progresses rapidly** (within a few hours to a few days) and presents with **fever, headache and altered sensorium**. Infants and young children may be highly irritable or drowsy on presentation. Neck rigidity and signs of meningism, i.e., Kernig's or Brudzinski's signs can be elicited.

The most common etiologic agents of acute illness are viruses and bacteria (Table 49.2).

Chronic Meningitis

Chronic meningitis has a more **indolent course (ranging from weeks to months)** with a persistent inflammation in the CSF. The presenting features are similar to those of acute meningitis. However, they are **gradual** in onset and progression. The longer duration may predispose the individual to cognitive changes. Most fungi, parasites, spirochetes and mycobacteria cause chronic illness, especially in immunocompromised individuals (Table 49.3).

Encephalitis

Encephalitis is the **inflammation of brain parenchyma**. In some cases, there may be concomitant involvement of

Table 49.1 Differential features of cerebrospinal fluid in CNS* infections

Feature	Normal	Bacterial meningitis	Viral meningitis	Fungal meningitis	Parasitic meningitis	Tuberculous meningitis	Encephalitis
WBC* count (per µl)	<5	>1,000	5–500	40–500	150–2,000	25–100	Mildly ↑ to grossly purulent
Differential leukocyte count	60–70% lymphocytes ≤30% monocytes/ macrophages No PMN	↑↑ PMNs* (≥80%)	Predominantly lymphocytes PMN in first 24–48 hrs	Lymphocytes or PMN, depending on specific organism	↑↑ Eosinophils (≥50%)	Predominantly lymphocytes	Predominantly lymphocytes
Gram stain	Negative	Positive (in >60% of cases)	Negative	Rarely positive	Negative	Occasionally positive	Negative
Glucose (mg/dl)	40–85	↓	Normal	↓	Normal to ↓	↓	Normal
Protein (mg/dl)	15–45	>100	20–80 Usually not ↑	150–300	50–200	100–200	50–100 (usually not ↑)
Common causes	–	*Streptococcus pneumoniae, Neisseria meningitidis, Haemophilus influenzae*	Enteroviruses Arboviruses	*Candida, Cryptococcus, Aspergillus*	*Angiostrongylus Gnathostoma Baylisascaris Naegleria*	*Mycobacterium tuberculosis*	Herpesviruses Enteroviruses Influenza virus Rabies virus *Acanthamoeba*

*CNS: central nervous system; WBC: white blood cell; PMN: polymorphonuclear neutrophils

Table 49.2 Infectious causes of acute meningitis

Protozoa	Helminths	Bacteria (pyogenic)	Viruses (aseptic)
• *Naegleria* • *Entamoeba histolytica* • *Toxoplasma gondii* • *Baylisascaris* • *Strongyloides stercoralis* (disseminated infection)	• Neurocysticercosis • *Angiostrongylus* • *Toxocara*	• *Streptococcus pneumoniae* • *Neisseria meningitides* • *Haemophilus influenzae* • Enteric gram-negative bacteria • Group B streptococcus • Rickettsiae • *Listeria* • Spirochetes (*Treponema, Borrelia burgdorferi*)	• Enterovirus • Arboviruses • Adenoviruses • Human immunodeficiency virus • Mumps • Measles • Herpes simplex virus • Influenza • Parainfluenza

Table 49.3 Infectious causes of chronic meningitis

Protozoa	Helminths	Bacteria	Viruses	Fungi
• *Toxoplasma gondii*, especially in AIDS patients • *Trypanosoma* • *Acanthamoeba* and *Balamuthia mandrillaris* (rare)	• Neurocysticercosis • *Angiostrongylus* • *Gnathostoma* • *Baylisascaris*	• Partially treated pyogenic meningitis • Tuberculosis • *Borrelia burgdorferi* • *Treponema* • *Actinomyces* • *Nocardia* • *Brucella*	• Mumps • Echovirus • Human immunodeficiency virus (acute retroviral syndrome) • Human herpesviruses • Rabies • Measles	• *Cryptococcus* (especially in immunocompromised patients) • *Coccidioides* • *Candida* • *Histoplasma* • *Blastomyces* • *Aspergillus* • *Sporothrix*

the meninges (meningoencephalitis), nerves and spinal cord. Patients with encephalitis predominantly have signs of meningeal inflammation and in addition, altered consciousness, confusion, stupor or coma. Seizures are common, and sometimes, cognitive changes are also seen (Table 49.4).

Table 49.4 Infectious causes of encephalitis

Parasites	Bacteria	Viruses	Fungi
• Malaria • *Trypanosoma* • *Toxoplasma gondii* in immunocompromised patients • *Naegleria* • *Acanthamoeba* • *Balamuthia mandrillaris* • *Baylisascaris*	• Tuberculosis • Rickettsiae • *Listeria* • *Treponema* • *Mycoplasma pneumoniae*	• Enterovirus • Arboviruses: Dengue, Japanese encephalitis, Zika virus, Chikungunya and other encephalitis-causing arboviruses • Herpesviruses: HSV, VZV, CMV, HHV - 6 • Rabies • Mumps • Measles • Rubella • Human immunodeficiency virus • Epstein-Barr virus (EBV) • Nipah virus	• *Cryptococcus* • *Aspergillus* • Mucormycosis • Black fungi

Focal Lesions/Brain Abscess

Focal lesions in the brain can lead to neurological deficits and seizures depending upon the area involved (Table 49.5). Sometimes, the organism develops a **space-occupying lesion** with minimal inflammation and the individual remaining asymptomatic (e.g., neurocysticercosis).

Table 49.5 Infectious causes of seizures

Protozoa	Helminths	Bacteria	Viruses	Fungi
• *Toxoplasma gondii* • Cerebral malaria • *Entamoeba histolytica* • *Acanthamoeba* • *Trypanosoma* • *Naegleria*	• Neurocysticercosis • *Onchocerca volvulus* • *Echinococcus* • *Schistosoma* • *Toxocara* • *Angiostrongylus*	• Tuberculosis • Any bacterial abscess	• Cytomegalovirus (CMV) • Enterovirus • Human herpesvirus - 6 • Herpes simplex virus • Japanese encephalitis virus	• *Cryptococcus* • *Candida* • *Aspergillus* • Mucormycosis • Black fungi

Chapter 50

Genitourinary System and Sexually Transmitted Infections

Sexually transmitted infections (STI) are infections transmitted predominantly by the sexual route, though they may be trasmitted by other modes also (Table 50.1). **Genitourinary tract infections**, on the other hand, may result from a wide range of infectious processes including sexually transmitted infections (Table 50.2). The treatment approach to STIs is **syndromic**—the common clinical signs and symptoms (e.g., urethral discharge or genital ulcer) are used in the management of the patient.

The disease manifestations range from localised genitourinary lesions depending on the organ involved (e.g., penile ulcer in syphilis) to systemic features (e.g., HIV and hepatitis virus), depending upon the infective agent, host immune status and disease duration (see box).

Genital Cutaneous/Mucocutaneous Infections

The skin or mucosa is exposed to microorganisms by direct sexual contact or secondary to infection elsewhere in the body (Table 50.3). The pathogen may invade the skin to cause a genital lesion (e.g., a syphilitic ulcer) or establish itself in its niche and cause chronic infection (e.g., *Trichomonas vaginalis*). Various types of lesions may be seen in the genital region such as **macules, papules, pustules, vesicles, warts, nodules and ulcers**. In lesions of **elephantiasis** (lymphatic filariasis), the scrotum, penis, labia and vulva may be enlarged due to the obstruction of the inguinal lymph nodes (e.g., *Wuchereria bancrofti* and *Brugia malayi*). Ectoparasites burrow subcutaneous tunnels in the inguinal area and genital organs (e.g., scabies and lice).

Disease manifestations of the genitourinary system and sexually transmitted infections

- Genital lesions
- Urethral discharge
- Urinary urgency
- Dyspareunia
- Scrotal swellings
- Fever
- Miscarriage
- Neonatal conjunctivitis
- Oro-labial lesions
- Vaginal discharge
- Chyluria
- Hematuria
- Inguinal swellings
- Abdominal/pelvic discomfort
- Still birth
- Ulcers – painful or painless
- Pruritus
- Dysuria
- Chyluria
- Lymphadenopathy
- Carcinomas
- Neonatal death

Table 50.1 Causative agents of STIs transmitted through sexual contact (with or without predilection for genital organs)

Parasites	Ectoparasites	Bacteria	Viruses	Fungi
• *Trichomonas vaginalis* • *Giardia duodenalis* (in MSM*) • *Entamoeba histolytica* (in MSM*)	• *Sarcoptes scabiei* (mite) • *Pthirus pubis* (lice)	• *Neisseria gonorrhoeae* • *Chlamydia trachomatis* (LGV) • *Treponema pallidum* (syphilis)	• Human immunodeficiency virus-1 and 2 • Human T cell lymphotropic virus • Herpes simplex virus-1 and 2 • Human papillomavirus • Hepatitis B virus • Hepatitis C virus • Molluscum contagiosum virus	• *Candida*

*MSM: Men who have sex with men

Table 50.2 Causative agents of genitourinary tract infections as part of systemic or anatomically contiguous infections

Parasites	Bacteria	Viruses	Fungi
• *Schistosoma* • Malaria • Filaria • *Enterobius*	• *Haemophilus ducreyi* (chancroid) • *Klebsiella granulomatis* (granuloma inguinale) • *Ureaplasma urealyticum* • *Gardnerella vaginalis* • *Mycoplasma genitalium* tuberculosis • Any cellulitis- or gangrene-causing bacteria	• Adenovirus • Cytomegalovirus	• *Candida* • *Malassezia* • *Trichophyton* • *Epidermophyton* • *Microsporum*

Table 50.3 Infectious causes of genital lesions

Parasites	Ectoparasites	Bacteria	Viruses	Fungi
• *Trichomonas vaginalis* • *Entamoeba histolytica* • *Wuchereria bancrofti* • *Brugia malayi*	• *Sarcoptes scabiei* (mite) • *Pthirus pubis* (lice)	• *Treponema pallidum* • *Haemophilus ducreyi* • *Chlamydia trachomatis* • *Klebsiella granulomatis* • *Mycobacterium tuberculosis* • *Francisella tularenesis*	• Herpes simplex virus-1 and 2 • Human papillomavirus • Molluscum contagiosum virus	• *Histoplasma* • *Candida* • Dermatophytes

Urethritis

Inflammation of the urethra is commonly due to **ascending infections** from the urethra, and may manifest as mild to severe dysuria or urethral discharge (Table 50.4).

Cystitis

Bladder infection causes cystitis which presents acutely with urinary urgency and frequency, hematuria or suprapubic bladder tenderness. It occurs generally due to **ascending bacterial infections** from the urinary tract (e.g., uropathogenic *Escherichia coli*) and sometimes, other pathogens (e.g., *T. vaginalis*). The bladder may also be affected by other modes of infections such as:

- **Indwelling catheters** colonised by microorganisms (e.g., fungal cystitis)
- **Parasites colonising the venous plexus** of the bladder release eggs which induce a granulomatous reaction in the surrounding tissues (e.g., *Schistosoma*)
- **Hematogenous spread** from another body site (e.g., HSV, CMV and adenovirus)

Kidney Infections

The kidney may be affected by several bacteria, parasites, fungi and viruses hematogenously in any systemic infection or by an ascending infection from the urinary tract.

- Parasites may affect the kidney either directly or through inflammatory mediators, and may cause **proteinuria, hematuria, nephrotic syndrome and renal failure** (e.g., malaria, schistosomiasis, kala-azar, *Toxoplasma*, filariasis, *Babesia* and *Trypanosoma*), **mass effect** (e.g., *Echinococcus*) or **abscesses** (e.g., *Entamoeba histolytica*).
- **Chyluria** is a condition in which the urine appears milky due to the leakage of lymphatic fluid in the urine. It occurs due to lymphatic obstruction caused by filarial worms (*Wuchereria bancrofti* and *Brugia* spp.) which reside the lymph nodes and lymphatics, and is not primarily a genitourinary infection.

Table 50.4 Infectious causes of urethritis

Parasites	Bacteria	Viruses
• *Trichomonas vaginalis*	• *Neisseria gonorrhoeae* • *Chlamydia trachomatis* • *Ureaplasma urealyticum* • *Mycoplasma genitalium*	• Adenovirus • Herpes simplex virus

Vulvovaginitis and Cervicitis

Normally, the vagina is protected by vaginal secretions and **lactobacilli** (which comprise 95% of the normal vaginal flora) which maintain a **healthy pH of 3.5–4.6** and prevent the colonisation of disease-causing microorganisms (Tables 50.5 and 50.6).

- When the normal physiological balance of the vagina gets disrupted, the lactobacilli in the vagina are replaced by anaerobic bacteria such as *Prevotella, Mobiluncus, Gardnerella, Ureaplasma* and *Mycoplasma,* causing **bacterial vaginosis (BV)**. The clinical manifestations of BV include malodorous, itchy vaginal discharge, dyspareunia or sometimes, abdominal discomfort. The vaginal discharge is typically profuse and watery in BV; thick white and curdy in *Candida* and frothy and green in *Trichomonas*. Typical features may sometimes be absent.

Table 50.5 Infectious causes of vaginitis

Parasites	Bacteria	Viruses	Fungi
• *Trichomonas vaginalis*	• Anaerobic bacteria causing BV	• HSV	• *Candida*

Table 50.6 Infectious causes of cervicitis

Parasites	Bacteria	Viruses
• *Trichomonas vaginalis*	• *Neisseria gonorrhoeae* • *Chlamydia trachomatis* • *Mycoplasma genitalium*	• Herpes simplex virus • Human papillomavirus

- The vagina and cervix, along with the other contiguous parts, may be affected in **vaginitis, vulvovaginitis, bartholinitis and cervicitis** by cytopathic effects, hemolytic enzymes and proteases of pathogens (e.g., *T. vaginalis* and *Candida*). The clinical features of cervicitis may be limited to a purulent vaginal discharge without vulvar irritation or pruritus. However, urethritis, endometritis or salpingitis may be associated conditions.
- Chronic infection with HPV may lead to **cervical cancer.**

Pelvic Inflammatory Disease (PID)

Pelvic inflammatory disease is an infection of the upper female genital tract that **ascends** from the cervix or vagina to involve the endometrium and/or fallopian tubes. The infection may extend beyond the reproductive tract to cause **pelvic peritonitis, generalised peritonitis, perihepatitis, perisplenitis or pelvic abscess**. PID is a common cause of **infertility**. The clinical features vary greatly but fever, lower abdominal and pelvic pain/tenderness are common.

- The agents most often implicated include the primary causes of cervicitis (*N. gonorrhoeae, C. trachomatis* and *M. genitalium*) and anaerobes associated with BV.
- Other gram-negative (e.g., enteric bacilli), gram-positive (*Streptococcus agalactiae*) and anaerobic bacteria may be involved.

Male Genitourinary System Infections

Infections of the male genital tract can lead to **epididymitis** (e.g., *C. trachomatis, N. gonorrhoeae and Pseudomonas*), **balanoposthitis** (e.g., *Candida*), **prostatitis** (e.g., *Escherichia coli*) and **orchitis** (e.g., mumps and *E. coli*).

Proctitis

The inflammation of the rectal epithelium is known as **proctitis**. It can occur due to anal intercourse (e.g., *N. gonorrhoeae*, *C. trachomatis*, syphilis and herpes simplex virus).

Chapter 51

Respiratory Tract Infections

A number of microbes are capable of affecting the lungs either directly or by indirect immunological mechanisms, causing associated clinical manifestations (see box). The infectious agents may gain entry to the lower respiratory tract by the following mechanisms:

- **Aspiration** of the upper airway resident flora
- **Inhalation** of aerosolised material
- **Metastatic seeding** of the lung through blood
- Helminths traversing the lungs in their **migratory pathway**; the passing larvae may affect the respiratory tract

Disease manifestations of lower respiratory tract infections

- Fever
- Cough
- Dyspnea
- Wheezing
- Hemoptysis
- Chest pain

The parasitic diseases of the lower respiratory tract may present as **pneumonia** or **lung abscess**. The upper respiratory tract is not usually infected by parasites except in the following cases:

- *Rhinosporidium seeberi* causes an obstructive **polypoidal pedunculated mass** in the mucosa of the nose and nasopharynx.
- The **roundworm may aberrantly crawl out** of the nares or cause respiratory distress by **obstructing** the airways.

Pneumonia

Pneumonia is one of the most significant causes of deaths attributed to infectious diseases. Several bacteria, viruses, fungi and parasites are implicated in the etiology of pneumonia. **Eosinophilic pneumonia, on the other hand, is more commonly caused by parasites** (Table 51.1).

The clinical presentations of pneumonia are non-specific and include fever, malaise, cough, dyspnea, chest pain, etc. The parasites affect the lung in many ways:

- Some parasites have a natural **predilection for the lung,** e.g., infections of the lung fluke *Paragonimus* present with cough, hemoptysis, fever and night sweats mimicking tuberculosis and lung cancer.
- **Migratory helminths:**
  - **Tropical pulmonary eosinophilia** is caused by the microfilariae of filarial worms (e.g., *Wuchereria bancrofti* and *Brugia malayi*) migrating through pulmonary blood vessels. These may induce immunological hyperresponsiveness, causing diffuse pulmonary infiltrates and eosinophilia.
  - **Loeffler's syndrome** is a **transient respiratory illness** associated with peripheral blood eosinophilia and radiographic shadows. It usually presents with mild symptoms like wheezing, dry or (less often) mucoid cough and dyspnea. Less commonly, the patient may present with myalgia, anorexia and urticaria. It may be associated with the helminth larvae (e.g., *Ascaris lumbricoides, Onchocerca volvulus*, hookworms and *Strongyloides stercoralis*) passing through the lungs. It is a benign, self-limiting disease without significant morbidity, and the symptoms usually subside within 3–4 weeks.
  - **Granulomatous pneumonia** may also be caused by the migratory larvae.
  - **Hemorrhagic eosinophilic pneumonia** may be associated with *S. stercoralis* hyperinfection in which the parasite's larvae mature in the lung itself and extensively invade the lung parenchyma and the airways.
- A lung **abscess may rupture** into the pleura or airways, leading to disseminated pulmonary infection (e.g., *Entamoeba histolytica*).

Table 51.1 Infectious causes of eosinophilic pneumonia

Parasites	Bacteria	Fungi
• *Ascaris lumbricoides* • *Onchocerca volvulus* • *Strongyloides stercoralis* • *Paragonimus westermani* • *Echinococcus* • *Toxocara* (larva migrans) • *Dirofilaria* • *Schistosoma* • Hookworms • *Wuchereria bancrofti* (tropical pulmonary eosinophilia)	• Tuberculosis • *Brucella*	• *Aspergillus* • *Coccidioides* • *Histoplasma*

- Rarely, pneumonia may be caused by *Toxoplasma gondii*, *Cryptosporidium* or microsporidia. Such cases are most often reported in **immunocompromised individuals.**
- **Aberrant ectopic localisation** of *Schistosoma* in the pulmonary vessels may cause an intense reaction to form pulmonary nodules, infarctions and necrotising or eosinophilic pneumonia.

Lung Abscess

A lung abscess results when an infection leads to **necrosis of the lung parenchyma,** producing one or more cavities (Table 51.2). Usually, it occurs as a complication of the aspiration of anaerobic and aerobic bacteria normally present in the oral cavity, either postoperatively or following certain procedures. Several parasites are also agents of lung abscesses.

- The granulomatous lesions (e.g., *Paragonimus*) or the cyst (e.g., *Echinococcus*) formed in response to the parasite may soften to form an abscess.
- Often, an abscess may form as a direct transdiaphragmatic extension from a contiguous site such as a liver abscess (e.g., *E. histolytica*).

Table 51.2 Infectious causes of lung abscesses

Protozoa	Helminths	Bacteria	Fungi
• *Entamoeba histolytica*	• *Paragonimus westermani* • *Echinococcus* • *Strongyloides stercoralis*	• Anaerobic and aerobic flora of the oral cavity • Tuberculosis • Rarely, *Staphylococcus aureus* • *Pseudomonas aeruginosa* • *Streptococcus pneumoniae*	• *Histoplasma* • *Blastomyces* • *Aspergillus* • *Pneumocystis* • *Zygomycetes*

Chapter 52

Musculoskeletal System, Skin and Soft Tissue Infections

SKIN INFECTIONS

The outermost layer of skin, the stratum corneum, provides robust protection to the body by acting as a mechanical barrier. However, because of its vast surface area, skin is always under attack by infectious and non-infectious agents. Therefore, skin and soft tissue infections are very commonly encountered with various clinical manifestations (see box).

Disease manifestations of skin infections

- Erythema
- Rash
- Swelling
- Macules
- Plaques
- Masses
- Ulcers
- Pruritius
- Nodules
- Papules
- Serpiginous tracts
- Polyps

Generally, the skin may be involved in infections in the following ways:

- **Primary skin infections** are caused by agents like streptococci and staphylococci.
- **The disruption of skin** by burns, abrasions, foreign bodies, surgery, vascular or pressure sores, animal bites and dermatologic disorders allows the penetration of microorganisms to the deeper parts of the skin or to the systemic organs of the body (e.g., tetanus and rabies).
- **Hair follicles** also serve as portals for the entry of microorganisms (e.g., staphylococcal and streptococcal infections and mites).
- **Insect bites** also disrupt the skin and are a mode of transmission for several microorganisms (e.g., malaria, filaria, kala-azar and scrub typhus).
- **Helminth L3-stage larval penetration** occurs through the skin (e.g., hookworm and *Strongyloides stercoralis*). Many helminths also **migrate** through the skin and induce skin lesions (e.g., *S. stercoralis* and cutaneous larva migrans).
- Conditions of the skin may develop as manifestations of **systemic infections** (e.g., bacteremia and septicemia). Some parasites disseminate widely in the body and encyst in the skin and soft tissues (e.g., cysticerci of *Taenia solium* and echinococcal cysts).
- Skin may also be affected due to a localised or generalised **allergic response.**

Various types of localised or generalised lesions may be produced with or without the involvement of the deeper tissues. The type of lesion often points towards the etiological agent. While macular, papular and vesicular lesions are commonly caused by viruses; bullae and pus-filled lesions are formed due to bacterial infections. Parasites and ectoparasites also infect the skin and soft tissues and may produce characteristic lesions.

Penetration of Worm Larvae and Subcutaneous Migration

- **Creeping eruptions** are caused by human **hookworms** and ***S. stercoralis*** larvae. The infective-stage larvae may provoke pruritic maculopapular dermatitis and rashes called **'ground itch'** at the site of skin penetration, while **serpiginous tracks** may be formed due to the subcutaneous migration of the larva. **Larva currens** is the term assigned to the fast-moving larvae of *S. stercoralis*.
- **Cutaneous larva migrans** is caused by the accidental penetration of the skin by the larvae of **non-human (zoonotic) hookworms**, which are unable to complete their life cycle in humans and die in the skin. These produce pruritic maculopapular dermatitis and rashes at the site of skin penetration; serpiginous tracks are produced during their aimless wandering.
- **Cercarial dermatitis or swimmer's itch** is a pruritic, erythematous and urticarial rash that develops on the affected areas of the skin due to the invasion of the cercariae of ***Schistosoma*** contracted by swimming or wading in infested freshwater lakes or ponds. This condition occurs when a person from a non-endemic area visits an area endemic for these schistosomes. The cercariae die in the skin and evoke severe allergic responses. The rash appears quickly while the person is still in the water.

Adult Worms Migrating Through Skin or Subcutaneous Tissues

- **Calabar swellings (fugitive swelling)** are seen in infections with ***Loa loa***. The adult worms migrate through the subcutaneous tissues, producing intermittent subcutaneous edematous swellings due to inflammatory reactions to the migratory worm. These infections are not prevalent in India.

- **Onchocercomas** are firm, non-tender nodules, especially over joints; they contain the coiled adult worms of ***Onchocerca volvulus.*** The disease is not prevalent in India.

Arthropod Bite and Inoculation of Parasite

- **Chagoma**, a feature of Chagas' disease, is caused by the bite of **kissing bugs** (*Reduviidae* family), the vectors for ***Trypanosoma cruzi***. The bug deposits its feces, which contains the parasite, on the skin. On scratching the site of deposition of feces, the parasite enters the skin and forms an erythematous, painful and subcutaneous nodule. This commonly occurs on the face.
- **Trypanosomal chancre** forms at the biting site of the **tsetse fly** (*Glossina*)—a vector of African trypanosomiasis which is caused by ***Trypanosoma brucei***. It occurs as a nodule or ulcer.
- **Cutaneous leishmaniasis (CL)** is caused by *Leishmania tropica* and *L. major* which are transmitted by the bite of the **sandfly** (genera *Lutzomyia* in the Americas and *Phlebotomus* in India). CL is also known as the **'oriental sore'**. It usually occurs on the face and hands, beginning as a papule, later becoming nodular and finally, ulcerating. However, it remains painless.
- **Diffuse cutaneous leishmaniasis (DCL)** is a rare form of leishmaniasis caused by *L. amazonensis* and *L. mexicana* in South and Central America (New World) and *L. aethiopica* in Ethiopia and Kenya (Old World). *L. mexicana* causes a specific form of CL called **'chiclero' ulcer (or bay sore)** characterised by persistent ulcerations in the pinna. It is seen in forest workers who harvest **chicle plants** to collect latex for chewing gum.
- **Mucocutaneous leishmaniasis (MCL) or espundia**, which is caused by *L. braziliensis*, involves the mucous membrane of the nose, oral cavity, pharynx or larynx. MCL is much more severe and disfiguring than CL or DCL.
- **Onchodermatitis is caused by *O. volvulus*.** Several dermatologic manifestations are produced as a result of the host's hyper-reactive immune response to the migrating larvae of *O. volvulus*; these include dermatitis, atrophy, depigmentation and lymphadenitis. The dermatitis may present as hypo- and hyper-pigmented lesions (**leopard skin**), lichenoid changes and hyperkeratosis.
- In ***Dirofilaria* (dog heartworm) infection**, the patient may complain of a sensation of movement under the skin.

Arthropod Infestation

- **Mite infestation** is common in humans as these parasites are widely distributed in the environment. The **itch mite** tunnels through the upper dermis (***Sarcoptes scabiei***), causing **scabies**. It presents as a rash and intense itching that worsens at night. The commonly affected sites in older children and adults include the interdigital spaces, flexor surfaces of the wrist and forearms, armpits, breasts, buttocks and the external genitalia. The **follicle mites** live in the hair follicles and sebaceous glands (***Demodex* spp.**).
- **Lice infestation (pediculosis)** refers to infestation by head and body lice (***Pediculus* spp.**) or pubic lice (***Pthirus pubis***). There may be intense itching, provoking scratching and finally resulting in excoriation.
- **Tungiasis** is an infestation of the skin with the burrowing flea ***Tunga penetrans*** or related species; this flea is commonly known as the chigger flea, sand flea, chigoe, jigger, nigua, etc. The chief habitat of *T. penetrans* is warm, dry soil and the sands of beaches, stables and farms. It causes painless ulcers, especially in the interdigital spaces.
- **Cutaneous myiasis** is caused by the deposition of **eggs (which hatch to release maggots) of flies** on the skin, which may burrow into the skin/wounds/sinuses and develop into mature larvae, producing foul-smelling exudative lesions.

Skin Manifestation of Parasitic Diseases

- **Post-kala-azar dermatitis (PKDL)** is characterised by non-ulcerative cutaneous lesions in about 5% of cases of kala-azar presenting months to years after the primary infection. These are disfiguring erythematous and nodular lesions on the face and depigmented macular lesions on the trunk and extremities. PKDL lesions harbour the parasite ***Leishmania donovani*** and are considered to be human reservoirs of the disease.
- **Filariasis** causes lymphatic obstruction due to adult filarial worms living in the lymph nodes and lymphatics, leading to hyperplasia of the skin and connective tissues. The affected parts are enormously enlarged (**elephantiasis**), and there may be secondary bacterial infections.

- The adult gravid female of the worm ***Dracunculus medinensis* (Guinea worm)** emerges near the surface of the skin to release its larvae from a blister. The initial presentation is a painful papule that enlarges over hours to days to form the blister, accompanied by local erythema, burning sensation, urticaria, fever, nausea and pruritus. To relieve the burning, the affected individuals immerse their feet in the water, whereupon the blister ruptures and the female worm releases thousands of larvae in water. The lesion may get secondarily infected with bacterial agents.
- **Cutaneous lesions** caused by ***Acanthamoeba*** are seen in immunosuppressed individuals and present as erythematous nodules, papules and non-healing ulcers.
- **Cysticerci** (larval form of ***Taenia solium***) may lodge in the subcutaneous tissue and appear as nodules.
- **Cutaneous rhinosporidiosis** presents with polypoidal, friable, tumour-like growths and is caused by ***Rhinosporidium seeberi***. Usually, the mucosa of the nose and oropharynx are involved. However, this condition may also affect the skin.
- **Ulcers caused by *Entamoeba histolytica*** are rarely seen in the genital and perineal area.

MYOSITIS AND MYONECROSIS

Muscle involvement is seen in numerous microbial infections (see box). Although myalgia develops in most of these infections, severe muscle pain is a characteristic of infections caused by coxsackievirus B, *Trichinella spiralis* and bacteria. *Streptococcus pyogenes* may induce primary myositis in association with severe systemic toxicity. Myonecrosis occurs concomitantly with necrotising fasciitis.

Disease manifestations of muscle infections

- Muscle pain
- Fever
- Fasciitis
- Nodules
- Abscesses
- Decreased muscle contractility

Myositis caused by parasitic agents is usually generalised, unlike localised pyogenic abscesses (bacterial) and is usually accompanied by an eosinophilic immune response (Table 52.1). However, some parasitic agents may encyst in the muscles without causing much inflammation (e.g., cysticercosis).

Table 52.1 Infections with muscle involvement

Parasites	Bacteria	Viruses	Fungi
• *Trichinella spiralis* • Cysticercosis • *Toxoplasma gondii* • Microsporidia • *Onchocerca volvulus* • *Trypanosoma* • *Echinococcus* • *Sarcocystis*	• *Staphylococcus aureus* • *Streptococcus pyogenes* • *Clostridium perfringens* (gas gangrene) • *Pseudomonas* • Mycobacteria • Gram-negative bacteria	• Coxsackievirus B • Influenza • Dengue	• *Mucor* • *Rhizopus*

Chapter 53

Ocular Infections

The eyes may be affected by microorganisms either directly (**exogenous**) or as part of a systemic illness (**endogenous**). The clinical manifestations depend on the part of the eye involved, i.e., whether the infection involves the conjunctiva, cornea, anterior or posterior chamber, uveal tract, retina or the ocular adnexa. However, multiple parts of the eyes are often involved (see box).

Disease manifestations of ocular infections

- Irritation of the eye
- Itching
- Discharge
- Tearing
- Decreased vision
- Subconjunctival nodules
- Floaters
- Foreign body sensation
- Redness
- Pain in the eye
- Photophobia
- Periorbital edema
- Blurred vision
- Ring of redness near corneoscleral border

Conjunctivitis

Conjunctivitis is the **inflammation of the conjunctiva** in response to an infection (Table 53.1). In severe cases, the cornea is also involved; this is called keratoconjunctivitis. Patients commonly present to the clinic with a red eye, itching, a foreign-body sensation and discharge, depending on the pathogen. The clinical features of the infections caused by different pathogens often overlap.

- Watery-mucoid (e.g., herpes simplex virus) or purulent discharge (e.g., *Neisseria gonorrhoeae*) or the formation of lymphoid follicles (e.g., *Chlamydia trachomatis,* adenovirus) may occur.
- Some helminths may penetrate and move around in the subconjunctival space, causing intense inflammatory damage (e.g., *Loa loa* and *Onchocerca volvulus*).
- The bite of the reduviid bug transmits *Trypanosoma cruzi* and leads to unilateral, painless and purplish edema associated with conjunctivitis (Romana's sign).
- In rare cases, vascular polypoidal growth may occur (e.g., *Rhinosporidium seeberi*).

Keratitis

In microbial keratitis, **epithelial defects are caused due to the necrosis of the corneal stroma** in response to an infection (Table 53.2). The pathogen is usually inoculated on an abrasion caused by trauma or contact lens use (e.g., *Acanthamoeba*). However, a few organisms can also invade the intact epithelium (e.g., *Neisseria* and microsporidia).

The migration of the larval forms of some parasites (e.g., *Onchocerca*) leads to the intense inflammation of the cornea or other parts and may lead to blindness (river blindness). This leads to corneal clouding, which may progress to scarring and perforation, resulting in a corneal ulcer. The usual presentation is severe pain in the eye, tearing, photophobia and decreased vision. It is potentially a vision-threatening condition.

Intraocular Involvement

Several pathogens have the ability to infect the aqueous and vitreous cavities, uveal tract (iris, ciliary body and choroid) and the retina; often, such infections involve multiple parts of the eye.

Table 53.1 Infectious causes of conjunctivitis

Parasites	Ectoparasites	Bacteria	Viruses	Fungi
• *Leishmania* • Microsporidia • *Trypanosoma* • *Loa loa* • *Onchocerca volvulus* • *Rhinosporidium seeberi*	• Mites *(Demodex)* • Lice	• *Chlamydia trachomatis* • *Chlamydophila pneumoniae* • *Staphylococcus aureus* • *Corynebacterium diphtheriae* • *Streptococcus pneumoniae* • *Haemophilus influenzae* • *Neisseria gonorrhoeae*	• Adenovirus • Herpes simplex virus (HSV) • Varicella zoster and herpes zoster	• *Candida* • *Blastomyces*

Table 53.2 Infectious causes of microbial keratitis

Protozoa	Helminths	Bacteria	Viruses	Fungi
• *Acanthamoeba* • Microsporidia • *Leishmania braziliensis* • *Trypanosoma* spp.	• *Onchocerca volvulus*	• *Staphylococcus aureus* • *Corynebacterium diphtheriae* • *Streptococcus pneumoniae* • *Haemophilus influenzae* • *Neisseria gonorrhoeae* • *Mycobacterium tuberculosis* • Non-tubercular mycobacteria • *Chlamydia trachomatis* • *Listeria monocytogenes* • Gram-negative bacilli	• Adenovirus • Herpes simplex virus • Varicella zoster and herpes zoster • Enterovirus	• *Fusarium* • *Candida* • *Aspergillus* • *Penicillium* • *Alternaria* • *Bipolaris*

- **Endophthalmitis** is the inflammation of the aqueous and vitreous fluids of the eye. It may occur either due to an exogenous infection (e.g., bacterial infection) following trauma/cataract surgery or an endogenous hematogenous seeding of the pathogen from a primary infection elsewhere (as with *Candida*). There may be accompanying necrosis of the uveal tract and retina and abscess formation.
- **Uveitis** is the inflammation of the uveal tract and is caused by many pathogens (Table 53.3).
  - **Anterior uveitis** (iridocyclitis) may present with blurred vision and floaters formed by inflammatory cells in the aqueous humour (e.g., HSV, *O. volvulus* and *M. tuberculosis*).
  - **Posterior uveitis** involves the vitreous humour and choroid and is associated with systemic disease (e.g., *Toxoplasma gondii*, *Candida*, cytomegalovirus and herpes simplex virus). It may also involve the retina.
- **The retina** may be affected in several ways by infectious agents.
  - **Retinochoroiditis** (primary infection of the retina with secondary spread to the choroid) causes focal necrotising lesions in the retina with chorioretinal scars (e.g., *T. gondii*).
  - **Chorioretinitis** (primary infection of the choroid with secondary spread to the retina) occurs mostly in viral infections with retinal necrosis and retinal vessel occlusion (e.g., HSV and CMV).
  - **Retinopathy** may be caused due to vascular changes, retinal hemorrhage and papilledema due to the sequestration of the parasites in the microvasculature of the retina (e.g., malaria retinopathy).
- Certain helminths occupying or migrating through the **intraocular chambers/subretinal space/optic nerve** may cause inflammatory reactions, disruption of the retina and optic nerve atrophy (e.g., *Taenia solium* cysticerci and *Toxocara*).

Ocular Adnexa and Periorbital Tissue Involvement

Infections may spread to the eye from adjacent sinuses and may involve the surrounding skin, subcutaneous tissue, muscles or bones.

- **Periocular subcutaneous nodules** may be found; these cause cellulitis or necrotising granulomas in response to microfilariae (e.g., *Dirofilaria*).
- Extraocular muscles may **harbour the cysts** of parasites (e.g., *Trichinella spiralis* and *Taenia solium* larva). A parasitic cyst in the orbit may lead to **proptosis** which may be progressive (e.g., *Echinococcus*).
- **Cellulitis** is an infection of the eyelid skin and orbit and may lead to the widespread destruction of the affected tissue (e.g., *Staphylococcus aureus, Streptococcus* and anaerobic bacteria).
- Invasive infections originating from the nasal cavity or sinuses may involve the orbits to cause significant **soft tissue and bone destruction** (e.g., mucormycosis), especially in immunocompromised individuals.
- Flies lay eggs in the host tissue (**myiasis**) in poor hygienic conditions. The emerging larvae may then invade the ocular tissues and the adnexa to cause significant damage.

Table 53.3 Infectious causes of uveitis

Protozoa	Helminths	Bacteria	Viruses	Fungi
• *Toxoplasma gondii*	• *Toxocara* (ocular larva migrans) • *Onchocerca volvulus* • *Taenia solium* larva	• Syphilis • Tuberculosis • *Borrelia burgdorferi*	• Cytomegalovirus • Herpes simplex virus	• *Candida* • *Cryptococcus* • *Aspergillus* • *Histoplasma*

Chapter 54

Opportunistic Infections

A practitioner of modern medicine should expect to encounter a large number of individuals with deficient immunities. Such individuals stand a higher risk of contracting **opportunistic infections** (see box).

Conditions that result in a deficient immune system

- Congenital immunodeficiency
- Human immunodeficiency virus infection
- Damaged integumental and mucosal barrier
- Solid organ transplantation
- Hematopoietic cell transplantation
- Malnutrition
- Cancer
- Cytotoxic therapy
- Irradiation
- Prolonged steroid intake

ROLE OF IMMUNITY

The human body is constantly exposed to microorganisms in the environment. The immune system of the body is responsible for combating the assault of these infectious pathogens at several stages. It does so by performing the following functions:

- **Preventing the establishment of infection** in the body
- **Controlling the disease** once infection is established
- **Limiting the severity and dissemination** of the disease

IMMUNODEFICIENCY

A defect in the immunity can occur due to several factors such as a functional or genetic abnormality in the immunity (humoral or cellular), a congenital or acquired illness (e.g., HIV infection, lymphomas, transplantation, high-dose steroids or other immune-suppressive medication and malnutrition) or a damaged integumental or mucosal barrier (e.g., central venous catheter in a hospitalised patient).

- **HIV infection** is characterised by the depletion of $CD4^+$ T cell lymphocytes. Cell-mediated (T cell) immunity plays a predominant role in controlling most parasitic infections. Once the $CD4^+$ T cell count drops <200 cells/μl, the patient is considered to have developed AIDS with the risk of acquiring an AIDS-defining illness or opportunistic infection. The condition can revert to normal with effective therapy and immune reconstitution.
- **Transplant recipients** are administered immunosuppressive drugs to facilitate the uptake of the transplanted solid organ or the hematopoietic cells by the body. In such individuals, the risk of parasitic infections differs based on the transplant type and organ and the degree or type of immunosuppression. There are four modes of parasite transmission in a transplant recipient:
  - **Reactivation** of a dormant/latent infection in the recipient
  - ***De novo*** infection in the recipient
  - **Donor-derived** disease
  - **Blood transfusion-**transmitted infection
- **Cancer patients** are predisposed to infections as there is local tissue dysfunction due to the tumour growth and mass effects such as obstruction of the natural excretory and secretory drainage of the affected organ, breach of the barriers to the normally sterile sites, creation of a fresh nidus for infection and facilitation of local invasion and spread of the infection. The side effects of chemotherapy further potentiate the infectious process.
- **Immunosuppressive therapy** (e.g., cytotoxic drugs, radiation therapy or corticosteroids) damages the cellular immunity by causing granulocytopenia or by decreasing the adherence, chemotaxis and phagocytic activity of inflammatory cells at the site of action. Humoral immunity is also compromised due to hypogammaglobulinemia.

IMMUNOCOMPROMISED HOST

The immune-suppressed host has **impaired defence mechanisms** and suffers greater morbidity and mortality as such an individual is more likely to:

- **Manifest the disease** after acquiring an infection
- **Fail to clear** the parasites, which results in advancement to a chronic carriage state
- **Undergo reactivation** of a latent infection
- **Have attenuated signs, symptoms and inadequate immune response** to the disease, thus making clinical suspicion as well as early diagnosis difficult

- **Develop more severe disease** with more chances of **dissemination and complications**

OPPORTUNISTIC INFECTIONS

Numerous microorganisms have the ability to act as opportunistic pathogens (Table 54.1).

- Microorganisms that typically **only** cause disease in an immunocompromised host while causing minimal or no disease in an immunocompetent individual are known as **opportunistic agents.** Such microorganisms are either **acquired from the environment** (e.g., *Cryptosporidium* and *Pneumocystis*) or are **reactivated from a pre-existing dormant/latent stage** in the body (e.g., *Toxoplasma gondii*). These are generally intrinsically low-virulence microorganisms.
- Some pathogens cause **more severe** disease in an individual with a weakened immune system than in a person with intact immunity (e.g., *Strongyloides stercoralis, Leishmania* and CMV). These pathogens are **virulent** and are agents of infectious disease in immunocompetent persons too.

DIAGNOSTIC ASPECTS

- As a rule, the **direct demonstration of the microorganism from the suspected site** by microscopy, culture or nucleic acid detection is most useful for the early diagnosis of an opportunistic infection in an immunocompromised host.
- Serological tests are usually dependent on the immune response of the body to the pathogen (e.g., an adequate rise in IgM antibodies detectable by a laboratory test) and are thus rendered **unreliable or inconsistent** in the context of immunodeficiency.

MANAGEMENT ASPECTS

- **Primary prevention** of infection should be practised by screening of donors and recipients, and through education, good hygiene practices and vaccines wherever possible.
- **Chemoprophylaxis** is the institution of drug therapy to **prevent** the development or spread of infection. The initiation of appropriate prophylaxis has saved a significant number of lives and is recommended for numerous infections as a standard regimen. Alternatively, it may be instituted for a specific infection based on epidemiological exposure as determined by serological or any other evidence (Table 54.2).
- **A longer duration of treatment** may be required for certain diseases.

Table 54.1 Important opportunistic infections in immunocompromised patients

Protozoa	Helminths	Bacteria	Viruses	Fungi
• *Cryptosporidium* • *Cystoisospora* • *Cyclospora* • *Toxoplasma gondii* encephalitis • *Leishmania* spp. (both visceral and cutaneous leishmaniasis) • *Giardia duodenalis* • *Plasmodium* spp. (malaria) • Microsporidia • *Entamoeba histolytica* • *Trypanosoma cruzi*	• *Strongyloides stercoralis*	• *Mycobacterium tuberculosis* • *Mycobacterium avium* complex • *Salmonella* septicemia • Recurrent bacterial pneumonia	• Cytomegalovirus • Herpes simplex virus • Herpes zoster (reactivation) • Adenovirus	• Candidiasis of bronchi, trachea, esophagus or lungs • *Coccidioides* • *Cryptococcus* • *Histoplasma* • Pneumocystis pneumonia

Table 54.2 Infectious agents commonly targeted for chemoprophylaxis in immunocompromised patients

Protozoa	Bacteria	Viruses	Fungi
• *Toxoplasma gondii*	• Latent tuberculosis • *Mycobacterium avium* complex • *Salmonella* • *Bartonella*	• Cytomegalovirus • Varicella zoster virus	• *Pneumocystis* pneumonia • *Cryptococcus* • *Penicillium* (talaromycosis) • *Histoplasma* • *Coccidioides*

CHAPTER 55

Medical Entomology

(*entomon* [Greek] = insect)

Learning Goals

- What are the various modes by which arthropods affect human health?
- What are the various categories of arthropods that cause human disease/transmit disease-causing pathogens?
- What are the different species of mosquitoes transmitting human diseases and what are the differences between them?

INTRODUCTION

Insects are an extremely diverse and successful group of the living world and are responsible for causing substantial morbidity and mortality in humans and animals. In this chapter, the medically important insects as well as other arthropods are briefly discussed to impart to the student of medicine an overview of the subject.

Medical entomology: The branch of entomology (the study of insects) that deals with insects and related arthropods that affect the health and well-being of humans and vertebrate animals is called medical entomology.

Agents of infectious agents: Arthropods act as **vectors** for the transmission of various protozoa, helminths, viruses and bacteria (Table 55.1). These vectors transmit microorganisms in the following ways:

- **Mechanical transmission:** *Musca domestica* (the common housefly) transmits agents of amoebiasis, giardiasis, bacillary dysentery, cholera and typhoid as well as the eggs of pinworms and tapeworms by carrying such pathogens on its sticky footpads.
- **Biological transmission:** In this mode, the microorganism spends some part of its life cycle in the vector, during which time, it passes through a few stages of its life cycle. The pathogen transmission may occur in many different ways as follows:
    - **Cyclo-propagative:** Some pathogens undergo complex cyclical changes as well as multiplication in the vector, e.g., malaria parasites.
    - **Cyclo-developmental:** Some pathogens undergo cyclical changes but do not multiply in the vector, e.g., filarial parasites.

Table 55.1 Classification of Arthropoda of medical importance and the diseases transmitted by them

Class	Order	Common names	Pathogens/disease transmitted
Insecta (3 pairs of legs)	Phthiraptera	Sucking lice	*Rickettsiae, Bartonella* and *Borrelia*
	Siphonaptera	Fleas	*Dipylidium caninum, Hymenolepis nana, Yersinia pestis* and scrub typhus
	Hemiptera	Bedbugs and kissing bugs	Chagas' disease
	Diptera (*di* = two, *ptera* = wings): Flies, mosquitoes, midges	Housefly	Giardiasis, *Salmonella, Shigella, Vibrio* and enteric viruses
		Deerfly	*Loa loa* and *Francisella*
		Sandfly	Leishmaniasis and *Bartonella*
		Tsetse fly	Sleeping sickness
		Blackfly	Onchocerciasis
		Mosquito	Malaria, filariasis and arboviral diseases
		Midge	*Dirofilaria perstans* and *Mansonella ozzardi*
Arachnida (4 pairs of legs)	Ixodida, Astigmata, Trombidiformes, Sarcoptiformes	Ticks, mites, chiggers	*Rickettsiae, Babesia, Ehrlichia, Borrelia, Anaplasma,* spirochetes and viruses
Crustacea (5 pairs of legs)	Copepoda	Copepods/cyclops	Guinea worm, *Diphyllobothrium latum, Sparganum* and *Gnathostoma spinigerum*
	Decapoda	Crabs, crayfish and prawns	*Paragonimus westermani, Clonorchis sinensis* and *Angiostrongylus cantonensis*

- **Propagative:** Some pathogens undergo no cyclical changes and simply multiply in the vector, e.g., plague bacilli.
- **Transovarian:** Some pathogens are transmitted from the adult female vector to its progeny, e.g., *Francisella* in ticks and Rickettsiae in mites.
- **Transstadial:** Some pathogens are transmitted from one life cycle stage of the vector to its next developmental stage, e.g., *Borrelia burgdorferi* in ticks.

Direct effect of insect infestation: There may be **tissue invasion** by way of infestation (e.g., scabies mites and maggots) or invasion (e.g., maggots), **blood loss** (e.g., bedbugs) or **hypersensitivity** reactions to the saliva/venom of wasps and bees resulting in local tissue reaction and life-threatening anaphylaxis; dust mites may exacerbate asthma and hay fever.

Entomophobia: Some patients develop an exaggerated fear of seeing or touching arthropods.

Delusory parasitosis: This is a condition characterised by a delusion of parasitic infestation despite there being evidence contrary to it.

INSECTS

These comprise >90% of all arthropods. However, only a few are responsible for human diseases. The body of an insect is typically divided into three parts—the head, thorax and abdomen. It is bilaterally symmetrical with a rigid, non-cellular chitinous exoskeleton. The sexes are separate. The various body structures of insects help in their morphological identification.

- The **head** is composed of a number of fused plates. It supports simple or compound eyes, diverse and specialised mouth parts, and a single pair of antennae covered with sensory hairs and bristles.
- The **thorax** is also composed of fused plates on which three pairs of jointed legs and one or two pairs of wings are attached; some insects have no wings. The arrangement of the wing veins ('venation') is important for the identification of different insects. These are the only arthropods in which the capacity for flight has developed.
- The **abdomen** has 8–11 segments on which various appendages may be present. The genitalia is situated on segment 8 or 9.
- The **alimentary canal** has a foregut that processes ingested food mechanically, a midgut for the storage of food and enzyme secretion and a hindgut for water resorption.

Metamorphosis: The process by which an insect develops from an egg into an adult is called metamorphosis. It is known as **simple metamorphosis** when there is very little change in morphology during development, i.e., a nymph stage similar to the adult but without wings precedes the winged adult (egg → nymph → adult as seen in kissing bugs and lice). Highly developed insects undergo **complete metamorphosis**, whereby the insect's life cycle consists of different stages of development which are significantly different from each other (egg → larva → pupa → adult as seen in flies, mosquitoes and fleas).

FLIES

Tabanid Fly, Mango Fly, Mangrove Fly and Deer Fly (*Chrysops* spp.)

There are more than 300 species of tabanid flies. These are vectors of *Loa loa* and *Francisella tularensis* (Fig. 55.1a).

Characteristic features:

- They are greyish-brown to yellow and measure 5–30 mm in size.
- They are stoutly built and their mouth parts can penetrate clothing.
- They are strong fliers.
- The blood meal is taken during the day; only females suck blood.
- They breed in wet mud beside streams or under the rain forest canopy and are attracted to the movement of people or vehicles and rising smoke.

Sandfly (Old World: *Phlebotomus* spp. and *Sergentomyia* spp.; New World: *Lutzomyia* spp.)

There are different genera of sandflies of human importance in the old and new worlds. These transmit agents of leishmaniasis and bartonellosis (Fig. 55.1b).

Characteristic features:

- They are brownish and very small, measuring 2–4 mm in size (45 meshes/square inch required to prevent their entry).
- They have long, hairy legs, hairy bodies and prominent eyes.
- Their proboscis is short and pointed downwards.
- Their wings are pointed upwards and the second vein bifurcates twice.
- They lay eggs in batches of 10–100 and the eggs are torpedo-like in shape.

- They are short hoppers (3 feet) and inefficient fliers.
- They are night biters, active at dawn and dusk; only the females suck blood.
- They breed indoors and require high humidity; hence they often breed in mud huts, tree barks, burrows and wall cracks.

Tsetse Fly (*Glossina* spp.)

This genus comprises 23 species. The tsetse fly transmits African trypanosomiasis and is not found in India (Fig. 55.1c).

Characteristic features:

- They are honey-brown and measure 6–15 mm in size.
- The proboscis is surrounded by piercing palpi.
- Their wings are tongue-shaped (gloss), folded and overlapping.
- They are day biters; both sexes feed on blood and can transmit the parasite.
- They live near rivers or in savanna forests and wet grounds.

Blackfly or Buffalo Gnat (*Simulium* spp.)

S. damnosum sibling species are found in Central and South America. These transmit onchocerciasis or river blindness (Fig. 55.1d).

Characteristic features:

- They are black to dark brown and measure 1–5 mm in size.
- The thorax is humped; the palpi are short and cigar-shaped.
- They bite in the day and cannot penetrate cloth; only females suck blood.
- These are **pool feeders**, i.e., they penetrate the skin, release saliva which contains anticoagulants and feed on the collected blood; their saliva contains substances that attract the skin-dwelling microfilariae.
- They lay eggs on immersed rocks. Fast-flowing streams are required for larval development.

Myiasis

Myiasis is the name given to **infections caused by the larvae of flies (maggots)** which feed on dead or living tissue of humans or animals (Fig. 55.1e). The flies may deposit their eggs on or close to a wound, following which the larvae hatch from the egg and burrow into the surrounding skin.

Myiasis depending on the location

- Superficial cutaneous (wound)
- Subcutaneous (furuncular or boil-like)
- Cavitary (orbits, aural or nasopharyngeal)
- Intestinal
- Genitourinary

Most species are of zoonotic origin. The human botfly, *Dermatobia hominis*, develops in boil-like subcutaneous lesions.

The association of the flies with mammalian tissues is of three types:

- **Accidental:** This group comprises rare accidental infections of an unusual host by fly eggs. For example, *Musca domestica* does not require mammalian tissue for development, yet it may be found in dead tissue or under plaster casts.
- **Facultative:** These associations are characterised by free-living maggots which normally feed on decaying or dead matter but can also feed on living tissue. For example, blowflies and flesh flies ordinarily feed on dead tissues and may move into adjacent viable tissues.
- **Obligatory:** This class comprises fly species which develop only in living tissues in the course of their life cycle and cannot survive without the living host.

Maggots can be recovered from a variety of body sites such as the eye, nose, sinuses, ear, skin wounds, feet, genitourinary tract, intestinal tract, etc. The specimens should be immersed in 70% alcohol and subjected to identification using morphological keys.

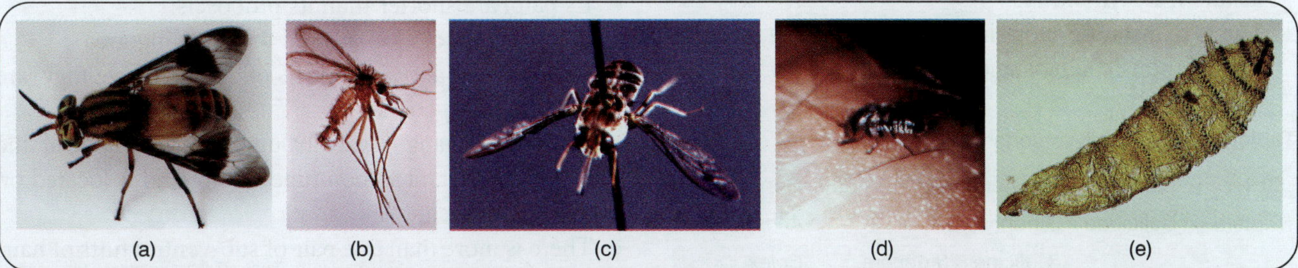

Fig. 55.1 Pictures of medically important arthropods: (a) tabanid fly, (b) sandfly, (c) tsetse fly, (d) blackfly and (e) maggot of rodent botfly (*Source:* Centers for Disease Control and Prevention [CDC], Public Health Image Library [PHIL], Image IDs 16012, 6274, 21024, 17562 and 1427)

Characteristic features:

- Maggots of different fly species can be differentiated on the basis of various specific features of their chitinous mouth parts, abdominal respiratory spiracles and cuticle structures.
- Alternately, live maggots may be allowed to hatch, and the adult flies may then be morphologically identified.

Treatment

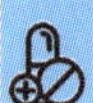

Extraction of fly larvae

- **Surgical removal**, followed by daily cleaning of the wound
- Occluding respiratory spiracles of maggots by coating wound with petroleum ointment (Vaseline)
- Tetanus prophylaxis
- Treatment of secondary bacterial infections
- Taking care of untreated and open wounds with proper hygiene

MOSQUITOES

There are 28 different genera of mosquitoes and >3,000 species worldwide. Only a few of these are medically important (Table 55.2).

Characteristic features:

- Males have a long, bushy antenna, while the females possess a sparsely hairy antenna.
- Generally, the life span of the males is about one week, whereas the females live for about one month. However, mosquitoes are known to hibernate for as long as six months to survive the extreme cold.
- The eggs are laid in water at night; the shapes, sizes and patterns of the eggs vary in different genera and species.
- The larvae are actively motile and feed on microbes. They have 10 abdominal segments with spiracles/a siphon tube on the 9th segment.
- The larvae undergo four moults which are called instars I, II, III and IV.
- The IVth instar develops into a pupa which is a comma-shaped, non-feeding stage.

Table 55.2 Medically important mosquitoes

Order	Family	Subfamily	Genus
Diptera	Culicidae	Anophelinae	*Anopheles*
		Culicine (20 genera, >2,000 species)	*Culex*
			Aedes
			Mansonia

- Males feed on plant juices (nectar), while females feed on plant juices and blood; blood is required for the development of eggs in the females.

Anopheles spp. (*A. stephensi, A. culicifacies, A. gambiae, A. fluviatilis, A. sundaicus* and *A. minimus*)

This genus comprises the vectors of malaria. The various species transmit **malaria** in different geographical areas (Fig. 55.2a–c).

Characteristic features:

- The adult sits at an angle of ~45° to feed.
- The males have a bushy antenna and long palpi with clubbed ends while females have sparsely hairy antennae.
- Eggs are laid one at a time in batches of 20–30 with characteristic lateral floats.
- The larvae are dorsoventrally flattened and do not have any siphon tubes; they lie parallel to the surface of the water.
- The pupa is comma-shaped and non-feeding.
- The respiratory trumpets are short and broad.
- These mosquitoes are known to bite throughout the night.
- They lay eggs in clean groundwater, rainwater collected in burrows and in pits, river margins, bed pools, canals, wells and ponds.

Brown House Mosquito (*Culex pipiens* Complex and *C. vishnui* Complex)

It is the most common and cosmopolitan mosquito and a major vector implicated in diseases such as **filariasis, Japanese encephalitis and West Nile encephalitis** (Fig. 55.2d–f).

Characteristic features:

- The adult rests parallel to the surface for feeding.
- It has white or dark and light brown markings on its thorax.
- Its palpi are shorter than its proboscis.
- It can fly up to 5 km around the breeding area.
- Eggs are laid at night in rafts of 200 or more; they are pale brown in colour.
- The larvae hang vertically under the surface of the water. The larval siphon tube is long and is located on the 8th segment.
- There is more than one pair of sub-ventral tufts of hair.
- These mosquitoes are night feeders.
- They lay eggs in water polluted with organic matter (ponds and ditches).

Aedes spp. (*Aedes aegypti* and *A. albopictus* or Tiger Mosquito)

There are more than 100 known species of *Aedes* in India. Only two of these—*A. aegypti* and *A. albopictus*—are vectors of diseases such as **dengue, chikungunya, West Nile encephalitis, yellow fever and zika virus disease** (Fig. 55.2g–i).

Characteristic features:

- The adults have silvery white stripes and bands.
- The eggs are shiny black, elongated and laid singly in more than one sitting with as many as 140 eggs laid in a batch.
- The mosquito can fly up to a distance of 50–100 meters.
- The larvae are bottom feeders. Their siphon tube is short and stumpy with one pair of sub-ventral tufts of hair.
- These mosquitoes are day biters and preferably feed at dawn and dusk.
- They breed in water collected artificially in vases, bottles, coolers or rainwater collected in tyres, stones, rocks, holes in trees, etc.

Mansonia spp.

These are agents of ***Brugia malayi* filariasis and Japanese encephalitis.**

Characteristic features:

- They look dusty and their wings and legs are speckled.
- They lay eggs in clusters on the undersurface of aquatic plants (*Pistia* and *Salvinia*).
- The larvae attach to the roots of plants by the hooks on their siphons.
- They are night biters.
- They breed in saline water (coastal areas).

MIDGES

Bloodsucking Midges or Gnats (*Culicoides*)

There are 800 known species of midges. Many species transmit disease pathogens such as *Mansonella*, *Dirofilaria* and arboviruses. No disease is transmitted by *Culicoides* in India.

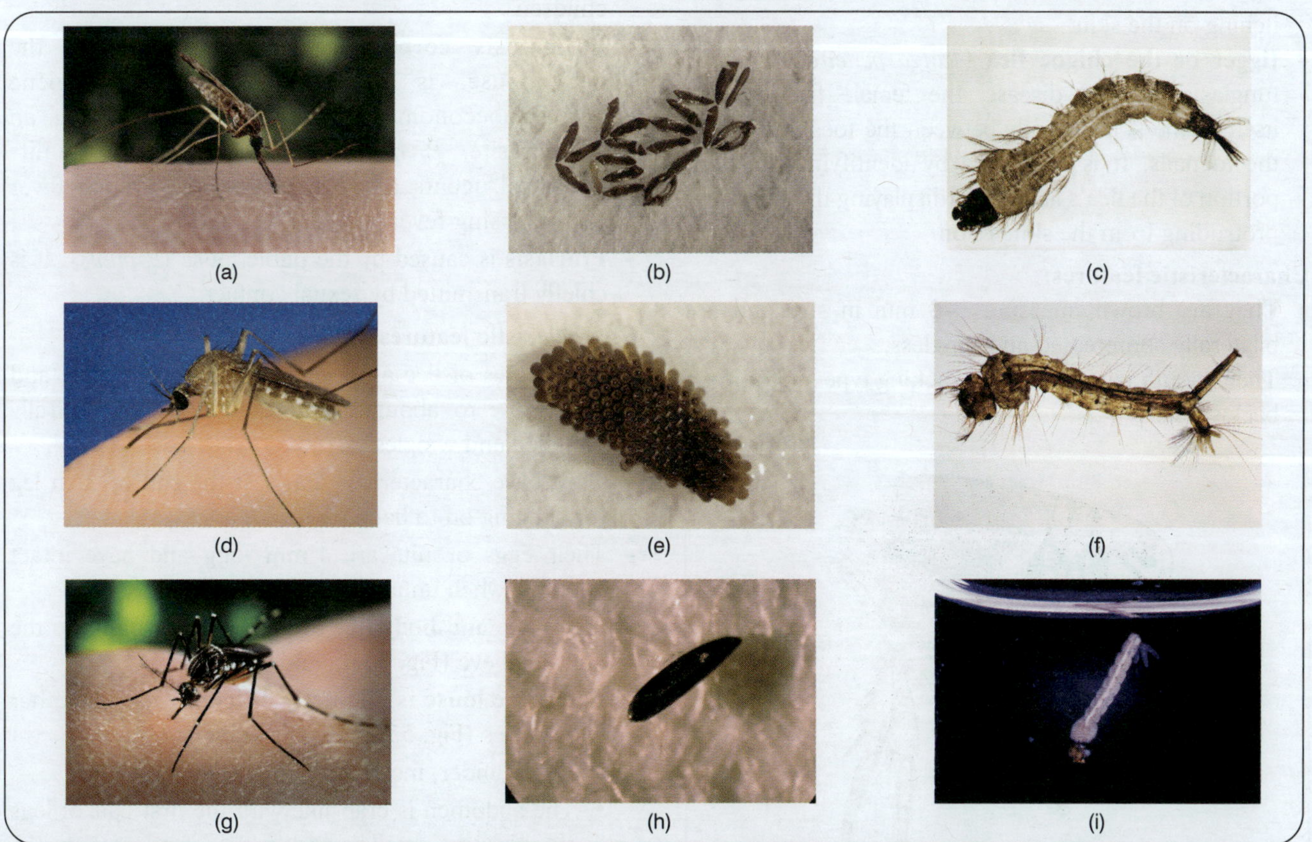

Fig. 55.2 Pictures of medical important mosquitoes: (a–c) *Anopheles stephensi* adult (sitting at a 45° angle), eggs (laid singly in batches with lateral floats) and a larva (without siphon); (d–f) *Culex quinquefasciatus* adult (brownish, sitting parallel to the surface), eggs (laid in rafts) and a larva (with siphon) and (g–i) *Aedes aegypti* adult (with white stripes and bands), an egg (shiny black, laid singly) and a larva (with short siphon) (*Source:* CDC, PHIL, Image IDs 18764, 12548, 12554, 4734, 12549, 12550, 9258, 688, and 1352)

Characteristic features:

- They are brown and measure 1–4 mm in size.
- They are robust, with a humped thorax and a beaded antenna with 13–15 segments.
- They usually feed at dusk; only females take the blood meal.
- They are cosmopolitan in distribution and found in a wide range of environments and altitudes.

FLEAS

Fleas are among the most pestiferous of insect species. Many of them are temporary ectoparasites of warm-blooded hosts such as dogs, cats and rats (Fig. 55.3). The following are the medical important fleas:

- **Cat fleas** (*Ctenocephalides felis*) **and dog fleas** (*Ctenocephalides canis*) are intermediate hosts for the tapeworm *Dipylidium caninum* and less frequently, *Hymenolepis diminuta* and *H. nana*.
- The **oriental rat flea**, *Xenopsylla cheopis*, transmits the plague bacillus and murine typhus.
- The **human flea**, *Pulex irritans*, infects human beings and other mammals. The flea bites cause rashes and itching on the skin.
- **Jigger or the chigoe flea** (*Tunga penetrans*) causes tungiasis. In this disease, the female flea embeds itself in the skin, usually between the toes and under the toenails. It is diagnosed by identifying the dark portion of the flea's abdomen (displaying the spiracles) protruding from the skin lesion.

Characteristic features:

- They are brown, measure 1–8 mm in size and are bilaterally compressed and wingless.
- Their mouth parts are of the sucking type and pointed backwards.

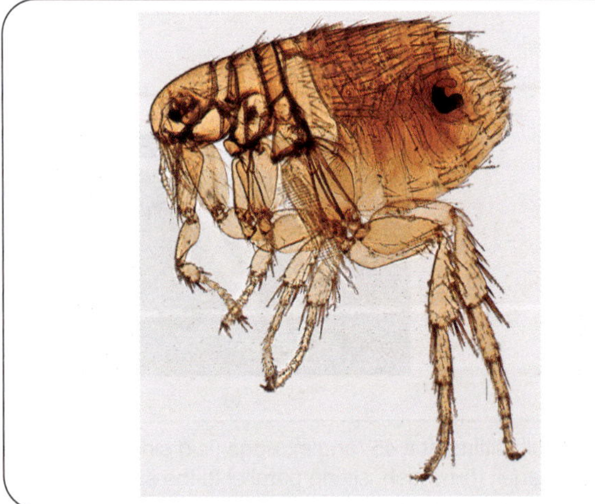

Fig. 55.3 A rat flea (*Source*: CDC, PHIL, Image ID 22259)

- The legs are long and highly developed, which enables them to jump up to a height of 10–15 cm.
- Fleas that affect humans are generally parasites of other mammals or poultry.
- These are domestic pests, which are generally found indoors. They are cosmopolitan in distribution.

LICE

Sucking Lice (Head Louse, *Pediculus humanus* var. *capitis*; Body Louse, *P. humanus* var. *humanus*; Pubic Louse, *Pthirus pubis*)

These are permanent ectoparasites of animals and humans and cause pediculosis. The species affecting humans are named for their primary site of attachment but do not always remain confined to that specific area.

- **Pediculosis capitis** is caused by the head louse (*P. humanus* var. *capitis*). It is the most common entity of the three types of human infections caused by lice. It affects millions of people every year, mostly children.
- **Pediculosis corporis**, which is caused by the body louse, is associated with poor hygiene and socioeconomic status. Apart from being an ectoparasite, *P. h.* var. *humanus* also transmits microbial agents of epidemic typhus, trench fever and relapsing fever.
- **Pthriasis** is caused by the pubic louse (*P. pubis*). It is chiefly transmitted by sexual contact.

Characteristic features:

- The bodies of lice are longer than they are wide and may grow to about 3 mm; they are dorsoventrally flattened and wingless.
- They have characteristic claws at the end of each leg for clinging on to hairs.
- Their eggs or nits are 1 mm long and have intact opercula when unhatched.
- **Head lice and body lice are indistinguishable** to the untrained eye (Fig. 55.4a and b).
- The **pubic louse is distinctly different** from the other two species (Fig. 55.4c) in the following ways:
  - It is rounder, measuring up to 2 mm in size.
  - The abdomen is crab-like with the first pair of legs significantly smaller and more slender than the other pairs; the claws are wider.
  - It is found primarily on pubic hair but may extend to the chest, armpit and facial hair.

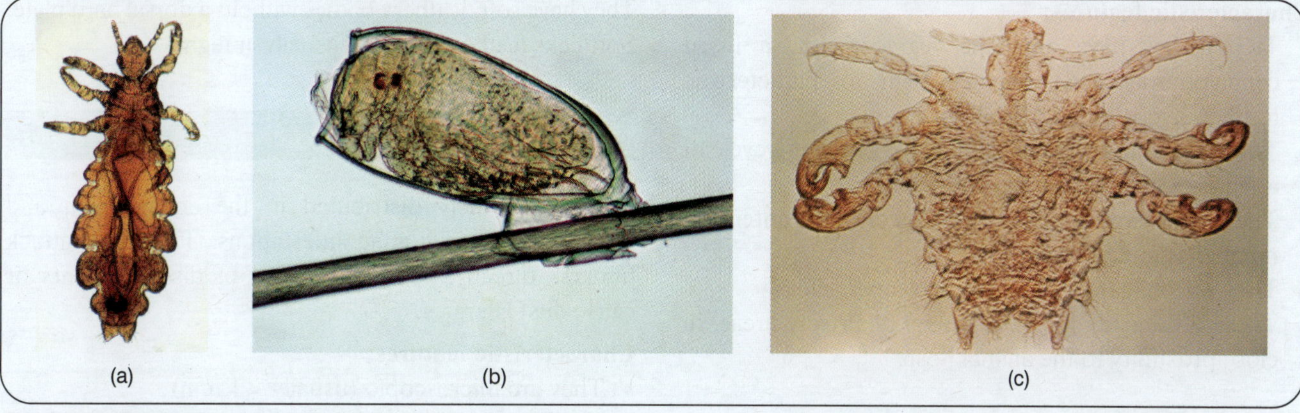

Fig. 55.4 Pictures of lice: (a) a head louse, (b) the egg (nit) of a head louse and (c) a pubic louse (*Source*: CDC, PHIL, Image IDs 377, 379 and 17331)

- It is chiefly transmitted during sexual intercourse but can also be transmitted between people sharing a bed.
- All the developmental stages of all species feed on blood intermittently.
- Lice are commonly found in settings of war, poverty and homelessness; irregular bathing and laundering practices are predisposing factors.

Treatment

Topical
- *Malathion:* 0.5% shampoo for persons above 6 months of age, applied topically and washed after 8 hours; second application after 7–10 days
- *Natural pyrethrins:* 0.33% pyrethrins plus 4% piperonyl butoxide shampoo for persons aged 2 years and above, applied topically and washed after 24 hours; second application after 7–10 days
- *Synthetic pyrethroids:* 1% permethrin cream for persons aged 2 years and above, topically applied and washed after 24 hours; second application after 7–10 days
- *Ivermectin:* 0.8% shampoo
- *Lindane:* 1% lotion/shampoo (only in those resistant to other regimens)

Systemic
- *Ivermectin:* 200 µg/kg orally as a single dose; repeated after 10 days

Supportive management
- Wet hair should be carefully combed with a fine-toothed nit comb.
- For body lice infestation, the body should be washed thoroughly with soap and water and then treated by applying the drug preparation.
- Close contacts should be checked carefully and treated if infested.

Reduviid Bug, Kissing Bug and Cone-Nosed Bug (*Triatoma*, *Rhodnius* and *Panstrongylus*)

These are responsible for transmitting *Trypanosoma cruzi* (which causes Chagas' disease) in its feces. These bugs are prevalent in Mexico and Central and South America (Fig. 55.5).

Characteristic features:
- The cone-shaped head sits on a narrow neck with a long, narrow proboscis folded underneath the body when not in use.
- The wings are well-developed.
- All species are blood-feeding. These are relatively painless feeders. The saliva they secrete while feeding contains irritants, which produce itching; scratching the skin facilitates the inoculation of the parasite, which is present in the bug's feces.
- They are night feeders and prefer to feed on sleeping individuals.

TICKS

Many families of hard and soft ticks are of human importance. These are vectors of various viruses, bacteria and protozoa.

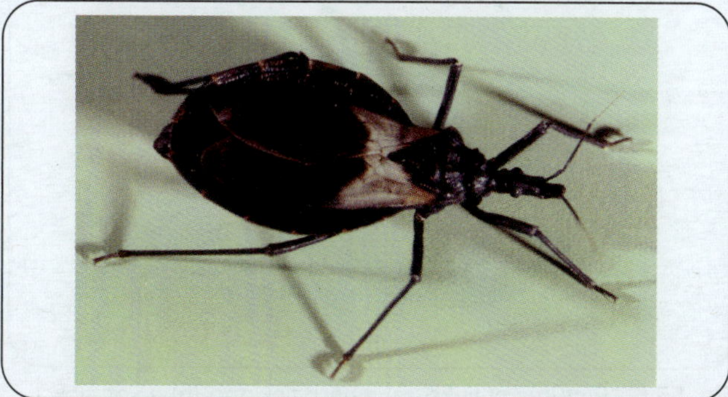

Fig. 55.5 A kissing bug (*Source:* CDC, PHIL, Image ID 21020)

Characteristic features:

- Tick bodies have only one segment, i.e., a fused cephalothorax and abdomen with a characteristic toothed hypostome for feeding.
- There are four developmental stages in the life cycle of a tick—egg, larva, nymph and adult.
- The larvae have three pairs of legs but lack antennae, mandibles and wings.
- They are obligate bloodsucking ectoparasites.
- These are mostly found in grassy or brushy areas, in close proximity to the animal hosts.

Hard Ticks (*Dermacentor, Ixodes* and *Amblyomma*)

Most of the ticks found on human skin are hard ticks. These have a hard dorsal plate (scutum) with various patterns enabling identification (Fig. 55.6a). These transmit many diseases.

- ***Dermacentor*** **ticks**: Rocky Mountain spotted fever, tularemia, Q fever, tick paralysis and Colorado tick fever
- ***Ixodes*** **ticks**: Lyme disease, babesiosis, anaplasmosis and ehrlichiosis and arboviruses
- ***Amblyomma*** **ticks**: Tularemia and ehrlichiosis

Soft Ticks (*Ornithodoros*)

These are vectors of spirochetes that cause relapsing fever, e.g., *Borrelia recurrentis* and related forms (Fig. 55.6b).

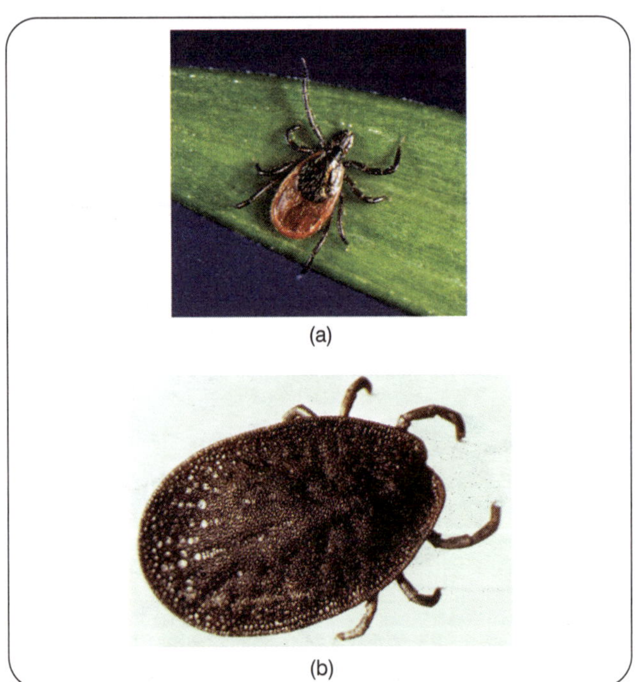

Fig. 55.6 Pictures of ticks: (a) a hard tick and (b) a soft tick (*Source:* CDC, PHIL, Image IDs 1669 and 5970)

They have soft, leathery bodies without a dorsal hard plate. Soft ticks feed only briefly, usually at night.

MITES

Mites are widely distributed in the environment and commonly cause human infestations. They may attack humans directly, serve as vectors of disease agents or cause dust allergies.

Characteristic features:

- They are microscopic (usually <1 mm).
- Their bodies have only one segment; the larvae have three pairs of legs but lack antennae, mandibles and wings.
- They are similar to ticks in their larval form, but lack the toothed hypostome.

Follicle Mite (*Demodex folliculorum* and *D. brevis*)

These may infest humans and cause mild dermatitis. Alternatively, they could be harmless saprophytes.

Characteristic features:

- They are minute (measuring 0.1–0.4 mm), elongate parasites with stubby legs.
- They are found in hair follicles and sebaceous glands.

Itch Mite or Mange Mite (*Sarcoptes scabei* var. *hominis*)

Scabies, which is caused by the itch mite, is a major public health problem worldwide. The mite tunnels through the upper epidermis and deposits its eggs and excreta there. This results in inflammation and generalised, intense nocturnal itching (Fig. 55.7). It is highly contagious. The transmission of the mite occurs by personal contact with an infected individual (such as sexual contact) or as a result of children playing close together or any interaction where there is direct contact. In its more severe form, it causes extensive hyperkeratotic papular lesions in older adults or immunocompromised individuals (crusted or Norwegian scabies). The lesions may be superinfected by bacteria.

The diagnosis is made by obtaining skin scrapings from tunnelled areas. The scrapings are covered with mineral oil and microscopically examined to look for the adult mites, eggs or fecal pellets.

Characteristic features:

- Eggs (170 × 90 μm), 6-legged larvae, 8-legged nymphs or adults (0.2–0.4 mm) can be seen in skin scrapings.

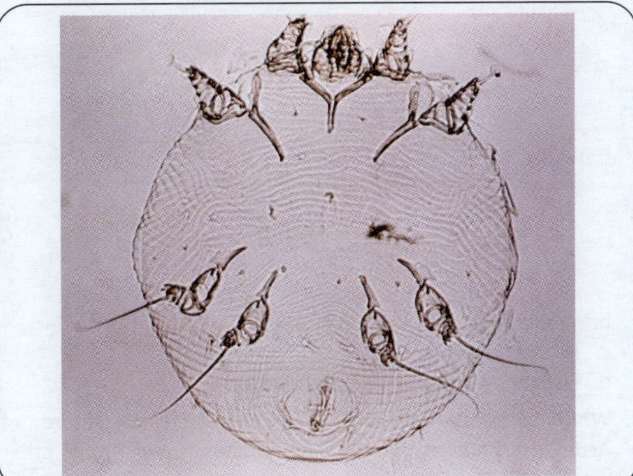

Fig. 55.7 A human itch mite (*Source:* CDC, PHIL, Image ID 6301)

- They live in tunnels in the upper epidermis.
- They are commonly found in interdigital spaces, flexor surfaces of wrists and forearms, and less commonly, in the skin of the breasts, buttocks and external genitalia.

Treatment

Topical

- *Permethrin:* 5% cream for persons aged 2 months and above, applied topically from neck downwards and washed after 8–14 hours; second application after 7 days
- *Alternate preparations:* 1% lindane, 10–25% benzoyl benzoate, 10% crotamiton, 5–10% sulphur ointment, 0.5–1% malathion and 0.8% ivermectin lotion

Systemic

- *Ivermectin:* 200 μg/kg orally as a single dose (can be considered in those with a severe burning sensation in response to permethrin); superior cure rates with a second dose after 15 days
- Recommended for epidemic scabies in institutions

Supportive management

- Close contacts should be treated simultaneously
- Clothing and bedding of infected persons must be discarded or machine washed at 60ºC or higher

Dust Mite (*Dermatophagoides farinae* and *D. pteronyssinus*)

These are commonly found in the dust and have a role in allergic rhinitis, asthma and eczematous conditions as a response to their secretions, excreta and body parts, which are all strong allergens.

CRUSTACEANS

Crustaceans are gill-breathing arthropods with shells. Some freshwater species are intermediate hosts for helminths.

Water Fleas or Copepods (*Cyclops* and *Diaptomus*)

Cyclops species are microscopic crustaceans. They are the first intermediate hosts for *Dracunculus medinensis*, *Diphyllobothrium latum*, *Gnathostoma spinigerum* and *Spirometra*. *Diaptomus* species are hosts of *D. latum* (Fig. 55.8). Infections transmitted by these vectors can be prevented by using filtration or boiling methods for treating drinking water.

Characteristic features:

- Copepods typically have elongated, pear-shaped and semi-transparent bodies measuring 0.5 mm in size.
- They have a single, central and pigmented eye.
- The copepod's abdomen has five segments with filaments present on the last segment.

Crabs and Crayfish

These larger crustaceans are intermediate hosts for the metacercariae of the lung fluke, *Paragonimus*. Crayfish also host *Clonorchis sinensis*.

Prawns

These are paratenic hosts of *Angiostrongylus cantonensis*.

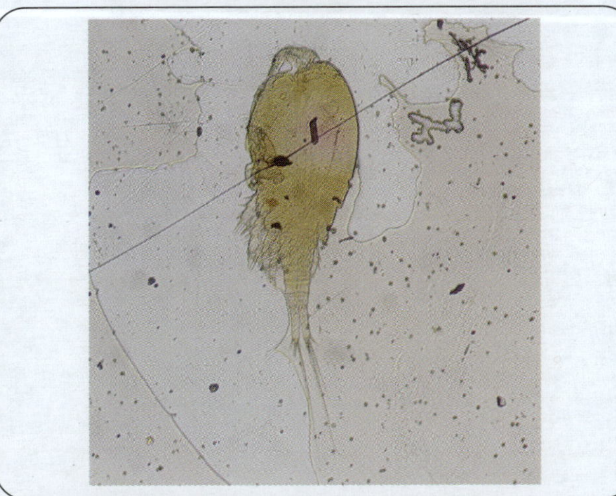

Fig. 55.8 A copepod

Questions

1. Discuss the diagnosis and management of scabies.
2. List the differential features of *Anopheles*, *Culex* and *Aedes* mosquitoes.

Multiple Choice Questions

1. Which of the following is true about mosquitoes?
   a. They are short hoppers.
   b. They have a single pair of wings.
   c. The antenna of females is conspicuously bushy.
   d. All mosquitoes suck blood.
2. Which of the following is the vector for the malaria parasite?
   a. Aedes mosquito
   b. Anopheles mosquito
   c. Culex mosquito
   d. Mansonia mosquito
3. Which of the following is TRUE about the sandfly?
   a. It is the vector for visceral leishmaniasis (kala-azar).
   b. It is bigger in size than mosquitoes.
   c. Both males and females suck blood.
   d. Its third vein of the wing bifurcates twice.
4. All the following are true about lice EXCEPT____________ :
   a. They are dorsoventrally flattened.
   b. They are wingless.
   c. They have three pairs of legs.
   d. They only cause mechanical irritation but do not serve as a vector for any disease.
5. Which of the following is true about soft ticks?
   a. They possess three pairs of legs.
   b. The entire body is covered with scutum.
   c. They possess no wings or antennae.
   d. The body is differentiated into a distinct head, thorax and abdomen.
6. *Cyclops* is an intermediate host for ____________ :
   a. Taenia solium
   b. Taenia saginata
   c. Hookworm
   d. Fish tapeworm (Diphyllobothrium)
7. Which of the following is a characteristic feature of *Aedes* mosquitoes which differentiates them from other mosquitoes?
   a. Both males and females are hematophagous.
   b. The body and legs have silvery and black scales.
   c. The mosquito lays eggs bound in rafts.
   d. The mosquito sits at an angle to the surface while feeding.
8. Myiasis is a term given to the disease caused by maggots of ____________ :
   a. Fleas
   b. Mites
   c. Ticks
   d. Flies
9. Phylum Arthropoda is characterised by all the following EXCEPT ____________ :
   a. Jointed legs
   b. Bilaterally symmetrical
   c. Sexes are separate
   d. Oxygen is carried to tissues by hemoglobin
10. All the following are characteristic features of the class Insecta EXCEPT ____________ :
    a. Body divisible into the head, thorax and abdomen
    b. Possess three pairs of legs
    c. Single antenna
    d. Metamorphosis into egg, larva, pupa and adult

Chapter 56 Zoonotic Infections and One Health

Zoonosis: Diseases that are naturally transmitted between animals and people are known as zoonotic diseases (Table 56.1).

One health: The concept of 'one health' essentially means that the health of people is connected to the health of animals and the environment. The **human–animal–ecosystem** interface plays an important role in the evolution and emergence of pathogens. It is estimated that among all the known infectious diseases prevalent worldwide, approximately 60% are zoonotic infections. Furthermore, zoonoses contribute to about 75% of the **emerging infectious diseases**.

Considering the major role of zoonoses and the environment in human health, it is clear that successful public health interventions require the cooperation of human, animal and environmental health communities. Therefore, public health organisations need to employ a multidisciplinary and multisectoral 'one health' approach by working in collaboration with physicians, veterinarians, parasitologists, microbiologists, geneticists, wildlife experts, ecologists, epidemiologists, urban planners, climatologists, environmental engineers, agriculturalists, botanists, policy makers and experts of other related fields. In collaboration, these experts can monitor and control threats to health and learn about the dynamics of disease maintenance and its spread among people, animals and their environments more effectively.

Modes of transmission: Human beings acquire zoonotic infections by the following modes:

- **Direct contact:** Humans acquire infections when they come in contact with the saliva, blood, urine, mucus, feces or other body fluids of an infected animal while petting or touching the animal or via bites or scratches.
- **Indirect contact:** Infections are also acquired through contact with habitats where animals live and roam, or objects or surfaces that have been contaminated with germs from the infected animals, e.g., cats' sandboxes, aquarium tank water, chicken coops, plants and soil, as well as pet food and water dishes.
- **Through vectors:** Vector-borne infections are transmitted by the bite of a mosquito, tick, sandfly, flea or other insects.
- **Through food or water:** The consumption of unpasteurised milk, undercooked meat or eggs, raw fruits or vegetables or water contaminated with the feces of an infected animal is also a common mode of transmission. These infections are known as foodborne or waterborne infections.

The classification of zoonoses based on the **reservoir host** (Table 56.2) is as follows:

- **Anthropozoonoses**: These infections are transmitted from lower vertebrate animals to humans. Examples of such infections include, *Toxoplasma gondii*, rabies, *Brucella* and *Yersinia*.
- **Zooanthroponoses**: These infections are transmitted from humans to the lower vertebrate animals. They are primarily of human origin. These infections are also called **reverse zoonotic diseases**. For example, infections caused by *Entamoeba histolytica*, *Giardia duodenalis*, *Cryptosporidium parvum* and *Trichuris trichiura* are transmitted in this manner.
- **Amphixenoses**: These infections are maintained between humans and lower vertebrate animals and

Table 56.1 Major zoonotic infections of human importance

Parasites	Bacteria	Viruses	Fungi
Cryptosporidiosis	Anthrax	Swine flu	Cryptococcosis
Giardiasis	Brucellosis	Bird flu	Histoplasmosis
Echinococcosis	Scrub typhus	Dengue	
Cysticercosis	Bovine tuberculosis	Ebola	
Plasmodium knowlesi malaria	Campylobacteriosis	Hepatitis E	
Toxocariasis (visceral larva migrans)	Glanders	Rabies	
Toxoplasmosis	Leptospirosis		
Trichinellosis	Listeriosis		
	Lyme disease		
	Plague		
	Q fever		

Table 56.2 Parasitic zoonoses and their reservoir hosts

Reservoir animal	Parasitic agent
Cattle	*Taenia saginata, Echinococcus granulosus, Toxoplasma gondii, Sarcocystis hominis, Trypanosoma brucei, Fasciola hepatica, Trypanosoma evansi, Cryptosporidium, Babesia,* microsporidia, *Giardia duodenalis*
Sheep and goat	*Echinococcus granulosus, Fasciola hepatica*
Pig	*Taenia solium, Taenia asiatica, Trichinella spiralis, Cryptosporidium, Fasciolopsis buski, Balantidium coli, Diphyllobothrium latum,* microsporidia, *Giardia duodenalis*
Dog	*Echinococcus granulosus, Diphyllobothrium latum, Toxocara canis, Leishmania* species, *Dipylidium caninum* (tapeworm of dog), *Trypanosoma cruzi, Dirofilaria* species, non-human hookworm species *(Ancylostoma caninum, Ancylostoma braziliense), Dracunculus medinensis, Spirometra, microsporidiosis, Giardia duodenalis*
Cat	*Toxoplasma gondii, Toxocara cati, Dracunculus medinensis, Trypanosoma cruzi, Spirometra,* microsporidia, *Giardia duodenalis*
Rodents	*Echinococcus multilocularis, Hymenolepis diminuta* (rat tapeworm), *Angiostrongylus, Babesia* species, *Trypanosoma cruzi, Giardia duodenalis*
Fish and shellfish	*Diphyllobothrium latum, Clonorchis sinensis, Opisthorchis viverrini, Heterophyes heterophyes, Capillaria philippinensis, Gnathostoma spinigerum, Anisakis*
Snails, freshwater fish, crayfish or crab	*Schistosoma* species, *Paragonimus westermani, Fasciola hepatica, Angiostrongylus cantonensis*
Non-human primates	*Plasmodium knowlesi*

may be transmitted in either direction. Examples include infections caused by *Staphylococcus* and *Streptococcus*.

The classification of zoonoses based on the **life cycle of the parasite** is as follows:

- **Direct zoonoses:** The infection is transmitted from the infected lower vertebrate host to humans either by direct contact (e.g., anthrax), fomites, secretions (as with rabies which is transmitted by dog bite), a mechanical vector or food (e.g., trichinellosis and brucellosis). Only a single vertebrate host is required for the infectious agent to complete its life cycle. During transmission, the agent undergoes no development or propagation (e.g., trichinellosis).
- **Cyclo-zoonoses:** The infection requires more than one vertebrate host species for the parasite to complete its life cycle. No invertebrate hosts are required (e.g., toxoplasmosis, echinococcosis, taeniasis, etc.).
- **Meta-zoonoses (vector-borne):** These infections are transmitted biologically by invertebrate vectors. The parasitic agent characteristically multiplies (**propagative**) or develops (**cyclo-developmental**) or does both (**cyclo-propagative**) in the invertebrate hosts. Sometimes, more than one vertebrate or invertebrate host may be required for the parasite to complete its life cycle. These parasites essentially show an extrinsic incubation period (pre-patency) before being transmitted to a suitable vertebrate host, e.g., leishmaniasis (sandfly → human), trypanosomiasis (tsetse fly → human), filariasis (mosquito → human), and paragonimiasis (snail → crab → human).
- **Sapro-zoonoses:** The infection is transmitted from inanimate substances or non-animal reservoirs such as food, soil (e.g., histoplasmosis and agents of visceral larva migrans) and plants (e.g., *Fasciolopsis buski*) to susceptible vertebrate hosts.

Chapter 57

Control Programmes for Parasitic Diseases

INTRODUCTION

The burden of parasites is highest in the tropical and subtropical regions of the world and disproportionately affects those belonging to the lowest socioeconomic groups. Most parasitic diseases can be controlled by preventing the transmission of the parasite between the susceptible host and the source of infection since most parasites require a living or non-living agent for their transmission.

A number of parasitic diseases have been targeted for control including dracunculiasis, malaria, kala-azar, lymphatic filariasis, etc. However, the successful control of an infectious disease requires sustained political will and active community participation. Till date, the most encouraging results for the control of any parasitic disease have been for dracunculiasis, which now exists only in a few foci in Africa. Other diseases like malaria have proven to be immensely challenging and prone to resurgence with the slightest of lapses in control.

The approach to the control of a disease depends on several factors such as the knowledge of the agent, the diagnostic and clinical modalities available and epidemiological knowledge about the mode of transmission (whether vector-borne, waterborne, foodborne, oro-fecal, sexual, vertical transmission, etc.).

DEFINITIONS

It is important to understand the concept of control versus elimination and eradication of infectious diseases.

Control: This refers to the reduction but **not absence** of disease incidence, prevalence, morbidity or mortality to an acceptable level which is achieved through deliberate efforts. However, continued intervention measures are essential to keep the disease under control.

- **Infection:** An infection is said to occur when a microorganism simply lodges itself in the tissues of the host and multiplies there. An infection may or may not cause any damage and thus is most often without any symptoms.
- **Disease:** A disease occurs when the infecting microorganism causes damage to the host tissues, leading to altered host physiology. It may lead to subclinical or clinical manifestations in the host which may be physiological or psychological.

Elimination of disease: The reduction of the incidence of a specified **disease to zero** in a defined geographical area as achieved by deliberate interventions is known as elimination. Continued intervention measures are required to maintain the status.

Elimination of infection: This refers to the reduction of the incidence of an **infection to zero** in a defined geographical area as a result of deliberate efforts. Continued measures are required to prevent the re-establishment of transmission.

Eradication: When the worldwide incidence of the infection caused by a specific agent is **permanently reduced to zero** as a result of deliberate efforts and when intervention is no longer required, the infection is said to be eradicated. Dracunculiasis is a parasitic infection on the verge of eradication.

Extinction: When a specific infectious **agent no longer exists** in nature or in the laboratory, it is said to be extinct.

GENERAL PRINCIPLES OF THE CONTROL OF PARASITIC DISEASES

Numerous factors are taken into account while planning the control of an infectious disease.

Establishing Priorities

The disease under consideration must be accepted as a public health problem internationally, and its control should be perceived as a worthy goal to achieve with specific reasons and sustained political commitment. There must be technically feasible intervention tools and strategies available for its control.

Disease Mapping, Estimation of Burden and High-Risk Populations

Different parasites exist in nature in different geographical and temporal patterns and hence their incidence rates vary across the world. Therefore, it is a challenging task to accurately develop a database of disease incidence, prevalence and the extent of the spread of a disease before a control programme can be initiated. For example, community-based surveys for soil-transmitted helminths are carried out to look for the presence of parasite eggs in stool samples collected from children in order to map the disease.

Interventions

The available tools for interventions to block the transmission of the targeted parasite should be easy to implement and adaptable to diverse conditions.

- **Case diagnosis and effective treatment:** The most direct methods of controlling and containing a disease are timely diagnosis and effective treatment of the affected persons. This intervention is an integral part of all control programmes.
- **Morbidity management:** In diseases such as lymphatic filariasis, where irreversible damage to tissues has already occurred, it is essential to provide adequate support for debilitation to improve the quality of the life of affected persons.
- **Mass prophylaxis:** This strategy relies on reducing the infected pool of individuals through chemoprophylaxis or vaccines. Chemoprophylaxis is employed in the form of mass drug administration to a wide stratum of the population in endemic regions, e.g., deworming all school-age children on specific days biannually has proven effective in controlling infections caused by soil-transmitted helminths. Vaccines, on the other hand, have been largely unsuccessful in controlling parasitic diseases.

Environment Management

- **Environmental modification:** Depending on the ecology of the parasite in context, the modification of environmental factors can sharply reduce the transmission of the parasite. For example, the elimination of the breeding sites of mosquitoes helps control malaria.
- **Hygiene and sanitation:** Millions of people lack access to safe drinking water, sanitation and hygiene (WASH) which renders them at-risk for many diseases. Therefore, the provision of WASH is a key intervention in the control and elimination of several parasitic diseases, e.g., infections caused by soil-transmitted helminths and schistosomiasis.

Management of Potential Reservoirs

- **Vector management:** A pathogen cannot be controlled if it persists in a reservoir or a vector. Such persistence of the pathogen may lead to the re-emergence of the disease despite all the control efforts. For example, malaria can be effectively controlled only by sustainably blocking transmission by the mosquito vector.
- **Food and water safety:** Diseases that spread through water, milk, vegetables, fruits or meat can be controlled by adequate chlorination of drinking water, pasteurisation of milk, washing, peeling and cooking of fruits and vegetables and adequate inspection, storage and processing of meat and meat products.

Health Education

- **Awareness and community participation:** It is crucial to provide education and awareness to individuals at risk so that they know how to protect themselves from mosquitoes, ticks, bugs, etc., ensure safe food and drinking water and seek timely medical attention.
- **Behavioural changes:** Diseases preventable by simple interventions without the use of drugs or vaccines are much easier to control provided the intervention can be implemented uniformly. For example, dracunculiasis can be controlled simply by filtering drinking water.

Operational Considerations

- **Monitoring and surveillance:** Effective surveillance is very important when control programmes are ongoing and also after the desired results have been achieved. This is because a few remaining cases may be concentrated in foci or clusters, may be asymptomatic or may be in the incubation period of the disease. These hidden cases may be the source of new outbreaks and continued transmission of the disease in that area. Therefore, control programmes require sensitive systems of surveillance, monitoring and evaluation to detect the presence of microbes within the environment, hosts and sub-clinical cases, and to define prevalence and trends of the disease.
- **Training and capacity building:** Regular learning and training activities must be offered to ensure that skilled staff is executing the programme objectives.
- **Operational research and evaluation of new tools:** The development of tools that improve diagnosis and treatment and directly affect the epidemiological parameters of the disease, evaluate the control strategies and optimise surveillance should be regularly undertaken.
- **Identifying challenges and threats:** A continuous evaluation of the control programme helps to identify hurdles in the way of disease control and answer questions such as the timeline of the implementation of control measures and when to scale up the interventions or stop them altogether.

- **Certifications:** The verification of the control status of the disease such as elimination or eradication is challenging since it is a rigorous task to determine the certainty of a negative finding recorded in a short period of time. Such certification is provided by competent bodies such as the World Health Organization (WHO). Once such certification is completed, the control measures can be curtailed as required.

CONTROL PROGRAMMES FOR PARASITIC DISEASES IN INDIA

Several National Health Programmes have been implemented in India by the government for various infectious diseases. Many of these are aided by international bodies such as the WHO, UNICEF, USAID, etc. **In India, the Directorate of National Vector-Borne Disease Control Programme (NVBDCP) is responsible for the prevention and control of vector-borne diseases caused by parasites (malaria, kala-azar and lymphatic filariasis [LF]) and viruses (Japanese encephalitis [JE], dengue and chikungunya).** Out of these six diseases, kala-azar and LF were targeted for elimination by 2015. This, however, could not be achieved, and the target date was extended to 2020 for kala-azar and to 2021 for LF. Malaria is now targeted for elimination by 2030. The states are responsible for the implementation of these programmes, while the NVBDCP provides technical assistance, policies and assistance to the states.

The important features of the control programmes for parasitic diseases in India are presented in Table 57.1. For detailed knowledge of the same, interested readers should refer to the disease-specific documents of the control programmes available on the websites of the WHO and NVBDCP.

Table 57.1 Important features of control programmes for parasitic diseases in India

Parasite/ programme	Important features
National Vector-Borne Disease Control Programme (NVBDCP): Malaria, kala-azar, lymphatic filariasis, Japanese encephalitis, dengue and chikungunya	The general strategy for the prevention and control of vector-borne diseases under the NVBDCP is: 1. **Integrated vector management:** This includes indoor residual spraying (IRS) of insecticides in selected high-risk areas, long-lasting insecticidal nets (LLINs), use of larvivorous fish, antilarval measures including bio-larvicides and minor environmental engineering including source reduction of larva breeding sites. 2. **Disease management:** This includes early case detection with active, passive and sentinel surveillance and complete effective treatment, strengthening of referral services, epidemic preparedness and rapid response. 3. **Supportive interventions:** This includes behaviour change communication (BCC), inter-sectoral convergence and human resource development, community participation and education. 4. **Vaccination:** Available for Japanese encephalitis only. 5. **Mass drugs administration (MDA) annually:** This modality is applicable only to lymphatic filariasis.
Malaria	**Goal** In line with the WHO Global Technical Strategy for Malaria 2016–2030 and the Asia Pacific Leaders Malaria Alliance's Malaria Elimination Roadmap, the goals of the **National Framework for Malaria Elimination in India 2016–2030** are: • To eliminate malaria (zero indigenous cases) across the entire country by 2030 • To maintain malaria-free status in areas where malaria transmission has been interrupted and prevent re-introduction of malaria **The framework has four objectives** • To eliminate malaria from all 26 low- (category 1) and moderate-transmission (category 2) states/union territories (UTs) by 2022 • To reduce the incidence of malaria to <1 case per 1,000 population per year in all states and UTs and their districts by 2024 • To interrupt indigenous transmission of malaria across the country, including all high-transmission states and union territories (UTs) (category 3) by 2027 • To prevent the re-establishment of the local transmission of malaria in areas where it has been eliminated and maintain national malaria-free status by 2030 and beyond **Key strategies under the NVBDCP** 1. **Early case detection and prompt treatment (EDPT)** • EDPT is the main strategy for malaria control. Radical treatment is necessary for all cases to prevent transmission. • Chloroquine is the main anti-malaria drug for uncomplicated malaria.

	• Drug distribution centres (DDCs) and fever treatment depots (FTDs) have been established in rural areas for easy access to anti-malarial drugs to the community. • Alternative drugs for chloroquine-resistant malaria are recommended as per the National Drug Policy of malaria. 2. **Vector control** i) **Chemical control** • Use of IRS with insecticides recommended under the programme • Use of chemical larvicides like abate • Aerosol space spray during daytime • Malathion fogging during outbreaks ii) **Biological control** • Use of larvivorous fish in ornamental tanks, fountains, ponds, etc. • Use of biocides iii) **Personal prophylactic measures that individuals/communities can take up** • Use of mosquito repellent creams, liquids, coils, mats, etc. • Prevention of mosquito entry into houses with wire meshes • Use of insecticide-treated bed nets (ITN)/LLINS • Wearing clothes that cover the maximum surface area of the body 4. **Community participation** • Sensitising and involving the community for the detection of *Anopheles* breeding places and their elimination • Involvement of NGOs in programme strategies and implementation 5. **Environmental management and source reduction methods** • Source reduction, i.e., filling of the breeding places • Proper covering of stored water 6. **Monitoring and evaluation of the programme** • Monthly computerised management information system (CMIS) • Field visits by State National Programme Officers • Field visits by Malaria Research Centres and other ICMR (Indian Council of Medical Research) institutes • Feedback to states on field observations for correction actions
Kala-azar	**Goal** To improve the health status of vulnerable groups and at-risk populations living in kala-azar endemic areas by eliminating the disease so that it no longer remains a public health problem **Target** To reduce the annual incidence of kala-azar and PKDL to less than 1 case per 10,000 population at block PHC level **Strategies to eliminate kala-azar** 1. Early case detection and complete case management 2. Integrated vector management and vector surveillance 3. Supervision, monitoring, surveillance and evaluation 4. Strengthening capacity of human resource in health 5. Advocacy, communication and social mobilisation of population at risk 6. Clinical and operational research to support the elimination programme **South-East Asia regional impact objectives** • Reducing kala-azar in all areas including vulnerable, poor and unreached populations in endemic areas • Reducing case fatality rates from kala-azar • Reducing cases of PKDL to interrupt transmission of kala-azar • Preventing the emergence of kala-azar/HIV/TB co-infections in endemic areas **Tools** • House-to-house active case detection • Index case-based screening • Fever camps • IRS spraying • Kala-azar fortnight: Annual awareness drive during the first fortnight of February • Miltefosine as monotherapy to be phased out and replaced by single-dose liposomal amphotericin B which is safer, more effective and ensures 100% compliance
Lymphatic filariasis	The National Filaria Control Programme (NFCP) is in operation since 1955. **Goal** • Interrupting transmission of lymphatic filariasis through MDA • Managing morbidity and preventing disability

	Strategies • **Vector control:** Recurrent anti-larval measures at weekly intervals, environmental methods including source reduction by filling ditches, pits and low lying areas, de-weeding, desilting, etc., and biological control of mosquito breeding through larvivorous fish • **Anti-parasitic measures:** Detection and treatment of microfilaria carriers and diseased persons with DEC (diethylcarbamazine citrate) at filaria clinics in towns covered under the programme • **Morbidity management** **Tools** • **Annual MDA** with a single dose of DEC and albendazole for 5 years or more to the eligible population (except pregnant women, children <2 years and seriously ill persons) to interrupt transmission of the disease, i.e., to reduce the number of parasites in the blood to levels that will prevent mosquito vectors from transmitting infection • Home-based management of lymphedema cases and up-scaling of hydrocele operations in identified CHCs/district hospitals/medical colleges **Recommended minimum package of care:** • Treating episodes of acute dermatolymphangioadenitis (ADLA) among people with lymphedema or elephantiasis • Preventing debilitating, painful episodes of ADLA and progression of lymphedema • Providing access to hydrocele surgery • Providing antifilarial medicines to destroy any remaining worms and microfilariae by mass drug administration or individual treatment
Soil-transmitted helminths (STH)	Since 2015, the national deworming day is observed in India on 10 February every year; on this day, annual deworming is implemented across the country in government, government-aided and private schools and *anganwadi* centres in all states and UTs; some states/UTs with higher prevalence of STH also conduct a second round of deworming on 10 August **Goal/objectives** To eliminate morbidity due to STH in children by regularly treating at least 75% of children in endemic areas **Principles/strategies** To control morbidity through the periodic treatment of at-risk people living in endemic areas. People at risk are: • Preschool children • School-age children • Women of the reproductive age (including pregnant women in the second and third trimesters and breastfeeding women) • Adults in certain high-risk occupations such as tea-picking and mining **Tools/actions** • WHO recommends periodic medicinal treatment (deworming) without prior individual diagnosis to all at-risk people living in endemic areas—single-dose albendazole (400 mg) is administered for this purpose • Treatment once a year when baseline prevalence is >20%, twice a year when it is >50%
Dracunculiasis	India launched the Guinea-worm eradication programme in 1984 when there were 40,000 cases reported from 12,840 villages. In 1996, only 9 Guinea-worm cases were documented in three villages from Jodhpur (Rajasthan), while the rest of the country continued to remain free from Guinea-worm. The last case in India was reported in 1996 from Jodhpur in Rajasthan. Since then, 'zero' incidence has been maintained. India was certified for the elimination of Guinea-worm disease by the WHO in February 2000 and declared 'Guinea-worm disease free' on 15 February 2001 **Current goals/objectives** • The WHO recommends active surveillance in a country and/or area that has recently interrupted Guinea-worm disease transmission to be maintained for a minimum of 3 consecutive years • Ongoing surveillance is essential to ensure that no cases have been missed and to prevent re-occurrence of the disease **Principles/strategies** • Heightening surveillance to detect every case within 24 hours of worm emergence • Preventing transmission from each worm by treatment, and regular cleaning and bandaging of the affected areas of the skin until the worm is completely expelled from the body • Preventing contamination of drinking water by advising patients to avoid wading into water • Ensuring wider access to improved drinking water supplies to prevent infection • Filtering water from open water bodies before drinking • Implementing vector control by using the larvicide temephos • Promoting health education and behavioural change **Challenges** • Finding and containing the last remaining cases are the most difficult and expensive stages of the eradication process as these usually occur in remote and often inaccessible rural areas • Lack of access to disease-endemic areas is a major constraint, especially in countries where cases and animal infections are still occurring • Canine infections with Guinea-worm pose a challenge to the programme particularly in Chad, Ethiopia and Mali

Approach to the Laboratory Diagnosis of Parasitic Infections

The diagnosis of parasitic diseases depends on the laboratory examination of appropriate clinical specimens in conjunction with the clinical presentation, associated comorbidities, physical examination, radiological findings, elicitation of the relevant history of exposure to parasites (through occupation or by being in contact with animals) or travel to regions endemic for certain parasites. In addition to case diagnosis, laboratory tests are also important tools to assess response to treatment on follow-ups with the patient, to study epidemiology and disease burden, to investigate the disease outbreak and to discover exotic agents or unsuspected agents for a timely intervention.

A variety of clinical samples can be subjected to investigations for the detection of parasites. These include blood, bone marrow, feces, perianal swabs or tapes, CSF and other body fluids such as aspirates from the lymph nodes, spleen, liver, abscesses, cysts, fragments of cysts, urine as well as cervical swabs, tissue biopsies and skin snips, sputum, bronchoalveolar lavage, worms and insects.

Universal precautions and occupational safety and health regulations should be mandatorily followed while handling any clinical specimen as **all samples are potentially infectious** and possible health hazards.

FECAL SPECIMENS

Collection of Fecal Specimens

Fecal or stool specimens are usually collected for the diagnosis of gastrointestinal parasites.

- Stool samples should be collected fresh and examined as soon as possible. Alternatively, they should be stored in preservatives to retain the morphology of parasites (see box).

> Freshly passed stool specimens are essential for the detection of the trophozoites of amoebae, flagellates and ciliates. Preferably, all liquid stools should be examined within 30 minutes of passage; if this is not possible, the samples must be preserved. Soft stool samples should be examined or preserved within one hour, whereas formed stool should be examined or preserved within 24 hours of passage.

- Fecal samples should be collected in a wide-mouthed, clean, leak-proof and screw-capped container. For most parasites, **at least three samples are required to be collected on three separate days** (preferably within a 10-day period) for reasonable diagnostic sensitivity, factoring in the intermittent shedding of parasites. With each additional sample, the yield of the investigation increases.
- Stool examination should be performed before oil emulsion or barium meal is given to the patient as these agents interfere with the detection of parasites. Contamination of the sample with urine or water should be avoided.
- Various preservatives, e.g., **5–10% formalin, polyvinyl alcohol (PVA), merthiolate-iodine-formalin (MIF) or Schaudinn's fixative** can be used to maintain the morphology of parasitic cysts and eggs (Annexure II). However, for most immunodiagnostic tests, only PVA or formalin preservation is suitable as other preservatives interfere with such tests. The recommended stool:fixative ratio is 1:3.
  [**CAUTION:** Given the toxicity of mercury, mercury-based preservatives should be handled and discarded carefully and as per the regulations.]
- Specimens other than stool are also routinely collected for the detection of certain parasites, e.g., perianal swabs for *Enterobius vermicularis* (scotch tape or NIH swab, see **Chapter 28**, *Enterobius*), duodenal contents by brush biopsy and entero test (gelatin capsule) for *Giardia duodenalis*.

Macroscopic Examination of Stool

- **Consistency:** The consistency of an unpreserved stool specimen is of importance as it may indicate the organism the specimen contains.
  - *Trophozoites:* The trophozoites of intestinal protozoa are usually found in liquid or soft stools but almost never in fully formed ones.
  - *Cysts:* Protozoan cysts are rarely seen in liquid stools and are usually found in solid specimens. On the other hand, coccidian cysts, microsporidian spores and helminth eggs are found in either liquid or formed stools.
- **Colour:** Dark red stool indicates upper GIT bleeding, whereas a bright red stool sample is suggestive of bleeding from the lower GIT. Bloody mucus in loose or liquid specimens is highly suggestive of amoebic ulcerations in the large intestine, though these could also be manifestations of other conditions. Occult blood in stool may be the result of intestinal bleeding caused by parasites but is more likely to be indicative of other gastrointestinal disorders.
- **Presence of worms or their segments:** Adult worms like pinworms, roundworms, hookworms, the larvae of *Strongyloides* or hookworms or the segments of tapeworms may be seen in stool samples.

Microscopic Examination of Stool

No single technique of stool examination is completely satisfactory. Hence a combination of techniques is desirable.

Direct wet film

Direct wet film examination is most useful for the detection of the trophozoites of amoebae and flagellates to observe the characteristic motility of the parasite. Both trophozoites and cysts appear as highly refractile structures. Helminthic eggs (Fig. AI.1) and larvae can be readily detected. In addition, the presence of pus cells and red blood cells can offer some clues about the disease pathology.

Saline mount: A small portion of fecal sample is mixed with a drop of normal saline on a clean glass slide and mounted with a coverslip. The film should be just thin enough for a newspaper print to be easily read through it; care should be taken not to make it thick. The mount is **first examined under the low-power objective (10×) and then under the high-power objective (40×) of the microscope.** The examination of a stool specimen may reveal:

- **Normal stool constituents:** These include vegetable and plant matter, fat globules, epithelial cells, pollen grains, yeast cells and bacteria.
- **Trophozoites and cysts of protozoa and eggs and larvae of helminths:** Some structures such as RBCs in trophozoites of *Entamoeba histolytica* and chromatoid bodies in cysts can be more easily appreciated. Moreover, bile staining can be observed—bile-stained helminth eggs appear golden brown, whereas non-bile-stained eggs appear colourless (see box).

> **Bile-stained eggs in stool samples**
> - *Ascaris lumbricoides*
> - *Trichuris trichiura*
> - *Fasciola hepatica*
> - *Taenia solium* and *T. saginata*
> - *Fasciolopsis buski*
> - *Clonorchis sinensis*

- **Cellular elements:** Pus cells, RBCs and epithelial cells may be seen.
- **Charcot–Leyden crystals:** They are the products of the breakdown of eosinophils and may be seen in stool or sputum samples.

Iodine mount: To prepare this, saline is augmented with Lugol's or D'Antoni's iodine during the preparation of the mount. Lugol's iodine must be diluted to a ratio of 1:5 for fecal preparations. It should be prepared fresh every day or else it fades.

Advantage: The nuclear details of cysts, ova and larvae are better visualised than they are in saline mounts, and the glycogen mass becomes prominent with iodine. The flagella may become prominent, especially if the specimen is visualised under dark-ground illumination.

Disadvantage: Iodine kills the organism, immobilising it.

Permanent stained smear

Often, it is not possible to accurately identify protozoa on wet mounts. Thus, fecal smears are stained with dyes to reveal the differential characteristics of the parasites. These stained smears can also be preserved for a long time to serve as a permanent record of the specimen. Specimens fixed in formalin may be unsuitable for permanent stain as the material does not adhere properly to slide. Thus, PVA-fixed material is better for this purpose. The stains commonly used for stool specimens are as follows (also refer to Annexure II):

- Trichrome stain and its modifications
- Iron-hematoxylin stain
- Modified acid-fast stain

Concentration techniques

When the organisms are few in number, they may not be detected on direct examination of the sample. In such cases, the parasitic cysts and eggs need to be **concentrated either by sedimentation or floatation** to increase the diagnostic sensitivity by 8–10 times. **However, trophozoites of protozoa get distorted or destroyed in the harsh process of concentration of stool.**

Sedimentation techniques

Fecal material is suspended in a solution with low specific gravity so that the eggs and cysts **sediment** at the bottom of

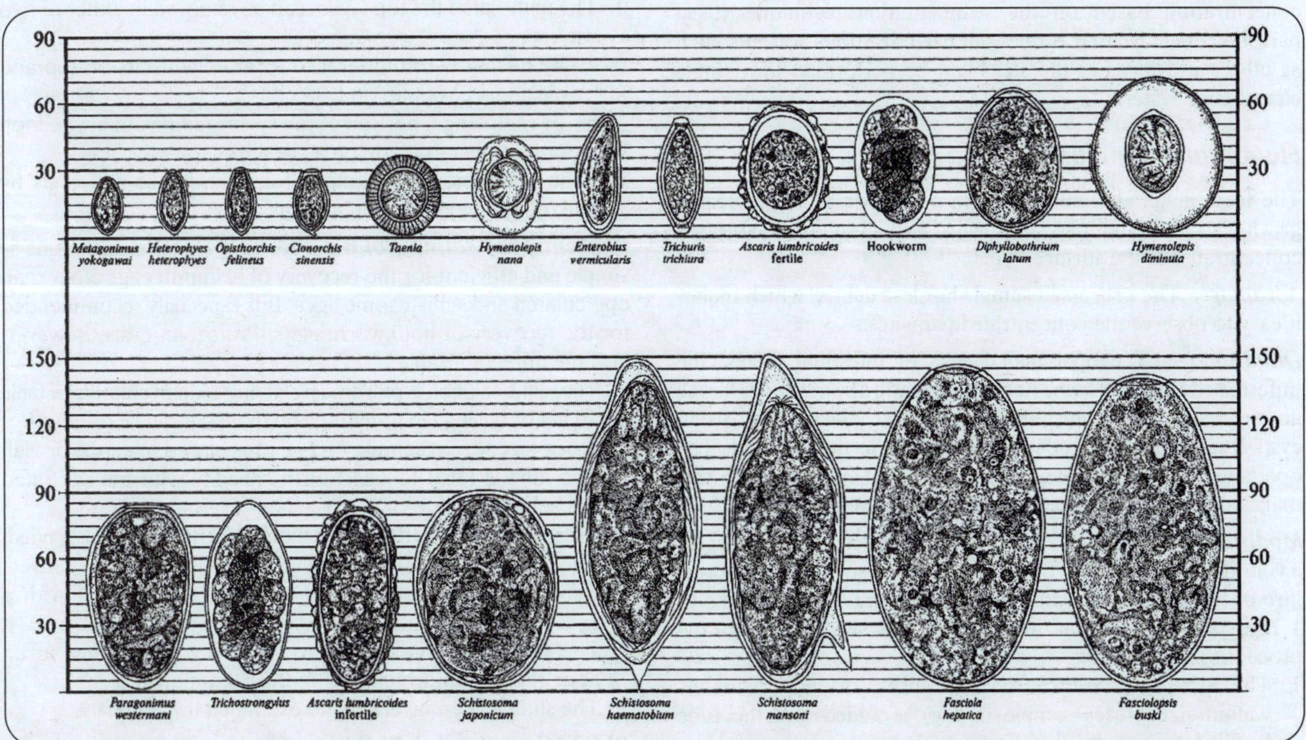

Fig. AI.1 Relative sizes (in μm) of different parasitic eggs (*Source:* Basic laboratory methods in medical parasitology, WHO, 1991)

the receptacle either by gravitation or by centrifugation. The commonly employed method is the **formol ether** method or **Ritchie's concentration method.** Ether was used in the original method but its use was discontinued because of its explosive nature. Instead, either ethyl acetate, acetone or the clearing agent Hemo-De can be used; these agents have similar efficacy and are much safer.

Formol-ether sedimentation technique: This is suitable for both preserved and unpreserved specimens. The procedure is as follows:

1. A walnut-sized fecal sample (~4 g) is transferred to a tube containing 10 ml of 5–10% formalin, mixed thoroughly and left to stand for 30 minutes. This step may be omitted if the sample is already preserved in formalin.
2. The mixture is filtered through two layers of gauze into a 15 ml conical centrifuge tube.
3. 0.85% saline (or 5–10% formalin) is added to this mixture until the tube is almost full. Then, the tube is centrifuged for 10 minutes at 500×g.
4. The supernatant is discarded. About 1 ml of the sediment is suspended in formalin and centrifuged again for 10 minutes at 500×g; this step is then and repeated once again.
5. Following this, about 4–5 ml of ethyl acetate is added to the tube and it is stoppered and shaken vigorously.
6. The stopper is removed, and the tube is centrifuged again for 10 minutes at 500×g.
7. Four layers are formed—the top layer consisting of ether or ethyl acetate. Below it, is a plug of debris. The third is a clear layer of formalin and the fourth is the sediment containing the parasites (Fig. AI.2).
8. The debris is removed with the help of a glass rod, and the supernatant is discarded.
9. The sediment is taken out with a pipette. A saline and iodine mount of the sediment is then made for microscopic examination.

Mini Parasep: It is a commercial method for fecal parasite concentration based on the sedimentation technique (fecal parasite concentrator). It does not use hazardous solvents such as ether, and most of the steps can be performed in a single closed-tube system.

Floatation techniques

The fecal material is suspended in a solution of high specific gravity so that the parasite's eggs and cysts **float** and get concentrated at the surface.

Advantage: The processed sample has less debris, which makes it easy to observe the concentrated parasites.

Disadvantage: The operculated eggs of intestinal flukes, the unfertilised eggs of *Ascaris lumbricoides* and *Strongyloides* larvae are not recovered because these are relatively heavy. Protozoan cysts lose their characteristic morphology in this method. The operculum of fluke eggs open up, allowing saline to enter; this makes them heavy and causes them to sink to the bottom.

Modified zinc sulphate centrifugal floatation technique: In a volumetric flask, 330 g of zinc sulfate is dissolved in about one litre of warm distilled water. The specific gravity is adjusted to 1.18 by adding water or zinc sulfate as needed. The rest of the procedure is as follows:

1. The mixture is transferred to a tube. An approximately walnut-sized feces sample (~4 g) is added and the tube is filled to two-third capacity with tap water to make a suspension.

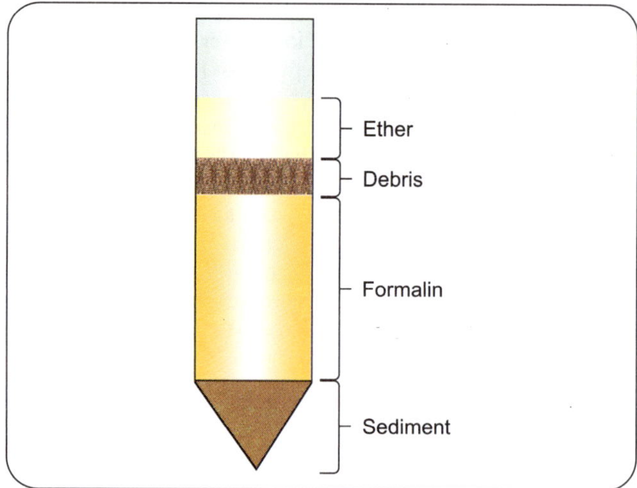

Fig. AI.2 Four layers formed in the formol-ether sedimentation technique

2. This preparation is centrifuged for one minute at approximately 650×g.
3. The supernatant is poured into a container filled with a disinfectant.
4. The washing is repeated only if the stool is very oily or contains excessive debris.
5. Zinc sulfate solution is added until the tube is half full.
6. Using an applicator, the sediment is mixed and suspended thoroughly in the solution.
7. Additional zinc sulfate solution is added to fill the tube within 1 cm of the top edge.
8. This suspension is centrifuged for one minute at 650×g. The tube is then placed carefully in a rack without shaking or spilling its contents.
9. The material in the top layers can be removed in either of two ways:
   a. By raising the fluid level to form a meniscus on top and placing a coverslip on it
   b. By removing a portion of the surface film with a wire loop or a capillary pipette on a slide
10. The suspension is examined for eggs, larvae and cysts by making saline and iodine mounts.

Concentrated saline flotation technique: This technique is simple and efficient for the recovery of helminth eggs other than operculated and schistosome eggs. It is especially recommended for the recovery of hookworm eggs. Protozoan cysts, however, become unrecognisable.

The saline solution is prepared by adding sodium chloride or table salt to hot or boiling tap water until no more salt can be dissolved.

1. A pea-sized feces sample (~1–2 g) is placed in a tube or vial.
2. The tube is filled to one-fourth capacity with the saturated salt solution.
3. Using an applicator, the feces is thoroughly mixed and suspended.
4. The vial is filled to the brim with salt solution.
5. Carefully, the surface of the suspension is touched with a grease-free glass slide.
6. The preparation is allowed to stand for 10 minutes to an hour (the optimum time being 20–30 minutes).
7. The slide is then inverted and examined immediately.

FLOTAC and mini-FLOTAC: These are semi-quantitative flotation methods that are available commercially. The advantage of these techniques is that they are less cumbersome and very useful if a large number of samples is to be examined.

Egg counting methods

Egg counting methods are used to estimate the worm burden by assuming the average egg-laying capacity of different worms. As a rule, **for nematode worms, 100 eggs/g of stool represents one female worm.** The egg count is an indirect approximate measure of the degree or intensity of infection as light, moderate or heavy. Several methods are available for counting eggs:

- **Standard smear technique (Beaver, 1949):** A wet mount is prepared by using approximately 1–2 g of feces. The number of eggs per gram of feces can be assessed if all the eggs in the mount are counted.
- **The Kato-Katz thick smear technique (Martin and Beaver, 1968):** A measured quantity (~50 mg) of stool can be examined in this technique. The feces is pressed between a slide and a cellophane coverslip soaked in glycerine-methylene blue which clears the fecal debris and facilitates easy counting of the eggs.

  [**NOTE:** Hookworm and schistosome eggs tend to collapse and disappear if left for a long time and therefore, should be examined immediately after clearing.]
- **Dilution egg counting technique (Stoll, 1923):** This method allows a defined quantity of fecal sample to be diluted in a defined quantity of saline and then examined for eggs which can be quantitated. However, the eggs per gram (epg or N) vary according to the consistency of the stool. For unformed feces, N is multiplied by the correction factor, viz. mushy formed (1.5N), mushy soft/pulpy (2N), mushy loose (3N), frankly diarrheic (4N) and watery (5N) stools.
- **McMaster's egg counting chamber:** A known volume of fecal suspension is transferred to a counting chamber and examined microscopically to count eggs.

Schistosomal hatching test

When feces containing viable schistosome eggs is diluted with water, the eggs hatch within a few hours, releasing miracidia which are positively phototrophic. The eggs of *S. haematobium* in urine may also be hatched in this manner but they are more easily concentrated by centrifugation or membrane filtration.

Disposal of Specimens

- If feces are collected in paper boxes, the best way to dispose of the specimens is by incinerating the box in its entirety. If it cannot be burnt or if the sample is collected in a plastic, metal or glass container, enough 10% formalin is added to cover the leftover specimen in the container. This will kill any parasites that might be present. The mixture is allowed to stand for one hour or more before discarding or washing.
- Slides used for wet mounts should be soaked in a container filled with disinfectant (e.g., sodium hypochlorite) for at least one hour before washing.
- An applicator is used to push the coverslip off into a beaker or a small container of disinfectant. The slide is soaked in another pan of disinfectant. Coverslips break easily; if soaked with the slides, they may break and cut the hands of the person washing them.
- Funnel stoppers and centrifuge tubes should also be soaked in disinfectant for one hour before washing.
- Applicator sticks and gauze pieces should be burnt or discarded after soaking them in a disinfectant.

BLOOD SPECIMENS

Parasites found in peripheral blood film
- Protozoa: *Plasmodium, Babesia, Leishmania* and *Trypanosoma*
- Helminths: *Wuchereria bancrofti, Brugia malayi, Loa loa, Mansonella perstans* and *M. ozzardi*

Collection of Specimens

Universal precautions must be observed at all times as a number of viral, bacterial and parasitological agents are transmitted by blood. Careful attention must be paid to the techniques used in the collection of blood and the preparation of blood films.

Collection time: The concentration of parasites in the peripheral blood depends on the time of collection. For example, for **malaria**, the highest number of parasites are found during episodes of fever and before treatment is started; for **microfilariae**, on the other hand, the collection time depends on the periodicity of the parasite. Blood should be collected at night between 10 p.m. and 4 a.m. for *Wuchereria bancrofti* and *Brugia malayi*.

Procedure for the collection of blood for smear:

1. The third finger of the patient's left hand or a ear lobe (the big toe can be used for infants) is selected. The thumb should never be used for adults or children.
2. A piece of cotton wool lightly soaked in alcohol is used to clean the finger and then the skin is allowed to dry.
3. The ball of the finger is pricked with a sterile lancet or needle.
4. By applying gentle pressure to the finger, the first drop of blood is expressed and wiped away with dry cotton. It should be ensured that no strands of cotton remain on the finger.
5. Gentle pressure is applied to the finger and a single small drop of blood is collected on the centre of a clean glass slide to prepare a thin film. Further pressure is applied to express more blood and collect two or three larger drops to prepare a thick film.
6. **Thin film:** A second clean slide is used as a 'spreader'. The small drop is touched with the spreader and the blood is allowed to run along its edge. The spreader is then firmly pushed along the first slide at an angle of 45° (Fig. AI.3b and c). The blood films should not extend to the edge of the slide (this is to protect those handling the slide from infection).

   Characteristics of a good thin film:
   - The blood film should be tongue-shaped, thin, uniform and should extend only a little over the centre of slide, tapering towards the end (tail end).
   - The smear should not touch the margins of the slide.
7. **Thick film:** Using the corner of the spreader, the larger drops of blood are swiftly combined and then spread in a circular or rectangular form with 3–6 movements to make an even, thick film (Fig. AI.3a and c). Since a thick smear has several layers, parasites cannot be visualised unless hemoglobin is removed

from the RBCs by performing **dehemoglobinisation** before the slide is fixed with methanol (see Annexure II).

The thick film is allowed to dry for 30 minutes to 2 hours, during which time it should be protected from flies, dirt and extreme heat.

8. The slide used for spreading the films must be disinfected; it may then be reused.

Direct Wet Mount

Wet mounts of fresh whole blood (or centrifuged blood) may be used for the detection of microfilariae and trypanosomes. However, this only provides evidence of infection. Stained films are necessary to confirm the species.

Stained Blood Smears

The most commonly used technique for the investigation of blood is the examination of stained blood films. **Romanowsky stains are used for most blood parasites.** Delafield's hematoxylin stain is used for microfilariae. Either thick films or thin films may be used depending on the circumstances.

Thick film: A thick blood film is **more sensitive** for detecting parasites and saves the time taken for examination. However, it may be difficult to identify the parasite species on a thick film. One microscopic field of thick film is equivalent to 50 microscopic fields of thin film. However, a thick film is **not** a substitute for a thin film.

Thin film technique: A thin blood film causes very little distortion of the parasite and **permits species identification** which may not be possible in thick films. However, it is less sensitive than a thick film. Thus many more fields may have to be examined to detect the parasite, especially if parasitemia is low.

Given the advantages and disadvantages of the two types of films, both thick and thin films must always be prepared when searching for plasmodia and trypanosomes. For the detection of microfilariae, thick films alone are sufficient. A combination of thick and thin smears may be made on a single slide as it is economical to do so, but such films must dry thoroughly (for 8–10 hours or overnight) before they can be satisfactorily stained.

Romanowsky stains (see Annexure II)

- **Giemsa stain:** This stain is available commercially as a concentrated stock solution. Each new batch should be tested for optimal dilution and staining time before using it on patient specimens. This is the most commonly used stain for malaria parasites.
- **Leishman's stain:** Prior fixation of the slide is not required as this stain is an alcoholic solution which fixes the smear while staining.
- **Jaswant-Singh-Bhattacharji (JSB) staining:** It is a rapid Romanowsky's staining method for malarial parasites.

Examination of Blood Films for Malaria

Thick films

- Malaria parasites should be looked for with the oil immersion objective.

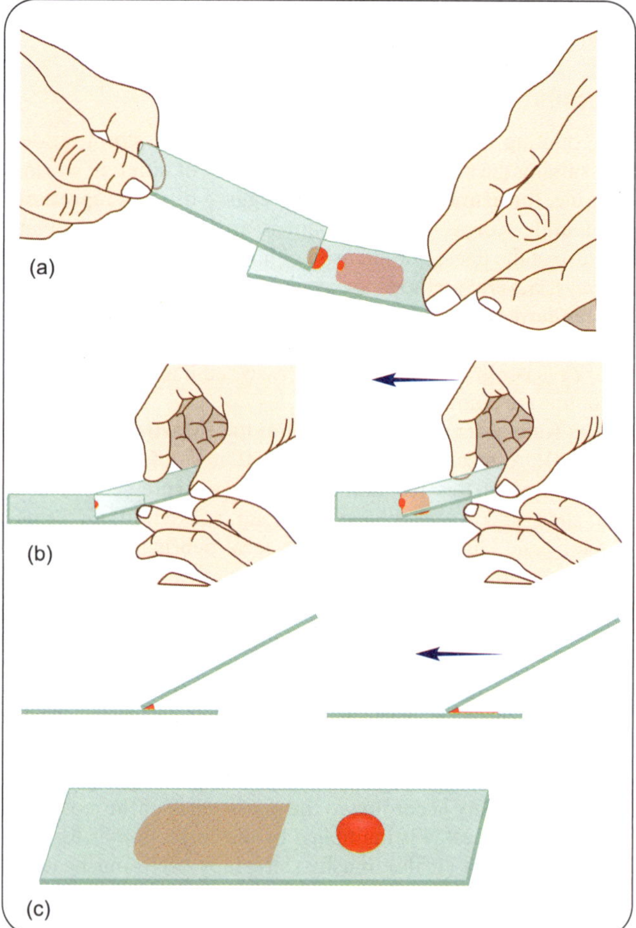

Fig. AI.3 Preparation of a blood film using two slides: (a) spreading a thick film, (b) spreading a thin film and (c) a single slide with both thin and thick blood films

- At least 100 fields should be examined.

Features of thick films:

- The background should be clean and free from debris, with a pale mottled grey colour from lysed erythrocytes.
- Leukocyte nuclei are stained a deep red chromatin with pale purplish-blue cytoplasm.
- Platelets stain purple and have a woolly outline.
- The ring forms of all species of *Plasmodium* appear as streaks of blue cytoplasm with detached nuclear dots or broken rings.
- Schizonts and gametocytes usually retain their appearance, and their hemozoin pigment is clearer.

Thin films

- The 10× objective should be focused on the thin tail end of the film where the red blood cells are arranged in a monolayer. The best area for parasite detection is along the upper and lower margins of the tail.
- Immersion oil should then be added to the slide, and the smear should be examined with the 100× objective. Around 200–300 fields of the thin smear should be examined for about 8–10 minutes for malaria parasites and trypanosomes.

Features of thin films:

- The background should be clean and free from debris; erythrocytes stain greyish pink.
- Neutrophils have deep purple nuclei and well-defined granules.
- The chromatin of malaria parasites is stained a deep purplish-red and cytoplasm, purplish-blue.
- Schüffner's dots can be seen as stippling in erythrocytes containing *P. vivax* or *P. ovale*. Maurer's dots appear as stippling in erythrocytes containing the ring forms of *P. falciparum*.

Examination of Blood for Microfilaria

Wet mount: Two or three drops of blood are collected on a clean glass slide and mixed with two drops of water to lyse the red cells. The drops are covered with a coverslip and examined for motile (wriggling) microfilariae.

Stained blood smears: A thick smear is made, as is done for malaria. It is then dehemoglobinised and stained with Romanowsky or Delafield's hematoxylin stain (better for staining the sheath).

Concentration techniques: When microfilariae are present in low numbers in blood, they may be concentrated by various techniques.

- **Tube centrifugation lysed blood technique:** Approximately 10 ml of venous blood is lysed in a solution of saponin saline (or 2% acetic acid). The microfilariae are then concentrated by centrifugation and observed under the microscope. The addition of a stain is helpful in identifying the species. The total number of microfilariae (mf) divided by 10 gives the number of mf/ml.
- **Microhematocrit tube technique:** Capillary blood is obtained from the ear lobe or finger in a heparinised or EDTA-coated capillary tube. It is then centrifuged in a microhematocrit centrifuge. The buffy coat layer obtained from this is then examined microscopically for motile microfilariae.
- **Knott concentration:** Approximately 1 ml of blood is mixed with 9 ml of 2% formalin in water. This solution lyses the RBCs, while the microfilariae are preserved by the formalin. The mixture is centrifuged at 120×g for 5 minutes, and the supernatant is removed. The sediment is then transferred to a glass slide and stained with Romanowsky stains for microscopic examination. Samples collected in this manner can be preserved for several weeks without loss of morphology of the microfilariae. For this reason, this method is useful for sampling in remote areas.
- **Gradient centrifugation:** About 4 ml of heparinised venous blood is mixed with 4 ml of Ficoll-Hypaque solution. The mixture is then centrifuged at 400×g for 30–40 minutes. This yields 3 distinct layers—the lower-most WBC layer, the middle Ficoll-Hypaque layer and the upper plasma layer. The middle layer is examined microscopically for microfilariae.
- **Membrane filtration:** 2–5 ml of blood is collected in an anticoagulant solution and passed through membrane filters (of 5 μm porosity) fixed to a syringe. The filter is removed, placed on a slide, stained with Giemsa stain and examined under a low-power microscope for microfilariae.
- **Diethylcarbamazine (DEC) provocation test:** The oral administration of a single dose of DEC 2 mg/kg (maximum 100 mg) induces the mobilisation of microfilariae into the peripheral blood in about 20–40 minutes. Thus, blood can be examined in the daytime even in nocturnally periodic microfilariae. This method is especially useful for field surveys.

The following characteristics are used for the differentiation of microfilariae (see **Chapter 33**, *Wuchereria and Brugia*):

1. The presence or absence of a sheath
2. The presence or absence of nuclei in the tip of the tail
3. The size of the microfilariae

Utility of microfilaria count: In heavy infections, especially in loiasis, severe reactions can occur during treatment. Thus it is useful to know whether the microfilarial concentration is high before starting treatment.

OTHER SPECIMENS

Examination of Urogenital Specimens

The eggs of *S. haematobium* and the microfilariae of *Wuchereria, Brugia, Loa* (chylous urine) and *Onchocerca* may sometimes be found in urine. These are best recovered by examining centrifuged or membrane-filtered urine samples.

Trophozoites of *Trichomonas vaginalis* with the characteristic jerky motility may be seen on a wet mount soon after urine or vaginal fluid has been collected. However, the parasites lose their motility rapidly and may become indistinguishable. Phase contrast microscopy is better to visualise the characteristic flagella. In stained preparations, these parasites get distorted and may not be recognisable.

Examination of Biopsy or Skin Tissue

All biopsy tissues must be submitted to the parasitology laboratory without adding a formalin fixative. Such specimens may be used for the examination of parasites, culturing and nucleic acid detection. A muscle biopsy may be obtained for the detection of the larval forms of *Trichinella spiralis*, *Taenia solium* (*Cysticercus cellulosae*) and the amastigotes of *Trypanosoma cruzi*.

Skin snips: Biopsy of skin may be required for the demonstration of parasites for the diagnosis of onchocerciasis, cutaneous leishmaniasis, etc.

- A skin snip can be obtained by grasping skin with forceps or elevating a portion of skin with the tip of a needle. The tip of the small cone of the skin is then sliced with a sharp blade or razor. These snips may be used for the demonstration of L-D bodies when cutaneous leishmaniasis is suspected or for the detection of microfilariae in suspected cases of subcutaneous filariasis or *Onchocerca volvulus*.

Examination of Cerebrospinal Fluid (CSF)

Direct wet mount examination of CSF is useful for:

- Assessing cellular response in the CSF
- Detection of free-living amoebae (*Naegleria, Acanthamoeba* and *Balamuthia*), trypanosomes and the larvae of *Angiostrongylus cantonensis*

- Sometimes, the tachyzoites of *Toxoplasma gondii* may be seen in AIDS patients with *Toxoplasma* encephalitis

Examination of Sputum

The examination of sputum is useful for the demonstration of the eggs of *Paragonimus* (lung fluke), the hooklets of *Echinococcus* in lung hydatid cysts and the trophozoites of *Entamoeba histolytica* in pulmonary amoebiasis. The migrating larvae of *Ascaris*, hookworms or *Strongyloides* may be seen rarely. *Cryptosporidium* and microsporidia can be found in sputum sometimes. *Trichomonas tenax* or *Entamoeba gingivalis* may be seen often but are oral contaminants (part of the normal flora).

Normally, sputum may be examined directly as a wet film but when the sputum is extremely viscous, it may be liquified by adding an equal volume of 3% N-acetyl cysteine or 3% sodium hydroxide. Such a sample is then centrifuged, and the sediment is examined.

Examination of Aspirates from Lymph Nodes, Spleen, Liver and Bone Marrow

These aspirates are most valuable for the diagnosis of visceral leishmaniasis but may also be useful for the diagnosis of other parasitic infections. Direct wet mount examination may be useful for the demonstration of *Entamoeba histolytica*, the components of hydatid cyst, etc. The aspirate is usually smeared on a glass slide, fixed and then stained with stains like Giemsa for the demonstration of trypanosomes or L-D bodies for the diagnosis of visceral leishmaniasis.

CULTURE METHODS

Parasites have complex life cycles but a few parasites can be grown in a culture. This, however, is not the usual modality for the diagnosis of parasitic infections.

- Culture techniques to isolate the disease-causing parasite, e.g., *Acanthamoeba, Trichomonas* and *Leishmania,* may be used for diagnosis.
- Culturing is sometimes used for the accurate identification of the parasite species by subjecting the cultured parasites to other investigations like zymodeme analysis for *Entamoeba* species.
- It is more often employed for obtaining large yields of the parasite as a source of antigen for in-house serological tests, animal inoculation and experimental or physiological studies.
- Drug sensitivity testing may be performed as in vitro tests on parasite cultures.
- Culturing is useful for studying mechanisms of pathogenesis, vaccine development, etc.

Culture Methods for Protozoa

The culture media used for protozoa are defined as **xenic** if they contain some microbial associates (e.g., *Escherichia coli, Crithidium,* etc.) for added nutrition or **axenic** if they do not contain any added microbial associates. Parasites usually grow in association with bacterial agents, which they require as supplements in culture media and have to be gradually axenised. The media that are commonly used for the culture of protozoans in clinical parasitology are described in Annexure II and listed below:

- **TYIS-33 medium** for axenic culture of *Entamoeba* and *Trichomonas*
- **Modified Boeck and Drbohlav's/Locke-egg-serum (LES) medium** for *Entamoeba* and *Giardia*
- **Novy-Nicolle-McNeal (NNN) culture medium** for in vitro cultivation of *Leishmania* and *Trypanosoma*
- **Non-nutrient agar (NNA) medium** for *Acanthamoeba* and *Naegleria*
- **Trager and Jensen medium** for the cultivation of *Plasmodium falciparum*

Protozoan parasites which may be cultured for laboratory diagnosis

Stool:
- *Entamoeba histolytica*
- *Giardia intestinalis*
- *Balantidium coli*

Vaginal secretions:
- *Trichomonas vaginalis*

Cerebrospinal fluid:
- Free-living amoebae: *Acanthamoeba* spp., *Naegleria fowleri*

Bone marrow:
- *Leishmania* spp.

Blood:
- *Trypanosoma* spp.
- *Plasmodium* spp.

Culture Methods for Helminths

Helminth parasites which may be cultured for laboratory diagnosis
- *Strongyloides stercoralis*
- Hookworm
- *Trichostrongylus*

Helminths such as hookworms or *Strongyloides stercoralis* can be cultured using a suitable medium. These methods rely on the migration of the worm's larvae from the stool samples towards water or observing the larval tracks on an indicator media. Some of the culture techniques used for the diagnosis of these helminths in a parasitology laboratory are described below.

Harada-Mori filter paper strip method: This test is performed to increase the chances of detecting the larvae of *S. stercoralis*, hookworms and *Trichostrongylus* larvae (Fig. AI.4a). This method is performed as follows:

1. Approximately 6 g of freshly passed feces is smeared on the middle portion of a strip of filter paper. The paper is then placed in a tube containing a small amount of water to keep it hydrated.
2. The tube is incubated at 25–28°C in an upright position to allow the larvae to moult and migrate to the water. A petri dish may be used in place of a tube and a glass slide may be used instead of the filter paper strip (**petri dish slant culture,** Fig. AI.4b).
3. A small amount of fluid from the bottom of the tube or the petri plate is examined every day for the helminth larvae. The cultures should be kept for 8–10 days before declaring them negative.

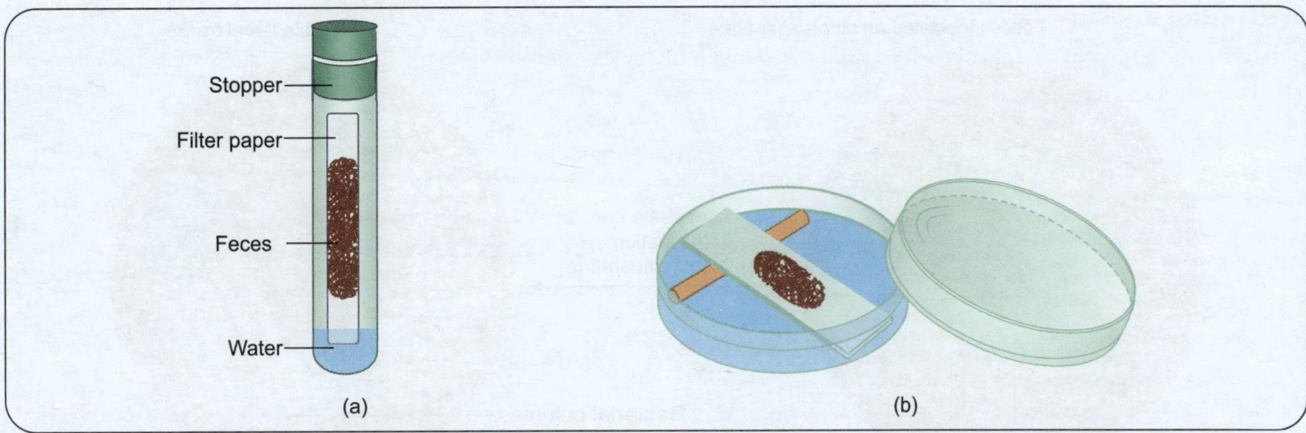

Fig. AI.4 Culture methods for the recovery of nematode larvae: (a) Harada-Mori filter paper strip and (b) petri dish slant culture

[**NOTE**: Gloves should be worn while handling these cultures as the filariform larvae of these helminths can penetrate skin.]

Baermann's funnel concentration method: For the examination of stool specimens suspected of having small numbers of *S. stercoralis* larvae, the Baermann's apparatus is used (Fig. AI.5). This method relies on the active migration of filariform larvae from the stool sample towards water. It can also be used to recover hookworm larvae hatched out of eggs.

1. Fresh feces are placed on a few layers of gauze placed on top of a wire mesh in a funnel containing warm tap water. The lower end of the funnel is clamped.
2. When left to stand at room temperature for about two hours or longer, the larvae migrate through the gauze into the water attracted by the warmth and settle at the bottom of the tube of the funnel. About 10 ml of this water can be collected in a beaker or test tube. It is then centrifuged for two minutes at 500×g, and the sediment is transferred onto a glass slide to be examined.

Charcoal culture: This method can be used to recover hookworms, *S. stercoralis* and *Trichostrongylus* larvae. The granulated charcoal and conditions of this culture provide an environment favourable for larval development. A charcoal culture is obtained as follows:

1. About 20–40 g of fresh feces is mixed with tap water to form a thick suspension.
2. This suspension is mixed with 5–10 parts of moist charcoal granules in a petri dish with a moistened filter paper at the bottom. Some water is added to maintain adequate moisture.
3. The larvae hatch out of the eggs and accumulate at the surface in 7–10 days. These can be collected by adding water to the mixture and exposing it to light for two hours. The water is collected in a test tube and centrifuged for 5 minutes at 2,000 rpm. The sediments are then examined under the microscope for larvae.

   [**NOTE:** The water condensed on the lid of the petri plate may contain larvae and should be handled carefully.]

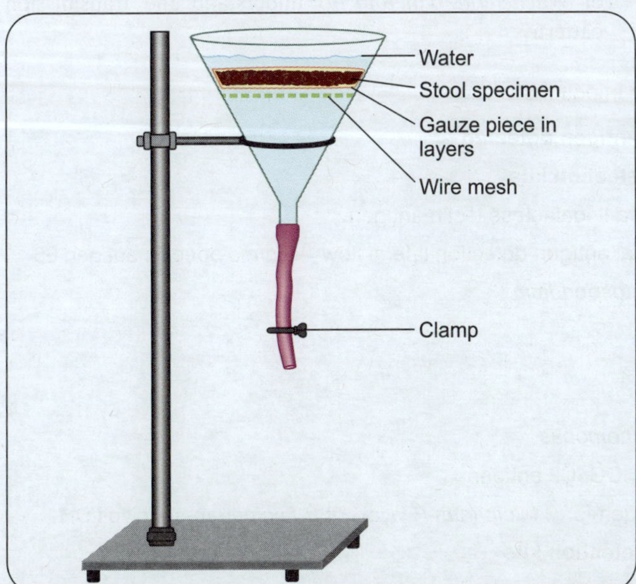

Fig. AI.5 Baermann's apparatus for the recovery of nematode larvae

Agar plate culture: These are used to recover the larvae of *Strongyloides stercoralis* or hookworm larvae from fecal samples (Fig. AI.6).

1. About 2 g of feces is inoculated onto agar or blood agar plates.
2. The plates are sealed with parafilm to prevent accidental infection and incubated at ambient temperature.
3. The filariform larvae crawl over the agar, making visible tracks in 2–3 days while hookworm larvae do so in about 5–7 days.
4. For further confirmation of larvae, the plates can be examined microscopically.

IMMUNODIAGNOSIS

Immunological tests are useful for the detection and surveillance of many parasitic infections. These tests may be based on the **detection of antigens or antibodies**. The antigens may be detected in serum or in other specimens like fecal samples, pus, cerebrospinal fluid, etc., depending upon the clinical condition. These tests may be available in various formats like ELISA, lateral flow assays, immunoblot, complement fixation, hemagglutination, etc. While ELISAs are available for most parasitic infections, a few point-of-care tests are also available for the rapid diagnosis of parasites (Table AI.1).

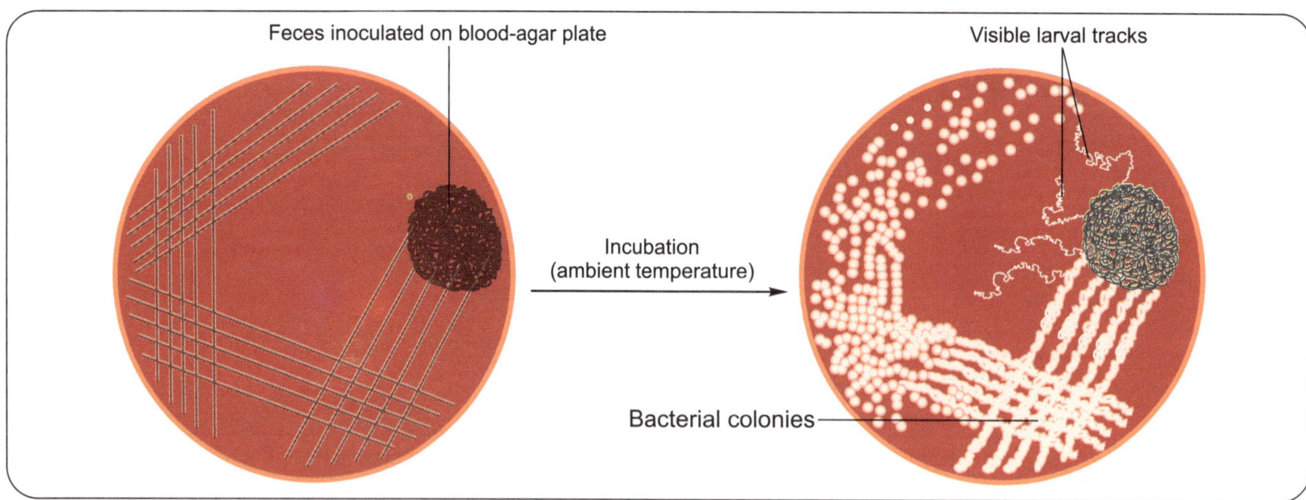

Fig. AI.6 Illustration of a blood agar plate showing streaks of larval movement

MOLECULAR METHODS

The deoxyribonucleic acid (DNA) of parasites present in clinical samples can be detected using molecular techniques such as **polymerase chain reaction (PCR)** which rely on identifying a specific DNA sequence of the parasite genome.

Parasites commonly targeted for molecular diagnosis

- *Entamoeba histolytica*
- *Cryptosporidium* spp.
- Microsporidia
- *Leishmania* spp.
- *Strongyloides stercoralis*
- Hookworms
- *Schistosoma* spp.
- *Giardia intestinalis*
- *Trichomonas vaginalis*
- *Toxoplasma gondii*
- *Plasmodium* spp.
- *Ascaris lumbricoides*
- *Trichuris trichiura*

Molecular tests have revolutionised the diagnosis of infectious diseases and have several uses in parasitology, some of which are as follows:

- Detection of parasites which are present in the human body in low quantities and are not detectable by conventional tests (e.g., asymptomatic malaria); PCR can even detect a single parasite per μl of blood
- Detection of parasites which are difficult to culture (e.g., *Toxoplasma*, helminths)
- Identifying parasite species/genotypes, e.g., differentiating various *Plasmodium* species in blood samples and rapid detection of new species such as *Plasmodium knowlesi*
- Differentiating morphologically similar parasites, e.g., *Entamoeba histolytica* from *E. dispar* and *E. moshkovskii*
- Detection of multiple pathogens at the same time using multiplex PCR
- Genetic characterisation of parasite strains, e.g., *Cryptosporidium* spp.
- Identification of genetic markers of drug resistance
- Identification of parasites in food and water
- Surveillance of vectors for the presence of parasites, e.g., several mosquitoes are collected and tested for the presence of *Wuchereria bancrofti* to understand the transmission pattern

Table AI.1 Rapid antigen/antibody detection assays for parasitic infections

Parasite	Kit name/antigen detected
	Rapid antigen detection kits
Entamoeba histolytica	*E. histolytica* II–galactose lectin antigen
Giardia duodenalis	*Giardia* fecal antigen detection lateral flow—*Giardia* specific antigen 65
Cryptosporidium spp.	Xpect *Cryptosporidium*
Cryptosporidium spp. and *Giardia duodenalis*	ColorPAC
Cryptosporidium spp., *Giardia duodenalis* and *Entamoeba histolytica*	Triage panel
Trichomonas vaginalis	OSOM *Trichomonas*
Wuchereria bancrofti	Binax Now, OG4C3 antigen
Plasmodium spp.	HRP-II antigen for *P. falciparum-P. vivax-* or *P. falciparum*-specific LDH
	Rapid antibody detection kits
Trypanosoma cruzi (Chagas' disease)	Chagas detect Plus
Leishmania spp. (visceral leishmaniasis)	rK39 antibody detection

Steps of a PCR assay: The three steps of the PCR—denaturation, annealing and extension—constitute one cycle of the reaction. PCR is carried out in a thermocycler which enables cycling between the different temperatures required for the three steps.

- **Denaturation:** First, the two strands of the double-stranded target DNA are separated (denatured) by heating the reaction mixture to 95°C.
- **Annealing:** The temperature is then reduced to 50–60°C to allow the primer pair to bind (anneal) to the 3′ ends of the separated DNA stands.
- **Extension:** Lastly, the temperature is raised to 72°C, and the complementary DNA sequence is synthesised by the enzyme *Taq* DNA polymerase using dNTPs as the building blocks.

In each PCR cycle, the target DNA doubles (2×). Therefore, at the end of *n* cycles, the quantity of the amplified DNA is 2^n of the original target DNA concentration in the sample. To produce sufficient copies of the target DNA required for detection, about 30–40 PCR cycles are generally required. Various modifications of PCRs are used in diagnostic microbiology (Table AI.2).

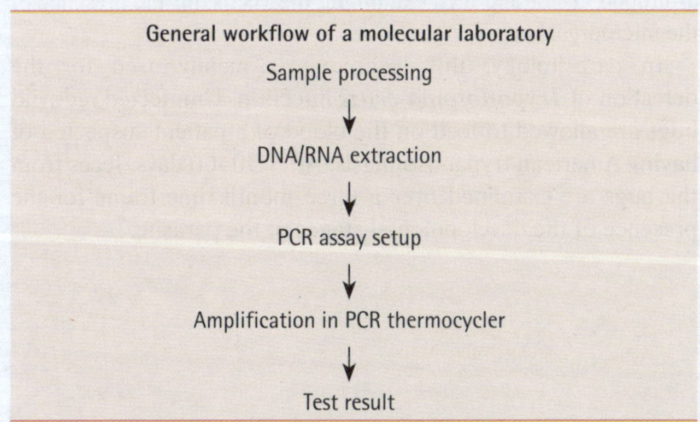

Though they have higher sensitivity and specificity than microscopy, the universal implementation of molecular diagnostics faces several challenges:

- Reagents and equipment for PCR are expensive and sophisticated compared to microscopy which is cheap and can be performed even in remote settings.
- Most molecular parasitology tests are based on in-house laboratory developed methods, and not available commercially. Recently, however, multiplex methods for gastrointestinal and respiratory infections and sepsis or fever panels have become available commercially.
- PCR is extremely sensitive and can detect the DNA of dead parasites also. Hence the results need to be interpreted cautiously.

INTRADERMAL TESTS

Intradermal skin tests have traditionally been used as an aid for indirect diagnosis of some helminthic and protozoan infections in the absence of reliable diagnostic tests (Table AI.3). These are generally based on **purified crude extracts of parasite proteins** which are inoculated intradermally, following which the immune response is read.

The test is performed by injecting the purified parasitic antigen intradermally, usually on volar aspect of the **test arm**, and observing the reaction. In an immediate hypersensitivity reaction, a wheal-and-flare reaction is observed within 30 minutes of injection, while for a delayed hypersensitivity reaction, erythema and induration are measured after 48 hours of injection. Normal saline injected on the other arm, which is used as the **control arm**, should not elicit any reaction.

ANIMAL INOCULATION

Animal models have a limited role in the diagnosis of parasitic diseases and are more commonly used for research on various microorganisms. The host specificity and complex life cycle of parasites make it even more difficult to use animals as models for parasitic diseases.

A number of animals like mice, rats, guinea pigs, hamsters, gerbils, etc., may be used for the isolation of parasites for diagnostic purposes.

1. **Leishmaniasis:** The hamster is the laboratory animal of choice for the isolation of *Leishmania* spp. from various

Table AI.2 Properties of polymerase chain reaction and its modifications

Type of PCR	Description
Conventional PCR	• Amplification of target DNA sequence using *Taq* polymerase, followed by detection of PCR product by agarose gel electrophoresis
Real-time PCR	• Real-time detection of the products of PCR amplification by detection of fluorescence signals • There is no requirement of post-amplification procedure; therefore there is less chance of cross-contamination • The specificity can be enhanced with the use of DNA probes specific to the amplified product • It can also be used for quantification of DNA in clinical samples
Nested PCR	• The first amplification of the target DNA is followed by the second amplification of an internal sequence of the amplified product • It is more specific and sensitive than conventional PCR
Reverse transcription PCR	• Amplification of RNA (RNA is first converted to a complementary DNA, which is then subjected to PCR)
Multiplex PCR	• Simultaneous amplification of two or more different target sequences of the same parasite or different parasites

Table AI.3 Intradermal skin tests to diagnose parasitic infections

Immediate hypersensitivity based	Delayed hypersensitivity based
• *Echinococcus* (Casoni's test) • *Wuchereria bancrofti, Brugia malayi* • *Trichinella spiralis* (Bachman's test) • *Schistosoma* (Fairley's test) • *Ascaris lumbricoides* (scratch test) • *Strongyloides stercoralis* • *Onchocerca volvulus* (Mazzotti's test)	• *Leishmania donovani* (Montenegro test) • *Trypanosoma*

clinical samples. The intraperitoneal inoculation of an infected specimen results in a generalised infection. Impression smears of the spleen should be examined for the presence of parasites.

2. **Toxoplasmosis:** Mice and rats are generally used for the isolation of *Toxoplasma gondii* from samples or for strain maintenance. The homogenised sample is generally inoculated intraperitoneally, which may result in a generalised fulminant infection within 5–6 days, following which the peritoneal fluid and spleen aspirates are harvested to demonstrate the tachyzoites. Alternatively, a chronic infection with persistence of tissue cysts develops, in which case, the parasites may be detected in the brain or an antibody response may be detected after 4–6 weeks.
3. **Trypanosomiasis:** A number of laboratory animals can be used for the isolation of trypanosomes. Organisms usually appear in the blood of the animals within the first week of inoculation. However, for negative samples, the animals should be re-tested at 2 and 4 weeks before the results are reported as negative.

XENODIAGNOSIS

Xenodiagnosis is a technique used to document the presence of an infectious agent by exposing the infected tissue or host to an arthropod vector and then examining the vector for the presence of the microorganism.

In parasitology, this technique is mainly used for the detection of ***Trypanosoma cruzi*** infection. Uninfected reduviid bugs are allowed to feed on the blood of a patient suspected of having American trypanosomiasis. After 30–60 days, feces from the bugs are examined over a three-month time frame for the presence of the developmental stages of the parasite.

Stains, Reagents and Culture Media

STAINS AND REAGENTS

Stains and Reagents for Fecal Specimens

Iodine solutions

Modified D'antoni's iodine	• Distilled water: 100 ml • Potassium iodide: 1 g • Powdered iodine crystals: 1.5 g 1. Grind the dry iodine and potassium iodide in a mortar. 2. Add water slowly and grind thoroughly until the iodine and iodide dissolve. 3. Store the solution in an amber glass bottle with the remainder of the distilled water. The solution is ready for use after 4–5 days. Sufficient quantity for daily use is decanted into a brown glass bottle and discarded after one day. The stock solution remains good as long as an excess of iodine remains in the bottle.
Lugol's solution	• Distilled water: 100 ml • Potassium iodide: 10 g • Iodine crystals: 5 g This stock solution of Lugol's iodine must be diluted to a 1:5 ratio for fecal wet mount examination.
Gram's iodine	• Lugol's solution: 1 part • Distilled water: 14 parts

Formalin-based preservatives for fecal specimens

10% formalin solution for preserving feces	• Formalin (neutral formaldehyde, at least 37%): 100 ml • Distilled water: 900 ml (Other concentrations can be prepared in a similar fashion directly or by diluting the 10% solution). 1. Measure the aqueous formalin solution in a graduated measuring cylinder and pour it into a bottle with a glass stopper or screw-cap. 2. Add the distilled water to the bottle and mix. **Warning:** Formalin is corrosive and poisonous.
Merthiolate-iodine-formalin (MIF)	**Solution I (stored in a brown bottle):** • Distilled water: 50 ml • Formaldehyde: 5 ml • Thimerosal (tincture of merthiolate, 1:1,000): 40 ml • Glycerine: 1 ml Combine 9.4 ml of solution I with 0.6 ml of Lugol's solution (solution II) just before use.

Modified Schaudinn's fixative

- Mercuric chloride crystals: 4.5 g
- 95% ethyl alcohol: 31 ml
- Glacial acetic acid: 5 ml

1. Dissolve the mercuric chloride in the alcohol in a 50/125 ml stoppered flask by swirling at regular intervals.
2. Add the acetic acid, stopper the bottle and mix by swirling.

Polyvinyl alcohol (PVA) fixative

- PVA powder: 5 g
- Glycerine: 1.5 ml
- Distilled water: 62.5 ml

1. In a small beaker, add the glycerine to the PVA powder and mix thoroughly with a glass rod until all particles appear coated with the glycerine.

2. Scrape the mixture into a 125 ml flask.
3. Add distilled water, stopper it and leave at room temperature for 3 hours or overnight. Swirl mixture occasionally to mix.

To obtain the full advantage of PVA fixative as a preservative, the specimen should be thoroughly mixed with the solution immediately after passage of stool before the organisms lose their characteristic morphology. Use approximately 3 parts of fixative to 1 part of feces or other material.

Sodium acetate formaldehyde (SAF) fixative

SAF can be used for both concentration and permanent stained smear.

SAF fixative:
- Sodium acetate: 1.5 g
- Acetic acid, glacial: 2 ml
- Formaldehyde (37–40% solution): 4 ml
- Distilled water: 92 ml

Mayer's albumin:
- Equal parts egg white and glycerine
  1. Put 1 drop of Mayer's albumin on a microscope slide to improve adhesion of fecal material.
  2. Add 1 drop of SAF-preserved fecal sediment from the concentration procedure.
  3. Allow the smear to dry at room temperature for 30 min prior to staining.

Advantage: Does not contain mercuric chloride as is found in Schaudinn's and PVA fixative.

Stains for intestinal parasites

Trichrome stain	The trichrome technique introduced by Wheatley (1951) is a rapid staining procedure for intestinal protozoa which gives good results for routine purposes. **Chromotrope stain:** • Chromotrope 2R: 6 g • Light green SF: 1.5 g • Fast green: 1.5 g • Phosphotungstic acid: 7 g • Acetic acid (glacial): 1 ml • Distilled water: 1,000 ml 1. Put the dry stains in a flask and add glacial acetic acid and shake to mix. 2. Allow the solution to stand for 'ripening' for 30 minutes. 3. Add distilled water. 4. The stain is good for use without diluting. **Acidified alcohol:** • 90% alcohol: 99.5 ml • Acetic acid: 0.5 ml **70% alcohol plus iodine:** This is made by adding iodine crystals to 70% alcohol until a dark colour is obtained. **Staining procedure for unpreserved specimens:** 1. Fix the smear in Schaudinn's fixative for 5 minutes at 50°C or 1 hour at room temperature. 2. Rinse in 70% alcohol plus iodine for 1 minute. 3. Rinse twice in 70% alcohol for 1 minute each. 4. Pour trichrome stain and leave for 2–8 minutes. 5. Dip in 90% acidified alcohol for 5–10 seconds. 6. Dip in 95% alcohol twice briefly. 7. Rinse with 100% alcohol for 1 minute. 8. Dip in xylene for 1–3 minutes. Step 1 may be omitted for PVA-fixed material. **Stain reactions:** • The cytoplasm of well-stained cysts and trophozoites is blue-green, tinged with purple. • The nucleus, chromatoid bodies, ingested red cells and bacteria stain red or purplish red. • Other ingested particles, such as yeasts or molds generally stain green, but variations frequently occur. • Background material usually stains green, thus contrasting with the protozoa.

	• Incomplete fixation may result in non-staining or red cysts. • Eggs and larvae stain red and contrast strongly with the green background. • Like the protozoa, the nuclei of pus cells and tissue cells stain red and the cytoplasm, green. However, the cytoplasm of these cells stain more greenish than that of the protozoa.
Modified trichrome stain for microsporidia	This staining method was developed at CDC to differentiate microsporidia spores from background fecal elements. This staining method is based on the fact that stain penetration of the microsporidial spore is more difficult. On using this stain, microsporidial spores appear as refractile, ovoid structures with bright pinkish spore walls. The polar tubule appears as a horizontal or diagonal stripe. Bacteria and debris usually take up a green colour. **Warning:** Glacial acetic acid is highly corrosive. • Absolute methanol • Chromotrope stain: Chromotrope 2R: 6 g Fast green: 0.15 g Phosphotungstic acid: 0.70 g Glacial acetic acid: 3 ml Put the dry stains in a flask and add glacial acetic acid and shake to mix. Allow the solution to stand for 'ripening' for 30 minutes. Add 100 ml of distilled water. This stain is good for use without diluting. • Acid alcohol: 90% ethanol: 995.5 ml Glacial acetic acid: 4.5 ml • 95% ethanol • 100% ethanol • Xylene or xylene substitute **Staining procedure:** 1. Prepare a smear by spreading the fecal material and air dry the smear. 2. Fix smear in absolute methanol for 5 minutes. 3. Place in chromotrope stain for 90 minutes. 4. De-stain with acid alcohol for only 1 to 3 seconds. 5. Rinse in 95% ethanol by dipping. 6. Place in two changes of 100% ethanol for 3 minutes each. 7. Place in two changes of xylene or xylene substitute for 10 minutes each. 8. Examine smear after drying with at least 100× objective oil immersion or higher. 9. Examine at least 200 to 300 oil immersion fields.
Iron-hematoxylin stain	This stain has been used to describe most of the original morphologic descriptions of intestinal protozoa. On using this stain, the cytoplasm of trophozoites appears bluish-grey, while the cysts appear darker. The nuclei and inclusions also take up a dark grey shade. **Solution 1:** • Hematoxylin (crystal or powder): 10 g • Absolute ethanol: 1 l Place solution in a stoppered clear flask or bottle, and allow to ripen in a lighted room for at least 1 week at room temperature. **Solution 2:** • Ferrous ammonium sulfate: 10 g • Ferric ammonium sulfate: 10 g • Hydrochloric acid (concentrated): 10 ml • Distilled water: 1 l **Working solution:** • Mix equal volumes of solutions 1 and 2. The working solution should be made fresh every week. **Staining procedure:** 1. Make a smear from stool fixed in Schaudinn's fixative/PVA. 2. Place slide in 70% ethanol for 5 min. 3. Place slide in 70% ethanol and iodine for 5 min. 4. Place slide in 70% ethanol for 5 min. 5. Rinse in running tap water for 10 min. 6. Place in iron hematoxylin working solution for 4–5 min. 7. Rinse in running tap water for 10 min.

	8. Place in 70% ethanol for 5 min. 9. Place in 95% ethanol for 5 min. 10. Place in 100% ethanol for 3–5 min. 11. Place slide in Xylene or xylene substitute for 5–10 min. 12. Allow slides to air dry with no coverslip.
Calcofluor white staining	This chemofluorescent technique is useful for the detection of microsporidia, *Acanthamoeba* spp. and *Pneumocystis jiroveci*. Chemifluorescent agents, such as Calcofluor, Fungi-Fluor or Uvitex 2B, also known as optical brightening agents, are rapid and inexpensive screening agents. However, these are non-specific since many objects and organisms other than parasites may fluoresce. This is usually used as a quick screening tool and not for specific identification. • Calcofluor white reagent 0.01% • Prepare a 0.01% solution in 0.1M Tris-buffered saline, pH 7.2 • Absolute methanol **Staining procedure:** 1. Prepare a thin smear of fecal culture or other sample material. 2. Heat fix on a slide warmer at 60°C until completely dry (5–10 minutes). 3. Fix the smear in methanol for 30 seconds. 4. Stain with 0.01% calcofluor white reagent for 1 minute. 5. Rinse with distilled water and let the smear dry and mount with a cover slip. 6. Examine with a fluorescent microscope equipped with a blue violet filter with a wavelength of 400 nm or less. 7. To screen for microsporidia, examine the smear with a 50× or 100× oil immersion objectives. The microsporidia spores will fluoresce a brilliant blue-white colour against a black background.
Modified Kinyoun's acid-fast stain	Coccidia (*Cryptosporidium, Cyclospora* and *Cystoisospora*) do not stain well with iron hematoxylin or trichrome, but they may be identified using a modified Kinyoun's acid-fast stain, in which they take up a pink to red colour, while yeasts and most other materials stain blue. **Kinyoun's carbol-fuchsin stain:** • Basic fuchsin: 4 g • Phenol (liquefied): 8 g • 95% ethyl alcohol: 20 ml • Distilled water: 100 ml • Dissolve fuchsin in alcohol, add liquefied phenol, mix well and then add water. **Counterstain:** • Alkaline methylene blue: 0.3 g • 95% ethanol: 30 ml • Potassium hydroxide 0.01%: 100 ml • Dissolve methylene blue in 95% ethanol and then add 100 ml of dilute potassium hydroxide. **Staining procedure:** 1. Make a fecal smear on a slide and allow it to air dry. 2. Fix with absolute methanol for 1 minute. 3. Flood the slide with Kinyoun's carbol fuchsin and stain it for 5 minutes. 4. Rinse the slide rapidly for 3–5 seconds with 50% ethanol. 5. Rinse the slide thoroughly with water. 6. Decolorise with 1% sulphuric acid for 2 minutes or until no more colour runs from the slide. 7. Rinse the slide with water. 8. Counterstain with methylene blue for 1 minute. 9. Rinse the slide with water and air dry and examine under 10×, 40× and oil immersion fields.

Stains and Reagents for Blood Specimens

Romanowsky stains

Romanowsky stains such as Giemsa, Wright and Leishman stains have been used since the 19th century to appreciate normal and pathological cells of blood and the bone marrow. This is attributed to the property of the highly polychromic effect of the stain components on different parts of the body cells. The formation of the purple colour, i.e., the Romanowsky-Giemsa effect, is peculiar to these stains.

The erythrocytes and eosinophil granules stain red, lymphocyte cytoplasm stains blue, nuclear chromatin, neutrophil granules, and platelets stain intensely purple with these stains. This differential staining is also useful for identifying parasites like *Plasmodium*,

Leishmania, *Trypanosoma* and microfilariae in the blood and bone marrow smears. Some other stains like Field's stain and Jaswant Singh and Bhattacharji stain (JSB) are also used, especially in the field setup as they are rapid, but they fade rapidly and do not stain Schüffner's dots very well.

Giemsa stain	Giemsa is the standard stain used for routine staining of blood films for malaria diagnosis. However, the quality of this stain in readymade solution or powder form varies according to its source of supply; hence it is advisable to obtain it from a reputed source. Even then, each batch should be tested for stain quality. **Stock solution:** • Giemsa powder: 3.8 g • Methanol: 250 ml • Glycerol: 250 ml • Glass beads (5 mm diameter): 50 approximately 1. Put the glass beads in a dark bottle, pour in the measured amount of methanol and add the stain powder. 2. Tightly stopper the bottle. Allow the stain to sink slowly through the methanol until it settles to the bottom. 3. Shake the bottle in a circular motion for 2–3 minutes. 4. Add the measured amount of glycerol and repeat the shaking process. 5. Continue to shake for 2–3 minutes at half-hourly intervals; do this at least six times. 6. Let the solution stand in the bottle for 2–3 days, shaking it 3–4 times a day until the stain is thoroughly mixed. Each newly prepared batch of stain should be properly labelled with the date of preparation. It should be tested for optimum dilution and staining time. The bottle should be kept tightly stoppered in a cool place and away from direct sunlight. Stock bottles should be covered with a thick dark paper to keep out the light. **Staining procedure:** **Thin blood smears** 1. Fix the smear by adding 3 drops of methanol or by dipping it in a container of methanol for a few seconds and allow to air dry. 2. Stain with Giemsa working solution (dilute the Giemsa stain 1:10 in neutral or faintly alkaline water, pH 7–7.2) for 30–45 minutes. 3. Rinse gently with phosphate buffer or tap water and air dry. **Thick blood smears** Since a thick smear is layered and thick, parasites cannot be visualised unless hemoglobin is removed from the RBCs by dehemoglobinisation before the slide is fixed with methanol. Dehemoglobinisation may be carried out with the following solution: • Mixture of glacial acetic and tartaric acid • Tap or distilled water • Saponin 1. Dehemoglobinise the slide for a few minutes till the smear becomes grey or white. 2. Allow the thick film to dry thoroughly; drying may be hastened by fanning or briefly exposing the slide to gentle heat such as that from the microscope lamp. 3. Care should be taken to avoid overheating, otherwise the thick film will be heat-fixed. 4. Other steps are same as those involved in staining a thin smear.
Leishman's stain	• Leishman's stain (powder): 150 mg • Methanol (pure): 100 ml 1. Dissolve stain in methanol. 2. Keep the stain in a glass, stoppered brown bottle. 3. Keep the stain in a place with plenty of sunlight or in an incubator (37°C) for 1 hour for 3 days for the maturation of the stain.
Jaswant-Singh-Bhattacharji (JSB) stain	It is a rapid Romanowsky's staining method for malarial parasites. **Solution I** • Methylene blue: 0.5 g • Potassium dichromate: 0.5 g • Sulphuric acid 1%: 3 ml • Potassium hydroxide 1%: 10 ml • Water: 500 ml **Solution II** • Eosin: 1 g • Tap water: 500 ml

	Staining procedure: **Thin blood smears** 1. Immerse the slide in methanol for a few seconds to 1 minute to fix the smear and then air dry. 2. Immerse the slide in solution I for 30 seconds and then wash with water for a few seconds. 3. Immerse the slide in solution II for 1 second, then wash with water (pH 6.2–6.6) for 4 seconds. 4. Immerse the slide in solution I again for 30 seconds, then wash with water till the smear develops a pink background. **Thick blood smears** 1. The smear is not fixed with methanol to permit dehemoglobinisation. 2. All other steps are same as those involved in staining a thin smear.

CULTURE METHODS

Some parasites can be grown in diphasic or monophasic media, media containing other microorganisms, or axenic cultures.

TYIS-33 medium for axenic culture	For *Entamoeba* and *Trichomonas* **Stock solution:** • TYI-S-33 broth base with 10% bovine serum: 1 bottle • Distilled water: 55 ml 1. Dispense 13 ml medium per tube into 16 × 125 mm screw-capped culture tubes. 2. Tubes may be stored at ambient temperature (25°C) for up to 90 days or at 2–8° C for longer. 3. Inoculate a small amount of the feces or vaginal fluid into the medium. 4. Add antibiotics, i.e., 100 international units (IU) of penicillin and 100 μg of streptomycin per ml of medium. Gentamicin, 50 μg/ml, may be used as a substitute for penicillin and streptomycin. 5. Incubate at 37°C and examine after 2, 3 and 4 days of incubation by removing small amount of sediment with a pipette. 6. Transfer the sediment onto a slide, cover it with a cover slip and examine under low-power.
Modified Boeck and Drbohlav's/Locke-egg-serum (LES) medium	For *Entamoeba* and *Giardia* This is basically an egg slant with an overlay of sterile serum or liver extract in buffered saline. **Locke's solution:** • Sodium chloride: 9 g • Calcium chloride: 0.2 g • Potassium chloride: 0.4 g • Sodium bicarbonate: 0.2 g • Glucose: 2.5 g • Distilled water: 1 l This solution should be autoclaved before storage. LES medium is prepared as follows: 1. Wash four eggs, brush with alcohol to sterilise, and break into a sterile flask containing glass beads. 2. Add 50 ml Locke's solution and shake until the mixture is homogenous. 3. Dispense sufficient quantities into test tubes to make 2.5 to 3.5 cm slants at the bottom of the tubes. 4. Plug the tubes and place the tubes in slanting position in an inspissator at 70°C until the slants are solidified. 5. Once the slants solidify, autoclave at 15 pounds pressure for 20 minutes. 6. Cover slants to a depth of about 1 cm with a mixture of 8 parts sterile Locke's solution and 1 part sterile inactivated human blood serum. Sterility of mixture of Locke's solution and serum should be ensured by filtration and followed by incubation at 37°C for 24 hours or longer before use. 7. Add a loopful of sterile rice starch or powder to each tube before inoculation. 8. Inoculate with a portion of pea-sized stool sample, break up well in the medium, and incubate at 37 °C. 9. Examine after 2, 3 and 4 days of incubation by removing a small amount of the overlay each time. Note: This is a xenic medium and antibiotics are not added.

Novy-Nicolle-McNeal (NNN) culture medium	In vitro cultivation of *Leishmania* or *Trypanosoma*. It is a biphasic medium, wherein the agar slant is the solid phase and the water of condensation forms the liquid phase of the medium. • Difco blood agar base: 8 g • Distilled water: 200 ml • Defibrinated rabbit blood: 0.6 ml in each 5 ml of medium Preparation of defibrinated rabbit blood: 1. Collect 20 ml of rabbit blood, preferably from the heart, in a flask containing 50–100 glass beads. 2. Defibrinate the blood by rotating the flask for 5 minutes. 3. Add antibiotics, i.e., 200 IU of penicillin, 200 mg of gentamicin and 2 mg of streptomycin per ml of blood. The medium should be prepared in aseptic conditions. 1. Pour 200 ml of water into a flask, add the agar to the water, mix and warm the flask in boiling water until the agar is completely dissolved. 2. Dispense the medium in 5 ml amounts into screw-capped bottles (of 20 ml capacity). 3. Sterilise by autoclaving (with caps loosened) at 121°C for 15 minutes and allow the agar to cool to 45–50°C. 4. Add 0.6 ml of sterile defibrinated rabbit blood to each bottle during cooling and mix gently. 5. Allow the medium to solidify as a slant by keeping it on an inclined surface. 6. Leave the bottles in an upright position at room temperature for 24 hours to allow fluid condensation to form. 7. The bottles should be stored at 4–6°C until required. **Culture method:** 1. Inoculate about 0.1 ml of specimen aseptically into the fluid of condensation in 2 bottles at room temperature. 2. Incubate the cultures at 24°C (±2°C) in the dark. 3. Examine every 4 days. 4. Transfer a drop of the culture using a sterile wire loop to a slide to examine for promastigotes. 5. Negative cultures must be sub-cultured weekly into fresh media and examined every 4 days for 4 weeks of incubation.
Non-nutrient agar (NNA) medium	For *Acanthamoeba* and *Naegleria* **Non-nutrient agar (NNA):** • Sodium phosphate: 0.0142 g • Potassium phosphate: 0.0136 g • Sodium chloride: 0.012 g • Magnesium sulfate: 0.0004 g • Calcium chloride: 0.0004 g • Agar: 15 g • Final pH 7.0+/–0.2 **Page's saline** • Sodium phosphate: 0.142 g • Potassium phosphate: 0.136 g • Sodium chloride: 0.12 g • Magnesium sulfate: 0.004 g • Calcium chloride: 0.004 g • Final pH 6.8+/–0.2 **Preparation of NNA *E. coli* plates:** 1. Place NNA plates in a 35–37°C incubator for approximately 30 minutes. 2. While the plates are incubating, prepare a heavy suspension (equivalent to a 4.0 McFarland turbidity standard or higher) of *E. coli* in Page's saline. 3. Pipette 2–3 drops of the suspension onto the surface of each warmed plate and spread using an L-shaped spreader. 4. If not used for testing at the time of preparation, these plates may be stored at 2–8°C and should be used for testing within 1 week of inoculation. **Preparation of sample:** **CSF samples:** 1. Centrifuge sample for 10 minutes at 250×g. 2. Inoculate the sediment in previously prepared NNA *E. coli* plates. Do not spread.

	3. Incubate the plates (inoculated media side down) overnight at 30–32°C and 35–37°C, allowing excess fluid to evaporate. 4. After initial incubation, seal NNA plates with a parafilm strip and continue incubation. 5. Beginning on the second day of incubation, examine the surface of the agar using an inverted or traditional microscope with a 10× objective for feeding tracks. Amoebae should be present at one end of each track. If no tracks are visible, continue to examine daily for up to 10 days before reporting the sample as negative for amebae. 6. Additionally, a loop can be used to scrape the agar where amoebae are located, and inoculate in 1 ml of Page's saline or water. 7. After incubation at room temperature for 3–20 hours, a wet mount can be made, viewed under oil-immersion using phase microscopy and observed for pear-shaped flagellates characteristic of *N. fowleri*.
Trager and Jensen medium	**For *Plasmodium falciparum* cultivation** Culture of *Plasmodium* remains fundamentally a research technique. It is difficult to establish and maintain *Plasmodium* spp. in vitro. The breakthrough in cultivation of malarial parasites came in 1976 when **Trager** and **Jensen** successfully maintained *P. falciparum* in continuous cultures in human erythrocytes using **Roswell Park Memorial Institute** (RPMI) 1640 medium. Other species of *Plasmodium* are difficult to maintain in vitro for long term. • This employs a HEPES-buffered RPMI 1640, a tissue culture medium supplemented with human serum, erythrocytes, and sodium bicarbonate. • Parasites are cultured in a continuous flow medium in an atmosphere of 7% CO_2, 1% O_2 and 92% N_2.

Drug Therapy for Parasitic Infections

Parasite (in alphabetical order)	Drug therapy
Acanthamoeba	**Granulomatous amoebic encephalitis** **Combination therapy:** • Cotrimoxazole: 20 mg/kg/day, rifampicin 10 mg/kg/day and ketoconazole 5 mg/kg/day until there is clinical improvement **Amoebic keratitis** **Drug of choice:** • Topical 0.02% polyhexamethylene biguanide **Alternate drug:** • 0.02% chlorhexidine in combination with 0.1% propamidine isethionate × 3–4 weeks or longer **Surgery:** Therapeutic penetrating keratoplasty
Angiostrongylus	**Drug of choice:** • No drug is 100% effective, but mebendazole 100 mg BDS × 5 days may be attempted • Symptomatic therapy should be given
Ascaris lumbricoides (roundworm)	• Albendazole: Adults and children >2 yr, 400 mg oral or 10 ml 4% suspension single dose; children 1–2 yr, 200 mg oral or 5 ml 4% suspension single dose • Mebendazole: 500 mg single dose or 100 mg BDS × 3 days • Pyrantel pamoate: 11 mg/kg (maximum 1 g) in a single dose
Balantidium coli	**Drug of choice:** • Metronidazole: Adults, 750 mg TDS oral × 5 days; children, 10–20 mg/kg body weight TDS × 5 days (maximum 2 g) **Alternate drug:** • Tetracyclines: Adults, 500 mg QID × 10 days; children, 10 mg/kg QID × 10 days
Clonorchis and *Opisthorchis*	**Drug of choice:** • Praziquantel: 25–75 mg/kg TDS × 2–3 days **Alternate drug:** • Albendazole: 10 mg/kg/day × 7 days **Surgery:** Complete resection for cholangiocarcinoma
Cryptosporidium parvum	**Drug of choice:** • Nitazoxanide: Adults, 500 mg BDS oral × 3 days, children >4 years, 200 mg BDS, and <4 years 100 mg BDS × 3 days **Alternate drug:** • Paromomycin: Oral 25–35 mg/kg/day × 14 days **HIV-AIDS patients:** • Anti-parasitic drugs not efficacious • HAART with a protease inhibitor in addition to nitazoxanide **Supportive management:** • Replacement of fluids and electrolytes
Cyclospora cayetanensis	**Drug of choice:** • Trimethoprim–sulphamethoxazole (TMP-SMX): Adults, 160/800 mg BDS × 7–10 days; children, 5/25 mg/kg BDS × 7–10 days • Recurrent symptomatic cyclosporiasis in AIDS patients may be administered secondary prophylaxis with TMP-SMX three times a week indefinitely **Alternate drug:** • Ciprofloxacin: 500 mg BDS × 7 days in patients allergic to sulfonamides **Supportive management:** • Electrolytes and fluids

Cystoisospora belli	**Drug of choice:** • Trimethoprim–sulphamethoxazole (TMP-SMX): Adults, 160/800 mg QID × 10 days followed by suppressive therapy with TMP-SMX 160/800 mg BDS × 21 days **Alternate drug:** • Pyrimethamine: 75 mg/day together with folinic acid 25 mg/day × 7–10 days • Ciprofloxacin: 500 mg BDS × 7 days
Diphyllobothrium latum	**Drug of choice:** • Praziquantel: 5–10 mg/kg body weight, single oral dose for both adults and children **Alternate drug:** • Niclosamide: Adults, single dose of 2 g (4 tablets chewed thoroughly); children <6 years, 50 mg/kg single dose **Supportive management:** • Parenteral vitamin B12 should be given if B12 deficiency is documented
Dirofilaria	**Surgery:** Removal of the worm is the only treatment
Dracunculus medinensis	• **Worm removal:** The affected body part is immersed in water every day to encourage more of the worm to come out. The exposed part of the worm is tied with a fine silk thread fastened to a rod or stick. By winding the thread around the rod/stick, the worm is slowly and gently pulled out over a period of 15–20 days. • **Anthelmintic drugs:** Drug therapy is not very useful. • **Supportive management:** Wet compresses may be applied to the affected skin, and anti-inflammatory drugs and topical antibiotics may be used to prevent secondary bacterial infections.
Echinococcus granulosus	**Drug treatment** **Drug of choice:** • Albendazole: Adults, 400 mg BDS; children, 10–15 mg/kg/day in 2 divided doses (maximum 800 mg) ×3–6 months has a cure rate of 30% **Alternate drug:** • Mebendazole: 40–50 mg/kg/day in 3 divided doses (if albendazole is not well-tolerated) **Surgery** • Total or partial cystectomy or hepatectomy for large or operable liver cysts **PAIR** (**p**uncture, **a**spiration, **i**njection and **r**e-aspiration) **Percutaneous thermal ablation** **Wait-and-watch**
Echinococcus multilocularis	**Surgery** • Resection of early lesions **Drug treatment** **Drug of choice:** • Albendazole: Adults, 400 mg BDS; children, 10–15 mg/kg/day in 2 divided doses (maximum 800 mg) × at least 2 years or even longer **Alternate drug:** • Patients monitored for side effects of prolonged administration of albendazole and switched to mebendazole, 40–50 mg/kg/day in 3 divided doses if not well-tolerated **Wait-and-watch**
Entamoeba histolytica	**Luminal agent (for amoebic dysentery; asymptomatic carriage or along with treatment with tissue-active agent in amoebic liver abscess (ALA) or colitis** **Drug of choice:** • Paromomycin: Adults, 30 mg/kg/day oral in divided doses TDS × 5–10 days; children, 25 mg/kg/day oral in divided doses TDS × 5–10 days **Alternate drugs:** • Diloxanide furoate: Adults 500 mg oral TDS ×10 days; children 20 mg/kg/day oral in divided doses TDS × 10 days • Iodoquinol: 650 mg TDS × 20 days **Tissue-active agent (for amoebic colitis and ALA)** **Drug of choice:** • Metronidazole: Adults, 750 mg TDS oral or IV × 5–10 days; children, 50 mg/kg/day oral in divided doses TDS × 10 days

	• Tinidazole: Adults, 2 g once daily oral × 3–5 days; children, 60 mg/kg/day oral in divided doses TDS × 5 days **Alternate drug:** • Nitazoxanide: Adults, 500 mg BDS oral × 3 days; children >4 yr, 200 mg BDS, <4 years 100 mg BDS × 3 days
***Enterobius vermicularis* (pinworm)**	• Albendazole: 400 mg single dose • Mebendazole: 100 mg single dose • Pyrantel pamoate: 11 mg/kg (maximum 1 g) single dose • A second course of treatment administered after 2 weeks; household contacts should also be treated
Fasciola hepatica	**Drug of choice:** • Triclabendazole: 10 mg/kg single dose. **Alternate drugs:** • Nitazoxanide: 500 mg/day BDS × 7 days • Bithionol: 30–50 mg/kg on alternate days × 10–15 doses **Surgery:** ERCP (Endoscopic retrograde cholangiopancreatography) for biliary obstruction
Fasciolopsis buski	**Drug of choice:** • Praziquantel: 25 mg/kg/day TDS × 1 day in both children and adults
Giardia duodenalis	**First-line:** • Tinidazole: Adults, 2 g oral single dose; children, 50 mg/kg single dose • Metronidazole: Adults, 250–500 mg oral TDS × 7–10–14 days or 2 g daily × 3 days; children, 5 mg/kg TDS × 10–14 days or 35–40 mg/kg daily for 3 days **Second-line:** • Albendazole: Adults, 400 mg QID × 5 days; children, 15 mg/kg × 5–7 days • Nitazoxanide: Adults, 500 mg BDS x 3 days; children, 200 mg BDS x 3 days • Paramomycin: Adults, 500 mg TDS × 5–10 days; children, 10 mg/kg TDS × 5–10 days
Hookworms (*Necator americana* and *Ancylostoma duodenale*)	• Albendazole: Adults and children > 2 yr, 400 mg oral or 10 ml 4% suspension single dose; children 1–2 yr: 200 mg oral or 5 ml 4% suspension single dose • Mebendazole: 500 mg BDS × 3 days • Pyrantel pamoate: 11 mg/kg × 3 days **Supportive treatment:** • Iron and nutritional supplements
Hymenolepis nana	**Drug of choice:** • Praziquantel: 25 mg/kg body weight single oral dose, both for adults and children; household contacts should also be treated
Larva migrans (cutaneous larva migrans, *Ancylostoma* spp.)	**Drug of choice:** • Ivermectin: 200 μg/kg once or twice **Alternate drugs:** • Albendazole: 400–800 mg/day × 3–5 days • Topical application of 10–15% thiabendazole is also used **Supportive management:** • Antihistaminics or topical anesthetics
Larva migrans (visceral, *Toxocara* spp.)	• Albendazole: 15 mg/kg × 5 days or mebendazole 20–25 mg/kg × 21 days are commonly used despite their limited efficacy against larvae in tissues • Surgery required in ocular larva migrans along with anthelmintic drugs
Leishmaniasis (visceral)	**Drugs of choice:** • Amphotericin: Liposomal amphotericin B 10 mg/kg in a single dose by infusion or 3 mg/kg daily on days 1 to 5, 14, and 21 (total dose 10–15 mg/kg) OR • Amphotericin B deoxycholate: 0.5–1 mg/kg per day by infusion, daily or on alternate days × 15–20 doses (this is currently the recommended first-line treatment in Bihar, India) • Miltefosine: Adults, 100 mg/day; children, 2.5 mg/kg/day × 28 days • Pentavalent antimonial sodium stibogluconate (SbV): 20 mg/kg/day IM or IV × 20–28 days • Combination (co-administered): Miltefosine, 2.5 mg/kg/day plus paromomycin, 11 mg/kg/day, both daily for 10 days

	Alternate drug: • Pentamidine: 2–4 mg/kg/day IV or IM up to 15 doses **Adjuvant immunotherapy:** IFNγ gamma in combination with pentavalent antimony has been used with success
Leishmaniasis (post-kala-azar dermal leishmaniasis)	Longer duration of treatment is required • Miltefosine: 150 mg/day orally × 12 weeks • Amphotericin B deoxycholate: 1 mg/kg/day by infusion, up to 60–80 doses over 4 months • Liposomal amphotericin B: 2.5 mg/kg/day IV × 20 days
Leishmaniasis (cutaneous)	**Topical:** • Intralesional injection of a pentavalent antimonial • Ointment containing 15% paromomycin sulfate • Adjuvant immunotherapy with topical imiquimod (5–7.5%) plus parenteral antimonials • Heat therapy with an FDA-approved radiofrequency generator • Cryotherapy with liquid nitrogen **Systemic:** • Pentavalent antimonial: 20 mg/kg × 20 days • Fluconazole: 200 mg/day orally × 4–6 weeks • Ketoconazole: 600 mg/day orally × 4–6 weeks • Miltefosine: 2.5 mg/kg × 4–6 weeks • Amphotericin B deoxycholate: 1 mg/kg IV on alternate days (a total of 25–45 mg/kg max.) • Liposomal amphotericin B: 2–3 mg/kg/day IV (a total of 6–10 doses)
Leishmaniasis (mucocutaneous)	**First-line:** • Pentavalent antimonial (SbV): 20 mg/kg IV or IM × 4 weeks **Second-line:** • Amphotericin B: 0.5–1mg/kg IV daily (a total up to 25–45 mg/kg) • Liposomal amphotericin B: 2–3 mg/kg/day × 20 days • Miltefosine: 2.5 mg/kg × 4 weeks
Lice infestation (human pediculosis, pthriasis)	**Topical:** • Malathion: 0.5% shampoo for persons above 6 months of age, applied topically and washed after 8 hours; second application after 7–10 days • Natural pyrethrins: 0.33% pyrethrins plus 4% piperonyl butoxide shampoo for persons of 2 years of age or above, applied topically and washed after 24 hours; second application after 7–10 days • Synthetic pyrethroids: 1% permethrin cream for persons of 2 years of age or above, topically applied and washed after 24 hours; second application after 7–10 days • Ivermectin: 0.8% shampoo • Lindane: 1% lotion/shampoo (only in those resistant to other regimens) **Systemic:** • Ivermectin: 200 μg/kg oral, single dose; repeated after 10 days **Supportive management:** • Wet hair should be carefully combed with fine-toothed nit comb • For body lice infestation, first bath with soap and water for body lice infestation, followed by application of drug preparation • Close contacts should be checked carefully and treated if infested
Loa loa	**Drug of choice:** • Diethylcarbamazine (DEC): 8–10 mg/kg/day in 3 doses × 3 weeks is effective against both the adult and microfilarial forms; multiple courses may be required **Alternate drug:** • Albendazole: 200 mg BDS × 3 weeks **Surgery:** Extraction of adult worms from the eye
Malaria (uncomplicated, *Plasmodium vivax*)	• Chloroquine: 25 mg/kg divided over 3 days (10 mg/kg on day 1, 10 mg/kg on day 2, 5 mg/kg on day 3) PLUS • Primaquine: 0.25 mg/kg daily for 14 days to prevent relapse Note: Primaquine is contraindicated in pregnant females, infants and those with G6PD deficiency

Malaria (uncomplicated, *P. falciparum*)	**Indian states other than North Eastern states** • Artemisinin combination therapy (ACT): Artesunate, 4 mg/kg/day × 3 days and sulphadoxine, 25 mg/kg + pyrimethamine 1.25 mg/kg × 1 day (ACT-SP) PLUS • Primaquine: 0.75 mg/kg administer single dose on day 2 **North Eastern states of India (due to resistance to SP)** • Artemether: 20 mg + lumefantrine 120 mg (ACT-AL) • Primaquine: 0.75 mg/kg; administer a single dose on day 2 **Pregnant women** • 1st trimester: Quinine, 10 mg/kg TDS × 7 days • 2nd and 3rd trimester: ACT as per geographical location
Malaria (severe and complicated)	**Initial parenteral treatment for at least 48 hours – CHOOSE ONE of following four options:** • Quinine salt: 20 mg/kg on admission IV infusion or divided IM injection, followed by maintenance dose of 10 mg/kg 8 hourly; infusion rate should not exceed 5 mg/kg per hour • Artesunate: 2.4 mg/kg IV or IM administered on admission, then at 12 hr and 24 hr, then once a day • Artemether: 3.2 mg/kg IM administered on admission, then 1.6 mg/kg per day • Arteether: 150 mg IM daily × 3 days, in adults only (not recommended for children) **Follow-up treatment** – when patient can take oral medication following parenteral treatment: • Quinine: 10 mg/kg TDS with doxycycline, 100 mg OD or clindamycin (in pregnant women and children under 8 years of age); to complete 7 days of treatment **Full oral course of area-specific ACT** In North Eastern states: • ACT-AL for 3 days + PQ single dose on 2nd day In other states: • ACT-SP for 3 days + PQ single dose on 2nd day
Mansonella	**Drug of choice:** • *Mansonella perstans:* Combination therapy of DEC plus mebendazole is preferred; thiabendazole is also found effective to reduce microfilaraemia; there are no definite guidelines • *Mansonella ozzardi:* Ivermectin 150 μg/kg single dose has shown good efficacy; optimal treatment not clear • *Mansonella streptocerca:* Ivermectin 150 μg/kg single dose is effective; DEC 6 mg/kg/day orally in 3 doses ×12 days has also been used effectively
Myiasis	**Extraction of fly larvae** • **Surgical removal** followed by daily cleaning of the wound • Occluding respiratory spiracles of maggots by coating wound with petroleum ointment (Vaseline) • Tetanus prophylaxis • Treatment of secondary bacterial infections • Taking care of untreated and open wounds with proper hygiene
Naegleria fowleri	**Drug of choice:** • Amphotericin B (AmB): 1–15 mg/kg/day IV × 3 days, followed by 1 mg/kg/day × 6 days; intrathecal AmB should be considered
Onchocerca volvulus	**Drug of choice:** • Ivermectin: 150 μg/kg orally in a single dose, either yearly or semi-annually; active against the microfilariae but not against the adult worms • Contraindicated in areas of Africa co-endemic for *O. volvulus* and *Loa loa*
Paragonimus westermani	**Drug of choice:** • Praziquantel: 25 mg/kg body weight orally TDS × 3 days **Alternate drug:** • Bithionol: 30–50 mg/kg on alternate days × 10–15 doses
Scabies	**Topical:** • Permethrin: 5% cream for persons aged 2 months or older; applied topically from neck downwards and washed after 8–14 hr; second application after 7 days • Alternate preparations: 1% lindane, 10–25% benzoyl benzoate, 10% crotamiton, 5–10% sulphur ointment, 0.5–1% malathion and 0.8% ivermectin lotion

	Systemic: • Ivermectin: 200 μg/kg oral, single dose (can be considered in those with severe burning sensation to permethrin); superior cure rates with a second dose after 15 days; recommended for epidemic scabies in institutions **Supportive management:** • Close contacts should be treated simultaneously • Clothing and bedding of infected persons must be discarded or machine washed at 60ºC or higher temperature
***Schistosoma* spp.**	**Drug of choice:** • Praziquantel: 40–60 mg/kg in single or 1–3 divided doses in 1 day
Strongyloides stercoralis	**Drug of choice:** • Ivermectin: 200 μg/kg oral for 2 days in uncomplicated strongyloidiasis, and for 7 days or more in hyperinfection syndrome • Thiabendazole: 25 mg/kg twice daily **Alternate drug:** • Albendazole: 400 mg twice a day for 10–14 days (less effective)
***Taenia solium* (intestinal taeniasis)**	**Drug of choice:** • Niclosamide: 2 g single dose for adults • Praziquantel: 5–10 mg/kg single dose for both children and adults
***Taenia solium* (cysticercosis)**	**Drug treatment** **Anti-parasitic agents:** • Albendazole: 15 mg/kg/day divided into 2 daily doses for 10–14 days for 1–2 viable parenchymal cysts • Praziquantel (in combination with albendazole): 50 mg/kg/day for 10–14 days for more than 2 viable parenchymal cysts **Symptomatic treatment:** • Anti-epileptic drugs for seizure control • Adjunctive corticosteroid therapy; methotrexate may be considered as a steroid-sparing agent when prolonged anti-inflammatory therapy is required **Surgery** • Removal of cyst is considered in severe extra-parenchymal disease, intraocular and spinal lesions • Shunt may be required for obstructive hydrocephalus
***Toxoplasma gondii* (pregnant women)**	**Infection <18 weeks of gestation:** • Spiramycin: 1 g TDS until delivery **Infection >18 weeks of gestation:** • Pyrimethamine: 50 mg BDS × 2 days followed by 50 mg daily PLUS • Sulfadiazine: 75 mg/kg initial dose, followed by 50 mg/kg BDS (maximum 4 g/day) PLUS • Folinic acid (leucovorin): 10–20 mg daily (during and 1 week after completion of pyrimethamine therapy)
***Toxoplasma gondii* (congenital toxoplasmosis)**	• Pyrimethamine: 1 mg/kg PLUS • Sulfadiazine: 100 mg/kg PLUS • Folinic acid Continued for at least one year
***Toxoplasma gondii* (ocular toxoplasmosis)**	• Pyrimethamine: 100 mg OD for 1 or 2 days and then 25–50 mg OD PLUS • Sulfadiazine: 1 g QID (OR Clindamycin: 1 mg intravitreal) PLUS • Folinic acid: 10–20 mg OD +/– • Prednisolone: 1 mg QID may be administered for a short time Continued for at least 1–2 weeks after resolution of symptoms

***Toxoplasma gondii* (AIDS)**	• Pyrimethamine: 200 mg loading dose, then 50–75 mg OD PLUS • Sulfadiazine: 1 g QID PLUS • Folinic acid: 10–25 mg OD Continued for at least 4–6 weeks after resolution of signs and symptoms followed by secondary prophylaxis **Secondary prophylaxis** **Drug of choice:** • Trimethoprim-sulfamethoxazole (cotrimoxazole): 160/800 mg daily
Trichinella spiralis	**Intestinal phase:** • Mebendazole: 200–400 mg oral TDS × 3 days, followed by 400–500 mg oral TDS × 10 days • Albendazole: 400 mg oral BDS × 8–14 days **Systemic disease:** • There is no data for efficacy of any drug regime in systemic illness. • Corticosteroids and anti-inflammatory agents administered in conjunction with mebendazole or albendazole in severe disease × 8–14 days.
Trichomonas vaginalis	**Oral therapy** **Drug of choice:** • Metronidazole: 2 g single dose or 500 mg BDS × 7 days OR • Tinidazole: 2 g single dose **Topical therapy** • Metronidazole: 500 mg vaginal tablets OD × 10 days or high-dose metronidazole, 750 mg with miconazole combination vaginal suppository BDS × 7 days
***Trichuris trichiura* (whipworm)**	• Albendazole: 400 mg oral daily × 3 days for light/moderate infections, 5–7 days for heavy infections • Mebendazole: 100 mg BDS × 3 days for light/moderate infections, 5–7 days for heavy infections **Supportive treatment:** • Iron and nutritional supplements
Wuchereria bancrofti* and *Brugia malayi	**Drug treatment** **First-line:** • Diethylcarbamazine (DEC): 6 mg/kg with or without albendazole, 400 mg, single-dose treatment; or 6 mg/kg/day × 12 days **Second-line:** • Doxycycline: 200 mg/day × 4 weeks with ivermectin, 400 μg/kg **Morbidity management** • **Lymphedema**: Hygiene, physiotherapy, doxycycline, 200 mg/day × 6 weeks • **Hydrocele**: Surgical hydrocelectomy • Prevention of secondary bacterial infections

Answer Key

Chapter 1 Introduction to Parasitology

1. (c) 2. (a) 3. (b) 4. (b) 5. (b)

Chapter 2 Immunology of Parasitic Infections

1. (c) 2. (a) 3. (c) 4. (a) 5. (b)

Chapter 3 Protozoa–Introduction and Classification

1. (b) 2. (a) 3. (a) 4. (d)

Chapter 4 Entamoeba histolytica

1. (a) 2. (b) 3. (b) 4. (a) 5. (b) 6. (b)
7. (c) 8. (c) 9. (c) 10. (b)

Chapter 5 Giardia

1. (b) 2. (d) 3. (b) 4. (a) 5. (b) 6. (c)

Chapter 6 Balantidium coli

1. (c) 2. (d) 3. (c) 4. (b) 5. (d)

Chapter 7 Cryptosporidium

1. (b) 2. (a) 3. (b) 4. (b) 5. (c)

Chapter 8 Cystoisospora

1. (b) 2. (a) 3. (c) 4. (d) 5. (b)

Chapter 9 Cyclospora

1. (c) 2. (c) 3. (a) 4. (b) 5. (b)

Chapter 10 Sarcocystis

1. (a) 2. (b) 3. (c) 4. (b) 5. (a)

Chapter 11 Microsporidia

1. (d) 2. (b) 3. (b) 4. (b) 5. (c)

Chapter 12 Trichomonas

1. (b) 2. (b) 3. (a) 4. (a) 5. (c)

Chapter 13 Plasmodium

1. (c) 2. (b) 3. (c) 4. (b) 5. (a) 6. (b)
7. (b) 8. (b) 9. (b) 10. (b) 11. (b) 12. (a)
13. (a) 14. (a) 15. (a) 16. (a) 17. (d) 18. (b)
19. (c) 20. (c)

Chapter 14 Babesia

1. (a) 2. (b) 3. (c) 4. (d) 5. (a) 6. (d)

Chapter 15 Trypanosoma brucei

1. (b) 2. (c) 3. (a) 4. (d) 5. (d)

Chapter 16 Trypanosoma cruzi

1. (c) 2. (d) 3. (a)

Chapter 17 Leishmania (Visceral Leishmaniasis)

1. (c) 2. (b) 3. (a) 4. (a) 5. (b) 6. (c)
7. (d) 8. (b) 9. (c) 10. (c)

Chapter 18 Leishmania (Cutaneous and Mucocutaneous Leishmaniasis)

1. (d) 2. (b) 3. (b) 4. (a) 5. (a)

Chapter 19 Toxoplasma

1. (c) 2. (b) 3. (a) 4. (b) 5. (b) 6. (a)
7. (b) 8. (b) 9. (d) 10. (d)

Chapter 20 Naegleria

1. (b) 2. (c) 3. (c)

Chapter 21 Acanthamoeba and Balamuthia

1. (b) 2. (b) 3. (c)

Chapter 22 Helminths–Introduction and Classification

1. (b) 2. (a) 3. (a) 4. (c) 5. (c)

Chapter 23 Soil-Transmitted Helminths (STH)

1. (d) 2. (a) 3. (d)

Chapter 24 Ascaris (Roundworm)

1. (b) 2. (b) 3. (d) 4. (d) 5. (b) 6. (d)

Chapter 25 Trichuris (Whipworm)

1. (c) 2. (b) 3. (c) 4. (c) 5. (b)

Chapter 26 Necator and Ancylostoma (Hookworms)

1. (a) 2. (c) 3. (c) 4. (b)
5. (a) 6. (a) 7. (d)

Chapter 27 Strongyloides

1. (c) 2. (d) 3. (a) 4. (d) 5. (a) 6. (c)

Chapter 28 Enterobius (Pinworm)

1. (c) 2. (a) 3. (b) 4. (c) 5. (b)

Chapter 29 Trichinella

1. (a) 2. (a) 3. (d) 4. (d) 5. (b)

Chapter 30 Toxocara and other Larva Migrans

1. (a) 2. (d) 3. (b) 4. (d) 5. (c)

Chapter 31 Angiostrongylus

1. (a) 2. (c) 3. (b)

Chapter 32 Dracunculus

1. (c) 2. (c) 3. (c) 4. (a) 5. (a)
6. (a) 7. (d)

Chapter 33 Wuchereria and Brugia

1. (b) 2. (a) 3. (d) 4. (a) 5. (b) 6. (b)
7. (b) 8. (b) 9. (c) 10. (b)

Chapter 34 Loa loa

1. (d) 2. (c) 3. (c) 4. (a) 5. (b)

Chapter 35 Onchocerca

1. (c) 2. (c) 3. (d) 4. (c) 5. (c) 6. (a)

Chapter 36 Mansonella and Dirofilaria

1. (c) 2. (d) 3. (a) 4. (a)

Chapter 37 Taenia

1. (c) 2. (c) 3. (c) 4. (b) 5. (c) 6. (c)

Chapter 38 Diphyllobothrium

1. (a) 2. (b) 3. (c) 4. (b) 5. (a)

Chapter 39 Hymenolepis

1. (c) 2. (b)

Chapter 40 Taenia solium - Cysticercosis

1. (b) 2. (c) 3. (b) 4. (d) 5. (d) 6. (d)

Chapter 41 Echinococcus

1. (a) 2. (b) 3. (b) 4. (a) 5. (d) 6. (a)
7. (a) 8. (c) 9. (c) 10. (c)

Chapter 42 Fasiolopsis and Other Intestinal Trematodes

1. (c) 2. (b) 3. (c) 4. (b) 5. (a) 6. (c)

Chapter 43 Fasciola

1. (c) 2. (a) 3. (a)

Chapter 44 Clonorchis and Opisthorchis

1. (b) 2. (a) 3. (b) 4. (a)

Chapter 45 Paragonimus

1. (b) 2. (c) 3. (d) 4. (a) 5. (a)

Chapter 46 Schistosoma

1. (b) 2. (a) 3. (c) 4. (b) 5. (c) 6. (c)
7. (b) 8. (d) 9. (a) 10. (b) 11. (b) 12. (b)

Chapter 55 Medical Entomology

1. (b) 2. (b) 3. (a) 4. (d) 5. (a) 6. (d)
7. (b) 8. (d) 9. (d) 10. (c)

Index

N

O